One of the essential qualities of the clinician is interest in humanity,
*for the secret in the care **of** the patient is in the caring **for** the patient.*

Francis Weld Peabody
1881–1927

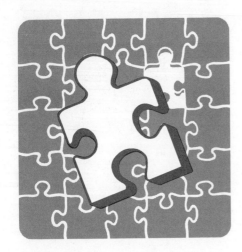

1989
W. B. SAUNDERS COMPANY

Harcourt Brace Jovanovich, Inc.
Philadelphia London Toronto Montreal Sydney Tokyo

Mark H. Swartz, M.D., F.A.C.P.

Associate Professor of Clinical Medicine
The Mount Sinai Medical Center
New York, New York

TEXTBOOK OF

Physical Diagnosis

HISTORY AND EXAMINATION

W. B. SAUNDERS COMPANY
Harcourt Brace Jovanovich, Inc.

The Curtis Center
Independence Square West
Philadelphia, PA 19106

Library of Congress Cataloging-in-Publication Data

Swartz, Mark H.
   Textbook of physical diagnosis.

   1. Physical diagnosis.   I. Title.   [DNLM:
1. Diagnosis.   2. Medical History Taking.   3. Physical
Examination.   WB 200 S973t]
RC76.S95   1989   616.07'54   87-35672
ISBN 0-7216-2475-8

Editor: Martin Wonsiewicz

Developmental Editor: David Kilmer

Designer: Dorothy Chattin

Production Manager: Carolyn Naylor

Manuscript Editor: Tom Stringer

Illustration Coordinator: Brett MacNaughton

Page Layout Artist: Dorothy Chattin

Indexer: Angela Holt

Textbook of Physical Diagnosis   ISBN   0-7216-2475-8

Last digit is the print number: 9   8   7   6   5   4   3   2   1

To **Vivian,**
my life's companion and best friend,
for her love, support, and understanding,

and

To **Phil** and to the memory of **Hilda,**
my parents.

PREFACE

Textbook of Physical Diagnosis offers a new approach and presentation to physical diagnosis. Through the use of a clear discussion of pathophysiology, illustrations, and a *humanistic* element, the importance of the "old fashioned" doctor's approach to the patient is emphasized. In this era of high technology, the doctor-patient relationship can suffer, and patient care can easily become *dehumanized*. Malpractice claims, resulting oftentimes from poor doctor-patient relationships, have risen at an alarming rate. The important basic skills of the "old-time" doctor have frequently fallen by the wayside. The *primary* aim of this textbook is to provide a framework for the clinical assessment of the patient in a *humanistic* manner.

There are many books on physical diagnosis. Why do we need another? This new text focuses on the patient: his needs, his problems, his hopes. Transcultural health care is discussed to illustrate the differences in the way patients of diverse ethnic backgrounds view their illnesses. Unlike many other books, this one focuses on the role of the patient as a person, *not* just a representative of a disease or a clinical state.

Textbook of Physical Diagnosis provides a practical approach to the patient with emphasis on the patient's physical and psychological condition. A step-by-step approach to the art of history taking is provided. It focuses at length on the problems that patients face when disease strikes. The impact of the disease and the behavioral and emotional interplay between patient and doctor are discussed throughout the chapters.

Each of the organ system chapters provides detailed information about the techniques of the physical examination. Each chapter addresses specific issues related to history taking of the organ system discussed in addition to discussing the science of performing the physical examination. Tables for easy reference are included in the chapters. When designing this book, I constantly kept in mind the need for an illustrated text to enhance the student's understanding of the techniques.

Writing a textbook of physical diagnosis is a difficult task. It should *not* be a textbook of medicine or pathology, but to omit pathologic states would provide the student with no frame of reference. Each chapter in *Textbook of Physical Diagnosis* starts with a fundamental review of the pathophysiology for that organ system. At the end of each chapter, there is a section that is specifically directed at clinicopathologic correlations related to the disease states of the organ system being discussed. This section serves to bridge the gap between the physical diagnosis program and the clinical clerkship in medicine. There are many tables with basic correlations of symptoms and signs in common diseases.

The vocabulary of medicine is quite difficult for the student. Instead of providing a glossary of terms at the end of each chapter, at the end of the book, or not at all, I have provided the most common prefixes, roots, and suffixes related to the subject area at the end of each chapter. In this manner, the student can learn the concepts of *word building*. The student's knowledge of technical terms and his spelling of terms will be enhanced far more than by mere memorization.

Over 500 original illustrations and photographs complement the text. Color photographs illustrate patients and their pathologic problems, whereas black and white photographs are included to demonstrate the basic diagnostic techniques. Almost all of the illustrations and photographs are original and were specifically prepared for this text. Over 400 patients were photographed for this work. Care was taken to include only those photographs of *common* conditions. Rare diseases are interesting but should not be part of a basic textbook of physical diagnosis.

Over the years, many techniques and physical signs have made their entry into textbooks of physical diagnosis. All too often, some of these maneuvers and findings are perpetuated despite high false positive and high false negative rates. This text attempts to evaluate the utility of various techniques and physical signs by addressing their sensitivity (true positive rate) and specificity (true negative rate) and by making the reader aware of this significant problem.

After the art of history taking and the skills involved in the physical examination are mastered, but before a definitive diagnosis and treatment plan can be made, *problem solving* must occur. One of the final chapters of the book deals with clinical problem solving and provides a basis for a logical, rational approach.

This single-authored textbook was written for students in an easy-to-read fashion. Every effort has been made to provide the "internist's" and *not* the "specialist's" approach to the patient and his disease. *Italics* have been used throughout the book to indicate the doctor's questions or the patient's responses. The use of italic print is also used to delineate those points that the *author* wishes to emphasize.

I recognize that there are an increasing number of women in medicine and that patients may be of either sex. After much consideration, I have decided to use "he" or "his" when referring to the interviewer, examiner, or patient. The use of "he/she" or "his/her" is cumbersome and would detract from the fluidity of the text. This decision was made for ease of reading *only,* and does not reflect any gender bias. Please understand that *every* time the word "he" or "his" appears in this generalized sense, it implies "he/she" or "his/her," respectively.

The doctor of today must be able to synthesize basic pathophysiology and provide humane medical care. The medical profession is under great scrutiny at the present time, owing mostly to the decline in the "old-time" doctor's approach. We must put more emphasis on the humanistic approach to patient care and use modern technology only to enhance our clinical assessment of the patient, *not* to replace it!

MARK H. SWARTZ, M.D.

ACKNOWLEDGMENTS

This textbook could not have been completed without the help of many individuals. I am indebted to the thousands of patients who have taught me about the human aspect of being a physician. I wish to thank my many mentors and students, all of whom have helped me continue to learn.

Peer review is a critical element in the development of a medical textbook. I would like to thank all of the reviewers who have aided in this process. To each of them, I express my appreciation and gratitude. I am particularly indebted to Wesley J. Miller, M.D., of the University of Minnesota; and Ellen M. Cosgrove, M.D., of Hahnemann University for their invaluable recommendations. Special thanks are given to Louis G. Monti, M.D., of The Mount Sinai Medical Center; and Marguerite M. Mayers, M.D., of The Albert Einstein College of Medicine for their valuable suggestions that helped me to ensure thoroughness and accuracy of the content of Chapter 20, The Pediatric Patient. I am grateful to Michael N. Mulvihill, Dr. P.H., of The Mount Sinai School of Medicine for his critical appraisal of Chapter 21, Clinical Decision Making. Louis L. Cregler, M.D., of The Bronx Veterans Administration Hospital was extremely helpful in providing me with greater insight into how to relate to the black patient.

I wish to express my deepest appreciation to Wendy B. Jackelow for providing all of the outstanding drawings that have complemented the text. It has been a real pleasure to be associated with such a fine artist who can make "one picture worth a thousand words." I also want to thank Lynne Cooper for her artistic rendition of the old Indian tale illustrated in Chapter 21.

It has taken over a year to produce all the photographs for this book. I am indebted to the fine Medical Arts Studio at The Mount Sinai Medical Center. I want to especially acknowledge the enormous help of Charles W. Silvey III, Richard E. Weinacht, and Judy Davis Goldman, whose expertise enhanced this book so greatly.

I want to thank Michael Hawke, M.D., of the University of Toronto Department of Otolaryngology for supplying the beautiful color slides of the tympanic membrane. Mark G. Lebwohl, M.D., of The Mount Sinai School of Medicine Department of Dermatology was kind to supply me with the wonderful photographs of the melanoma and squamous cell carcinoma of the skin. Joyce E. Shriver, Ph.D., of The Mount Sinai School of Medicine was helpful in reviewing the neuroanatomic illustrations. I am grateful to the many members of the house staff, attending physicians, and nurses at The Mount Sinai Medical Center for their help and cooperation.

Writing this book has been made easier because of the efforts of David P. Guest and

Wanda M. Volpe of Beaman Porter, Inc. The entire manuscript was prepared using their product, the PowerText Formatter. I thank both of them for their constant availability and help.

I would also like to express my appreciation to Mr. Martin J. Wonsiewicz and Mr. David H. Kilmer of the W.B. Saunders Company for their editorial assistance. I am grateful to Ms. Karen O'Keefe for her tremendous help in coordinating all the design aspects. I would like to acknowledge Ms. Carolyn Naylor for her unfailing efforts to ensure the smooth production of this book.

Last, but certainly not least, the publication of this textbook would not have been possible without the tireless efforts of my wife, Vivian Hirshaut, M.D. She painstakingly read and reread every word of this text. She is my best critic, editor, and proofreader. She guided me through all aspects of this book, and the structure and philosophy of this book were greatly influenced by her. She spent countless hours making valuable suggestions, always with good humor and patience. I want also to thank my 10 year old daughter Talia for her forbearance in allowing me the time to write this book.

MARK H. SWARTZ, M.D.

FOREWORD

Ours is an age of technology and continued scientific achievement. Medicine has been at the forefront. Consequently, the medical student is constantly bombarded with new information, new biological concepts, and ever new methods for diagnosis and treatment.

The physician must achieve certain goals that precede and may supersede all that is "new." First, he must know how to apply his skills to determine what is the patient problem. Only this allows application of all the new knowledge and technology. Second, the physician has a role that transcends discrete treatment and depends on his ability to understand and thereby manage the patient and his disease.

Textbook of Physical Diagnosis fills a remarkably evident void. Dr. Mark Swartz has chosen to deal with perhaps the most difficult yet most fundamental of all subjects: the encounter with the patient. It is much easier to describe how to interpret an echocardiographic image than how to take a complete systematic and revealing history!

This book deals with the most challenging and sensitive issues of doctor-patient communication. The student learns how to put the patient at ease, how to discuss sensitive topics such as sexual behavior and substance abuse in ways acceptable to the patient but in a style no different from the approach to the family history. Dr. Swartz has characterized not only the various responses of patients but also different "kinds" of patients, both by psychological and by cultural criteria. He points out how one can prepare himself for an interview with an Asian patient as well as with a physically handicapped person. The reactions of the interviewer to the patient are carefully explained as well as the effect of this reaction in turn on the patient and on the relationship.

There are excellent sections devoted to the physical examination with ample illustrations, and these are integrated with pathophysiology when appropriate. Dr. Swartz tries to quantify the utility of the various parts of the history and physical examination. This certainly is an attempt to provide a scientific basis for the evaluation of the patient.

The book is rich in "how to" methodology. The history sections contain question after question, particularly in sensitive areas. The attitude and posture of the interviewer and the subtle clues given by the patient's body language are described in detail. A sample patient interview is given in depth. Great detail is provided for the techniques of the physical examination.

The ultimate value of this book is in its uniqueness for the beginning student of medicine. Few other texts deal in specifics or present the entire panorama of the communication that is required to effect a meaningful encounter with the patient.

The ideas and suggestions given herein can form the matrix for a uniform, effective, and dignified approach to the patient — and thereby a basis for the intelligent application of biomedical skills for the patient's welfare.

RICHARD GORLIN, M.D.
Murray M. Rosenberg Professor of Medicine
Chairman of the Department of Medicine
The Mount Sinai Medical Center
New York City

CONTENTS

PLATE I

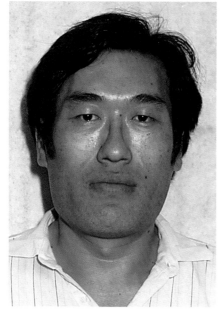

A. Acromegaly.

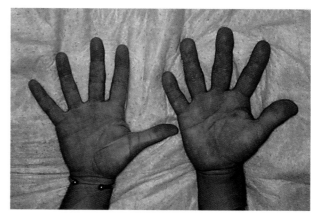

B. Acromegaly.

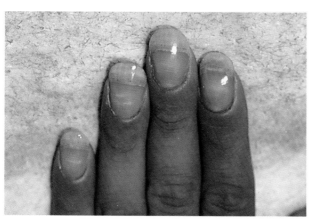

C. Mees' bands.

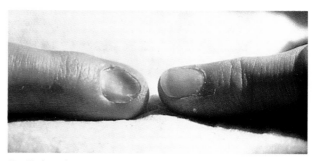

D. Koilonychia.

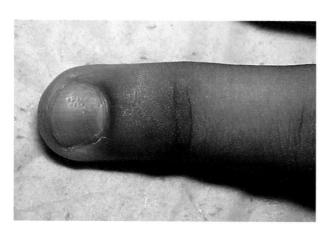

E. Psoriasis.

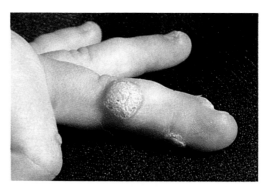

F. Wart. (From Lookingbill DP, Marks JG Jr: Principles of Dermatology. Philadelphia, WB Saunders Co, 1986, p 56.)

PLATE II

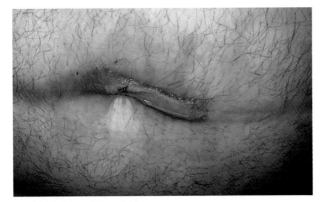

A. *Squamous cell carcinoma in scar.*

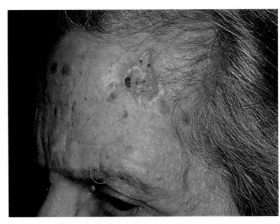

B. *Basal cell carcinoma.*

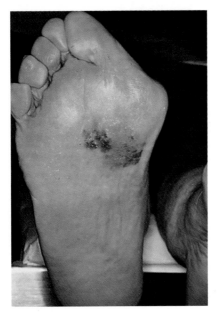

C. *Acral-lentiginous melanoma.*

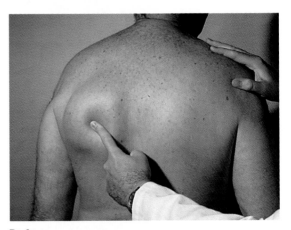

D. *Lipoma.*

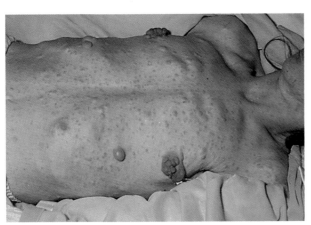

E. *Neurofibromatosis.*

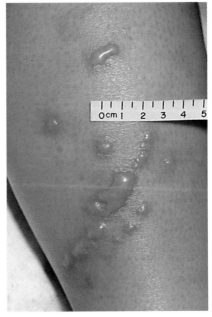

F. *Poison ivy.*

PLATE III

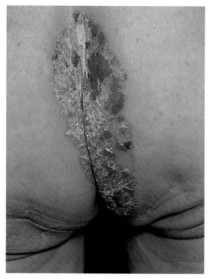

A. Psoriasis.

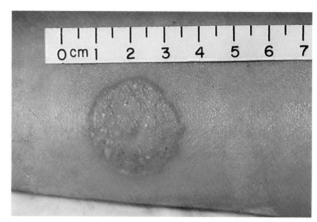

B. Tinea corporis.

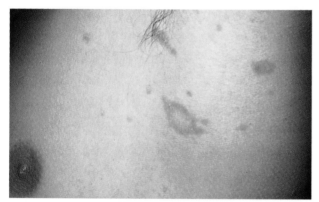

C. Pityriasis rosea.

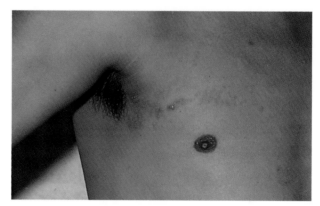

D. Herpes zoster.

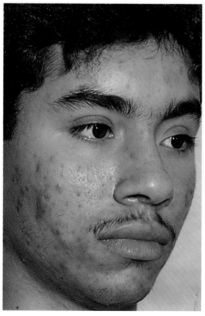

E. Acne.

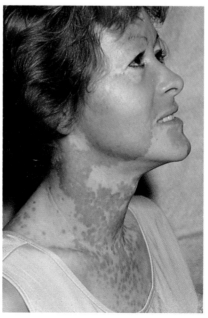

F. Vitiligo.

PLATE IV

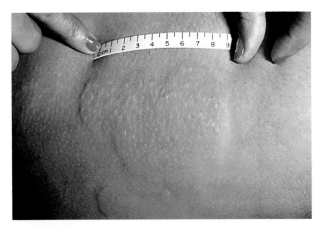

A. Giant urticaria.

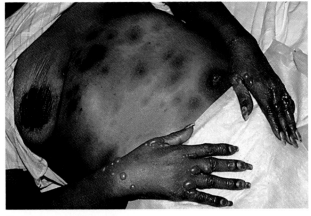

B. Erythema multiforme.

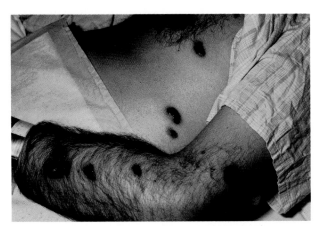

C. Kaposi's sarcoma.

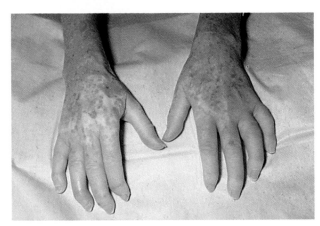

D. Scleroderma.

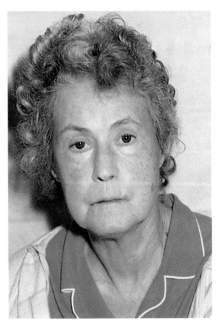

E. Scleroderma.

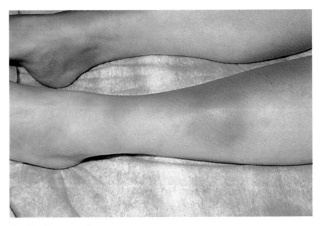

F. Erythema nodosum.

PLATE V

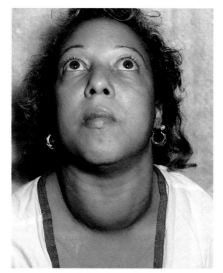

A. Graves' disease.

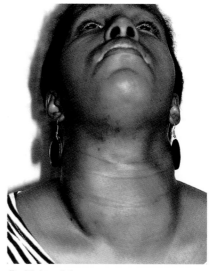

B. Multinodular goiter.

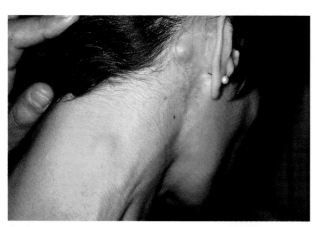

C. Posterior auricular and posterior cervical adenopathy.

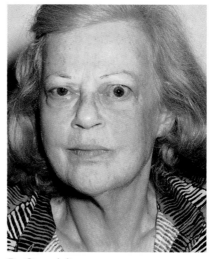

D. Graves' disease.

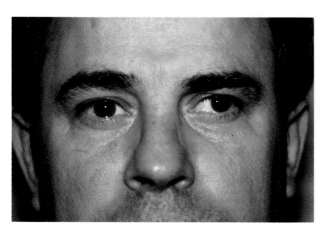

E. Left exotropia.

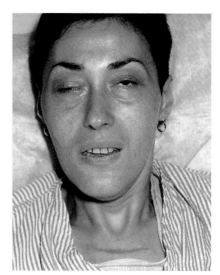

F. Myasthenia gravis.

PLATE VI

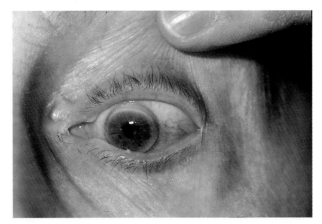

A. Arcus senilis.

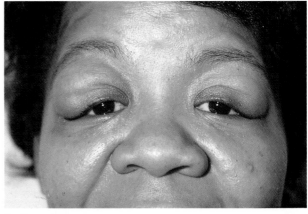

B. Sarcoidosis.

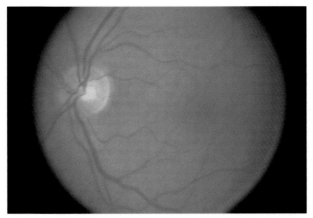

C. Retina: normal.

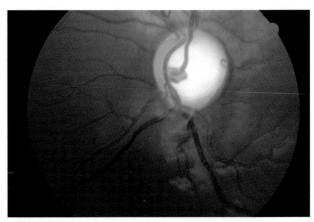

D. Retina: glaucomatous cupping.

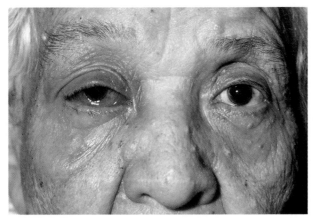

E. Red eye.

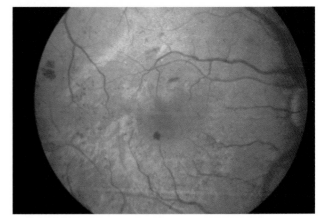

F. Retina: diabetes.

PLATE VII

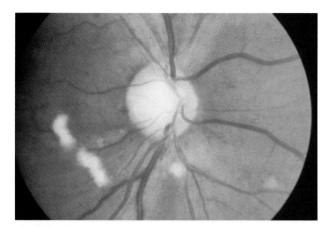

A. *Retina: hypertension.*

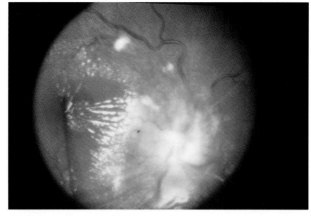

B. *Retina: chronic papilledema.*

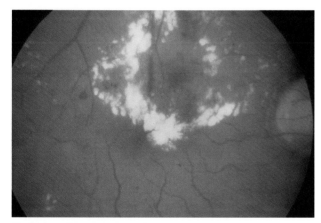

C. *Retina: circinate retinopathy.*

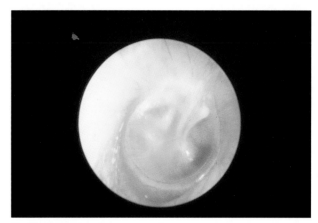

D. *Tympanic membrane: normal.*

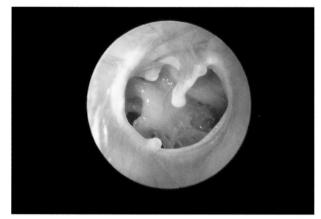

E. *Perforated tympanic membrane.*

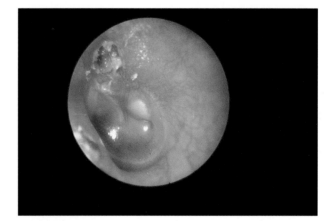

F. *Cholesteatoma.*

PLATE VIII

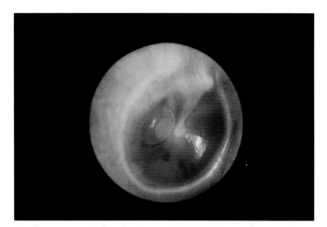

A. Tympanic membrane: serous otitis media.

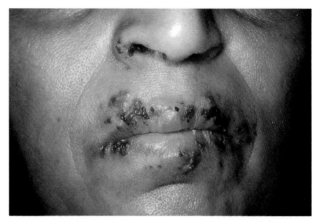

B. Herpes simplex labialis.

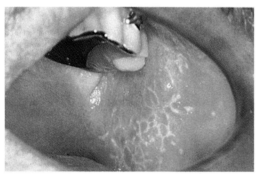

C. Oral lichen planus. (From Lookingbill DP, Marks JG Jr: Principles of Dermatology. Philadelphia, WB Saunders Co, 1986, p 241.)

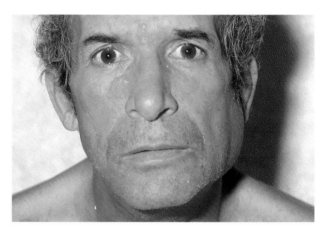

D. Left parotid enlargement.

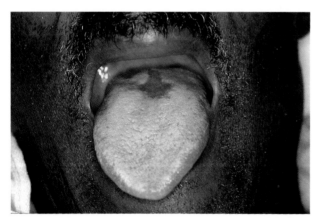

E. Oral candidiasis.

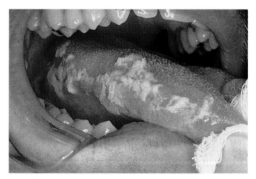

F. Hairy leukoplakia. (From Silverman S Jr: JADA 112:192, 1986. Copyright by the American Dental Association. Reprinted by permission.)

PLATE IX

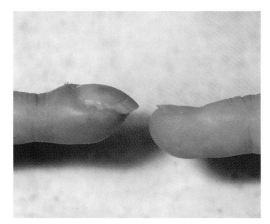

A. Clubbing.

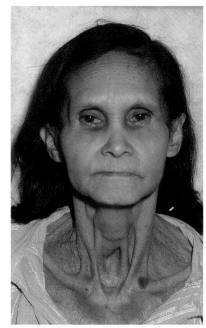

B. Tracheal deviation.

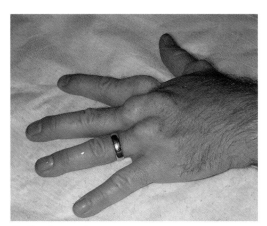

C. Tendon xanthomata.

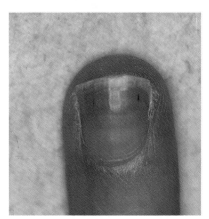

D. Splinter hemorrhages.

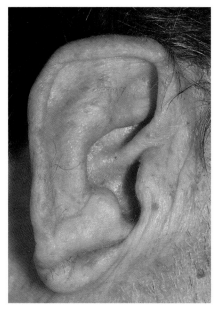

E. Ear lobe creases.

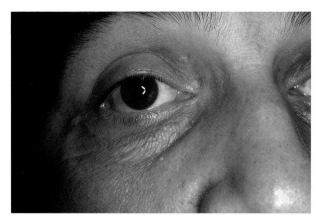

F. Xanthelasma.

PLATE X

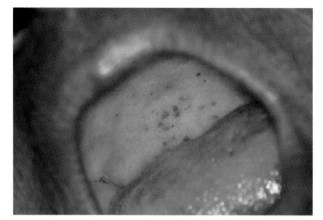

A. Palatal petechiae.

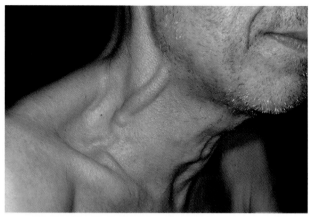

B. Neck vein distention.

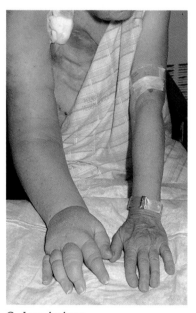

C. Lymphedema.

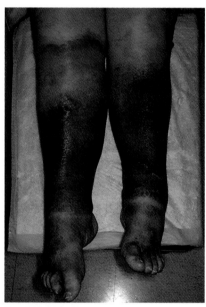

D. Chronic venous stasis.

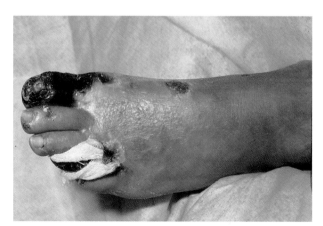

E. Diabetic gangrene.

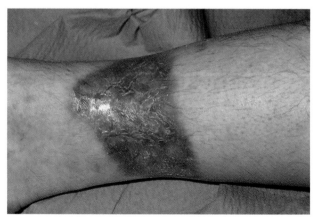

F. Necrobiosis lipoidica diabeticorum.

PLATE XI

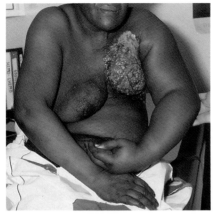

A. *Inflammatory breast carcinoma.*

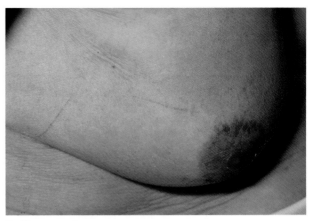

B. *Breast carcinoma.*

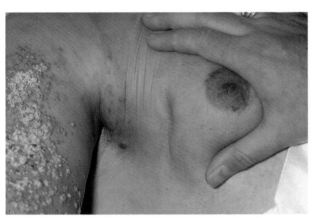

C. *Breast dimpling.*

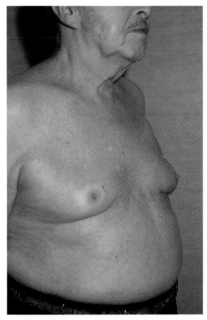

D. *Gynecomastia.*

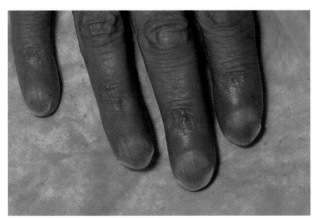

E. *Lindsay's nails.*

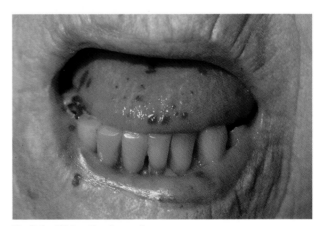

F. *Osler-Weber-Rendu syndrome.*

PLATE XII

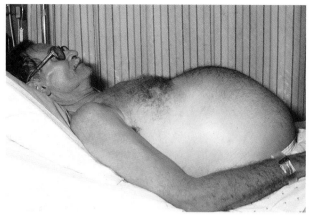

A. Ascites.

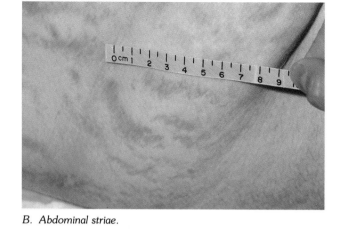

B. Abdominal striae.

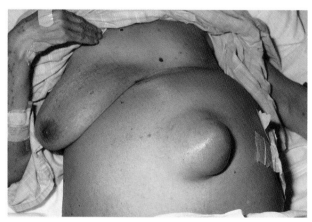

C. Ascites with umbilical hernia.

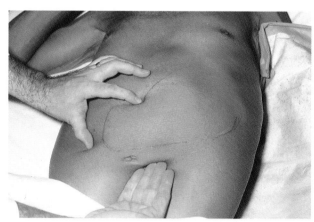

D. Splenomegaly.

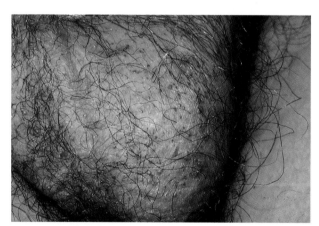

E. Angiokeratomas.

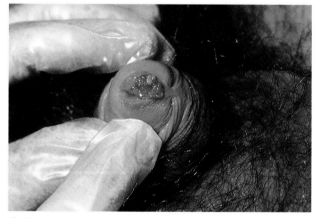

F. Condylomata acuminata.

PLATE XIII

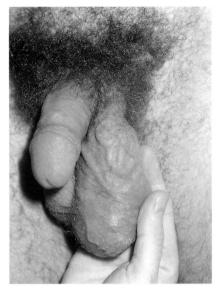

A. Varicocele.

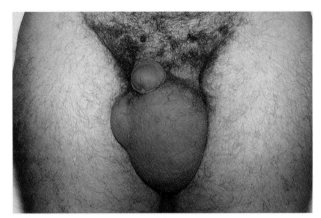

B. Hydrocele.

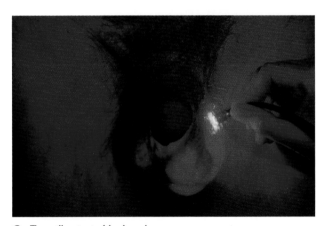

C. Transilluminated hydrocele.

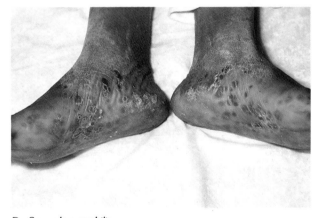

D. Secondary syphilis.

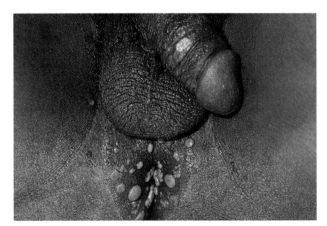

E. Condylomata lata.

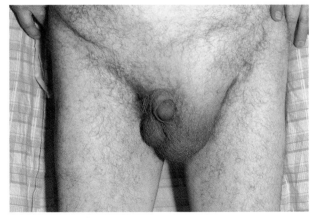

F. Left indirect inguinal hernia.

PLATE XIV

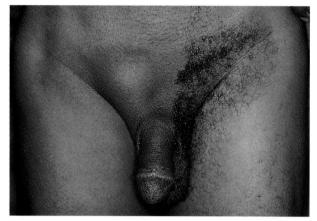

A. Right direct inguinal hernia.

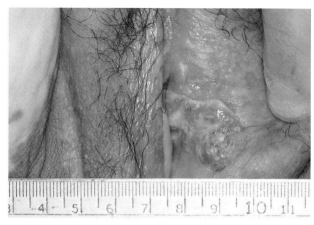

B. Vulvar carcinoma.

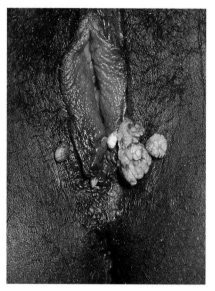

C. Condylomata acuminata.

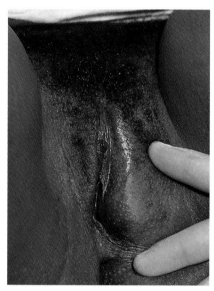

D. Bartholin's cyst.

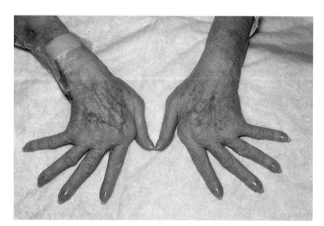

E. Rheumatoid arthritis.

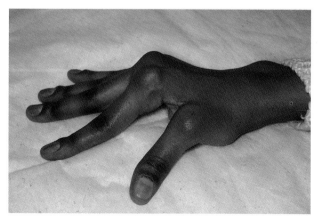

F. Rheumatoid arthritis.

PLATE XV

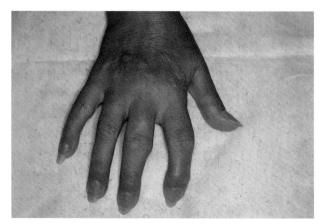

A. Osteoarthritis.

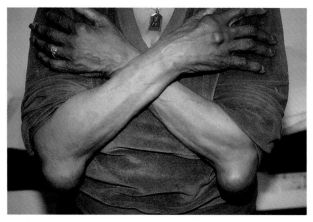

B. Gout.

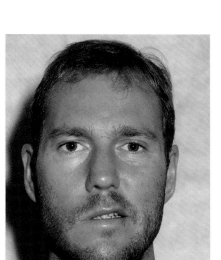

C. Right facial palsy.

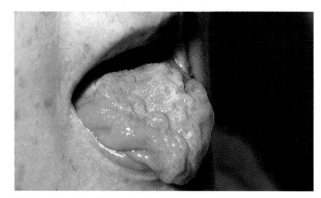

D. Amyotrophic lateral sclerosis.

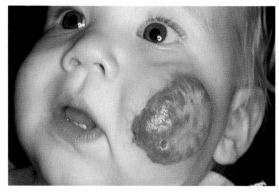

E. Cavernous hemangioma. (From Hurwitz S: Clinical Pediatric Dermatology: A Textbook of Skin Disorders of Childhood and Adolescence. Philadelphia, WB Saunders Co, 1981, p 192.)

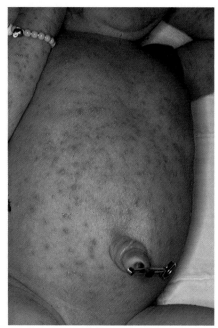

F. Erythema toxicum. (From Hurwitz S: Clinical Pediatric Dermatology: A Textbook of Skin Disorders of Childhood and Adolescence. Philadelphia, WB Saunders Co, 1981, p 11.)

PLATE XVI

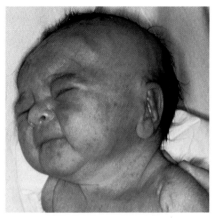

A. Congenital rubella. (From Hurwitz S: Clinical Pediatric Dermatology: A Textbook of Skin Disorders of Childhood and Adolescence. Philadelphia, WB Saunders Co, 1981, p 18.)

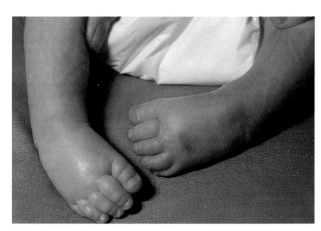

B. Talipes equinovarus.

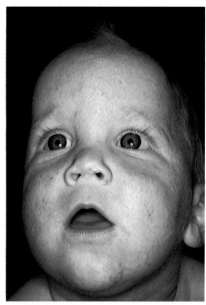

C. Atopic pleat. (From Hurwitz S: Clinical Pediatric Dermatology: A Textbook of Skin Disorders of Childhood and Adolescence. Philadelphia, WB Saunders Co, 1981, p 40.)

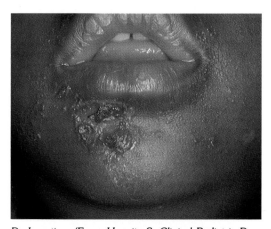

D. Impetigo. (From Hurwitz S: Clinical Pediatric Dermatology: A Textbook of Skin Disorders of Childhood and Adolescence. Philadelphia, WB Saunders Co, 1981, p 216.)

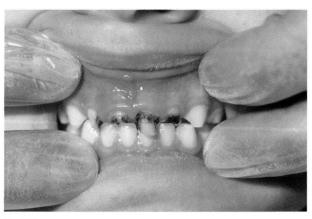

F. Milk caries.

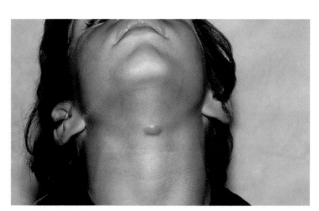

E. Thyroglossal cyst.

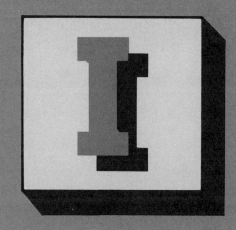

THE ART OF
INTERVIEWING

THE INTERVIEWER'S QUESTIONS

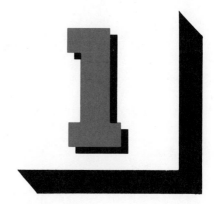

What is spoken of as a "clinical picture" is not just a photograph of a man sick in bed; it is an impressionistic painting of the patient surrounded by his home, his work, his relations, his friends, his joys, sorrows, hopes and fears.

Francis Weld Peabody
1881–1927

BASIC PRINCIPLES

The main purpose of an interview is to gather all basic information pertinent to the patient's illness and the patient's adaptation to illness. An assessment of the patient's condition can then be made. An experienced interviewer considers all the aspects of the patient's presentation and then follows the leads that appear to deserve the most attention. The interviewer should also be aware of the influence of social, economic, and cultural factors in shaping the nature of the patient's problems.

Communication is the key to a successful interview. The interviewer must be able to ask questions of the patient freely. These questions must always be easily understood and keyed to the medical sophistication of the patient. If necessary, slang words describing certain conditions may be used in order to facilitate communication and avoid misunderstanding. For any patient who speaks another language, it is important to seek a translator. The interviewer should master a number of key words in that language in order to gain the respect and confidence of the patient. Family members who translate for the patient may alter the meanings of what has been said. It is therefore advantageous to have an objective observer act as translator.

In the beginning, the patient will bring up the subjects that are easiest to discuss. The more painful experiences can be elicited by tactful questioning. The neophyte interviewer will need to gain experience to feel comfortable asking questions about subjects that are more painful, delicate, or unpleasant. Timing of such questions is critical.

A cardinal principle of interviewing is to permit the patient to express his story in his own words. The manner in which the patient tells his story reveals much about the nature of the patient's illness. Careful observation of the patient's facial expressions as well as body movements may provide valuable nonverbal clues. The interviewer may also use body language such as a smile, a nod, silence, a hand gesture, or a questioning look to encourage the patient to continue his story.

Listening without interruption is important and requires skill. If given the chance, patients will often disclose their problems spontaneously. The interviewer needs to *hear* what is being said. The interviewer should be attentive as to how the patient uses his words to conceal or reveal his thoughts and history. The interviewer should be wary of quick, very positive statements such as, "Everything's fine!," "I'm very happy," or "No problems." If the interviewer has reason to doubt these statements, he may respond by saying, "Is everything really as fine as it could be?"

If the history given is vague, the interviewer may use direct questioning. Asking "How," "Where," or "When" is generally more effective than questions such as "Why," which tend to put the patient on the defensive. One must be particularly careful not to disapprove of certain aspects of the patient's story. Different cultures have different mores, and one must listen without any suggestion of prejudice.

Always treat the patient with respect. Take care not to contradict the patient. You should refrain from trying to impose your own moral standards upon the patient. Knowledge of the patient's social and economic background will make the interview progress more smoothly.

The interviewer's own appearance will influence the success of the interview. Patients have a role model for physicians. Neatness counts. The slovenly interviewer might be considered immature or careless, and his competence may be questioned from the start. Provocative dressing or uncleanliness will impede a fruitful interview. Surveys of patients have indicated that patients prefer medical personnel to dress in white coats and to wear shoes instead of sneakers.

The future physician must be compassionate and interested in the patient's story. He must create an atmosphere of openness in which the patient will feel comfortable and will be encouraged to describe his problem. These guidelines will set a foundation for effective interviewing.

As a rule, patients like to respond to questions in a way that will satisfy the physician in order to gain approval. This may represent fear on the part of the patient. The interviewer should be aware of this phenomenon.

The interviewer must be able to question the patient about subjects that may be distressing or embarrassing to the interviewer or the patient or both. Frequently, the young interviewer may have more of a problem than the patient with questions related to sexuality, alcoholism, death, or secrets. Answers to many of the routine questions may cause embarrassment to the interviewer and leave him speechless. Therefore, there is a tendency to avoid such questions.

The interviewer's ability to be open and frank about such topics will promote the chances of discussion in these areas.

Very often, patients will feel comfortable discussing what the interviewer would consider antisocial behavior. This may include drug addiction, unlawful actions, or "aberrations" of sexual behavior. The interviewer must be careful not to pass judgment on this "unusual" behavior. One must accept the patient's values, behavior, or beliefs without imposing his own standards. Should the interviewer pass judgment, the patient may reject him as an unsuitable listener. The acceptance will indicate to the patient a feeling that the interviewer is sensitive. It may be appropriate for the interviewer to nod his head and say, "I understand." Some patients might interpret the *"I understand"* statement as a signal that the interviewer has heard enough. It should be used with care. It is also important not to imply approval of behavior, since this may reinforce behavior that is actually destructive.

Although there are few hard and fast rules to interviewing, there is the *"rule of five vowels,"* which is useful to remember in conducting an interview. The rule states that a good interview contains elements of *a*udition, *e*valuation, *i*nquiry, *o*bservation, and *u*nderstanding. *Audition* reminds the interviewer to listen carefully to the patient's story. *Evaluation* refers to the sorting out of relevant from irrelevant data and the importance of the data. With *inquiry,* the interviewer probes into the significant areas requiring more clarification. *Observation* refers to the importance of nonverbal communication, regardless of what is said. Finally, *understanding* the patient's concerns and apprehensions will allow the interviewer to play a more empathetic role.

Speech patterns are relevant to the interview. By manipulating the intonation, rate, emphasis, and volume of speech, both the interviewer and the patient can convey significant emotional meaning to their dialogue. Because many of these features are not under conscious control, they may provide an important statement about the patient's personal attributes. These audible parameters are useful in detecting a patient's anxiety or depression, as well as other affective and emotional states. The interviewer's use of a warm, soft tone is soothing to the patient and enhances the communication.

In the past few years, a broad interest in body language has evolved. This type of nonverbal communication in association with the spoken language can provide a more total picture of the patient's behavior. A patient who strikes his fist on a table while talking is dramatically emphasizing what has been said. A patient who moves about in a chair and looks embarrassed is uncomfortable. A frown indicates annoyance or disapproval. The patient who slips his wedding band on and off may be ambivalent about his marriage. A palm placed over the heart asserts sincerity or credibility. People often rub or cover their eyes when they refuse to accept something that is pointed out. When a patient disapproves of a statement made by the interviewer but restrains himself from speaking, he may start to remove dust or lint from his clothing. Lack of comprehension is indicated by knitted brows. Full interpretation of body language can only be made in the context of the patient's cultural and ethnic background. An Arabic or Asian patient often speaks with dropped eyelids. This type of body language would be inappropriate and indicate depression or lack of attentiveness in a patient from the United States. The interviewer may use his facial expression to facilitate the interview. An appearance of attention demonstrates an interest in what the patient is describing. Attentiveness on the part of the interviewer is also indicated by his leaning slightly forward in his chair toward the patient. Touching the patient can also be very useful. The appropriate placing of a hand on a patient's shoulder provides support. The interviewer who walks with good posture to a patient's bedside can hope to gain the patient's respect and confidence. The interviewer who alternately looks into each of the patient's eyes conveys interest in the patient. The interviewer is soul-searching.

In this age of rapid scientific and biomedical advancements, a new problem has arisen. With the advent of the latest technology in the medical world, there has been a depersonalization of the doctor-patient relationship. Both may feel increasingly neglected, rejected, or abused. A patient may feel dehumanized upon admission to the hospital. He frequently finds himself in a strange environment. He may be apprehensive because he has a problem that his physician considers too serious to be treated on an outpatient basis. The future is filled with uncertainty. The patient admitted to the hospital is stripped of his clothing and many times dentures, glasses, hearing aid, and whatever other personal belongings he has. This serves to lower the morale of the patient. The physician at the same time may be pressed for time, overworked, and sometimes unable to cope with everyday pressures. He may become irritable and pay inadequate attention to the patient's story. He may eventually come to rely on the technical results and reports. This failure to communicate undermines the doctor-patient relationship.

The inexperienced interviewer (medical student, nurse, or physician) not only must learn about the patient's problems, but also must gain insight into his *own* feelings, attitudes, and vulnerabilities. This introspection will enhance the self-image of the student and will result in the student being perceived by the patient as a more careful and compassionate human being, to whom the patient may turn in time of crisis.

A good interviewing session will determine what the patient comprehends about his own health problems. What does the *patient* think is wrong with him? Do not accept merely the diagnosis. Inquire specifically as to what the patient thinks is happening. What kind of impact does the illness bear on work, family, or financial situation? Is there a feeling of loss of control? What is the patient's guilt about his own illness? Does the patient think he will die? By pondering these questions, you will learn much about the patient, and the patient will realize that you have an interest in him as a whole person, not merely as a statistic among the admissions to the hospital.

The literature indicates that malpractice suits are increasing at an alarming rate. The good doctor-patient relationship is probably the single most important factor in preventing malpractice claims. Most malpractice litigation is the result of a deterioration of the traditional doctor-patient relationship rather than the result of true medical negligence. The patient is dissatisfied with and may have lost respect for the physician. From the patient's point of view, the most serious barriers to a good relationship are the physician's lack of time, seeming lack of concern, and failure to inform the patient what he needs to know about his illness. Failure to discuss the patient's illness and treatment in understandable terms is viewed as a rejection by the patient. A doctor-patient relationship based on honesty and understanding is thus recognized as essential for good medical practice and the well-being of the patient.

In summary, the medical interview is a blend of the cognitive and technical skills of the interviewer and the feelings and personalities of both the patient and the interviewer. The interview should be flexible, spontaneous, and not interrogating. When utilized correctly, it is a powerful diagnostic tool.

SYMPTOMS AND SIGNS

The physician must be able to elicit and recognize a wide variety of symptoms and signs. The word *symptom* refers to what the patient feels. Symptoms are used by the patient to describe the nature of his illness. Shortness of breath, chest pain, nausea, diarrhea, and double vision are all symptoms. These labels help the patient to describe the discomfort or distress that he is experiencing. Symptoms are *not* absolute. They are influenced by culture, intelligence, and socioeconomic background. As an example, consider the symptom of pain. Patients have different thresholds of pain.

The term *constitutional* refers to those symptoms commonly occurring with problems in any of the body systems, such as fever, chills, weight loss, or excessive sweating.

The word *sign* refers to that which the examiner finds. Signs can be observed and quantified. Certain signs are also symptoms. For example, a patient may describe episodes of wheezing. This is a symptom. In addition, an examiner may hear wheezing during a patient's physical examination. This is a sign.

The major task of the interviewer is to sort out those symptoms and signs associated with a specific illness. A major advantage the seasoned interviewer has over the beginner is a better understanding of the pathophysiology of disease states. The novice operates under the limitation of not knowing all the signs and symptoms of the associated diseases. With experience and education, the novice will recognize the combination of symptoms and signs as they relate to the underlying illness. For any given disease, there usually is a clustering of symptoms and signs that tend to occur together. When there is only an isolated symptom, the interviewer must be careful in making a definitive assessment.

CONDUCTING AN INTERVIEW

Getting Started

The diagnostic process begins at the first moment of meeting. The interviewer should greet the patient by name, make eye contact, shake hands firmly, and smile. He may wish to say,

> *"Mr. Smith, I'm John Jones, a medical student (or student doctor) at this hospital. I've been asked to interview and examine you."*

It is appropriate to address the patient by his correct title, e.g., Mr., Mrs., Dr., Ms. A formal address clarifies the professional nature of the interview. Terms such as "Dear" or "Grandpa" are *not* to be used.

The patient may address the interviewer as Mr. Jones, or could elect to call the interviewer by the first name. The interviewer now has two choices. The preferred choice would be to disregard the patient's casual form of address. It is not correct at this time for the interviewer to address the patient by his first name. Alternately, the interviewer might say,

> *"I would prefer if you would call me Mr. Jones."*

This approach would tend to formalize the interview, but might make the patient ill at ease.

If the patient is having a meal, ask him if you may return when he is finished eating. If the patient is using a urinal or bedpan, allow him his privacy. Do not begin an interview in this setting. If the patient has a visitor, you may inquire whether or not the *patient* wishes him to stay. Don't assume that the visitor is a family member. Allow the patient to introduce the person to you.

If possible, the interview should take place in a quiet, well-lit room. Unfortunately, most hospital rooms do not afford such luxury. The teaching hospital with four patients in a room is rarely conducive for good human interactions. Therefore, one must make the best of the existing environment. The curtains should be drawn around the patient's bed to create privacy. You may request that the volume of neighboring patients' radios or televisions be turned down. Lights and window shades can be adjusted to eliminate excessive glare or shade. Arrange the patient's bed light so that he does not feel under interrogation.

You should make the patient as comfortable as possible. If the patient has had his eyeglasses, hearing aid, or dentures removed, ask him if he would like to use them. It is often useful to use your stethoscope as a hearing aid for those hearing-impaired individuals without other devices. The eartips should be placed in the ears of the patient, and you can use the diaphragm as a microphone. The patient may be in a chair or lying in bed. Allow the patient his choice of position. This makes the patient feel that you are interested and concerned about him while it allows him some control over the interview. If the patient is in bed, it is a nice gesture to ask if the pillows should be arranged to make him more comfortable.

The interviewer should sit in a chair directly facing the patient in order to make good eye contact. Sitting on the bed is too familiar and not appropriate. It is generally preferred that the interviewer sit at a distance of about 3 feet from the patient. Distances greater than 5 feet are impersonal, and distances closer than 3 feet interfere with the patient's "private space." The interviewer should sit in a relaxed position without crossing his arms across his chest. The crossed arms position is not appropriate, as this body language projects an attitude of superiority and may interfere with the progress of the interview.

Once the introduction has been made, one may begin the interview by asking a very general open-ended question such as, "What problem has brought you to the hospital?" This type of opening remark allows the patient to speak first. The interviewer can then determine the patient's *chief complaint*, or that problem that is regarded as paramount. If the patient says "Haven't you read my records?" it is correct to say, "No, I've been asked to interview you without any prior information." Alternately, the interviewer could say, "I would like to hear your story in your own words."

The Narrative

Novice interviewers are often worried about remembering the patient's history. It is poor form to write extensive notes during the interview. Attention should be focused more on what the person is saying and less on the written word. In addition, one cannot observe the facial expressions and body language that are so important to the patient's story. A pad of paper may be used to jot down important dates or names during the session.

After the introductory question, the interviewer should proceed to questions related to the chief complaint. These should naturally evolve into questions related to the other formal parts of the medical history, such as the present illness, past medical illnesses, social and educational history, and review of systems. The patient should largely be allowed to tell his narrative in his own way. The interviewer must select certain aspects about which further details must be explored and guide the patient toward them. Overdirection is to be avoided, as this will stifle the interview and prevent important points from being clarified.

"Small talk" is a very useful method of enhancing the narrative. Small talk is neither random nor pointless, and studies in conversation analysis have indicated that it is actually useful in communication. It has been shown that during conversations, the individual who tells a humorous anecdote is the one who is in "power." For example, if an interviewer interjects a humorous remark during an interview and the patient laughs, the interviewer is "in control." If the patient does not laugh, he may take control.

Be aware of the patient who asks, "Let me ask you a hypothetical question" or "I have a friend with _____, what do you think about _____?" In each case, the question is probably related to the patient's own concerns.

A patient often uses words such as "Uh . . .," "Ah . . .," and "Well . . ." to avoid unpleasant topics. It is natural for a patient to delay talking about an unpleasant situation or condition. Pauses between words as well as the use of the words cited provide a means for the patient to put off discussing a painful subject.

When patients use terms such as "somewhat," "a little," "fair," "reasonably well," "sometimes," "rarely," or "average," the interviewer must ask for clarification. Precise communication is always desirable, and these words have been shown to have significant variations in meaning.

The interviewer should be alert for subtle clues from the patient to guide the interview further. There are a variety of techniques to encourage and sustain the narrative. These guidelines consist of verbal and nonverbal facilitation, reflection, confrontation, interpretation, and directed questioning. These techniques are discussed later in this chapter.

The Closing

It is important that the interviewer pace the interview so that adequate time will be left for any patient questions and the physical examination. About 5 minutes before the end of the interview, the interviewer should begin to close the important issues that were discussed.

By the conclusion of the interview, the interviewer should have a clear impression of the reason(s) why the patient sought medical help, the history of the present illness, the patient's past medical history, and an understanding of the patient's social and economic position. At this time, the interviewer may wish to say, "You've been very helpful. I would now like to take a few notes." If any part of the history needs further clarification, this is the time to do so. The interviewer may actually wish to summarize for the patient the most important parts of the history to help illuminate the important points made.

If the patient asks for an opinion, it is prudent for you as a novice interviewer to answer, "I am a medical student. I think it would be best to ask your doctor that question." You have not provided the patient with the answer he was seeking. On the other hand, you have not jeopardized the existing doctor-patient relationship by possibly giving either the wrong information or a difference of opinion.

At the conclusion, it is polite to encourage the patient to discuss any additional problems or ask any questions. "Is there anything else that you would like to tell me that I have not already asked?" "Are there any questions you might like to ask?" Usually, all possible avenues of discussion have been exhausted, but these remarks allow the patient "the final say." At this time, you, the interviewer, can thank the patient and tell him that you are ready to begin the physical examination.

BASIC INTERVIEWING TECHNIQUES

The successful interview is smooth and spontaneous. The interviewer must be aware of subtleties and be able to pick up on these clues. Just as the accomplished pianist appears to play without a conscious effort, so does the successful interviewer sustain the interview. There are several techniques that one uses every day to encourage someone to continue speaking. This section discusses the various interviewing techniques. It should be remembered that each of these techniques has its limitations and not all of them are used in every interview. They are outlined here to be used as a guide and may be incorporated, where appropriate, into the narrative.

Types of Questions

The secret of effective interviewing lies in the art of questioning. The wording of the question is often less important than the tone of voice used to ask it. In general, questions that stimulate the patient to talk freely are preferred.

Open-Ended Questions

Open-ended questions ask the patient for general information. This type of question is most useful in opening up the interview or for changing the area to be discussed. An open-ended question allows the patient to tell his story spontaneously. It can be very useful to allow the patient to "ramble on." Too much rambling, however, must be controlled by the interviewer in a sensitive but firm manner. This freedom of speech should obviously be avoided with the overtalkative patient, whereas it should be utilized often with the silent patient. Examples of open-ended questions are the following:

"What kind of problem are you having?"
"You are having stomach pain? Tell me about it."
"How was your health before your heart attack?"
"Can you describe your feelings when you get the pain?"

Direct Questions

After a period of open-ended questioning, the interviewer should direct the attention to specific facts learned during the open-ended questioning period. These direct questions serve to clarify the areas and add detail to the story. A direct question can usually be answered in one word or a brief sentence. For example:

"Where does it hurt?"
"When do you get the burning?"
"How do you compare this pain with your ulcer pain?"

Care must be taken to avoid asking direct questions in a manner that might bias the response.

Symptoms are considered in the classic seven dimensions, which include *bodily location, quality, quantity, chronology, setting, aggravating* (or *alleviating*) *factors,* and *associated manifestations*. These dimensions may be used as a framework to clarify the illness. Examples include the following:

Bodily Location:
"Where in your back?"
"Can you tell me where you feel the pain?"
"Do you feel it anywhere else?"

Quality:
"What does it feel like?"
"What do you mean by 'a sticking pain'?"
"Was it sharp, dull, or aching?"

Quantity:
"How many pads do you use?"
"What do you mean by 'a lot'?"
"What kind of effect does the pain have on your work?"
"How does the pain compare with the time you broke your leg?"
"How does it compare with childbirth?"

Chronology:
"When did you first notice it?"
"How long did it last?"
"Have you had the pain since that time?"
"Then what happened?"
"Have you noticed that it is worse during your period?"
"When you get the pain, is it steady, or does it change?"

Setting:
"Does it ever occur at rest?"
"Do you ever get the pain when you are emotionally upset?"
"Where were you when it occurred?"

Provocative:
"What seems to bring on the pain?"
"Have you noticed that it occurs at a certain time of day?"
"Is there anything else besides exercise that makes it worse?"

Palliative:
"What do you do to make it better?"
"Does lying quietly in bed help you?"

Associated   "Do you ever have nausea with the pain?"
Factors: "Have you noticed other changes that happen when you start to sweat?"
    "Before you get the headache, do you ever get a strange taste or smell?"

Question Types to Be Avoided

There are several types of questions that are to be avoided. The "yes-no" question is one that when answered with a "yes" leaves the interviewer unsure of its true meaning. For example,

Interviewer: "Have you been taking the medicine?"
Patient: "Yes."

The "Yes" can mean (1) he *is* taking the medicine, (2) he wants to please the interviewer even if he has not been taking the medicine, (3) he takes it but not according to the directions, or (4) he wants to avoid the subject.

Another type of question to avoid is the *suggestive* one. This type provides the answer to the question. For example,

"Do you feel the pain in your left arm when you get it in your chest?"

A better way to ask the same question would be,

"When you get the pain in your chest, do you notice it anywhere else?"

The "Why" questions carry tones of accusation. This type of question almost always asks a patient to account for his behavior and tends to put him on the defensive. For example,

"Why haven't you taken the medication?"
"Why did you wait so long to call me?"

The use of multiple questioning is likewise to be avoided. In this type of question, there is more than one point of inquiry. The patient can easily become confused and respond incorrectly. For example,

"How many brothers and sisters do you have, and has any one of them ever had asthma, pneumonia, or tuberculosis?"

Questions should be concise and easily understandable. The context should be free of medical jargon. Frequently, the novice interviewer tries to use his new vocabulary of medicine. He may at times respond to the patient with technical terms, leaving the patient feeling confused or put down. This use of technical terms is sometimes called "doctorese." For example,

"You seem to have a homonymous hemianopsia."
"We perform Papanicolaou smears to check for carcinoma in-situ."

Medical terminology, as a rule, should not be used in conversations with patients. Technical terms scare patients. Every medical and nursing student understands the term "heart failure." A patient might interpret this term as failure of the heart to pump: i.e., cardiac standstill, or death. Although patients should be given only as much information as they can handle, adequate explanations must always be given. A partial explanation will leave the patient confused and fearful.

A leading or biased question carries a suggestion of the kind of response the interviewer is looking for. For example, "You haven't used any types of drugs, have you?" suggests that the interviewer disapproves of the patient's use of drugs. If the patient has used drugs, he may not admit to it under this line of questioning.

In addition to avoiding certain types of questions, the interviewer should avoid certain situations. Patients may respond to a question in a manner not expected by the interviewer. This could potentially leave a period of unexpected silence. This "stumped silence" can be interpreted by the patient in a variety of ways. The interviewer must be able to respond quickly in such instances, even if it means broaching another topic.

False reassurances restore a patient's confidence but ignore the reality of the situation. Informing a patient that "surgery is always successful" clearly discounts the known morbidity and mortality associated with it. The patient *wants* to hear what has been said, but this may be a false reassurance.

If a patient suggests that a test not be performed, perhaps because of an underlying fear of the test, the interviewer should never respond defensively by stating, "I'm the doctor. I'll make the decisions." He should recognize the anxiety and handle the response from that point of view.

Silence

This technique is most useful for the silent patient. Silence should never be used with the overtalkative patient, as letting him "have the floor" would not allow the interviewer to control the interview. This difficult type of communication, when used correctly, can indicate interest and support. Silence on the part of the patient can be related to hostility, shyness, or embarrassment. The interviewer should remain silent with direct eye contact and attentiveness. The interviewer may lean forward and even nod his head. After no more than 2 minutes of silence, the interviewer may say,

> *"What are you thinking about?"*
> *"You were saying . . ."*
> *"These things are hard to talk about."*
> *"You were about to say . . ."*

If the patient remains silent, another method of sustaining the interview will have to be chosen.

The interviewer must utilize silence when the patient becomes overwhelmed by emotion. This act will allow the patient to release some of the tension evoked by the history and will indicate to the patient that it is "OK" to cry. Handing the patient a box of tissues is a supportive gesture. It is inappropriate for the interviewer to say, "Don't cry" or "Pull yourself together," as these statements imply that the patient is wasting the interviewer's time or that it is shameful to show emotions.

It is important to use silence correctly. The interviewer who remains silent, becomes fidgety, reviews his notes, or makes a facial expression of evaluation will inhibit the patient. The patient may perceive the frequent use of silence on the part of the interviewer as aloofness or a lack of knowledge.

Facilitation

Facilitation is a technique of verbal or nonverbal communication that encourages a patient to continue speaking but does not direct him to a topic. A common verbal facilitation that we all use is "Uh, huh." Other examples of verbal facilitations include "Go on," "Tell me more about that," "And then?," and "Mmmm."

Not all types of facilitations are verbal. An important nonverbal facilitation is nodding of the head, or a hand gesture to continue. Moving toward the patient connotes interest. These nonverbal motions convey to the patient, "Continue."

One must be careful not to use the head nodding too much, as this may convey approval in situations in which approval may not be intended.

Often a puzzled expression can be used as a nonverbal facilitation to indicate, "I don't understand."

Confrontation

Confrontation is a response based on an observation by the interviewer that points out to the patient something striking about his behavior or previous statement. This interviewing technique directs the patient's attention to something of which he may or may not be aware. The confrontation may be either a statement or a question. For example,

> *"You look upset."*
> *"Is there any reason why you always look away when you talk to me?"*
> *"You're angry."*
> *"You sound uncomfortable about it."*
> *"Why are you so silent?"*

Confrontation is particularly useful in encouraging the narrative when there are subtle clues given. By confronting the patient, the interviewer may be able to permit the patient to expound upon the problem further. Confrontation is also useful to clarify discrepancies in the history.

Confrontation must be used with care, as excessive use will be considered impolite and overbearing. If correctly utilized, however, confrontation can be a very powerful technique. Suppose a patient is describing a symptom of chest pain. By observing the patient, you notice that there are now tears in his eyes. By saying sympathetically, "You look very upset," you are encouraging the patient to express his emotions.

Interpretation

Interpretation is a type of confrontation that is based on inference rather than on observation. The interviewer "interprets" the patient's behavior, encouraging the patient to observe his own part in the problem. The interviewer must first fully understand the clues that the patient has given before he can offer his interpretation. He must look for signs of underlying fear or anxiety that may be indicated by other symptoms, such as recurrent pain, dizziness, headaches, or weakness. Once these underlying problems have surfaced, the patient may be led to the recognition of the inciting event in future interviews. Interpretation frequently will open new lines of communication previously not recognized. Examples are the following:

"You seem to be quite happy about that."
"Sounds like you're scared."
"Are you afraid you've done something wrong?"
"Your dizziness appears to be aggravated by your arguments with your wife."

Interpretation can demonstrate support and understanding if used correctly.

Reflection

Reflection is a response that mirrors or echoes that which has just been expressed by the patient. The tone of the voice is important in reflection. The intonation of the words may indicate entirely different meanings. For example,

Patient: "I was so sick that I haven't worked since January 1986."

Response: "Haven't worked since *1986?*"

In this example, the emphasis should be on "1986?." This asks the patient to describe further the conditions that did not allow him to work. If the emphasis is incorrectly placed on "worked," the interviewer immediately puts the patient on the defensive, implying "What did you do with your time?" Though generally very useful, reflection can hamper the progress of the interview if used improperly.

Support

Support is a response that indicates an interest in or an understanding of the patient. Supportive remarks promote a feeling of security in the doctor-patient relationship. A supportive response might be, "I understand." An important time to use support is immediately after a patient has expressed strong feelings. The use of support when a patient suddenly begins to cry cements the good doctor-patient relationship. Two important subgroups of support are reassurance and empathy.

Reassurance

Reassurance is a response that conveys to the patient that the interviewer understands what has been expressed. It may also indicate that the interviewer approves of something the patient has done or thought. It can be a very powerful tool, but false reassurance can be devastating. Examples of reassurance are the following:

> *"That's wonderful. I'm delighted that you started in the rehabilitation program at the hospital!"*
> *"You're improving steadily!"*

The use of reassurance is particularly helpful when patients seem upset or frightened. Reassurance must always be based on fact.

Empathy

Empathy is a response that recognizes the patient's feeling and does not criticize it. It is *understanding,* not an emotional state of sympathy. The empathetic response is saying, "I'm with you." The use of empathy can strengthen the doctor-patient relationship and allow for the interview to flow smoothly. Examples of empathy are the following:

> *"I'm sure your daughter's problem has given you much anxiety."*
> *"The death of someone so close to you is hard to take."*
> *"I guess that this has been kind of a silent fear all of your life."*
> *"You must have been very sad."*
> *"I know it's not easy for you . . . I'm delighted to see that you're trying to eat everything on your tray."*

The last example illustrates a very important point: giving credit to a patient to encourage *his* role in his own improvement.

Empathetic responses can also be nonverbal. An understanding nod is an empathetic response. The interviewer who hands a box of tissues to a crying patient is saying, "I understand your emotions. It's all right to cry." The interviewer who places his hand on the shoulder of an upset patient communicates support. The interviewer understands and appreciates how the patient feels without himself showing any emotion.

FORMAT OF THE HISTORY

The information obtained by the interviewer is ultimately organized into a comprehensive statement about the patient's health. The interviewer should proceed through each of these major sections in a logical sequence and direct his questions relevantly to each area. The format of this history is as follows:

- Source and reliability
- Chief complaint
- History of the present illness
- Past medical history
- Occupational and environmental history
- Biographical information
- Family history
- Psychosocial history
- Review of systems

Source and Reliability

The *source* is usually the patient. If the patient requires a translator, the source is the patient and the translator. If family members help in the interview, their names should be included in a single sentence statement. The reliability of the interview should be assessed.

Chief Complaint

The *chief complaint* is the patient's brief statement explaining why he sought medical attention. It is the answer to the question, "What is the problem that brought you to the hospital?" In the written history, it is frequently a quoted statement of the patient; for example,

"Chest pain for the past 5 hours"
"Terrible nausea and vomiting for 2 days"
"Headache for the last week, on and off"
"Routine examination for school"

Patients sometimes use medical terms. The interviewer must ask the patient to define such terms to ascertain what the individual means by them.

History of Present Illness

The *history of the present illness* refers to the recent changes in his health that led the patient to seek medical attention at this time. It describes the information relevant to the chief complaint. It should answer the questions what, when, how, where, which, who, and why.

Chronology is the most practical framework around which to organize the history. It enables the interviewer to comprehend the sequence of the development of the underlying pathologic process easily. It is in this section that the interviewer gathers all necessary information, starting with the first symptoms of the present illness and following its progression to the present day. It is important to verify that the patient was entirely well before the earliest symptom in order to establish the beginning of the current illness clearly. Patients often may not remember when a symptom developed. If the patient is uncertain about the presence of a symptom at a certain time, the interviewer may be able to relate it to an important or memorable event. For example, "Did you have the pain during Christmas vacation?" In this part of the interview, mainly open-ended questions are asked of the patient, as these afford him the greatest opportunity to describe his history.

Past Medical History

The *past medical history* constitutes the overall assessment of the patient's health prior to the present illness. It includes all of the following:

- General state of health
- Past illnesses
- Injuries
- Hospitalizations
- Surgery
- Allergies
- Immunizations
- Substance abuse
- Diet
- Sleep patterns
- Current medications

As an introduction to the past medical history, the interviewer may ask, "How has your health been in the past?" If the patient doesn't elaborate about specific illnesses but only says, "Excellent" or "Fair," for example, the interviewer might ask, "What does excellent (fair) mean to you?" Direct questioning is appropriate and allows the interviewer to focus on pertinent points that need further elaboration.

The *past illnesses* should include a statement of both childhood and adult problems. The recording of childhood illnesses is obviously more important for the pediatric and young adult interview. All patients should nevertheless be asked about measles, mumps, whooping cough, rheumatic fever, chickenpox, polio, and scarlet fever. Older patients may respond, "I really don't remember." It is important to remember that a "diagnosis" given to the interviewer by a patient should never be considered absolute. Even if the patient had been evaluated by a competent physician in a reputable medical center, the patient may have misunderstood the information given.

The patient should be asked about any prior *injuries* or accidents. The type of injury and the date are important to record.

All *hospitalizations* must be indicated, if not already described. These include admissions for both medical and psychiatric illnesses. The interviewer should not be embarrassed to ask specifically about psychiatric illness. Psychiatric illness *is* a medical problem. Embarrassment on the part of the interviewer will inevitably lead to patient embarrassment and will reinforce the "shame" associated with a psychiatric illness. Students should learn to ask direct questions in a sensitive manner.

All *surgical procedures* should be specified. The type of procedure, date, hospital, and surgeon's name should be obtained, if possible.

All *allergies* should be described. These include environmental, ingestible, or drug related. The interviewer should seek specificity and verification of the patient's allergic response. "How do you know you're allergic?" "What kind of problem did you have when you took _____?" The symptoms of an allergy (e.g., rashes, itching, anaphylaxis) should be clearly indicated.

One should determine whether the patient has been *immunized* against tetanus, diphtheria, polio, measles, pertussis, influenza, pneumococcal pneumonia, mumps, or rubella.

A careful review of any *substance abuse* by the patient is included in the past medical history. Substance abuse includes cigarette smoking, alcohol, and "street drugs." The interviewer should determine whether the patient smokes, and for how long. A *pack-year* is the number of years a patient has smoked cigarettes multiplied by the number of packs per day. A patient who has smoked two packs of cigarettes a day for the past 25 years has a smoking history of 50 pack-years.

The history of *alcoholic consumption and dependency* should be integrated into the history immediately after inquiring about less threatening subjects such as the consumption of cigarettes. It is acceptable to broach the topic of alcoholism by asking directly, "Do you drink alcohol?" The interviewer should *not* focus on the quantity of alcohol consumed but rather on the adverse effects of drinking. By asking, "How much do you drink?," the interviewer may put the patient on the defensive. This type of question may also create an unnecessary power struggle between patient and physician. Most individuals who drink will also underestimate the quantities they consume. The interviewer will often learn more about the quantity of alcohol consumed by asking about the patient's feelings and his interpersonal relationships than by asking directly about the amount consumed. One must determine if the patient drives while intoxicated, if he has suffered amnesia of events while drinking, if he neglects or abuses his family, and if he has missed work as a result of his alcohol consumption.

Ewing and Rouse (1970) have suggested the CAGE questionnaire as a tool for helping to make the diagnosis of alcoholism. The acronym CAGE helps the interviewer to remember the four clinical interview questions. Once it is established that a patient drinks alcohol, the following questions should be asked:

"Have you ever felt the need to Cut down on your drinking?"
"Have people Annoyed you by criticizing your drinking?"
"Have you ever felt bad or Guilty about your drinking?"
"Have you ever taken a morning 'Eye-opener' to steady your nerves or get rid of a hangover?"

Since its introduction, the CAGE questionnaire has been shown to be one of the most efficient and effective screening devices to detect alcoholism. Four positive responses are pathognomonic for alcoholism. Two or three positive answers should create a high level of suspicion. If neither the answers nor the nonverbal responses to these questions are positive, the diagnosis of alcoholism can be generally excluded. One study by Bush (1987) has indicated that one or more affirmative responses to these questions has a sensitivity of 85% and a specificity of 89%.

The history of alcoholic consumption and dependency can be further assessed by using the sets of questions referred to by the acronyms HALT, BUMP, and FATAL DT. The HALT questions include the following:

"Do you usually drink to get High?"
"Do you drink Alone?"
"Do you ever find yourself Looking forward to drinking?"
"Have you noticed that you seem to be becoming Tolerant to alcohol?"

The BUMP questions are as follows:

"Have you ever had Blackouts?"
"Have you ever used alcohol in an Unplanned* way?"
"Do you ever drink alcohol for Medicinal† reasons?"
"Do you find yourself Protecting‡ your supply of alcohol?"

The final acronym will remind the interviewer about other major associations with alcoholism. The FATAL DT questions are as follows:

"Is there a Family history of alcoholic problems?"
"Have you ever been a member of Alcoholics Anonymous?"
"Do you Think you are an alcoholic?"
"Have you ever Attempted or had thoughts of suicide?"
"Have you ever had any Legal problems related to alcoholic consumption?"
"Do you ever Drive while intoxicated?"
"Do you ever use Tranquilizers to steady your nerves?"

---

* Drink more than you intended or have an additional drink after you have decided you have had enough.
† As a cure for anxiety, depression, or the "shakes."
‡ Buying enough alcohol just in case "company" arrives.

These questions will provide the interviewer with a useful, thoughtful, and organized approach to the interview strategy designed to uncover the patient with a drinking problem.

The interviewer must ask all patients about the use of street drugs. People who use street drugs often engender negative feelings and/or anger in their health care professionals. These feelings are almost unavoidable. The interviewer must not allow these feelings to interfere with his empathetic interviewing. A useful way of approaching the topic of street drugs is to ask,

> *"Have you ever used drugs other than those required for medical reasons?"*
> *"Have you abused prescription drugs?"*

If the answer to either of these questions is in the affirmative, it is important to determine the types of drugs used, the route(s) of administration, and the frequency of use. In contrast to the alcoholic, the drug abuser is more likely to magnify his use. The interviewer must ask all patients with a history of drug abuse the following questions:

> *"What type of drugs do you use?"*
> *"At what age did you start using drugs?"*
> *"What was your period of heaviest use?"*
> *"What is your recent pattern of use?"*
> *"Are larger doses necessary to get the same effect now?"*
> *"What do you feel when you take the drug?"*
> *"Have you ever tried to quit?. . .What happened?"*
> *"Have you ever had any convulsions after taking the drug?"*
> *"Do you use more than one drug at a time?"*
> *"Do you abuse drugs on a continuous basis?"*
> *"Have you been in trouble at work because of drug use?"*
> *"Have you ever had withdrawal symptoms as a result of your use of drugs?"*

It is important to use simple words and expressions when inquiring about street drugs. It may also be more appropriate to use the slang than to use the more formal terms. For example, "Do you ever shoot up or snort coke?" This may be more acceptable than saying, "Have you ever taken cocaine intravenously or by insufflation?" With experience, the interviewer will acquire relevant knowledge about recreational drugs. Knowing the local "street names" is often as important as knowing the pharmacology. The knowledge of these names may provide a means for better communication. It should be recognized that these street names do change often from place to place and from time to time. The appendix at the end of this book summarizes some commonly abused drugs, their street names, and the major symptoms and signs associated with each of them.

When questioning a patient about his *diet,* it is useful to ask him to describe what he ate the day before, including all three meals plus any snacks. How many fish meals does he have each week? Has his diet changed recently? What kinds of foods does the patient like or dislike and why? Are there any food intolerances? Does the patient eat foods with high fiber content, such as whole grain breads and cereals, bran, fresh fruits, and vegetables? High fiber snack foods include sesame bread sticks, date nut bread, oatmeal cookies, fig bars, granola bars, and corn chips. What is the consumption of sodium? Pickled foods, cured meats, snack foods, and prepared soups have high sodium content. One should ascertain the amount of exercise the patient gets. The consumption of caffeine containing products, such as coffee, tea, or chocolate, is important to determine.

It is important to know a patient's *sleep history,* as this may provide information about the patient's psychological problems. When does he go to bed? Does he have trouble falling asleep? Does he stay asleep the whole night, or does he awaken in the middle of the night, unable to go back to sleep?

All *current medications* should be noted. If possible, ask the patient to show you the bottles and have him tell you how he takes the medications. It is important to note if the patient is taking them according to the directions on the bottle. Ask the patient if he is taking any other medicines. Frequently, patients will consider over-the-counter medications such as vitamins, laxatives, antacids, or cold remedies not worth mentioning. Ask specifically about each of these types of drugs. It is also important to determine the type of contraception used, if any, and if a woman has used or uses birth control pills.

Occupational and Environmental History

The *occupational and environmental history* concerns exposure to potential disease-producing substances or environments. It is important to inquire about all occupations and the duration of each. The history should include more than just a listing of jobs. The duration and precise activities must be sought. The use of protective devices and cleanup practices as well as work in adjacent areas *must* be determined. The job title (e.g., electrician, machine operator) is important, but actual exposure to hazardous materials may not be reflected in these descriptions. Industrial work areas are complex, and the actual location of work in relationship to other areas where hazardous materials are used is important to ascertain. It is well known that just living near areas of industrial toxins can produce disease many years later. It is therefore relevant to inquire if the patient resides or ever resided near mines, farms, factories, or shipyards. The following questions regarding occupational and environmental exposure should be asked of all patients:

"*What type of work do you do?*"
"*How long have you been doing this work?*"
"*Describe your work.*"
"*Are you exposed to any hazardous materials? Do you ever use protective equipment?*"
"*What kind of work did you do before you had your present job?*"
"*What was your wartime employment, if any?*"
"*Where do you live? . . . For how long?*"
"*Have you ever lived near any factories, shipyards, or other potentially hazardous facilities?*"
"*Has anyone in your household ever worked with hazardous materials that could have been brought home?*"
"*What type of hobbies do you have? What type of exposures are involved?*"

Biographical Information

Biographical information is a statement of the date and place of birth, sex, race, and ethnic background.

Family History

The *family history* provides information about the health of the entire family, living or dead. One should pay particular attention to possible genetic and environmental aspects of disease that might have implications for the patient. The age and health of all the immediate family members should be determined. If a family member is deceased, the age of the person and the cause of death should be recorded. It is important to inquire how a family member's illness affects the patient.

Psychosocial History

The *psychosocial history* includes information on the education, life experiences, and personal relationships of the patient. This section should include the patient's lifestyle, other people living with the patient, schooling, military service, and marriage. A statement regarding the patient's knowledge of his symptoms and illness is important. Has the illness caused the patient to lose time from work? What kind of insight does the patient have regarding the symptoms? Does he think about the future?

The *sexual history* is a normal part of the psychosocial history. The interviewer must inquire about sexual relationships in a nonjudgmental fashion. Sexual drive is a sensitive indicator of general well-being. Direct questions regarding oral and anal sex, sexual contacts, and sexual problems are very important. Patients frequently have less of a hang-up about discussing their sexual behavior than does the young interviewer in asking about it. When in doubt regarding sexual preference, the term *partner* rather than a gender-specific term is appropriate. Asking the patient if he has had any contact with individuals with AIDS or AIDS-related illness is appropriate. The term "homosexual" should be avoided, as it is generally perceived to be demeaning.

There are several general questions that can help broach the topic of sexual activity. Some of the following suggested questions may be helpful in your questioning:

> *"Most people experience some disappointment in their sexual function. Can you tell me what disappointments you might have?"*
> *"Are you satisfied with your sexual performance?" "Do you think your partner is?"* If not, *"What is unsatisfactory to you (your partner)?"*
> *"Have you had any difficulty with achieving orgasm?"*
> *"How frequently, on the average, do you have intercourse?"*
> *"How frequently does it occur that your partner desires sexual intercourse and you do not?"*
> *"What activities and positions does your sex include?"*
> *"Are there any questions pertaining to your sexual performance that you would like to discuss?"*
> *"Many people experience what others may consider unusual sexual thoughts or wish to perform sexual acts that others consider abnormal. We often are bothered about these thoughts. What has been your experience?"*

Review of Systems

The *review of systems* summarizes in terms of body systems all the many symptoms that may have been overlooked in the history of the present illness or in the past medical history. By reviewing in an orderly fashion the list of possible symptoms, the interviewer can specifically check each system and uncover additional symptoms of "unrelated" illnesses not yet discussed. The review of systems is best organized from the head down to the extremities. Patients are told that they are going to be asked if they have ever had a particular symptom, and they should answer just "yes" or "no." If they answer in the affirmative, further direct questioning is appropriate. The interviewer need not repeat questions that were previously answered, unless clarification of the data is necessary.

Table 1–1 is the review of systems that should be asked of all patients. The questions should be asked of the patient in a way in which he will understand

TABLE 1–1. Review of Systems

General
Usual state of health
Fever
Chills
Usual weight
Change in weight
Weakness
Fatigue
Sweats
Hot or cold intolerance
History of anemia
Bleeding tendencies
Blood transfusions and
  possible reactions
Exposure to radiation

Skin
Rashes
Itching
Hives
Easy bruisability
History of eczema
Dryness
Changes in skin color
Changes in hair texture
Changes in nail texture
Changes in nail appearance
History of previous skin
  disorders
Lumps
Use of hair dyes

Head
"Dizziness"
Headaches
Pain
Fainting
History of head injury
Stroke

Eyes
Use of eyeglasses
Current vision
Change in vision
Double vision
Excessive tearing
Pain
Recent eye examinations
Pain when looking at light
Unusual sensations
Redness
Discharge
Infections
History of glaucoma
Cataracts
Injuries

Ears
Hearing impairment
Use of hearing aid
Discharge
"Dizziness"
Pain
Ringing in ears
Infections

Nose
Nosebleeds
Infections
Discharge

Frequency of colds
Nasal obstruction
History of injury
Sinus infections
Hay fever

Mouth and Throat
Condition of teeth
Last dental appointment
Condition of gums
Bleeding gums
Frequent sore throats
Burning of tongue
Hoarseness
Voice changes
Postnasal drip

Neck
Lumps
Goiter
Pain on movement
Tenderness
History of "swollen glands"
Thyroid trouble

Chest
Cough
Pain
Shortness of breath
Sputum production (quantity,
  appearance)
Tuberculosis
Asthma
Pleurisy
Bronchitis
Coughing up blood
Wheezing
Last x-ray
Last test for tuberculosis
History of BCG vaccination

Cardiac
Pain
High blood pressure
Palpitations
Shortness of breath with
  exertion
Shortness of breath when
  lying flat
Sudden shortness of breath
  while sleeping
History of heart attack
Rheumatic fever
Heart murmur
Last ECG
Other tests for heart function

Vascular
Pain in legs, calves, thighs, or
  hips while walking
Swelling of legs
Varicose veins
Thrombophlebitis
Coolness of extremity
Loss of hair on legs
Discoloration of extremity
Ulcers

Breasts
Lumps
Discharge

Pain
Tenderness
Self-examination

Gastrointestinal
Appetite
Excessive hunger
Excessive thirst
Nausea
Swallowing
Constipation
Diarrhea
Heartburn
Vomiting
Abdominal pain
Change in stool color
Change in stool caliber
Change in stool consistency
Frequency of bowel move-
  ments
Vomiting up blood
Rectal bleeding
Black, tarry stools
Laxative or antacid use
Excessive belching
Food intolerance
Change in abdominal size
Hemorrhoids
Infections
Jaundice
Rectal pain
Previous abdominal x-rays
Hepatitis
Liver disease
Gall bladder disease

Urinary
Frequency
Urgency
Difficulty in starting the stream
Incontinence
Excessive urination
Pain on urination
Burning
Blood in urine
Infections
Stones
Bed wetting
Flank pain
Awakening at night to urinate
History of retention
Urine color
Urine odor

Male Genitalia
Lesions on penis
Discharge
Impotence
Pain
Scrotal masses
Hernias
Frequency of intercourse
Ability to enjoy sexual
  relations
Fertility problems
Prostate problems

History of venereal disease
  and treatment

Female Genitalia
Lesions on external genitalia
Itching
Discharge
Last Pap smear and result
Pain on intercourse
Frequency of intercourse
Birth control methods
Ability to enjoy sexual rela-
  tions
Fertility problems
Hernias
History of venereal disease
  and treatment
History of DES exposure
Age at menarche
Interval between periods
Duration of periods
Amount of flow
Date of last period
Bleeding between periods
Number of pregnancies
Abortions
Term deliveries
Complications of pregnancies
Description(s) of labor
Number of living children
Menstrual pain
Age at menopause
Menopausal symptoms
Postmenopausal bleeding

Musculoskeletal
Weakness
Paralysis
Muscle stiffness
Limitation of movement
Joint pain
Joint stiffness
Arthritis
Gout
Back problems
Muscle cramps
Deformities

Neurologic
Fainting
"Dizziness"
"Blackouts"
Paralysis
Strokes
"Numbness"
Tingling
Burning
Tremors
Loss of memory
Psychiatric disorders
Mood changes
Nervousness
Speech disorders
Unsteadiness of gait
General behavioral change
Loss of consciousness
Hallucinations
Disorientation

them. For example, a question regarding paroxysmal nocturnal dyspnea should be asked,

> *"Do you ever awaken in the middle of the night with sudden shortness of breath or sudden difficulty in breathing?"*

Each of the organ and system specific chapters that follow discusses a review of specific symptoms that further elaborates on the symptoms related to that specific organ system. Hints about specific questioning and the pathophysiology of the symptoms are also provided in each chapter.

Not infrequently, a patient may answer in the affirmative to *all* the questions. If one detects that this is occurring, it may be useful to ask a question about a physiologically impossible condition. If when asked "Do your stools glow in the dark?" the patient answers in the affirmative, the interviewer should not continue with the review of systems. The interviewer can state in his written history or in his verbal presentation that, "The patient has a positive review of systems."

Because the goal of the medical history is to acquire as much information about each patient's illness as possible, other specific questions related to that particular patient may be indicated. Look at the patient shown in Plate I A. If you were to see such a patient, you may wish to try to determine when the facial changes occurred. In such a case, it is important to ask the man if he has noticed a change in his hat size and when he first noticed it.

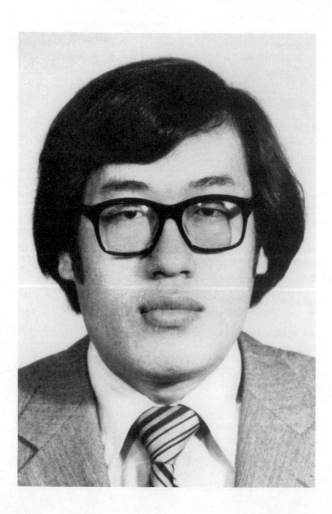

FIGURE 1–1. A photograph of the patient shown in Plate I *A* taken 20 years earlier. Compare the facial features with those shown in the color illustration.

Look at Plate I B, which compares the right hand of the same patient with the right hand of a normal individual. Asking about a change in glove size is also useful in this particular patient. It would also be appropriate to inquire whether there has been a change in shoe size as well.

A useful bit of information may be an old photograph of the patient to help determine when the suspected changes occurred. Compare the photograph in Figure 1–1 of the same patient taken 20 years earlier with Plate I A. Notice the bulging forehead and the prominent jaw in the later photograph. This is a patient with acromegaly, a condition of abnormal growth hormone excess secreted by a pituitary tumor. The changes are insidious over many years. The photograph was helpful in determining the change in bone and soft tissue structure.

The important point to remember is that a medical history must be dynamic. Every history is different. All patients are asked the "standard" questions, but each patient should be evaluated individually. There is no limit to the questions to be asked.

The *written history* is a permanent, legal document of the patient's health history. The information that is recorded must be accurate and objective. Based upon all the information gleaned from the patient's history, the interviewer carefully summarizes all the data into a readable format. It is important to remember that anything that is written in a patient's record may someday be presented to a court of law. Only objective data should be included. Opinions or statements about previous care and therapy must be avoided.

By convention, when the review of systems is stated or written, all symptoms that the patient has experienced are indicated first. Those symptoms never experienced are indicated afterwards. The *pertinent positive* symptoms are those symptoms that have possible relevance to the present illness. *Pertinent negative* symptoms are those symptoms that are not present but that may often be related to the present illness.

If information in the review of systems has been described previously in the history of present illness, for example, it is correct to indicate under the systems review of that symptom, "See History of Present Illness."

As you proceed with the interview, you may sense that it is not going well. Is the patient comfortable? Is there a language barrier? Did you say or do something to interfere with the rapport? Is the patient intimidated? Is the patient concerned about confidentiality? Is the patient reluctant to talk in the presence of family members? Is the patient able to express his feelings? These are just a few of the common reasons for lack of progression of an interview. If you can alleviate the problems, do so. Perhaps interviewing the patient on another day using the same approach will be more successful.

BIBLIOGRAPHY

Adler G, Buie DH: The misuses of confrontation with borderline patients. Int J Psychoanal Psychother 1:109, 1972.

Bernstein J: Conversations in public places. J Communication 25:85, 1975.

Brown BL, Strong WJ, Rencher AC: Perceptions of personality from speech: Effects of manipulation of acoustical parameters. Acoust Soc Am J 54:29, 1973.

Bush B, Shaw S, Cleary P, Delbanco TL, Aronson MD: Screening for alcohol abuse using the CAGE questionnaire. Am J Med *82*:231, 1987.

Chafetz ME: No patient deserves to be patronized. Med Insight *2*:68, 1970.

Clark WD: The medical interview: Focus on alcohol problems. Hospital Practice *11A*:59, 1985.

Ewing JA, Rouse BA: Identifying the hidden alcoholic. Presented at the 29th International Congress on Alcohol and Drug Dependence, Sydney, Australia, Feb 3, 1970.

Francis V, Korsch BM, Morris MJ: Gaps in doctor-patient communication. N Engl J Med *280*:535, 1969.

Gregg D: Reassurance. Am J Nurs *55*:171, 1955.

Hall ET: The Silent Language. Garden City, NY, Doubleday and Co, Inc, 1959.

Kahn A: The Dynamics of Interviewing. New York, John Wiley and Sons, Inc, 1957.

Larsen KM, Smith CK: Assessment of nonverbal communication in the patient-doctor relationship. J Fam Pract *12*:48, 1981.

Lief HI, Karlen A (eds): Sex Education In Medicine. New York, Spectrum Publications, 1976.

Matthews D, Hingson R: Improving patient compliance: A guide to physicians. Med Clin North Am *61*:879, 1977.

Payne SL: The Art of Asking Questions. Princeton, Princeton University Press, 1951.

Peabody FW: The care of the patient. JAMA *88*:877, 1927.

Rosenthal RS: Malpractice: Cause and its prevention. Laryngoscope *88*:1, 1978.

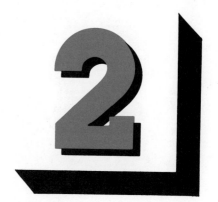

THE PATIENT'S RESPONSES

It is our duty to remember at all times and anew that medicine is not only a science, but also the art of letting our own individuality interact with the individuality of the patient.

Albert Schweitzer
1875 – 1965

RESPONSES TO ILLNESS

Health is characterized by a state of well-being, enthusiasm, and an energetic pursuit of life's goals. Illness is characterized by feelings of discomfort, helplessness, and a diminished interest in the future. Once a patient recognizes that he is ill and possibly faces his own mortality, a series of emotional reactions occur. These include anxiety, fear, anger, frustration, denial, depression, withdrawal, projection, and an exaggeration of symptoms. These psychological reactions are general and are not specific to any particular physical illness. The patient must learn to cope not only with the symptoms of the illness but also with life as it is altered by the illness.

Anxiety

Anxiety is a state of uneasiness in which the patient has a sense of impending danger. It is the fundamental response to stress of any kind, such as separation, injury, social disapproval, or decreased self-esteem. Anxiety and fear are common reactions to the stress of illness. The feelings of loss of control, guilt, and frustration contribute to the patient's emotional reaction. Illness makes patients feel helpless. Recognizing the body's mortality leads patients to an intense feeling of anxiety. In addition to the emotional reaction, fear can be manifested physiologically by restlessness, gastrointestinal problems, or headaches. Other

27

common symptoms of anxiety include difficulty in falling asleep, nightmares, frequency of urination, palpitations, fatigue, vague aches and pains, paresthesias, and shortness of breath. Not uncommonly, the patient may feel that he is "falling apart."

The young man who has been stricken with a heart attack feels helpless. As he lies in his intensive care unit bed, he begins to recognize how mortal he really is. Being confined to bed makes him feel helpless. The patient feels that he must be dependent upon everyone and everything: the nurse, the doctor, the intravenous line, even the monitor. His anxiety, based on helplessness, is a normal response to his illness. His sudden illness and the threat of possible death oppose his belief that he is indestructible.

A 72 year old man who has lived alone for years since his wife died is admitted to a hospital for a transurethral prostatectomy. He is anxious that he may become dependent upon his children. He may be more threatened by his fear of dependency than by the illness itself.

The hospitalized patient who is brought to the radiology department for a routine chest x-ray and is forced to wait 2 hours for a transporter to bring her back to her room suffers anxiety. She is angry to have been left waiting and perhaps missed some visitors. But she says nothing. Her anxiety is based on the fear of expressing anger to the nurses and staff members on the floor. She feels that if she were to express her anger, the hospital personnel might interfere with her medical care.

Some hospitalized patients cannot accept the love and care expressed by family or friends. This inability to accept tenderness is a common source of anxiety. The patient is threatened by these affectionate acts because they serve to reinforce his dependency.

There is anxiety in all patients admitted to a hospital. The patient must put his most important commodity, his life, into the hands of a group of strangers who may or may not be competent to assume responsibility for his survival. This is the fear of strangers.

Depression

Depression is a psychological reaction to the loss of health, a loved one, or one's own self-esteem. Certain degrees of depression probably accompany every chronic illness. There are many types of depression: reactive, neurotic, manic, melancholic, and agitated, to name only a few. In general, the patient with depression has pessimistic tones in his speech and a downcast facial expression. He may express feelings of futility and self-accusation. The patient will respond to questions with brief answers. His speech is slow; his volume is low; his pitch is monotonous. Typically, the speech pattern tends to put the interviewer to sleep. The depressed patient feels that he is inadequate, worthless, and defeated. He also suffers profound feelings of guilt. A confrontation such as *"You look sad"* allows the patient to talk about his depression. Crying allows relief of severe depressive feelings and permits the patient to continue his story. Although crying may be brought on by a patient's concern for his own illness, crying usually occurs when a patient thinks of an illness or death of a loved one or of a potential loss. He often has much hostility and resentment and suffers from rejection and loneliness. Self-accusative and self-depreciative delusions can occur in the severely depressed patient. When these delusions are present, such overwhelming feelings of worthlessness are present that the patient may feel that suicide is the only way out.

The 23 year old law student is engulfed with anxiety when he learns that he has AIDS. When his friends and family learn of the illness, he is immediately excluded from all relationships. He has violent feelings of guilt. His depression is worsened when he learns that his university has asked him to leave his studies. He is found later hanged in his parent's attic. His only way of coping with his illness was through suicide.

Depression may be the most common reaction to illness seen in medicine, as well as the most frequently overlooked. The most important diagnostic symptoms of depression are the following:

- Insomnia
- Poor appetite or weight loss
- Fatigue or loss of energy
- Agitation
- Loss of interest
- Feelings of guilt or self-reproach
- Decreased ability to think or concentrate
- Thoughts of death or suicide

Denial

Denial is acting and thinking as if a part of reality were not true. Denial is one of the most common psychological mechanisms of defense in medicine and is seen in both patients *and* physicians. Denial is often an emotional response to inner tension and prevents a painful conflict from producing overt anxiety. It is actually a form of *self-deception*. Denial is often seen in terminal illnesses or in chronic incurable diseases. In general, the more acute the illness, the greater is the patient's insight; the more insidious, the greater the denial.

A patient dying slowly from cancer can observe his weight dropping and the side effects of his medications. His frequent visits to the hospital for chemotherapy or radiotherapy confirm the severity of his illness; yet, in spite of all this, he will continue to deny his illness. He will make plans for the future and talk about when he will be cured. Denial is the psychological mechanism that keeps this patient going. The interviewer should not confront his denial despite its apparent absurdity. Telling such a patient to "face the facts" is cruel punishment. Breaking down denial in such a patient only serves to add to the dying patient's misery. However, the patient's family must recognize and understand the poor prognosis.

Denial can sometimes obstruct proper medical care. A woman presents for the first time to a breast clinic with an orange-sized mass in her breast. The mass has already started to ulcerate, with a resultant foul smelling infection. When asked how long she has had the mass, she responds that she noticed it just yesterday. It is often best to interview a reliable informant when the patient with denial is recognized.

Projection

Projection is another common defense mechanism by which a person unconsciously rejects an unacceptable emotional feature in himself and "projects" it onto someone else. It is the major mechanism involved in the development of paranoid feelings. For example, the hostile patient may say to the interviewer, "Why are you being so hostile to me?" In reality, the patient is projecting *his* hostility onto the interviewer.

Patients commonly project their anxieties onto their physicians. Patients who use projection are constantly watching a doctor's face for subtle signs of their own fears. Take, as an example, the 42 year old woman with a strong family history of death from breast cancer. She has intense fears of developing cancer. During the inspection portion of the physical examination, the patient may be watching the physician's face for information. If the physician frowns or makes some type of negative gesture, the patient may interpret this as "He *sees* something wrong!" The physician may have made this expression only because he was thinking of how much work he still has to do that day, or what type of medication he should prescribe for another patient. The patient has projected her anxiety onto the physician. The physician must be aware of these silent "conversations."

In some instances, projection may have a constructive value, saving the patient from being overwhelmed by the illness.

Regression

Regression is a common, primitive defense mechanism by which the patient with extreme anxiety attempts unconsciously to return to earlier, more desirable stages of development. During these periods, the individual enjoyed full gratification and freedom from anxiety. The patient with regression becomes dependent upon others and frees himself of the complex problems that have created his anxiety.

For example, take the middle-aged married man who has recently been told that he has inoperable lung cancer that has already spread to his bones. He is stricken with grief and intense anxiety. There are so many unanswered questions. How long will he live? Will his last months be plagued with unremitting pain? How will his wife be able to raise their young son by herself? How will she manage financially without his income? By regression, the patient can flee this anxiety by becoming childlike and dependent. The patient becomes withdrawn, shy, and often rebellious; he now requires more affection.

A teenager learns that the cause of his 6 month history of weakness and bleeding gums has been diagnosed as acute leukemia. He learns that he will spend what little time he has left in the hospital undergoing chemotherapy. His reaction to his anxiety may be regression. He now needs his parents at his bedside around the clock. He becomes more desirous of his parent's love and kisses. His redevelopment of enuresis, or bed wetting, is part of his psychological reaction to his illness.

The 25 year old woman with inflammatory bowel disease has had many admissions to hospitals for exacerbations of her disease. She fears the future and the possibility that a cancer may have already started to develop within her. She is engulfed by an overwhelming feeling of terror and apprehension. She fears that some day she may require a colostomy and she will be deprived of one of her most important functions: bowel control. She acts inappropriately, has temper tantrums, and is indecisive. Her dependency on her parents is a manifestation of regression.

RESPONSES TO THE INTERVIEWER

Much of the enjoyment of medical practice comes from talking with patients. Each patient brings a challenge to the interviewer. Just as there are no two interviews that are alike, there are no two people who would interview the same patient in the same manner. This section distinguishes several common clinical types of patients and illustrates how the interview may be modified in each case.

The Silent Patient

Some patients have a lifelong history of shyness. Some of these individuals lack self-confidence. They are very concerned about their self-image and do not want to say or do the wrong thing. These patients are embarrassed easily. Other individuals become hostile or silent as fear of illness develops. The silent patient frequently is seriously depressed. This may be primary to an illness or a secondary response to it. Commonly these patients have many of the other signs of depression as seen in their attitude, facial expressions, and posture. The use of open-end questions with these patients is generally of little value. Carefully directed questioning may provide some of the answers.

The Overtalkative Patient

The overtalkative patient presents a real challenge to the novice interviewer. These patients dominate the interview. The interviewer can hardly "get a word in edgewise." Every question has a long answer. Even the answers to "yes-no" questions seem endless. There is usually an aggressive quality to these patients' communications. Every answer is overdetailed. A courteous interruption followed by another direct question will focus on the subject of the interview. The use of open-ended questions, facilitations, or silence is to be avoided, as these techniques will only encourage the patient to continue speaking. If all else fails, the interviewer should try to relax and accept the problem.

The Seductive Patient

One of the most difficult patients for the novice to interview and examine is the seductive patient. In many ways, the seductive patient is more difficult than a hostile patient. Many of these patients are hysterics who have fantasies of developing an intimate relationship with their physician. Characteristically, these patients tend to expose themselves early in the interview. The interviewer may elect to cover the patient, but usually this is unsuccessful. Coping with one's own feelings when one finds himself attracted to such a patient is difficult. The feeling of attraction is a natural one, and the interviewer must accept it. However, the interviewer must always maintain a strictly professional demeanor. Empathy and reassurance must be kept to a minimum, as these supportive techniques will stimulate further fantasies on the part of the patient. The interviewer should never become involved in a relationship that may sacrifice his professional self-respect or effectiveness. If necessary, he should get the advice of someone he trusts.

The Angry Patient

Very commonly, one interviews the angry, obnoxious, or hostile patient. Some are demeaning or sarcastic, whereas others are demanding, aggressive, and blatantly hostile. Some patients may remain silent during most of the interview. At other times, they may make inappropriate remarks that are condescending to the novice or even to the experienced physician. The interviewer may feel resentment, anger, threatened authority, impatience, or frustration. Reciprocal hostility and a power struggle can develop.

The interviewer must realize that these reactions are the patient's responses to his *illness* and not necessarily a response to the interviewer. These reactions may be deep-rooted in the patient's past. Every interviewer should be aware that the same emotions such as rage, envy, or fear are present in both the patient and interviewer. A patient may express feelings toward the interviewer, who must act in a detached, professional way and not feel offended or become defensive.

How should we deal with such a patient? The interviewer immediately feels animosity toward the angry patient. But hating our patients is against everything we have been taught. The student has always been taught that he must like his patients in order to treat them appropriately. This ambivalence in the interviewer is the problem. Why *should* we like the patient? We must treat the patient medically correctly and with respect, but we *don't* have to like him. Because of illness, the patient may have feelings of loss of control, threatened authority, and fear. His anger is the mechanism by which he can handle his fears. Once the interviewer gains this insight and becomes aware of his own feelings, he can better treat such a patient. The interviewer must accept and restrain his own negative feelings toward the patient so that his professional judgment will not be distorted. The interviewer's awareness of his own anxieties and feelings will aid in a more productive interview. Conscious expression of one's own feelings in a frank and non-insulting manner will facilitate the interviewing process. Regulation and control of *our* feelings is the goal.

Confrontation may be a useful technique for interviewing such patients. By saying "You sound very angry," you allow the patient to vent some of his fears. Another confrontational approach is to say, "You're obviously angry about something. Tell me what you think is wrong." You must maintain your equanimity and avoid becoming defensive. If at the beginning of the interview you detect that the patient is angry, try to disarm him. Proceed with your questions slowly, avoid interpretations, and ask questions that are confined to the history of the present illness.

The Paranoid Patient

The paranoid patient is the patient who constantly asks, "Why are you asking me that? Do I have _____?" When the interviewer asks the many questions in the review of systems, the patient responds, "Who told you about that?" The paranoid patient thinks that there is some devious plan and that people are constantly talking about him. The air of suspiciousness on the part of the patient can sometimes be handled by the interviewer saying, "These are routine questions that are asked of all my patients." Reassurance tends to be threatening to these patients and should not be used, as it tends to produce more paranoia. The patient's delusion is beyond reason. The interviewer should therefore complete the questioning and not try to convince the patient about his false ideations. Avoidance of any anger on the part of the interviewer is of paramount importance.

The Insatiable Patient

Insatiable patients are never satisfied. They have many questions, and despite adequate explanations, they feel that the interviewer has not answered all their questions. They tend to be very sensitive, anxious individuals. These patients are best handled with a firm, non-condescending approach. A definite closing statement is helpful, such as, "We have reached the end of our time for today, but I will be back." Alternately, the interviewer could say, "We have reached the end of our time for today. I will refer your concerns to Dr. _____."

The Ingratiating Patient

The ingratiating patient is the patient who attempts to please the interviewer. The patient believes that everything he answers must satisfy the interviewer. He thinks that if he answers a question to the disapproval of the interviewer, the interviewer will abandon him. Intense feelings of rejection are present in this type of patient. The interviewer must recognize that anxiety is the cause of the patient's behavior and should try not to respond to it. The interviewer should recognize the patient's tendency of trying to please and should stress to the patient how important it is to be accurate.

The Aggressive Patient

The aggressive patient is a patient with a personality disorder. This individual is easily irritated and often flies into a rage when dealing with the normal stresses of daily life. He is domineering and tries to control the interview. However, if allowed to have his way, he may be quite pleasant. Very frequently, the aggressive patient has intense dependency needs that he cannot consciously handle. He masks the primary problem by becoming aggressive and hostile to disguise his anxiety and feelings of inadequacy and inferiority. The aggressive patient is very difficult to interview. One must try carefully to stay away from areas provoking anxiety early in the interview. Once a rapport is established, the interviewer may attempt to delve into the deeper areas. In general, the aggressive patient will refuse any type of psychotherapy.

The Help-rejecting Patient

The help-rejecting patient, commonly known as a "crock," is not generally hostile. He describes having been seen by many "expert" physicians for help and is smug in telling you that no one can find out what's wrong with him. He returns over and over again to the doctors' offices, indicating that the physicians' suggestions "didn't work." Commonly, when a symptom appears relieved, another suddenly appears in its place. These patients use their symptoms to enhance their relationship with their doctors. Such patients are often very depressed, although they will deny it. They feel that they have made many self-sacrifices and have had countless disappointments, which they attribute to their "illness." The best approach to these individuals is strong emotional support and gentle reasoning. Despite the need for psychiatric help, these patients generally refuse to accept it.

The Demanding Patient

The demanding patient makes demands of everyone: the physician, the nurse, the student, the aide. This patient uses intimidation and guilt to force others to take care of him. The patient views himself as being neglected and abused. The patient may have outbursts of anger toward the physician, who may fear for his own reputation. A power struggle may result.

INFLUENCE OF BACKGROUND AND AGE ON PATIENT RESPONSE

Although disease is universal, patients respond to their illnesses differently. A particular question asked to different patients will be answered in a style that is governed by the patient's ethnic background, emotions, customs, age, social history, and family history. These factors determine the way in which a patient perceives and responds to a question. This section illustrates the importance of understanding a patient's background as an aid to better communication.

Ethnic Background

The socioeconomic status as well as ethnicity influences the way in which patients perceive their symptoms, illness, and health care. The novice interviewer must learn some of the values and cultural patterns of the minority groups he will be treating so that he will be better equipped to care for them. It is dangerous to view the lifestyle of another ethnic group by one's own "standards." Competence and compassion are important factors in administering good patient care.

Black Americans comprise a very heterogeneous ethnic group. Most black Americans are of African, West Indian, or Southern descent, each group having both common and distinct cultural values. The family and religious beliefs are extremely important to most black Americans. Strong kinship bonds are common.

The range of responses of black Americans is similar to that of the general population, but certain fears and disenfranchisements may be more common. Socioeconomic status as well as ethnicity plays an important role in the way black patients perceive their illness, symptoms, and health care in general. Some black Americans delay their medical care despite the availability of subsidized health care. Some don't know how to get into the health care system, whereas others simply mistrust it. Some blacks have a great fear of being hospitalized and may believe in herbal remedies, spiritualism, and religious cures. Preventive medical care is not available to many blacks because of inadequate financial resources. Many seek attention only when their symptoms become unbearable and frequently when it is too late to effect a change in their prognosis.

In obtaining information from the black patient, the most important qualities that the interviewer should project are competency, empathy, and a sense of compassion. In order to gain the confidence of the black patient, the interviewer must treat the patient with respect, and the individual should always be allowed to maintain his dignity.

The incidence of hypertension and diabetes in the black patient is high. Dietary patterns are particularly important to investigate in the black patient. There are certain ethnic foods that have deep cultural roots and should not be totally eliminated from the diet, if possible.

Many *Hispanic* patients still believe in witchcraft, spiritualism, and mediums. Mediums are the persons through which the spirits communicate with the visible world. Mediums treat illness by means of herbal remedies, magic, and religion. The remedies often include herbal teas and salves. Never try to belittle the patient's belief; work *with* the belief. By using medical knowledge and adapting it to the patient's beliefs, you can gain the patient's confidence.

Some Hispanic patients believe in the "hot-cold" theory of disease. In this belief, which is intuitive and widespread in much of Latin America, the body is regulated by hot or cold "humors." Health is the balance of these "hot" and "cold" body fluids. Illness is defined by a humoral imbalance. Foods, herbs, and medications are also classified as to "hot" and "cold" and serve to restore the body to its natural balance. In this theory, conditions that are "hot," such as ulcer disease, should be balanced by and treated with "cold" foods, such as coconut or avocado. "Cold" illnesses, such as arthritis, are treated with "hot" therapy, such as aspirin or cinnamon. A patient may be on diuretic therapy and require potassium supplementation. The physician may advise the patient to eat foods that are high in potassium, such as oranges or bananas. If the patient gets an upper respiratory infection, which is a "cold" disease, he may stop taking these fruits, which are classified as "cold," as they will only worsen the imbalance. This belief should be recognized, as it contributes significantly to a patient's noncompliance with drug therapy. Problems can arise when the physician prescribes a "hot" medication for a "hot" disease, or vice versa. The "hot-cold" theory is even more complex when one recognizes that the assignment of the "hot" and "cold" qualities varies from culture to culture.

Most Spanish speaking patients have a great fear of being hospitalized, because of isolation from their families. As a rule, modesty is common among the Chicanos. Those individuals who speak only Spanish are concerned that they will not be able to communicate with the medical personnel when help is necessary. Though many Spanish American patients prefer to speak Spanish, never assume that they cannot speak English. Usually, the family is very close. It is, therefore, not uncommon for a 90 year old woman who speaks no English to be accompanied to the hospital by her children, grandchildren, great-grandchildren, and even great-great-grandchildren. Not infrequently, as many as 15 to 20 family members may want to sleep in the halls or television room waiting to take their relative home. Decision making is likewise a *family* matter. Never pressure the patient into making a decision. Allow the patient time to discuss an issue with his family.

The *Asian* patient places much emphasis on obligation, authority, and honor. Those individuals who have disgraced their families consequently suffer guilt. This guilt can then be transformed into psychosomatic disease, which is very common in this culture. The Asian patient rarely complains of pain. He may suffer from it, but his complaints are few. If the interviewer suspects that the patient is having pain, it is fitting to ask if pain is present. Generally, *after* being asked, the patient will acknowledge the pain. Another very important reality in dealing with Japanese patients relates to the "yes-no" question and the infrequent use of the word "No." Most Japanese people feel that to answer "No" will put an individual on the defensive. Therefore, they may answer "Yes," meaning that they understand, not necessarily answering in the affirmative to the question. In some Japanese, giggling is often a sign of embarrassment.

Many Asians believe in folk medicine. The "hot-cold" theory of disease, which was discussed previously, is still accepted by some Asian Americans. Another example of the balancing of internal forces is seen in the Chinese culture. The balance of *yin* and *yang* is comparable with the "hot-cold" principle. In this belief, *yin* represents the feminine, cool, empty, and negative force. *Yang* represents the masculine, hot, full, and positive force. Everything in the world consists of both *yin* and *yang*. Health is the perfect balance of these forces. Diseases caused by excesses of *yin* are treated by hot foods or medications. Illnesses caused by *yang* excesses are treated by cold foods or medications. For example, a sore throat, caused by *yang* excess, should be treated with a cold food such as watermelon. Unless contraindicated, the patient's family should be encouraged to bring in the foods that they believe will be helpful.

A common problem in the Chinese patient is related to medication. In folk medicine, one dose of an herbal remedy will usually "cure" an illness. Prescriptions of Western medications require multiple doses over longer periods of time. The Chinese patient may have difficulty in complying with this schedule. It is incumbent upon the physician to explain this difference in "medical" therapy carefully. The interviewer must respect this patient's belief, and, by attempting to understand it, the physician will be more able to provide better care.

The Holocaust Survivor Patient

The holocaust survivor patient is a patient with complex problems that have affected his life for the past 45 years. He is a *survivor;* therefore, he never stops fighting for survival. He is frightened of becoming sick. To survive in the past meant to be in good health; the alternative was to face doom. This patient is afraid of losing control over his life as well as losing his dignity.

The holocaust survivor patient may have many psychosomatic complaints, commonly related to the gastrointestinal tract. Chest pain, often relieved by belching, may be related to frequent air swallowing. This patient experiences vivid dreams and nightmares. The survivor is suspicious and doesn't trust people readily. He has many reasons for his mistrust, for he suffered so much in the past. The interviewer must be very kind and understanding. The majority of the survivors of the Nazi death camps are now over the age of 65 and suffer from the delayed stress syndrome, which is now taking its toll. Many are suffering from severe depression, panic attacks, and anxiety. The interviewer must be careful when asking about the family and background. Most of the survivors lost entire families; many lost their first spouse and children. The wounds are deep, and anything can trigger an outpouring of grief. It is frequently difficult to find out anything about the family history, as parents and grandparents were killed at young ages. The patient should be reassured that he will be gently and competently treated.

The Aged Patient

The aged patient can be a delight if he is the jovial, friendly type or a nuisance if he is bitter and angry; in either case, he requires a lot of attention. Depression is prevalent among the elderly. The aged patient must frequently cope with the loss of loved ones and other important persons in his environment. He is also stressed by changes in his own self-image and the way he is perceived by others. A deterioration in bodily function also contributes to the depression seen in the aged patient.

The patient's depression may be so severe that he may consider suicide a reasonable alternative to living with a severe chronic illness or living alone after the death of a spouse. Among this bereaved population, more deaths from suicide occur within the first 4 years following the spouse's death than from all other causes (McMahon and Puch, 1965).

The interviewer must never assume that the older patient's complaints are natural for his age. People don't die of old age; they die of illnesses. Most of these patients are alert and capable of independent living. The ones who are unable to care for themselves are usually accompanied by a family member or an attendant. The interviewer must obtain as much information from these sources as possible. The interviewer should also refrain from using patronizing mannerisms that belittle the individual. A friendly, respectful approach will reassure the patient. The aged patient should be advised about everything that will be done to him. This makes the patient confident that no unpleasant surprises are in store for him. Because of his advanced age, the aged patient may be afraid of dying. The individual who is afraid should be reassured that everything possible will be done to make him better. Many times people survive an illness because of their desire to live and, therefore, fight to stay alive. Overzealous reassurance is not appropriate in all aged patients, as death is a reasonable outcome for many.

The Widowed Patient

There is something special about the widowed patient. He comes to the hospital, many times alone, with the thought that because his spouse is gone, nobody really cares about him. He may be suffering from depression as a result of loneliness. The interviewer has to inquire gently if there are any children, relatives, or friends who can be contacted or will come to visit. The patient may be at odds with his children and may prefer that they not know he has entered a hospital. At other times, the family may live far away. The patient doesn't want them to worry, so he doesn't tell them. In these cases, it is advisable for the physician to alert the social worker to the particular situation. Volunteers visiting the patient as well as members of the clergy can bring soothing counsel. A warm handshake and reassurance are effective ways of putting this patient in a relaxed state of mind. Many widowed patients are quite active. The physician should not presume that all widowed individuals are isolated.

The Child Who Is Ill

Children tend always to be "on guard." The ill child is especially vulnerable and wary. First of all, the child is taken from his "friendly" home environment. Second, doctors, nurses, and students are constantly staring at him with a wide variety of facial expressions. Many older children believe that the physician has some sort of "magical eye" that can see through them and know everything about them. All of this adds up to a frightening experience for the youngster. Frequently, tests that may cause discomfort may have to be performed by the "persons in white." The physician becomes a symbol of danger and pain. The white coat is soon awaited with terror and anxiety. The child cannot understand the reason for his being taken from his own environment.

When the physicians, nurses, or technicians take the youngster for a test, the child experiences his greatest fear: separation from his parents. This separation produces an intense emotion of fear and anxiety, manifested by wailing, irritability, and aggressive behavior. The child's fear stems from his concern that he will not see his parents again. This fear may actually be subconscious. The physician should explain to the child, if old enough, that he knows why the child is crying and should assure him that he will see his parents soon. The parents should be urged to talk to the child, informing him that the doctor is going to help him. The parent should be careful *not* to indicate that the doctor will *not* hurt the child, because if the child has pain as a result of a test, the child-parent relationship may be jeopardized. The parent should be encouraged to stay with the child in the hospital as long as possible and even sleep in the child's room at night, if permitted. Studies have shown that when parents are permitted to stay with the child, the recovery is quicker and there is less emotional trauma. An important part of caring for children is talking to the parents. If they comprehend the situation, they can go a long way toward helping the doctor-child relationship.

The disabled child, as the disabled adult, is even more apprehensive of the atmosphere in the hospital. It reminds him of his previous experiences. The interviewer must take time to play with the child while talking to the parent or the person accompanying the child. Complimenting the youngster with statements such as "How pretty you are" or "What a nice outfit you're wearing" seems to foster good will. These children crave love, affection, and attention. The parent has to be reassured that the staff members are reliable and caring. This will give the parent peace of mind. If a child wishes to keep his favorite toy or blanket, there should be no restrictions. Separation from home and family is a terrible experience for any child, but even more so for the disabled one, who functions better in familiar surroundings.

The Sick Doctor

Perhaps the hardest of all patients to take care of is the sick doctor. The anxiety of sick physicians should not be underestimated. The old expression "A little knowledge is a dangerous thing" applies to the sick doctor. Every medical or nursing student goes through the "student syndrome," which is the suspicion that he has been stricken with the disease about which he is learning. Imagine the anxiety that occurs when the physician *is* stricken. In addition to his anxiety about his health, there is the new role identification of being the patient. He feels helpless, and he has great difficulty divorcing himself from the role of physician. He constantly asks what the electrocardiogram shows and the results of his blood tests. He tries to suggest additional tests or even disagrees with the tests that have been ordered. The novice interviewer should provide ample time for the sick doctor to express his fears and anxieties. By the interviewer being supportive to his needs, the sick physician will eventually recognize and accept his new role as patient.

INFLUENCE OF DISEASE ON PATIENT RESPONSE

Just as background and age govern a patient's response, so do the patient's present illness and past medical illneses. This section illustrates the influence of disease on the type of response.

The Disabled Patient

The disabled patient may come to the hospital with great apprehension and mistrust. He is usually familiar with the shortcomings of hospitals, because he has probably been hospitalized previously for painful tests or surgery. He may be burdened with an inferiority complex and may feel unattractive. The interviewer must take all this into consideration and assure the patient that every-thing will be done to make him comfortable. The interviewer must sort out the emotional problems of the disabled person from the physical ones that brought him to the hospital. A friendly smile or a few kind words can go a long way in making this patient cooperate and thereby secure a better doctor-patient rela-tionship.

Many disabled people have developed their own routines that work for them. They often don't want medical personnel to impose their way of doing some-thing if the patient's way works.

The individual with a hearing impairment is a special type of disabled patient. You should sit directly in front of the patient to allow him to benefit from lip reading. Make sure that the lighting in the room is correct so that your face is well illuminated. It is important to speak slowly with appropriate gestures and expressions to punctuate the question. Ask these patients if it is necessary for you to raise your voice. If they wear a hearing aid, raising your voice may not be necessary. If all else fails, the use of written questions can be helpful.

Another special type of disabled patient is the visually impaired patient. Because the patient with limited or no vision has no reference for you in the room, it is useful for you to occasionally touch the patient on his arm or shoulder. This can be used in place of the more standard nonverbal facilitations, which are of no value in this patient.

The severely mentally retarded patient must be accompanied by a family member or guardian in order to provide a proper history.

The Cancer Patient

The cancer patient has five major concerns: loss of control, pain, alienation, mutilation, and mortality. Loss of control makes the cancer patient feel helpless. The knowledge of something growing within a patient's body without control creates frustration, fear, and anger. Suffering with pain is one of the most feared aspects of the patient with cancer. The feeling of alienation stems from the reactions of people around him.

Fears of mutilation are common among cancer patients. The fear of being perceived as lacking "wholeness" contributes to the patient's depression and anxiety. The young woman with breast cancer who requires a mastectomy fears that she will be rejected as no longer being a complete woman. Supportive family members are the key in reassuring this patient that they will love her just as before her surgery. A diagnosis of cancer makes a patient aware of her mortality and leads to intense fears of unremitting pain.

Family members and friends often express grief before death occurs. Resentment and anger may be directed toward the cancer patient. The physician often harbors feelings of inadequacy with this type of patient and has difficulty speaking with him. The patient is rejected now by his own physician. On ward rounds, the patient is skipped over and avoided. The physician is afraid that the patient may ask some questions, perhaps about death, that he cannot handle. The physician must recognize his emotional and behavioral reaction and be realistic about the limitations of medical science.

The interviewer should allow the patient to vent his anxieties and promote dialogue. Listening to the patient aids in the doctor-patient relationship.

The AIDS Patient

The patient with acquired immune deficiency syndrome (AIDS) is fearful for his life and of being stigmatized as a member of an undesirable group. He is aware that his chance of survival is slim. The fear and misunderstanding common in such high risk groups result in delayed medical treatment. Denial is the important factor in most of these patients. The patient has an intense fear of physicians, nurses, students, and paramedical personnel, who may have strong emotions related to this disease and its risk groups. The patient's fear is paralleled by the anxiety on the part of the hospital workers who have to treat an individual with this deadly disease. Their fear of contracting the disease, even by casual contact, is formidable. These fears are also present among the patient's friends and family, who often banish the patient from all activities. The patient may have been fired from his employment, as his employer is afraid of catching the disease. Owing to the lack of knowledge concerning the spread of the disease, there is an unsympathetic rejection of the AIDS patient. He suffers inner turmoil, which contributes to intense anxiety, hostility, and depression. He may have to die alone.

The interviewer should be as supportive as possible without giving false reassurances. Most patients with AIDS recognize their prognosis. The patient should be given as many facts as appropriate, and the staff members tending to him must be educated concerning the disease.

The Dysphasic Patient

The dysphasic patient is an individual who has an impairment of speech and cannot arrange words correctly. Dysphasia is usually caused by a cerebral lesion, such as a stroke. The degree of dysphasia can vary enormously, almost to complete aphasia. Although the patient may appear relatively unresponsive, he may be totally aware of all conversation. Therefore, it is stressed that all discussions conducted in the presence of the patient must be made with the assumption that the patient can understand. During an interview of a patient with dysphasia, the interviewer may give the patient a pen and paper to detemine if he can respond by writing. "Yes" or "No" answers may be given by a nod of the head.

The Psychotic Patient

In general, interviewing psychotic patients presents a difficult task for the inexperienced interviewer. Some of these patients tend to be inarticulate and preoccupied with fantasies, whereas others are reasonably lucid. The symptoms and signs of their psychosis are not clearly evident at first assessment. There are several clues to the existence of a psychosis. One should pay particular attention to the speech pattern and its organization. Is there a flight of ideas? The psychotic patient is easily distracted, and the interviewer must constantly remind him of the subject in question. The patient fails to complete any train of thought and cannot follow any idea to its completion. Such patients often have illusions, which are the misinterpretations of a sound, sight, or other sensory data. Illusions are, however, common in normal individuals under emotional stress and strain. In addition, delusions, feelings of persecution, and hallucinations are characteristic of the psychotic patient. These patients can have bizarre impressions about their bodies. They may complain that they have noticed that one arm has recently shortened, or that their external genitalia have suddenly shrunk or enlarged. In addition, they may have evidence of an inappropriate affect. The patient may laugh while telling about the death of a friend or relation.

A special type of psychotic personality disorder is found in the patient with *Münchausen's syndrome*. This is the classic hospital malingerer. The patient is a pathologic liar and travels from physician to physician, from hospital to hospital. He complains of a wide variety of symptoms and, in fact, *creates* signs of illness in order to seek an advantage. His history is well rehearsed, and he has a masochistic perpetuation of self-injury. The Münchausen patient may actually prick the skin under his fingernail so it will not be obvious, drop some blood into his urine, and call his physician, stating that he has blood in his urine. He will frequently seek out painful diagnostic and therapeutic procedures. At times, he may even undergo surgical procedures.

The Demented Patient

The patient with an organic mental syndrome presents a special problem. At times these patients seem perfectly lucid, while at other times they are disoriented to person, place, or time. If the patient is able to answer some of the questions, you should record the answers. The same questions should be asked at a later time to determine if the patient will respond similarly. Patients with an organic mental syndrome have defects in attention span, memory, and abstract thought. You should be alert to inconsistent and slow, hesitant responses. Occasionally, patients may interject some humor to try to cover up for their difficulty in memory. A careful mental status examination will indicate the problem. It may be useful to remind the patient of your name and tell him that you will ask him for the name in a few minutes. Frequently such patients will have forgotten it. Once you have recognized that the patient has an organic mental syndrome, it is very important to understand that the history he gives may not be reliable.

The Patient Who Is Acutely Ill

The acutely ill patient demands prompt attention. In these situations, a concise history and physical examination are in order. A careful history of the present and past illnesses must be taken expeditiously so that the diagnosis may be made and treatment begun. It may be appropriate in this setting to actually interview the patient at the same time you are doing the physical examination. Time is of the essence. However, patients who are acutely ill may respond to questions slower than normally because of their pain, nausea, or vomiting. Don't rush them. Be considerate of their problems and allow them time to answer your questions. After the patient has been stabilized, there will be plenty of time to go back and take a more complete history.

The Surgical Patient

The patient faced with a surgical procedure is scared despite a possible calm outward appearance. He may be helpless and out of control. The fear of anesthesia, disfigurement, disability, or death is always present. The fear that he will not awaken from the anesthesia can be devastating. When he awakens, will he find that his body is no longer "whole"? Did the surgeon find something that was not expected? The bottom line is the fear of the unknown. The question "He's a good surgeon, isn't he?" is an expression of the patient's anxiety. Often patients have tests and are told they are normal "except" for a small area: they'll need surgery to "check it out." This lack of communication on the part of the physician adds to the patient's anxiety. A surgeon's schedule is frequently erratic. Surgery may be delayed or postponed, which adds to the surgical patient's anxiety and anger. Many possible communication difficulties exist. The best way to avoid the unnecessary anxiety-provoking situations is for there to be a free line of communication maintained among the patient, the physician, and the patient's family. In the postoperative period, the relief of having lived through surgery may be displayed in a variety of ways. The patient may be apathetic and show a general lack of interest. He may be moody, irritable, aggressive, angry, or tearful. These are various mechanisms by which the surgical patient can now finally vent his anxiety. Subconsciously the patient may wish to harm the surgeon for "cutting" into his body, whereas consciously he wants to thank the surgeon. This dichotomy may be the root of the anger so commonly seen in the postoperative patient. In other patients, depression may be seen as a result of the loss of part of the body. The best example of this is the "phantom limb." Patients who have had an amputation of their leg frequently claim sensation in their lost limb. Some of this may be physiologic, but certainly some of the phantom leg pain is related to depression. The caring interviewer should allow the patient time to release these tensions and feelings of loss.

The Alcoholic Patient

The alcoholic patient has a physiologic and/or psychological dependence on alcohol. Most of the time, the interviewer conducts the session when the patient is not inebriated. Excessive drinking is often an attempt to deaden feelings of guilt and failure. The more the patient drinks, the more he is abandoned by his family and friends. He feels castigated and alone. He is left to his only friend: alcohol. Speaking with the alcoholic patient is fascinating. He is often ready to talk, and his account of his drinking habits may be interesting. Alcoholics generally have a low opinion of themselves. They may even be upset about their persistent drinking habits. Their hatred of themselves may be a manifestation of a self-destructive wish. The alcoholic patient may also have fears about sexual inadequacy or homosexuality. It is not easy to open up such topics, as this patient is likely to respond explosively. The sensitive interviewer should approach these issues in a manner that is neither condescending nor moralistic.

The Psychosomatic Patient

Just as physical illness can produce psychological problems, so can psychological problems create physical ailments. The intimate interaction of the mind and body is clearly demonstrated in the psychosomatic disorder. Anxiety, fear, and depression are the main psychological problems associated with the psychosomatic patient. The list of associated, common symptoms and illnesses is long and includes chest pain, headaches, peptic ulcer disease, ulcerative colitis, irritable bowel syndrome, nausea, vomiting, anorexia nervosa, urticaria, tachycardia, hypertension, asthma, migraine, muscle tension syndromes, obesity, rashes, and dizziness. Answers to an open-ended question such as "What's been happening in your life?" often provide insight into the inner problems. Giving the patient the freedom to discuss his hopes and fears will often be more beneficial than a written prescription for medications.

The Dying Patient

Many physicians have a dread of death that can be so intense that they can behave irrationally. They avoid patients who are dying or those with incurable diseases. The emotional needs of the dying patient may be largely ignored. Many patients have a greater fear of dying than of death itself. The fear of living as a chronically ill patient can be almost as intolerable (and often more so) as the fear of death.

The dying patient suffers from the pain, nausea, or vomiting caused by his disease or treatment. He may be rejected by his family, hospital staff members, or even his own physician. Many patients have strong feelings of anger, guilt, resentment, and frustration. "Why me?" "It should have been diagnosed earlier." They are envious of healthy individuals. They will actively deny their imminent death. This is the first stage of dying. Not uncommonly, a dying patient will be interviewed and not tell the interviewer about his illness. Even when asked specifically about the disease, the patient will deny any knowledge of having a fatal disease. This mechanism of denial allows the patient to cope with his life as it is. Each person faces death differently. Some can deal with it "head-on"; others cannot. Some approach it with fear and tears, whereas others grow to accept it as an inevitable event. Given sufficient time and the necessary understanding, most dying patients can arrive at the final stage of dying: acceptance. This stage is characterized by apathy and social withdrawal. Counselors specifically trained in the grieving process are often helpful to the patient, family, and physician.

The dying patient needs to speak to someone. The physician should be alert for subtle clues that the patient actually wishes to discuss the topic of death. For example, if the patient remarks that his "wife is well provided for," it is correct to pursue this point by making an interpretive statement such as, "I sense that you are very worried about your illness." Although the conversation that ensues might be emotionally draining for the interviewer, it is incumbent upon him to allow the dying patient to speak. Sometimes the most appropriate response to an expression of grief is a thoughtful period of silence.

BIBLIOGRAPHY

Adler G: The physician and the hypochondriacal patient. N Engl J Med 304:1394, 1981.

Cassem NH, Hackett TP: Psychological aspects of myocardial infarction. Med Clin North Am 61(4):711, 1977.

Chang B: Asian-American patient care. In Henderson G, Primeaux M (eds): Transcultural Health Care. Menlo Park, CA, Addison-Wesley, 1981.

Clark M: Health in the Mexican American Culture. Los Angeles, University of California Press, 1970.

Cousins N: Anatomy of an illness (as perceived by the patient). N Engl J Med 295:1458, 1976.

Currier RL: The hot-cold syndrome and symbolic balance in Mexican and Spanish American folk medicine. In Martinez RA (ed): Hispanic Culture and Health Care: Fact, Fiction, Folklore. St. Louis, CV Mosby, 1978.

Dombro RH: The surgically ill child and his family. Surg Clin North Am 50:759, 1970.

Dunn FL: Transcultural Asian medicine and cosmopolitan medicine as adaptive systems. In Leslie C (ed): Asian Medical Systems: A Comparative Study. Berkeley, CA, University of California Press, 1975.

Gorlin R, Zucker HD: Physician's reactions to patients: A key to teaching humanistic medicine. N Engl J Med 308:1057, 1983.

Groves JE: Taking care of the hateful patient. N Engl J Med 298:883, 1978.

Harwood A: A hot-cold theory of disease: Implications for treatment of Puerto Rican patients. JAMA 216:1153, 1971.

Kornfield DS: Psychiatric problems of an intensive care unit. Med Clin North Am 55(5):1353, 1971.

Kübler-Ross E: On Death and Dying. New York, Macmillan, 1969.

Lipsett DR: Medical and psychological characteristics of "crocks." J Psychiatry Med 1:15, 1970.

Lock M: The relationship between culture and health or illness. In Christie-Seely J (ed): Working with the Family in Primary Care. New York, Praeger, 1984.

McMahon B, Puch G: Suicide in the widowed. Am J Epidemiol 81:23, 1965.

Murillo-Rohde I: Hispanic American patient care. In Henderson G, Primeaux M (eds): Transcultural Health Care. Menlo Park, CA, Addison-Wesley, 1981.

Rainwater L: The lower class: Health, illness, and medical institutions. In Millon T (ed): Medical Behavoral Science. Philadelphia, WB Saunders Co, 1975.

Reichel W: Care of the elderly. In Taylor RB (ed): Family Medicine: Principles and Practice. New York, Springer-Verlag, 1983.

Senescu RA: The development of emotional complications in the patient with cancer. J Chron Dis *16*:813, 1963.

Stern M, Pascale L, Ackerman A: Life adjustment postmyocardial infarction. Arch Intern Med *137*:1680, 1977.

Sue S, Sue DW: Understanding Asian-Americans: The neglected minority. Personnel Guid *51*:387, 1973.

Tseng WS: The nature of somatic complaints among psychiatric patients: The Chinese case. Compar Psychiatry *16*:237, 1975.

Williams JGL, Jones JR, Workman MC, Williams B: The psychological control of preoperative anxiety. Psychophysiology *12*:50, 1975.

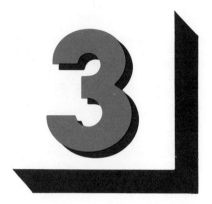

PUTTING THE HISTORY TOGETHER

The doctor may also learn more about the illness from the way the patient tells the story than from the story itself.

James B. Herrick
1861 – 1954

In the previous two chapters, the interviewer's questions and the patient's responses have been discussed. At this time, it would be useful to put these sections together to shape a mock interview.

In the ensuing interview, note carefully the way in which the interviewer allows the patient to speak and how the various techniques are incorporated.

The footnotes refer to the type of technique used or to some other important aspects of the interview.

INTERVIEW OF MR. JOHN DOE

Mr. John Doe, the patient, is lying comfortably in a four-bedded room in Mount Hope Hospital. He is a white man appearing slightly obese and in his mid-forties. Mr. Doe is watching television. The interviewer enters the room, wearing a white coat.

Interviewer	*(smiling, extending hand for a firm hand-shake)* Good morning, Mr. Doe. I'm Susan Smith, a second year medical student. I've been asked to interview and examine you today.
Patient	*(smiling, appearing friendly)* Dr. James, my resident, told me you'd be coming to see me.
Interviewer	*(draws curtain around bed; pulls up a chair at the patient's bedside and sits down; legs crossed, arms in lap)* Would you mind if we turn off the TV?
Patient	*(turns off television)* Not at all.
Interviewer	How are you today?
Patient	OK. No pain for the past 2 days.
Interviewer	What was the problem that brought you to the hospital, Mr. Doe?*
Patient	I've been having terrible chest pain for the past 6 months . . . *(pause)* . . . I guess I should start at the beginning . . . About 4 years ago, I started having this strange sensation in my chest. It wasn't pain exactly . . . it was a dull aching discomfort. I didn't pay any attention to it. I guess I should have . . . Well, anyway, I was able to go to work, play tennis, and have fun. Occasionally when I had an argument at work, I would get this sensation. *(looking sad)*

---

* Inquiring about the chief complaint by using an open-ended question.

My wife never knew anything about it. I never told her. No one knew. I didn't want to upset them. Then all of a sudden on July 15th, 1987, it happened . . .

(silence)

Interviewer

It happened?*

Patient

Yeah. I had my first heart attack.† I was playing tennis when I got this God-awful pain. I never had anything like that before. I was just getting ready to serve when this pain hit me. All I could do was lie down on the court. My partner ran over to me, and all I remember was that pain . . . I woke up in Kings Hospital.

(pause)

They told me I lost consciousness and was taken to the hospital by ambulance. I remember that when I came to in the hospital, I still had the pain. I was there for 2 weeks.

Interviewer

How did you feel when you left the hospital?

Patient

I really felt fine. No more chest pain. My doctor there had given me some pills and said I would be fine.‡

Interviewer

Then what happened?§

Patient

I went back to work after about 3 weeks. I really felt great!

(smiles)

Interviewer

What type of work do you do?

Patient

I'm a lawyer.

---

* This is an example of reflection.
† The patient is now telling the history of the present illness.
‡ Possibly false reassurance from the physician, or the patient heard what he wanted to hear.
§ Continues obtaining information with another open-ended question about the present illness.

| Interviewer | You mentioned that this was your *first* heart attack. Have you had others? |

| Patient | Unfortunately . . .

(looking down)

. . . yes |

| Interviewer | Tell me about it.*

(leaning forward†) |

| Patient | Six months later, I had my second attack.

(pause) |

| Interviewer | What were you doing? |

| Patient | Playing tennis.

(silence)

. . . This time I don't remember anything . . . not even the pain. I remember being on the court and waking up in the intensive care unit of Kings Hospital. They said I had a massive heart attack and had some irregularity of my pulse that made me faint. But I left the hospital in 3 weeks feeling much better. I went back to work after 3 weeks. |

| Interviewer | Did you have any tests while you were in the hospital? |

| Patient | No . . .

(pause, hand over mouth)

. . . the doctor just gave me some pills to strengthen my heart and for the irregularity . . .

(silence) |

---

* An example of verbal facilitation.
† An example of nonverbal facilitation.

Interviewer	*(silence, then after 10 seconds)*
	Your silence makes me think that you want to tell me something.*
Patient	I should have listened to him.
	(pause, shaking head)
Interviewer	To whom?
Patient	My doctor suggested after my first heart attack that I should have cardiac catheterization. I told him that I was fine . . . I didn't need it . . . Even after my second attack, I didn't listen to him . . .
	(pause)
	. . . I hope it's not too late.
Interviewer	Too late?
Patient	Yeah. That's why I'm here. I'm going to have the cardiac catheterization tomorrow. Emily finally convinced me to have it . . .
	(pause)
	. . . I've really not been able to do anything for the past 6 months . . .
	(pause, looking down)
	. . . I had to give up my work at the office . . . Sure they still call me for advice, but it's not the same . . .
	(pause, almost tearful)
	. . . The commuting by car just got to me . . .
	(pause)
	. . . My son and his friends yelling around the house . . .
	(longer pause)
	. . . I just can't take it anymore.

---

* An example of confrontation.

Interviewer	What did your doctor tell you about the test?*

Patient	The doctor told me if I have some blockage, he'll operate or fix it. Will I be normal again?

Interviewer	*(pause)*
	. . . After the study your doctor will be in the best position to answer that question.†
	(pause)
	Tell me about the pain you've been having.

Patient	It seems I have the pain all the time. I can hardly walk up the stairs at home without getting the pain.

Interviewer	What's the pain like now?

Patient	It's an awful tightness, like a vise . . .
	(closes fist over chest‡)
	right here . . .

Interviewer	When you get the pain, do you feel it anywhere else?

Patient	Yeah. It goes straight to my back and my left arm . . . The arm feels so heavy.

Interviewer	Are there any other times when you get the pain?

Patient	It seems I get it with the slightest effort or emotion.

* Inquiring about the patient's understanding of the test.

† The interviewer does not want to give false reassurances. Therefore, she elects not to answer the question directly. Notice how the interviewer gets the narrative back on course.

‡ This example of body language has been termed Levine's sign. It is discussed in Chapter 11, The Heart.

Interviewer	Do you get the pain during sexual intercourse?
Patient	I had to stop even that 6 months ago. I'd get the pain just when I'm about to come . . . and . . . and . . . I'd have to stop.
Interviewer	Have you had any difficulty breathing?
Patient	When I get the pain, I get short of breath.
Interviewer	Do you ever get short of breath without the pain?
Patient	I find I just can't walk far any more without getting winded.
Interviewer	How many level blocks can you walk now without getting short of breath?
Patient	About 1 block.
Interviewer	How much could you walk 6 months ago?
Patient	I guess about 2 to 3 blocks.
Interviewer	Since your heart attack, have you had any skipped beats or fluttering of your heart?
Patient	No, never.
Interviewer	Has anyone ever told you that your cholesterol or fats in your blood were high?*

---

* The interviewer is now starting to ascertain if the patient has any risk factors for coronary artery disease.

Patient	No.
Interviewer	Have you ever smoked?
Patient	I stopped after my first heart attack.
Interviewer	How much did you smoke?
Patient	About 2 packs a day.
Interviewer	For how long?
Patient	Oh . . . since I was about 18.
Interviewer	May I ask your age?*
Patient	I'm 42.
Interviewer	Have you ever had high blood pressure?
Patient	Yep . . . My doctor gave me some medications for it but . . . but . . . I never refilled the pills after they ran out . . . I felt fine.
Interviewer	Do you know how high your pressure was? †
Patient	Not really.

---

* Notice that the interviewer has just now decided to ask the patient's age.
† Notice that the interviewer ignores the statement that the patient didn't take his medications. Questioning the patient "Why not" would only put the patient on the defensive.

Interviewer	Do you have diabetes?
Patient	Thank goodness, I don't . . . My father does though . . . He's been pretty sick lately . . . He's got some sort of a problem with his eyes. The doctor said that it's from his diabetes. He's going to see a specialist in a couple of weeks . . . He's had a lot of problems. He broke his hip a few years ago when he was walking our dog. Some big guy came pulling a cart out of supermarket and knocked my father over. He was hospitalized for several weeks since he really couldn't take care of himself. His hip is fine now. He would
Interviewer	*(interrupting)* I'm glad his hip is well healed. Is there anyone else in your family who has diabetes?*
Patient	No.
Interviewer	Anyone with a heart attack?
Patient	I think my mother's father died of a heart attack.
Interviewer	How old was he?
Patient	About 75.
Interviewer	What about your mother?†
Patient	She died when she was age 64 . . . right after my first heart attack. She had stomach cancer. She really suffered . . . I guess it's a blessing.

---

* Notice that the patient was beginning to ramble. The interviewer politely interrupted and redirected the interview. She is now inquiring about the family history.

† Notice that the interviewer does not assume anything about the mother's well-being or health. Because the patient approached the family's health history, the interviewer is now directing her questions to that history.

Interviewer	Do you have any brothers or sisters?
Patient	My sister is 37 and she's fine . . . *(pause)*
Interviewer	Any other siblings?
Patient	My brother is 45 . . . He had a heart attack when he was 40.*
Interviewer	Do you have any children?
Patient	One boy who's 10.
Interviewer	How's your son's health?
Patient	No problem except he's a little overweight.
Interviewer	Are you married?†
Patient	To a great gal. Emily's the one who convinced me to have the test.‡
Interviewer	Does anyone in your family have high blood pressure?
Patient	No.

---

* Notice that the patient did not mention his brother when first asked about other family members with heart attacks or when asked about other brothers or sisters. The patient has even denied to acknowledge his brother's cardiac problem!

† Notice that the interviewer does not assume that Mr. Doe is married *now*, even though he referred to his wife at the beginning of the interview and has acknowledged "Emily" previously. "Emily" may *not* be his wife!

‡ In this case, "Emily" *is* the patient's wife. It is extremely important for the patient to identify family members. Never make an assumption that another person with the patient or described in the history is related to the patient.

Interviewer	Asthma?
Patient	No.
Interviewer	Tuberculosis?
Patient	No.
Interviewer	Birth defects or congenital diseases?
Patient	Not that I know of.
Interviewer	Have you ever been hospitalized previously here at Mount Hope Hospital?
Patient	No.*
Interviewer	Have you ever been hospitalized at any time other than for your heart attacks?
Patient	I had my appendix taken out when I was 15.
Interviewer	Do you remember the surgeon's name and the hospital?
Patient	I think it was a Dr. Meyers at Booth Hospital. We were then living in Rochester.
Interviewer	Any other operations?

---

* Had the patient answered in the affirmative, the interviewer would have asked when, and the patient's record would have been reviewed later.

Patient	No.
Interviewer	Have you ever been hospitalized for any other reason?*
Patient	No, what do you mean?
Interviewer	Just a routine question. Do you have any allergies?
Patient	No.
Interviewer	How was your health as a child?
Patient	I guess OK. I had the usual sore throats and earaches that most kids get.
Interviewer	Did anyone ever tell you you had rheumatic fever?†
Patient	No.
Interviewer	Did you have any of these illnesses:‡ chickenpox? . . . measles? . . . diphtheria? . . . polio? . . . mumps? . . . whooping cough? . . .
Patient	*(shakes head "no")*
Interviewer	Do you take any medications?
Patient	Just Inderal and Isordil.

---

* The interviewer is specifically asking about nonmedical hospitalizations, e.g., for psychiatric reasons. This type of question is not offensive. If the patient has had such admissions to hospitals, he can generally describe them at this time. If not, as in this case, watch how the interview progresses. (Notice how the interviewer continues directly with the next question.)

† This question can follow nicely after the history of sore throats.

‡ The interviewer slowly asks about each illness, after which she pauses for the patient to respond.

Interviewer   Do you know the dosages?

Patient   I take Inderal 40 mg and Isordil 20 mg, both four times a day.

Interviewer   Do you think the medications help you?

Patient   I guess so. I think I feel better with them.

Interviewer   Any other medications?

Patient   *(pause)*

Nitroglycerin . . . when I get the pain.

Interviewer   How long does the nitroglycerin take to work?

Patient   Real quickly.

Interviewer   How long is that?

Patient   About 4 to 5 minutes.

Interviewer   Do you take any other medications . . .

(pause)

cold medicine? . . . vitamins? . . . anything else?

Patient   *(thinking)*

I take Chlor-Trimeton when I get a cold . . . but that's about it.

Interviewer   Have you ever had any other health problems?

Patient	No.

Interviewer	Any problems with your liver? . . . kidneys? . . . stomach? . . . lungs? . . .*

Patient	*(shakes head "no")*

Interviewer	How's your appetite?

Patient	Pretty good. I haven't been real hungry lately.

Interviewer	Starting with breakfast yesterday, what did you eat?

| Patient | Toast, coffee, and juice for breakfast . . . |

(pause)

A ham sandwich with a Tab for lunch . . .

(pause)

Oh yeah, blueberry pie for dessert . . .

(pause)

and . . . uh . . . steak with a baked potato and salad for dinner.

Interviewer	Any snacks between meals?

Patient	I had a cupcake with milk before I went to bed.

Interviewer	Do you eat fish?

---

* Because this patient has demonstrated so much denial, the interviewer wishes to ask specifically about the major organs. Each question is asked slowly, and the interviewer pauses after each question, waiting for a response.

Patient	Sometimes.

Interviewer	How often?*

Patient	Maybe . . .
	(pause)
	Once every 2 weeks. I enjoy shrimp, but I hear it's not good for me.†

Interviewer	Have you had any weight change recently?

Patient	I lost about 10 pounds in the past 3 months . . .
	(pause)
	. . . but I wanted to . . .

Interviewer	Were you on a diet?

Patient	No . . . not exactly . . . I just haven't been too hungry lately.

Interviewer	How well do you sleep? ‡

Patient	Like a baby . . .
	(pause)
	although I've been getting up pretty early recently.

Interviewer	Mmmm?

---

* The interviewer is not satisfied with qualitative statements. She pursues each question to quantify as best as possible.

† Despite the fact that he knows that shrimp is not as healthy as fish, he still eats it. Further denial of his illness!

‡ The interviewer has now picked up some other somatic element of depression and will now pursue it.

Patient

Yeah . . . recently I go right to sleep . . . but seem to get up about 3 in the morning . . . and can't go back to sleep . . .

(pause)

. . . I guess I've got a lot on my mind . . .

(pause, looking down, hand to mouth)

Interviewer

You seem depressed.*

Patient

(pause)

. . . I guess I am . . . What's going to happen to me? . . . I really want to live . . .

(beginning to cry)

. . . I've been so stupid . . .

(pause)

. . . My kid's only 10 . . . He's a great kid . . . He needs me . . . What's the test gonna show? . . . I hope I can have the surgery to get relief from this pain.†

Interviewer

(silent, handing a box of tissues to the patient)‡

Patient

(sobbing, trying to control his emotions)

I'm sorry doc . . . I can't help it . . .

(wiping his tears)

. . . I guess we'll have to wait till tomorrow.

Interviewer

I just have a few more questions for you. Do you drink alcohol?

---

* An example of an interpretation.

† The interviewer could have elected to ask the patient his reactions if surgery cannot be performed. How will he face life? Is there a possibility of suicide? The interviewer chose not to create further anxiety at this time.

‡ An example of empathetic support. The interviewer can't answer the patient's questions, but she allows the patient to express his emotions. She is, in essence, saying, "I'm with you."

Patient	*(shaking head "no")*
	Just socially . . . one drink . . . maybe after work, sometimes.
Interviewer	Do you ever feel that you have a need for a drink as the day goes on?
Patient	Yeah . . . I sure do!
Interviewer	Have you ever felt the need to cut down on your drinking?
Patient	No.
Interviewer	Have people annoyed you by criticizing your drinking?
Patient	Never . . . but my wife doesn't like me drinking.
Interviewer	Have you ever felt bad or guilty about your drinking?
Patient	Yeah . . . once about 10 years ago my friend's father made some wine . . . We got really drunk . . . It was terrible . . . But never again!
Interviewer	Do you drink in the morning?
Patient	Never.
Interviewer	Do you ever drive while intoxicated?
Patient	No! That's suicide.
Interviewer	Do you drink coffee or tea?

Patient

About 3 cups of coffee a day at work. I only have tea when I'm sick with a cold.

Interviewer

Have you *ever* used street drugs?

Patient

I've tried pot a couple of times . . . Never did anything to me . . . Nothing else.

Interviewer

What's your usual day like?*

Patient

Before I stopped working at the office, I got up about 5:30, dressed, and was at my desk in the office by 7:30. I usually left the office about 7 and got home by 8:15. We'd have dinner, and I'd be in bed by 11:30, after the news.

Interviewer

Sounds like you have a pretty busy day.

Patient

Yeah . . . I enjoy my work . . . Or at least I used to . . .

Interviewer

How long have you been working with your present office?

Patient

I started right after law school. I guess I've been there . . . about . . . 17 years. I'm one of the senior partners . . .

(pause)

. . . I was just promoted . . . A lot of good that will do now . . .

Interviewer

I now have several questions that I would like to ask you. You can just answer "yes" or "no" to each.†

(pause)

Have you had any recent fevers?

---

* Interviewer is inquiring about the patient's lifestyle and psychosocial history.
† The interviewer will now begin asking the *review of systems*. She will ask about each symptom. If the patient answers in the affirmative, further questioning will be appropriate.

Patient	No.
Interviewer	Chills?
Patient	No.
Interviewer	Sweats?
Patient	No.
Interviewer	Rashes?
Patient	No.
Interviewer	Changes in your hair or nails?
Patient	No.
Interviewer	Headaches?
Patient	Rarely, about once every 2 to 3 months.
Interviewer	For how long have you been having headaches?
Patient	Years . . . I guess about 20 to 25 years.
Interviewer	Can you describe them to me?
Patient	That's hard. They're right here. *(pointing to the center of his forehead)* . . . They last about 1 to 2 hours.

Interviewer	What relieves them?
Patient	Usually aspirin.
Interviewer	Have you noticed a change in the pattern or severity of your headaches?
Patient	No.
Interviewer	Have you had any head injuries?
Patient	Never.
Interviewer	Have you ever fainted?
Patient	No.
Interviewer	Do you have any problems with . . .*
Interviewer	*(After the review of systems has been completed, the interviewer asks,)* Is there anything else you would like to tell me that I haven't asked about?
Patient	No . . . you've certainly been very thorough.
Interviewer	I'd like to summarize your history briefly to make sure I have the details correct before I proceed with your physical examination. This is your first time here at Mount Hope Hospital. You had your first heart attack on July 15, 1987, while playing tennis. You were hospitalized in Kings Hospital for 2 weeks. Your second heart attack was 6 months later. You

---

* The interviewer continues through the entire review of systems, asking further questions when necessary.

were again hospitalized in Kings Hospital. Your medications since then have been Inderal 40 mg and Isordil 20 mg both four times a day. Because of a worsening of your chest pain and an increase in your shortness of breath in the past six months, you're now being admitted for cardiac catheterization. Is that correct?

Patient

Exactly!

Interviewer

Do you have any questions for me before I begin your physical examination?

Patient

No, doc . . . I can't think of any.

Interviewer

(The interviewer stands up, sets up the equipment on the night table, and goes to the sink to wash her hands. The physical examination then commences.)

Interviewer

(Concluding the physical examination)

I want to thank you for your time.

Patient

Well . . . what do you think? . . . Will I make it? . . .

Interviewer

(opening curtain around patient's bed)

. . . I'm now going to meet with my preceptor. Afterwards, we'll be back.*

The preceding interview has certainly revealed much about this 42 year old lawyer. Superficially, he is a patient with coronary artery disease. Just as important as his physical illness is his emotional reaction to it. As the interview progressed, the interviewer recognized that the patient is scared and anxious. What will happen "after tomorrow"? Will he need surgery? Can surgery be performed? Is he a good candidate for bypass surgery? Will he *live*? The anxiety from these questions has resulted in his depression, which must be dealt with as well.

---

* By indicating to the patient that the interviewer and her preceptor will be back, the patient is less likely to press the interviewer for *her* opinion at this time. The interviewer should never provide an answer at this point. False reassurances can be dangerous!

The written history is a summary of the information obtained during the interview. It is usually written after the interview and the physical examination have been completed. The following is an example of the written history of Mr. Doe, based on the preceding interview.

- **Chief Complaint.** "Chest pain for the past 6 months."

- **History of Present Illness.** This is the first Mount Hope admission for Mr. John Doe, a 42 year old lawyer with coronary artery disease. His history dates back to approximately 4 years prior to admission, when he started to experience a vague discomfort in his chest. He describes it as "a dull ache," provoked by emotional upsets at work. He suffered his first heart attack on July 15, 1987, while playing tennis. He was hospitalized for 2 weeks in Kings Hospital. After 3 weeks at home, he returned to work. Six months later, he suffered his second heart attack, again while playing tennis. At this time he was again hospitalized at Kings Hospital and was told that he had "irregularity" of his heart. He was started on some medications for same. The patient denies any palpitations since then.

Over the past 6 months, the patient has had increasing chest pain with radiation down his left arm despite Inderal 40 mg qid and Isordil 20 mg qid.* The patient's chest pain is produced by exercise, emotion, and sexual intercourse. The patient takes nitroglycerin as needed, with relief within 5 minutes. One block dyspnea on exertion is also present. This has worsened in the past 6 months, before which he could walk 2 to 3 blocks. The patient's risk factors for coronary artery disease include a history of untreated hypertension, a 40 pack-year history of smoking (2 packs per day for 20 years), and a brother with a myocardial infarction at the age of 40 years. The patient's brother is now 45 years old. The patient denies any history of diabetes or hyperlipidemias. At his physician's and wife's request, he now enters the hospital for elective cardiac catheterization. The patient has a significant denial of his illness and a secondary depression.† Although cardiac catheterization was suggested after the patient's first heart attack, he has refused to accept it until this admission.

- **Past Medical History.** The patient was hospitalized at age 15 for a appendectomy in Booth Hospital in Rochester, New York. The surgery was performed by a Dr. Meyers. The only other hospitalizations were for the patient's two heart attacks, as indicated previously. The patient is predominantly a red meat eater with little fish in his diet. Recently, presumably owing to depression, there has been a loss of appetite with a 10 pound weight loss. The patient admits to a sleeping problem. He falls asleep normally but awakens early and cannot go back go sleep. His only medications are indicated in the history of present illness. There is no history of renal, hepatic, pulmonary, or gastrointestinal disease. There is no history of allergy.

- **Family History.** The patient's father is 75 years old and has a history of diabetes. He apparently has some ocular problem, cataracts or retinopathy. The patient's mother died at age 64 from stomach cancer. The patient's older brother, as indicated previously, is 45 years old and has coronary artery disease. The patient has a younger sister who is 37 years old and is well. There is

---

* Four times a day.
† Notice that the history of the present illness summarizes all the information related to the present illness chronologically, regardless of when the information was obtained during the interview.

no history of congenital disease. The patient is married and has a 10 year old son, who is well.

■ **Psychosocial History.** The patient is a type "A" personality. He admits to having a need to drink alcohol occasionally after work. He drinks coffee about three times a day. He has only used marijuana on rare occasions, and he denies the use of other street drugs.

■ **Review of Systems.** There is a 20 – 25 year history of headaches without any recent change in their pattern or severity. The patient denies any head injury. There is. . . . * There is no history of claudication.† The remainder of the review of systems is noncontributory.‡

BIBLIOGRAPHY

Bird B: Talking with Patients. Philadelphia, JB Lippincott, 1973.

Cassell EJ: Talking with Patients: The Theory of Doctor-Patient Communication. Cambridge, MA, MIT Press, 1985.

Cassell EJ: Talking with Patients: Clinical Technique. Cambridge, MA, MIT Press, 1985.

Enelow AJ, Swisher SN: Interviewing and Patient Care. New York, Oxford University Press, 1979.

Enelow AJ, Wexler M: Psychiatry in the Practice of Medicine. New York, Oxford University Press, 1966.

Feinstein AR: Clinical Judgement. Baltimore, Williams and Wilkins Co, 1967.

Morgan WL Jr, Engel GL: The Clinical Approach to the Patient. Philadelphia, WB Saunders Co, 1969.

---

* The review of systems would then indicate any of the other symptoms that may be present.

† Notice that the positive symptoms are indicated first. The important, or pertinent, negatives are then listed. A pertinent negative in this patient is the lack of claudication. Coronary artery disease is often associated with peripheral vascular disease. The absence of a major symptom of peripheral vascular disease, claudication, makes claudication in this patient a pertinent negative. Chapter 21 has a further discussion on pertinent positives and negatives.

‡ This statement indicates that none of the other symptoms is present or does not contribute to the patient's present illness.

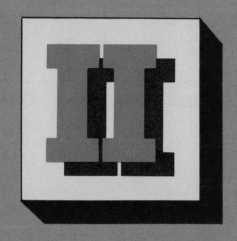

THE SCIENCE OF THE PHYSICAL EXAMINATION

THE PHYSICAL EXAMINATION

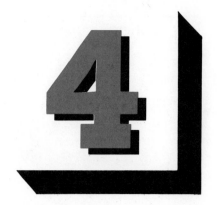

Don't touch the patient — state first what you see; cultivate your powers of observation.

Sir William Osler
1849–1919

THE BASIC PROCEDURES

In the previous chapters, the general rules for mastering the art of history taking have been discussed. The specific skills necessary to perform a proper physical examination will now be introduced. The four cardinal principles of physical examination are the following:

- Inspection
- Palpation
- Percussion
- Auscultation

In order to achieve competence in these procedures, the student must, in the words of Sir William Osler, "teach the eye to see, the finger to feel, and the ear to hear." The ability to coordinate all this sensory input is not inborn; it is learned with time and practice.

Even though the examiner will not use all these techniques for every organ system, he should think of these four skills before moving on to the next area to be evaluated.

Inspection

Inspection can provide an enormous amount of information. Proper technique requires more than just a glance. The examiner must train himself to look at the body using a systematic approach. All too often, the novice examiner will rush to use his ophthalmoscope, stethoscope, or otoscope before he has used his naked *eyes* for inspection.

An example of what is meant by "teaching the eye to see" can be demonstrated in the following illustration.* Read the sentence in the box. Afterwards, go back and count the number of "F's" in the sentence.

> **Finished files are the result of years of scientific study combined with the experience of years.**

How many did you count? The answer is in a footnote at the end of this chapter. This example clearly shows that we have to train our eyes to see!

While taking the history, the examiner should have already noticed certain things about the patient:

- General appearance
- State of nutrition
- Body habitus
- Symmetry
- Posture and gait
- Speech

The *general appearance* includes the state of consciousness and personal grooming. Does the patient look well or sick? Is he comfortable in bed, or does he appear in distress? Is he alert, or is he groggy? Does he look acutely or chronically ill? The answer to this last question is sometimes difficult to determine from inspection. There are some useful signs to aid the examiner. Poor nutrition, sunken eyes, temporal wasting, and loose skin are associated with chronic disease. Does the patient appear clean? Although the patient is ill, he does not have to appear unkempt. Is his hair combed? Does he bite his nails? The answers to these questions may provide useful information about the patient's self-esteem and mental status.

Inspection will provide an evaluation of the *state of nutrition*. Does the patient appear thin and frail? Is he obese? Most individuals with chronic disease are *not* overweight. These patients are cachectic. Longstanding ailments such as cancer, hyperthyroidism, or heart disease can result in a markedly wasted-looking individual.

---

* This test has been circulated widely in the medical community. The original writer is unknown.

The *body habitus* is useful to observe, because certain disease states are more common in different body builds. The asthenic, or ectomorph, has the classic "lean and hungry look." He is thin, with poor muscle development and small bone structure, and appears malnourished. The sthenic, or mesomorph, is the athletic type. He has excellent development of his muscles with a large bone structure. The hypersthenic, or endomorph, is the short, round individual with good muscular development, but this individual frequently has a weight problem.

Because the body is a *symmetrical* structure, any asymmetry should be noted. Many systemic diseases provide clues that can be uncovered on inspection. An obvious unilateral supraclavicular swelling or a less obvious unilateral miotic pupil: each clue serves to aid the examiner in reaching a final diagnosis. The left supraclavicular swelling in a 61 year old man may represent an enlarged supraclavicular lymph node and could be the only sign of gastric carcinoma. The miotic pupil in a 43 year old woman may be a manifestation of interruption of the cervical sympathetic chain by a tumor of the apex of the lung. The recent onset of a left-sided varicocele in a 46 year old man could be related to a left hypernephroma.

The patient is usually in bed when introduced to the examiner. If the patient were walking about, the examiner could use this time to observe the patient's *gait* and *posture*. The ability of a person to walk normally involves the coordination of the nervous and musculoskeletal systems. Does the patient drag a foot? Is there a shuffling gait? Does the patient limp? Are the steps normal?

The examiner can learn much about the patient from his *speech patterns*. Is the speech slurred? Does the patient use words appropriately? Is the patient hoarse? Does he have an unusual high- or low-pitched voice?

Is the patient oriented to person, place, and time? This can easily be evaluated by asking the patient, "Who are you?"; "Where are you?"; "What is the date, season, or month?"; and "What is the name of the President of the United States?" These questions certainly do not have to be asked at the beginning, but they should be asked at some time during the interview and examination. These questions provide an insight into the mental status of the patient. The mental status examination is discussed further in Chapter 18.

The examiner must be able to recognize the cardinal signs of inflammation: swelling, heat, redness, pain, and disturbance of function. Swelling results from edema or congestion in local tissues. Heat is the sensation that is due to an increased blood supply to the involved area. Redness is a manifestation of the increased blood supply. Pain often results from the swelling that exerts an increased pressure on the nerve fibers. Because of the pain and swelling, a disturbance of function occurs.

Palpation

Palpation is the use of the tactile sense to determine the characteristics of an organ system. For example, an abnormal impulse may be felt in the right chest that could be related to an ascending aortic aneurysm. A pulsatile mass in the abdomen might be an abdominal aneurysm. An acutely tender mass in the right upper quadrant of the abdomen that descends upon inspiration is probably an inflamed gallbladder.

Percussion

Percussion relates to the tactile sensation and sound produced when a sharp blow is struck to an area being examined. This provides valuable information about the structure of the underlying organ or tissue. The difference in the sensation compared with normal may be related to fluid in an otherwise nonfluid containing area. A collapse of a lung will change the percussion note, as will a solid mass in the abdomen. Percussion of a dull note in the midline of the lower abdomen probably represents a distended urinary bladder.

Auscultation

Auscultation involves listening to sounds produced by internal organs. This technique furnishes information about an organ's pathophysiology. The examiner is urged to learn as much as possible from the other techniques before using the stethoscope. This instrument should corroborate those signs that were suggested by the other techniques. One should not use auscultation alone to examine the heart, chest, and abdomen. This technique should be used together with inspection, percussion, and palpation. Listening for carotid, ophthalmic, or renal bruits can provide lifesaving information. The absence of normal bowel sounds could indicate a surgical emergency.

PREPARATION FOR THE EXAMINATION

The physical examination generally begins after the history has been completed. The examiner should have a portable case designed to contain his equipment, which should include the items listed in Table 4–1.

The examiner should place the equipment on the patient's night table or bedstand. By presenting all the "tools," the examiner will be less likely to forget

TABLE 4–1. Equipment for Physical Examination

Required	Optional	Available in Most Patient Care Areas
Stethoscope	Nasal illuminator†	Sphygmomanometer
Oto-ophthalmoscope	Nasal speculum	Tongue blades
Pen light	Tuning fork:	Applicator sticks
Reflex hammer	512 Hz	Gauze pads
Tuning fork: 128 Hz		Gloves
Safety pins or a box of straight pins*		Lubricant gel
Tape measure		Guaiac card for occult blood
Pocket visual acuity card		Vaginal speculum

* A new pin should be used in examining each patient as a precaution against transmission of the AIDS and hepatitis viruses.
†Attachment for the otoscope handle.

to perform a specific examination. It is preferable to use daylight for illumination, because skin color changes may be masked by artificial light. The patient's curtains should be drawn at the start of the interview.

Before you examine the patient, wash your hands, preferably while the patient is watching. Washing with soap and water is an effective way to reduce the transmission of disease.

The patient should be wearing a gown that opens at the front or back. Pajamas are also acceptable. It is most important for you to consider the comfort of the patient. You should allow the patient the use of pillows if requested. There are few relationships in which an individual will expose himself to a stranger after only a brief contact.

It is important that you become facile in each organ system examination. Incorporate the individual evaluations into the complete examination with the least amount of movement of the patient. Patients, regardless of age, tire quickly when asked to "sit up," "lie down," "turn on your left side," "sit up," "lie down," etc. You should perform as much of the examination as possible with the patient in one position. It is also important that the patient never be asked to sit up in bed without support for any extended period of time. Try this position yourself.

By convention, the examiner stands to the *right* of the patient as the patient lies in bed. The examiner uses his right hand for most maneuvers of the examination. It has been a common experience that even left-handed individuals will learn to perform the examination from the right side using their right hand. Each of the forthcoming organ system chapters pays particular attention to the placement of hands.

Although it will be necessary for the patient to disrobe completely, the examination should be carried out by exposing only those areas that are being examined at that time, without undue exposure of other areas. When one is examining a woman's breasts, for example, it is necessary to check for any asymmetry by inspecting both breasts at the same time. After inspection has been completed, the physician may use the patient's gown to cover the breast not being examined. The examination of the abdomen may be done discreetly by placing a towel or the bedsheet over the genitalia. Examination of the heart in the supine position may be performed with the right breast covered. This caring for the patient's privacy will go a long way in establishing a good doctor-patient relationship.

While performing the physical examination, the examiner should continue speaking to the patient. The examiner may wish to pursue various parts of the history, as well as to tell the patient what he is doing. The examiner should always refrain from comments such as, "That's good" or "That's normal" or "That's fine," in reference to any part of the examination. Although this is initially reassuring to the patient, if the examiner fails to make such a statement during another part of the examination, the patient will automatically assume that there is something wrong or abnormal.

The chapters that follow discuss the individual organ system examinations. After they have all been presented, Chapter 19 will summarize a method of putting all of the individual evaluations together into one smoothly continuous examination.

PRECAUTIONS TO TAKE DURING THE EXAMINATION

The medical student and physician are frequently exposed to patients with hepatitis and/or AIDS. The fear that exists in many regarding these diseases frequently interferes with the development of a good doctor-patient relationship. Once clearly defined procedures are maintained to ensure the safety of the health-care worker, this fear can be better handled.

It is known that the virus identified as the most likely causative agent of AIDS, human immunodeficiency virus* (HIV), is easily inactivated by several common germicides, such as 25% ethanol and standard household bleach.

There are several precautionary guidelines established by the Centers for Disease Control (1986) that should be followed routinely by all health-care workers whenever there is a possibility of exposure to potentially infectious materials such as blood or other bodily secretions.

1. The use of gloves should provide adequate protection when performing the physical examination or when handling blood-soiled or body fluid–soiled sheets or clothing.
2. Gloves should be worn when examining any individual with exudative lesions or weeping dermatitis.
3. When a procedure is performed, the use of gowns, masks, and eye covers is indicated if aerosolization of blood or saliva is anticipated.
4. Hands or other contaminated skin surfaces should be washed thoroughly and immediately if accidentally soiled with blood or other body fluids.
5. All sharp items, such as needles, scalpel blades, and other pointed items, must be handled with extraordinary care to prevent injuries.
6. To prevent needlestick injuries, needles should *not* be recapped. They should be disposed of in clearly marked, puncture resistant containers.
7. If mouth-to-mouth contact is necessary, mouth pieces, resuscitation bags, or other ventilatory devices should be used.
8. Blood specimens must be clearly labeled "BLOOD PRECAUTIONS."
9. Areas that have been soiled with blood or other body fluids should be cleaned with an appropriate disinfectant.
10. All reusable items should be processed according to current recommendations by autoclave or gas sterilization.

A patient may be in isolation, indicating that he is suffering from a contagious disease, such as tuberculosis or chickenpox. Proper protection for the health-care worker should include a gown and mask. Gloves may also be indicated. A patient in reverse isolation has a decreased immunologic response and is susceptible to infection, including opportunistic ones. The health-care worker should wear a gown, mask, and gloves to prevent infecting the patient with common germs.

---

* Formerly known as human T-cell lymphotropic virus type III (HTLV-III) or lymphadenopathy-associated virus (LAV).

THE GOAL OF THE PHYSICAL EXAMINATION

The goal of the physical examination is to determine valid information concerning the health of the patient. The examiner must be able to identify, analyze, and synthesize the accumulated knowledge into a comprehensive assessment.

The validity of a physical finding is dependent upon many factors. Clinical experience and reliability of the examination techniques are most important. False positives or false negatives reduce the precision of the techniques. Variance can occur when techniques are performed by different observers, with different equipment, on different patients. The concepts of validity and precision are further discussed in Chapter 21.

Unconscious bias is an important concept to understand. It is well known that unconscious bias in an examiner can influence the evaluation of the physical finding. For example, in patients with rapid atrial fibrillation, the ventricular rate is irregular and varies from 150 to 200 beats per minute. The radial pulse rate is significantly less, owing to a pulse deficit (explained in Chapter 11). If an examiner records the apical heart rate first, he will find that the rate varies from 150 to 200 beats per minute. If that observer then checks the radial pulse, he will detect a radial pulse rate that is a faster pulse rate than if he had measured the radial pulse first. The first observation, therefore, biases the second observation. Contrariwise, if the observer starts determining the radial pulse first and the heart rate second, the apical heart rate will be slower but the chance of bias is lower because observer error is less at the apex (Chalmers, 1981).

The concepts of *sensitivity* and *specificity* are important to review. Sensitivity relates to the reliability of a technique to give a positive result when the finding is present. Specificity relates to the reliability of a technique to successfully rule out that a finding is present.

An example is breast palpation, which is a sensitive but nonspecific technique for detecting breast cancer:

An examiner palpates a stony hard mass in the breast of a woman and suspects that a tumor is present. Further testing indicates that the mass is cancer. The technique has a high degree of sensitivity. If another examiner fails to palpate a mass in the breast of another woman, he may rule out that cancer is present. Further testing shows that a malignant mass is actually present. The technique of breast palpation, therefore, has a low degree of specificity.

On the other hand, the finding of microaneurysms at the macula of the eye is a specific but insensitive finding for diabetes:

If an examiner fails to visualize microaneurysms at the macula, he cannot exclude diabetes in a patient with symptoms of increased thirst, increased urination, and increased appetite. Many patients with diabetes do not have this macular finding. Further testing may actually indicate that the patient has diabetes. Therefore, the finding of macular microaneurysms has a low degree of sensitivity. A second examiner visualizes macular microaneurysms in another patient with similar symptoms. The physician suspects that the patient has diabetes. Normal individuals without diabetes do not have macular microaneurysms. Further testing indicates that the patient does have diabetes. Therefore, the presence of microaneurysms at the macula has a high degree of specificity.

Unfortunately, a technique can rarely be both very sensitive and very specific. One must apply several techniques together to be able to make an appropriate assessment. A test of high sensitivity is useful as a screening test, although there may be several false positives. A test of high specificity will fail to determine a finding in many patients and will have many false negatives.

USEFUL VOCABULARY

The vocabulary of medicine is difficult and broad. Memorization of a term is less useful than trying to determine the meaning by understanding its etymology, or roots. The spelling of terms will also be easier.

Listed here are some general roots that are important to understand. At the end of the following chapters, there is a section on specific roots and terminology for that area of the body. The following list should not be memorized at this time. It should be used in conjunction with the roots of the subsequent chapters.

	PERTAINING TO	EXAMPLE	DEFINITION
PREFIX/ROOT			
ab-	away from	*ab*duction	Away from the body
ad-	toward	*ad*duction	Toward the body
aden-	gland	*aden*opathy	Glandular disease
an-	without	*an*osmia	Without the sense of smell
aniso-	unequal	*aniso*coria	Unequal pupils
asthen-	weak	*asthen*opia	Eye fatigue
contra-	against; opposite	*contra*lateral	Pertaining to the opposite side
diplo-	double	*diplo*pia	Double vision
duc-	lead	ab*duc*tion	Turning outward
dys-	bad; ill	*dys*uria	Painful urination
eso-	in	*eso*tropia	Eye deviated inward
eu-	good; advantageous	*eu*pnea	Easy breathing
exo-	out	*exo*tropia	Eye deviated outward
hemi-	half	*hemi*plegia	Paralysis of one side of the body
hydro-	water	*hydro*philic	Readily absorbing water
hyper-	beyond	*hyper*emia	Excess of blood
hypno-	sleep	*hypno*tic	Inducing sleep
idio-	separate; distinct	*idio*pathic	Of unknown causation
infra-	below	*infra*hyoid	Below the hyoid gland
intra-	within	*intra*cranial	Within the skull
ipsi-	self	*ipsi*lateral	Situated on the same side
leuko-	white	*leuko*cyte	White cell
lith-	stone	*lith*otomy	Incision of an organ to remove a stone
neo-	new	*neo*plasm	Abnormal new growth
pedia-	child	*pedia*trics	Branch of medicine involved with treating diseases of children
poly-	many	*poly*cystic	Many cysts
retro-	situated behind	*retro*bulbar	Behind the eye
soma-	body	*soma*tic	Pertaining to the body
sten-	narrowed	*sten*osis	Narrowed duct or canal
trans-	through	*trans*urethral	Through the urethra
SUFFIX/ROOT			
-ectomy	removal of	append*ectomy*	Removal of the appendix
-gnosis	recognition	stereo*gnosis*	Recognizing an object by touch
-gram	something written	myelo*gram*	X-ray of the spinal cord
-ism	state; condition	gigant*ism*	State of abnormal overgrowth
-itis	inflammation of	col*itis*	Inflammation of the colon
-lysis	dissolution	hemo*lysis*	Liberation of hemoglobin into solution
-malacia	softening	osteo*malacia*	Softening of bones
-megal-	enlargement	cardio*megaly*	Cardiac enlargement
-mycosis	fungus	blasto*mycosis*	A specific fungal infection
-ologist	specialist in study of	cardi*ologist*	A specialist in heart disease
-oma	tumor; growth	fib*roma*	A tumor of fibrous tissue
-orrhaphy	suture	herni*orrhaphy*	Suture of a hernia

	PERTAINING TO	EXAMPLE	DEFINITION
SUFFIX/ROOT			
-osis	diseased state	endometri*osis*	Disease state of abnormally located uterine tissue
-pathy	disease	uro*pathy*	Disease of the urinary tract
-phobia	fear	photo*phobia*	Abnormal intolerance of light
-plasty	repair	valvulo*plasty*	Surgical repair of a valve
-plegia	paralysis	hemi*plegia*	Paralysis of one half of the body
-ptosis	drooping	blepharo*ptosis*	Drooping eyelids
-scope	instrument for examining	ophthalmo*scope*	Tool for examination of the eye
-spasmos	spasm	blepharo*spasm*	Twitching of the eyelids
-stom	opening	ileo*stom*y	Surgical creation of an opening into the ileum
-tome	cut	micro*tome*	An instrument for cutting thin slices

The preceding list represents the more common prefixes, roots, and suffixes. Each chapter will further enhance your knowledge with more organ specific roots.

BIBLIOGRAPHY

Centers for Disease Control (CDC): Recommendations for preventing transmission of infection with human T-lymphotrophic virus type III lymphadenopathy-associated virus during invasive procedures. MMWR *35*:221, 1986.

Chalmers TC: The clinical trial. Milbank Mem Fund Q *59*:324, 1981.

Answer to puzzle: How many "F's" did you count? There are *six* in the sentence in the box. Go back and count them. Most individuals count only three. Don't forget the "F's" in the three "of"s!

5

THE SKIN

*What is the hardest of all? That which you hold the
most simple; seeing with your own eyes what is
spread out before you.*

Johann Wolfgang von Goethe
1749 – 1832

GENERAL CONSIDERATIONS

The skin, which is the largest organ in the body, is one of the best indicators of general health. Even the untrained person is capable of detecting changes in skin color and texture. The trained examiner can detect these changes and at the same time evaluate more subtle cutaneous signs of systemic medical disease.

Diseases of the skin are common. Approximately one third of the population in the United States has a disorder of the skin that warrants medical attention. Nearly 8% of all adult outpatient visits are related to dermatologic problems. Skin cancer is the most common malignancy, with over 400,000 new cases diagnosed annually. Although most of these patients are treated and cured, skin cancer still causes over 4000 deaths a year.

The most important function of the skin is to protect the body from the environment. The skin has evolved in humans to be a relatively impermeable surface layer that prevents the loss of water, protects against external hazards, and insulates against thermal changes. It is also actively involved in the production of vitamin D. The skin appears to have the lowest water permeability of any naturally produced membrane. Its barrier to invasion retards potentially noxious agents from entering the body and causing internal damage. This barrier protects against many physical stresses while it prohibits the invasion of microorganisms. Only when one has observed patients with extensive skin problems, such as burns, can one appreciate the importance of this organ.

STRUCTURE AND PHYSIOLOGY

The three tissue layers of the skin are as follows:

- Epidermis
- Dermis
- Subcutaneous tissue

These layers are shown in Figure 5–1.

The *epidermis* is the thin, outermost layer of the skin and is composed of several layers of keratocytes, or keratin producing cells. Keratin is an insoluble protein that provides the skin with its protective properties. The stratum corneum is the outermost layer and serves as a major physical barrier. The stratum corneum is composed of keratinized cells, which appear as dry, flattened, anuclear, and adherent flakes.

The *basal cell layer* is the deepest layer of the epidermis. The basal cell layer forms a single row of rapidly proliferating cells that slowly migrate upward, keratinize, and are ultimately shed from the stratum corneum. The process of maturation, keratinization, and shedding takes approximately 4 weeks. The cells of the basal layer are intermingled with melanocytes, which produce melanin. The number of melanocytes is approximately equal in all people. The difference in skin color is related to the amount and type of melanin produced as well as to its dispersion in the skin.

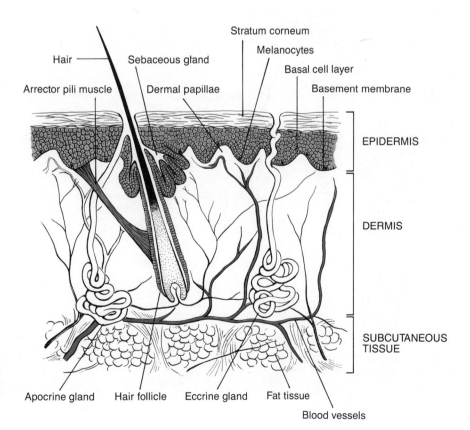

FIGURE 5–1. Cross-section through the skin, showing the structures in the epidermis, dermis, and subcutaneous tissues.

Beneath the epidermis is the *dermis,* which is the dense connective tissue stroma forming the bulk of the skin. The dermis is bound to the overlying epidermis by finger-like projections that project upward into the corresponding recesses of the epidermis. In the dermis, blood vessels branch and form a rich capillary bed in the dermal papillae. The deeper layers of the dermis also contain the hair follicles with their associated muscles and cutaneous glands. The dermis is supplied with both sensory and autonomic nerve fibers. The sensory nerves end either as free endings or as special end-organs that mediate pressure, touch, and temperature. The autonomic nerves supply the arrector pili muscles, blood vessels, and sweat glands.

The third layer of the skin is the *subcutaneous tissue,* which is largely composed of fatty connective tissue. This highly variable adipose layer is a thermal regulator as well as a protection for the more superficial skin layers from bone prominences.

The sweat glands, hair follicles, and nails are termed *skin appendages.* The evaporation of water from the skin by the sweat glands provides a thermoregulatory mechanism for heat loss. Figure 5–2 illustrates the types of sweat glands.

Within the skin, there are two to three million small, coiled *eccrine glands.* The eccrine glands are distributed over the body surface and are particularly profuse on the forehead, axillae, palms, and soles. They are absent in the nail beds and in some mucosal surfaces. These glands are capable of producing over 6 L of watery sweat in one day. The eccrine glands are controlled by the sympathetic nervous system.

The *apocrine gland* is larger than the eccrine gland. The apocrine glands are found in close association with hair follicles but tend to be much more limited in

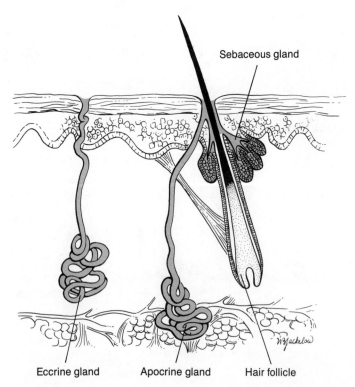

Sebaceous gland

Eccrine gland   Apocrine gland   Hair follicle

FIGURE 5–2. Types of sweat glands.

distribution than the eccrine glands. The apocrine glands occur mostly in the axillae, the areola, the pubis, and the perineum. They reach maturity only at puberty, secreting a milky, sticky substance. Apocrine glands are adrenergic mediated and appear to be stimulated by stress.

The *sebaceous glands* are also found surrounding hair follicles. The sebaceous glands are distributed over the entire body, with the largest glands found on the face and upper back. They are absent on the palms and soles. The secretory product, sebum, is discharged directly into the lumen of the hair follicle, where it lubricates the hair shaft and spreads to the skin surface. Sebum consists of sebaceous cells and lipids. The production of sebum is dependent upon gland size, which is directly influenced by androgen secretion.

Nails are derived by keratinization of cells from the nail matrix, which is located at the proximal end of the nail plate. The nail plate consists of the nail root embedded in the posterior nail fold, a fixed middle portion, and a distal free edge. The whitish nail matrix of proliferating epithelial cells grows in a semilunar pattern. It extends outward past the posterior nail fold and is called the lunula. The structural relationships of the nail are shown in Figure 5–3.

Hair is a dead, keratinized structure that grows out of the hair follicle. Its lower end, called the hair matrix, consists of actively proliferating epithelial cells. Hair is present over the entire body except on the palms, soles, glans penis, and labia minora. The arrector pili muscles attach to the follicle below the opening of the sebaceous gland. Contraction of this muscle erects the hair and causes "goose bumps." The structure of the hair follicle is shown in Figure 5–4.

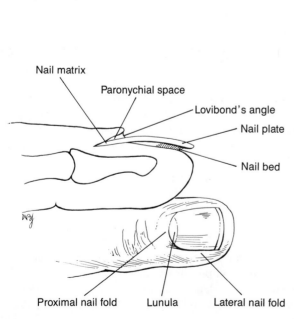

FIGURE 5–3. Structural relations of the nail: cross-section and from above.

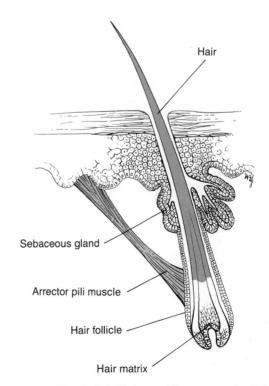

FIGURE 5–4. The hair follicle and its surrounding structures.

REVIEW OF SPECIFIC SYMPTOMS

The main symptoms of disease of the skin, hair, or nails are the following:

- Rash or skin lesion
- Changes in skin color
- Itching (pruritus)
- Changes in hair
- Changes in nails

Rash or Skin Lesion

There are some very important points to elucidate when interviewing a patient about a new rash or new skin lesion. The specific time of onset and location of the rash or skin lesion are critical. A careful description of the first lesions and any changes is vital. The patient with a rash or skin lesion should be asked the following questions:

"Was the rash initially flat? . . . raised? . . . blistered?"
"Did the rash change in character with time?"
"Have there been new areas involved since the rash began?"
"Does it itch or burn?"
"Is the lesion tender or numb?"
"What makes the rash better? . . . worse?"
"Was the rash initiated by sunlight?"
"Is the rash aggravated by sunlight?"
"What kind of treatment have you tried?"
"Do you have any joint pains? . . . fever? . . . fatigue?"
"Does anyone near you have a similar rash?"
"Have you traveled recently?" If so, *"To where?"*
"Have you had any contact with anyone who has had a similar rash?"
"Is there a history of allergy?" If so, *"What are your symptoms?"*
"Do you have any chronic disease?"

It is important to note whether the patient has used any medications that may have changed the nature of the skin disorder.

Inquire whether the patient uses any prescription medications or any over-the-counter drugs. Ask specifically about aspirin and aspirin-containing products. Patients can suddenly develop a reaction to medications that they have taken for many years. Do not ignore a long-standing prescription! Has the patient had any recent injections or taken any new medications? Does the patient use "recreational" drugs? Ask the patient about the use of soaps, deodorants, cosmetics, and colognes. Has the patient changed any of these items recently?

A family history of similar skin disorders should be noted. The effect of heat, cold, and sunlight on the skin problem is important. Can any contributing factor be brought to bear, such as occupation, specific food allergies, alcohol, or menses? Is there a history of gardening or household repair work? Has there been any contact with animals recently? The interviewer should also remember to inquire about psychogenic factors that may contribute to a skin disorder.

It is very important to determine the patient's occupation, if not already known. Avocations and recreational activities are important to ascertain. The information is important even if the patient has been exposed to chemicals or similar agents for years. Manufacturers frequently change the basic constituents without notifying the consumer. Patients may also need years to become sensitized to a substance.

Changes in Skin Color

Patients may complain of a *generalized* change in skin color as the first manifestation of an internal illness. Cyanosis and jaundice are examples of this type of problem. It is important to determine whether the patient is aware of any chronic disease that may be responsible for these changes. *Localized* skin color changes may be related to aging or to neoplastic changes. Certain medications can be responsible for skin color changes as well. The examiner should inquire whether the patient is taking, or has recently taken, any medications.

Pruritus

Pruritus, or itching, may be a symptom of a generalized skin disorder or an internal illness. Ask the following questions of any patient with pruritus:

> *"When did you first notice the itching?"*
> *"Did the itching begin suddenly?"*
> *"Is the itching associated with any rash or lesion on your body?"*
> *"Are you taking any medications?"*
> *"Has there been any change in the sweating or dryness of your skin?"*
> *"Have you been told that you have a chronic illness?"*
> *"Have you traveled recently?"* If so, *"To where?"*

Diffuse pruritus is seen in biliary cirrhosis and in cancer, especially lymphoma. Pruritus in association with a diffuse rash may be dermatitis herpetiformis. It is important to determine whether the pruritus has been associated with a change in perspiration or dryness of the skin, as both of these conditions may be the cause of the pruritus.

Changes in Hair

The interviewer should inquire whether there has been a loss of hair or an increase in hair. A change in distribution or texture is also important to ascertain. The interviewer should ask the following questions:

> *"When did you first notice the changes?"*
> *"Has the change occurred suddenly?"*
> *"Is the hair loss symmetrical?"*
> *"Has the change been associated with itching? . . . fever? . . . recent stress?"*
> *"Are you aware of any exposure to any toxins? . . . commercial hair compounds?"*
> *"Have you changed your diet?"*
> *"What medications are you taking?"*

Changes in diet and medications are frequently responsible for changes in hair patterns. Hypothyroidism is frequently associated with loss of the lateral third of the eyebrows. Vascular disease in the legs often causes hair loss on the legs. On the other hand, ovarian and adrenal tumors can cause an increase in body hair.

Changes in Nails

Changes in nails may be splitting, discoloration, ridging, thickening, or separation from the nail bed. Ask the patient these questions:

"When did you first notice the nail changes?"
"Have you had any acute illness recently?"
"Do you have any chronic illness?"
"Have you been taking any medications?"
"Have you been exposed to chemicals at work or at home?"

Fungal disease will cause thickening of the nail. Acute illnesses are associated with lines and ridges in the nail bed and nail. Medications and chemicals are notorious for causing nail changes.

General Suggestions

All patients should be asked whether there have been any changes in moles, birth marks, or spots on the body. Any color changes, irregular growth, pain, scaling, or bleeding are important to determine. Any recent growth of a flat, pigmented lesion is relevant information.

Ask all patients whether there are any red, scaly, or crusted areas of skin that do not heal. Has the patient ever had skin cancer? If the patient has had skin cancer, further questioning regarding the body location, treatment, and description is appropriate.

IMPACT OF SKIN DISEASE ON THE PATIENT

Diseases of the skin play a profound role in the way the affected patient interacts socially. If located on visible skin surfaces, long-standing skin diseases may actually interfere with the emotional and psychological development of the individual. The attitude of a person toward himself and others may be markedly affected. Loss of self-esteem is very common. The adult with a skin disorder often faces limitation of sexual activity. This disruption of intimacy will increase the patient's hostility and anxiety. Skin is a sensitive marker of an individual's emotions. It is known that blushing can reflect embarrassment, sweating can indicate anxiety, and pallor or "goose bumped" skin may be associated with fear.

Patients with rashes have always evoked feelings of revulsion. Since time immemorial, rashes have been associated with impurity and evil. Even today, friends and family may reject the individual with a skin disease. Patients with skin that is red, oozing, discolored, or peeling are rejected not only by family members but also perhaps even by their physicians. At other times, skin lesions cause others to stare at the patient, causing further discomfort. Some skin disorders may be associated with such extreme physical or emotional pain that marked depression may result, occasionally leading to suicide.

Skin diseases are often treated palliatively. Because numerous skin disorders have no cure, many patients go through life helpless and frustrated, as do their physicians.

The role of anxiety as a natural stressor in producing rashes is frequently observed. Stress tends to worsen certain skin disorders, such as eczema. This creates a vicious cycle, because the rash then serves to exacerbate the anxiety. Rashes are common symptoms and signs of psychosomatic disorders.

Medical personnel should attempt to discuss with the patient his anxieties in an attempt to break the cycle. The interviewer who tries to elicit the patient's feelings about his disease will allow the patient to "open up." The fears and fantasies can then be discussed. The examiner should also be comfortable to touch the patient to reassure him. This will tend to allow a better doctor-patient relationship, as the patient will have less of a sense of isolation.

PHYSICAL EXAMINATION

> The only equipment necessary for the examination of the skin is a penlight.

The examination of the skin consists of

- Inspection
- Palpation

The patient and the examiner must be comfortable during the examination of the skin. The lighting should be adjusted to produce the optimal illumination. Natural light is preferable. Even in the absence of complaints related to the skin, a careful examination of the skin must be performed on all patients because the skin may provide subtle clues of an underlying systemic illness. Examination of the skin may be performed as a separate system approach, or preferably the skin should be examined when the other parts of the body are evaluated.

If there is a possibility of an infectious disease, gloves should be worn.

General Principles

The examiner should be suspicious of any lesion that the patient describes as having increased in size or changed in color. In addition, the development of any new growth warrants attention.

When you examine the skin, the initial evaluation is made to determine the general aspects of the skin. Evaluate the *color, moisture, turgor,* and *texture* of the skin.

Note any *color* changes, such as cyanosis, jaundice, or pigmentary abnormalities.

Red vascular lesions may be either extravasated blood into the skin, known as petechiae or purpura, or angiomas. Angiomas are malformed elements of the vascular tree. When pressure is applied by a glass slide over an angioma, it will blanch. This is a useful test to differentiate an angioma from petechiae, which will not change when pressure from a glass slide is applied.

Excessive *moisture* may be seen in normal individuals, or it may be associated with fevers, emotions, neoplastic diseases, or hyperthyroidism. Dryness is a normal aging change, but it may also be seen in myxedema, nephritis, and certain drug-induced states. Look for excoriations, which might indicate the presence of pruritus as a clue to an underlying systemic illness.

When you palpate the skin, evaluate its *turgor* and *texture*. Tissue turgor provides a mechanism for roughly estimating the patient's general state of hydration. If the skin over the forehead is pulled up and released, it should promptly reassume its normal contour. A patient with decreased hydration will show a delayed response.

The texture of the skin is often difficult for the inexperienced examiner to evaluate because texture is a more qualitative parameter. Softness has occasionally been likened to the texture of skin over a baby's abdomen. ''Soft'' textured skin is seen in secondary hypothyroidism, hypopituitarism, and eunuchoid states. ''Hard'' textured skin is associated with scleroderma, myxedema, and amyloidosis. ''Velvety'' skin is associated with Ehlers-Danlos syndrome.

Examination with Patient Seated

When the patient is seated, the examiner should examine the hair and the skin on the hands and upper extremities.

Inspect the Hair

The hair and scalp are evaluated for any lesions. Is alopecia or hirsutism present? You should pay close attention to the pattern of distribution and texture of hair over the body. In certain diseases, such as hypothyroidism, the hair becomes sparse and coarse. In contrast, patients with hyperthyroidism have hair that is very fine in texture. Loss of hair occurs in many conditions: anemia; heavy metal poisoning; hypopituitarism; and some nutritional disease states, such as pellagra. Increased hair patterns are seen in Cushing's disease; Stein-Leventhal syndrome; and several neoplastic conditions, such as tumors of the adrenals and gonads.

Inspect the Nail Beds

Evaluation of the nails is next and can provide important clues about systemic diseases. Nail bed changes are usually not pathognomonic for a specific disease. Disorders stemming from renal, hematopoietic, or hepatic conditions may be

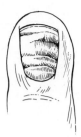
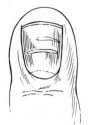
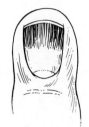
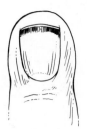

BEAU'S LINES   MEE'S BANDS   LINDSAY'S NAILS   TERRY'S NAILS

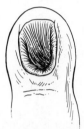
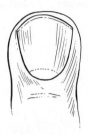
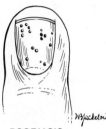

FIGURE 5–5. Common nail findings associated with medical diseases.

KOILONYCHIA   CLUBBING   PSORIASIS

evident from the nails. Inspect the nails for color, brittleness, hemorrhages under the nail, transverse lines or grooves in the nail or nail bed, and an increased white area of the nail bed. Figure 5–5 illustrates some typical nail changes associated with medical diseases.

Beau's lines are transverse grooves parallel to the lunula, often associated with significant infections or renal or hepatic diseases. This abnormality is caused by diseases that cause the nail to grow slowly or even cease to grow for short intervals. The point of arrested growth is seen as a transverse groove in the nail. Beau's lines may also result from coronary occlusion, surgical procedures, and anti-cancer agents. Occasionally, a white transverse line or band, instead of a groove, will result from poisoning or an acute systemic illness. These lines, called *Mee's bands*, are historically associated with chronic arsenic poisoning. These lines or bands are also parallel to the lunula. By measuring the width of the line and approximating nail growth at 1 mm per week, it may be possible to determine the duration of the antecedent acute illness. Plate I C shows the fingernails of a patient who was ill with pneumonia 6 weeks earlier.

Lindsay's nails are also called "half-and-half nails." The proximal portion of the nail bed is whitish, whereas the distal part is red or pink. Chronic renal disease and azotemia are associated with this type of nail abnormality. Plate XI E shows a patient with Lindsay's nails secondary to hypoalbuminemia. *Terry's nails* are white nail beds to within 1–2 mm of the distal border of the nail. These nail findings are most commonly associated with cirrhosis and hypoalbuminemia.

Is *koilonychia* present? Koilonychia, or spoon nail, is a dystrophic state in which the nail plate thins and a cup-like depression develops. Spoon nails are most commonly associated with iron deficiency anemia but may be seen in association with thinning of the nail plate from any cause, including local irritants. Plate I D shows a normal fingernail compared with a nail showing koilonychia secondary to iron deficiency anemia.

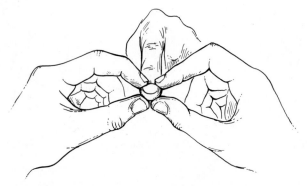

FIGURE 5–6. Technique for assessing whether clubbing is present.

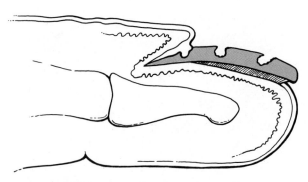

FIGURE 5–7. A cross-section of pitting.

Inspect the Nails for Clubbing

The patient's finger is placed on the pulp of the examiner's thumbs, and the base of the nail bed is palpated by the examiner's index fingers. Figure 5–6 illustrates the technique for assessing whether early clubbing is present. If *fluctuation* is found, clubbing is said to be present. If the fluctuation is marked, there may be an impression that the nail is *floating*.

As clubbing progresses, there is an increase in the angle between the nail fold and the nail plate, known as *Lovibond's angle,* to greater than 180°. A fusiform enlargement of the distal digit may also occur. Look at Plate IX *A,* in which a normal finger is compared with a clubbed finger.

Clubbing of the nails is associated with congenital cyanotic heart disease, cystic fibrosis, and acquired pulmonary pathology. The most common acquired pulmonary causes are bronchogenic carcinoma and chronic obstructive lung disease. The initial manifestation of clubbing is a softening of the tissue over the proximal nail fold.

Inspect the Nails for Pitting

Pitting of the nails is commonly associated with psoriasis and psoriatic arthropathy. Involvement of the nail bed and nail matrix by psoriasis causes the nail plate to be thickened and pitted. Nail involvement occurs in about 50% of all patients with psoriasis. Multiple pits in the nail are produced by discrete psoriatic lesions in the nail matrix. Minor degrees of pitting are also seen in persons with no other skin complaints. A patient with psoriatic nail pitting is shown in Plate I *E.* Figure 5–7 illustrates a cross-section of pitting.

Inspect the Skin of the Face and Neck

The eyelids, forehead, ears, nose, and lips are evaluated carefully. The mucous membranes of the mouth and nose should be evaluated for ulceration, bleeding, or telangiectasia. Is the skin at the nasolabial fold and mouth normal?

Inspect the Skin Over the Back

Walk to the patient's back and examine the skin in this area. Are any lesions present?

Examination with Patient Lying

Inspect the Skin of the Chest, Abdomen, and Lower Extremities

Ask the patient to lie down in order to complete the examination of the skin. Inspect the skin of the chest and abdomen. Particular attention should be paid to the skin of the inguinal and genital area. Inspect the pubic hair. Elevate the scrotum. Inspect the perineal area. The pretibial areas are evaluated for the presence of ulcerations or waxy deposits.

The feet and soles (see Plate II C) are carefully examined for any skin changes. The toes should be spread to evaluate the webs between them thoroughly.

The patient is asked to roll on his left side so that the skin on the back, gluteal, and perianal areas may be examined.

DESCRIPTION OF LESIONS

If a skin lesion is found, it should be classified as a *primary* or *secondary* lesion, and a careful description of its shape and its distribution should be given. Primary lesions arise from normal skin. They result from anatomic changes in the epidermis, dermis, or subcutaneous tissue. The primary lesion is the most characteristic lesion of the skin disorder. Secondary lesions result from changes in the primary lesion. They develop during the natural history of the cutaneous disease.

The first step in identifying a skin disorder is to characterize the appearance of the primary lesion. In the description of the skin lesion, it is important to note whether the lesion is flat or raised, and whether it is solid or contains fluid. A penlight is often useful to determine whether the lesion is slightly elevated. If a penlight is directed to one side of a lesion, a shadow will be appreciated according to the height of the lesion.

In addition to the type of lesion present, its location on the body is very important. Therefore, the distribution of the eruption is crucial in helping to make a diagnosis. It may be rewarding to inspect a patient's clothing when contact dermatitis or pediculosis (infestation with lice) is suspected. Occasionally, occupational exposure may leave traces of contamination with oils or other materials that may be visible on the clothing and help in the assessment.

The three specific criteria for a dermatologic diagnosis are based on *morphology, configuration,* and *distribution,* morphology being the most important. The purpose of the following section is to acquaint the reader with the morphology of the primary and secondary lesions and the vocabulary associated with them.

Primary and Secondary Lesions

In order to facilitate reading, the primary lesions are listed with respect to being flat or elevated and being solid or fluid-filled (Figs. 5 – 8 to 5 – 11). There is no "standard" size of a primary lesion. The dimensions indicated are therefore only approximate. The secondary lesions are grouped according to their occur-

PRIMARY LESIONS
Flat, Nonpalpable

FIGURE 5–8.

Lesion	Description	Example
Macule	A circumscribed area of color change flush with the skin plane less than 1 cm in diameter	Freckle
Patch	A macule measuring over 1 cm in diameter	Vitiligo

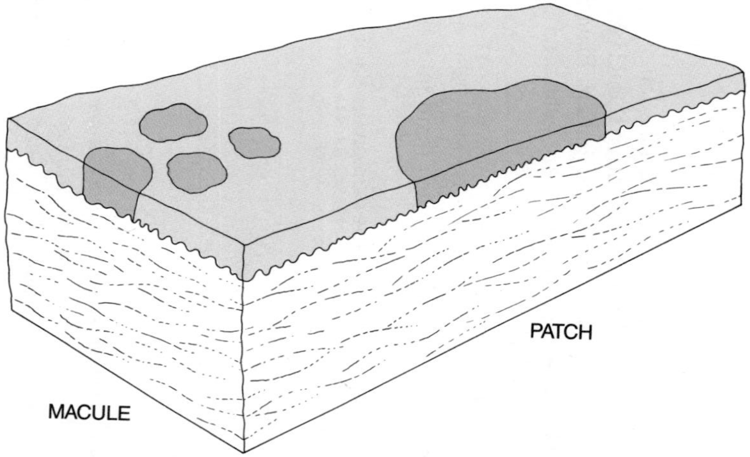

PRIMARY LESIONS
Palpable, Elevated, Solid Masses

FIGURE 5–9.

Lesion	Description	Example
Papule	A circumscribed, solid elevation less than 1 cm in diameter	Acne, lichen planus
Nodule	A palpable, solid lesion that is greater than 1 cm in diameter and that may extend above or below the plane of the skin	Nevus, or birthmark
Tumor	A large, solid lesion that is greater than 2 cm in diameter	Lipoma
Plaque	A palpable lesion that has a large surface area in relation to its height	Psoriasis
Wheal	A temporary elevation of the skin caused by leakage of fluid into the dermis	Hives, dermatographism*

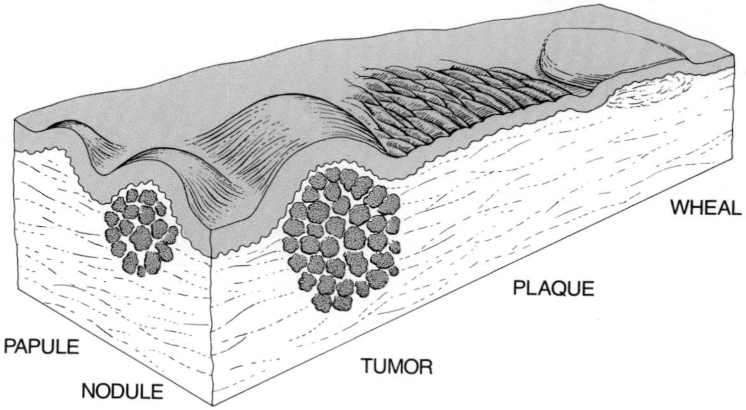

* Firm striking of the skin produces erythema and wheal formation.

PRIMARY LESIONS
Palpable, Elevated, Fluid-Filled Masses

FIGURE 5 – 10.

Lesion	Description	Example
Vesicle	A circumscribed elevation of skin less than 1 cm in diameter that contains fluid	Cold sore, chickenpox
Bulla	A circumscribed elevation of skin that is greater than 1 cm in diameter and contains fluid	Poison ivy dermatitis, bullous pemphigoid
Pustule	A vesicle that contains purulent exudate	Acne

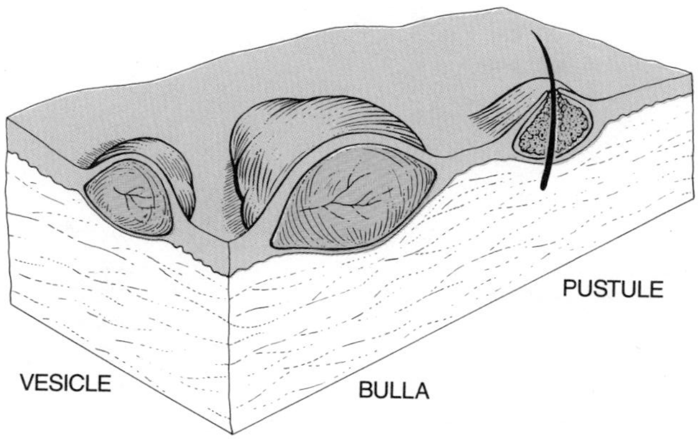

SPECIAL PRIMARY LESIONS

FIGURE 5 – 11.

Lesion	Description	Example
Comedo	A plug of secretion and horny material retained in a hair follicle	Blackhead, acne
Burrow	A characteristic linear lesion that is a tunnel under the epidermis produced by an animal parasite	Scabies
Cyst	A sac containing liquid or semisolid material	
Abscess	A specific type of primary lesion with localized accumulation of purulent material in the dermis or subcutis. Generally, the accumulation is so deep that the pus is not visible from the skin's surface	
Furuncle	A specific type of primary lesion that is a necrotizing form of inflammation of a hair follicle	
Carbuncle	A coalescence of several furuncles	
Milia	Tiny, keratin-filled cysts representing an accumulation of keratin in the distal portion of the sweat gland	

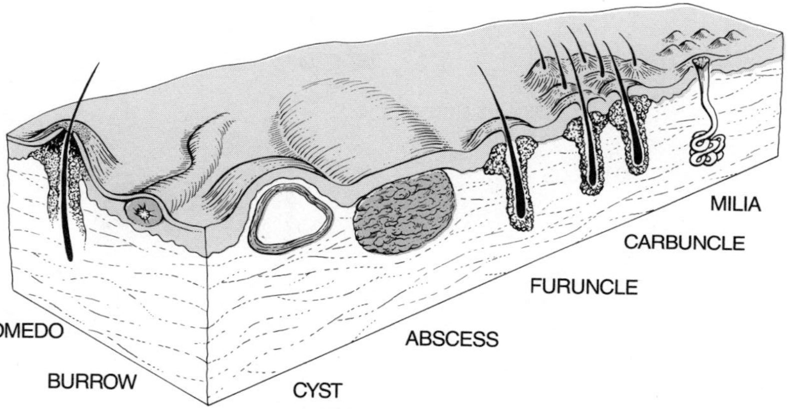

SECONDARY LESIONS BELOW THE SKIN PLANE

FIGURE 5–12.

Lesion	Description	Example
Erosion	Loss of the epidermis. Healing occurs without scarring	From rupture of a fever blister vesicle
Ulcer	Loss of the epidermis and part of the dermis. Healing occurs with scarring	Chancre
Fissure	A crack in the skin extending through the upper cutis with fibrotic replacement. This results from marked drying or chronic inflammation	
Excoriation	A superficial linear, or "dugout," traumatized area, usually self-induced	A scratch mark
Atrophy	Changes resulting in a whitish and slightly sunken epidermis. May be severe when associated with a decrease in collagen	
Sclerosis	Diffuse or circumscribed hardening of the skin	

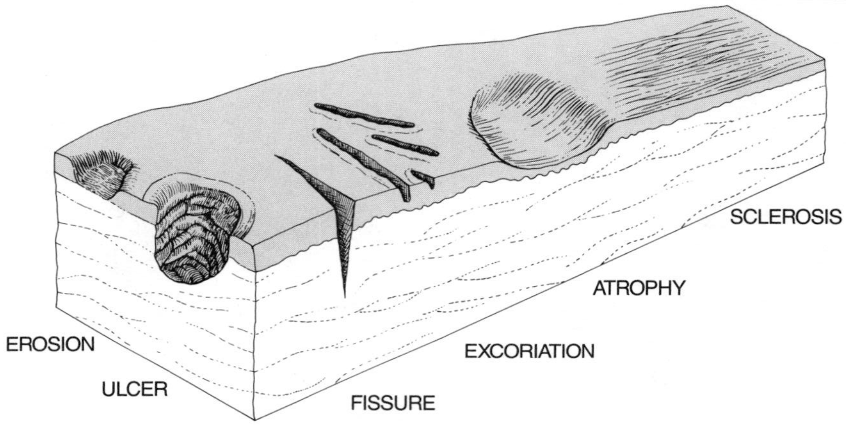

SECONDARY LESIONS ABOVE THE SKIN PLANE

FIGURE 5–13.

Lesion	Description	Example
Scaling	Excessive shedding of cells from the stratum corneum, manifested by flaking of the skin	Dandruff, psoriasis
Crusting	Dried serum, blood, and/or purulent material on the surface of the skin (a scab)	Impetigo

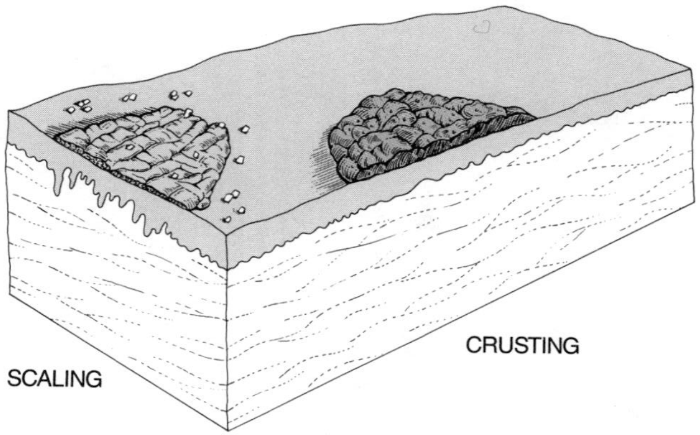

OTHER IMPORTANT DERMATOLOGIC TERMS

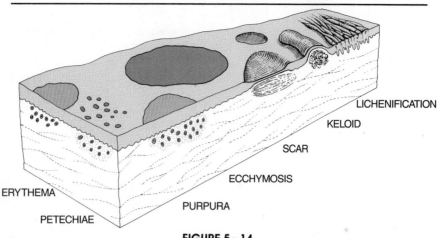

LICHENIFICATION
KELOID
SCAR
ECCHYMOSIS
ERYTHEMA
PURPURA
PETECHIAE

FIGURE 5–14.

Lesion	Description	Example
Erythema	Pink or red blanchable discoloration of the skin secondary to dilatation of blood vessels	
Petechiae	Purplish-red, nonblanchable, pinpoint flat spots caused by intradermal or submucosal hemorrhage	
Purpura	Purple, nonblanchable discoloration of the skin as a result of extravasation of blood	
Ecchymosis	Large purpuric lesions, generally greater than 1 cm	"Black and blue mark"
Scar	Connective tissue replacement following dermal tissue loss	
Alopecia	Loss of hair	
Keloid	Hypertrophied scar tissue	
Lichenification	A thickening and roughening of skin with accentuation of the normal skin lines	

rence below or above the plane of the skin (Figs. 5–12 and 5–13). Other important lesions are shown and described in Figure 5–14.

Configuration of Skin Lesions

It is not essential for the examiner to make a definitive diagnosis of all skin disease. A careful description of the lesion, the pattern of distribution, and the arrangement of the lesion will often lead the examiner to a group of related disease states with similar presenting dermatologic signs (e.g., confluent macular rashes, bullous diseases, grouped vesicles, papular rashes on an erythematous base). For example, grouped urticarial lesions with a central depression suggest insect bites. Listed in Figure 5–15 are the terms used to describe the configurations of lesions.

DESCRIPTIVE DERMATOLOGIC TERMS

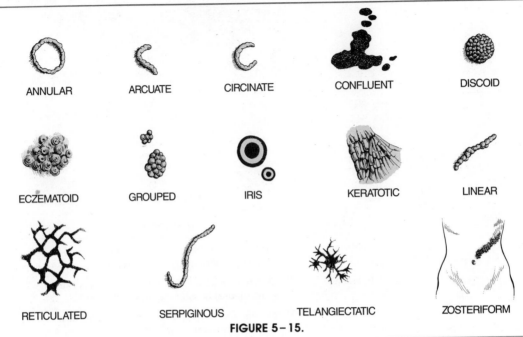

ANNULAR ARCUATE CIRCINATE CONFLUENT DISCOID

ECZEMATOID GROUPED IRIS KERATOTIC LINEAR

RETICULATED SERPIGINOUS TELANGIECTATIC ZOSTERIFORM

FIGURE 5–15.

Lesion	Description	Example
Annular	Ring shaped	Ringworm
Arcuate	Partial rings	Syphilis
Bizarre	Irregular or geographic pattern *not* related to any underlying anatomic structure	Factitial dermatitis
Circinate	Circular	
Confluent	Lesions run together	Childhood exanthems
Discoid	Disc shaped without central clearing	Lupus erythematosus
Discrete	Lesions remain separate	
Eczematoid	An inflammation with a tendency to vesiculate and crust	Eczema
Generalized	Widespread	
Grouped	Lesions clustered together	Herpes simplex
Iris	Circle within a circle; a bull's-eye lesion	Erythema multiforme (iris)
Keratotic	Horny thickening	Psoriasis
Linear	In lines	Poison ivy dermatitis
Multiform	More than one type of shape or lesion	Erythema multiforme
Papulosquamous	Papules or plaques associated with scaling	Psoriasis
Reticulated	Lace-like network	Oral lichen planus
Serpiginous	Snake-like, creeping	Cutaneous larva migrans
Telangiectatic	Relatively permanent dilatation of the superficial blood vessels	Osler-Weber-Rendu disease
Universal	Entire body involved	Alopecia universalis
Zosteriform*	Linear arrangement along a nerve distribution	Herpes zoster

* Also known as dermatomal.

CLINICOPATHOLOGIC CORRELATIONS

Skin disorders are frequently perplexing to the examiner. When one sees a rash, the common thought is, "Where do I begin?" All too often, the examiner may become frustrated and not even attempt to make a diagnosis. Dermatologic terms are complicated, and the names of dermatologic disorders may be intimidating. Often the descriptions of skin disorders in textbooks are more confusing than helpful.

There are over 2500 separately named dermatologic diagnoses. When one considers the low frequency of most of these diseases, one is left with only 10 – 15 common conditions that compose about 50% of all dermatologic diagnoses. If one were to consider the 50 most common conditions, over 95% of all patients could be diagnosed.

In approaching a skin lesion, it is important to

- First, identify the primary lesion.
- Second, identify its distribution.
- Third, identify any associated findings.
- Fourth, consider the age of the patient.

There are many common skin disorders or lesions with which the examiner should be familiar. Illustrated in the color plates at the front of the book are examples of some of these conditions; the cross-sectional diagrams shown in this chapter illustrate the locations of these abnormalities in the skin. These color figures and diagrams illustrate the involvement of the various skin layers in the pathogenesis of the conditions, and the text gives a description of the primary lesions.

A *wart* is a common, benign growth caused by an infection of an epidermal cell by a virus. This results in a thickening and vacuolation of the epidermis with scaling and an upward growth of the dermal papilla. Figure 5 – 16 and Plate I *F* illustrate a wart.

A *squamous cell carcinoma* is a malignant neoplasm of keratocytes in the epidermis and is locally invasive into the dermis. The tumor results in a scaling, crusting nodule or plaque that can ulcerate and bleed. Plate II *A* shows a patient

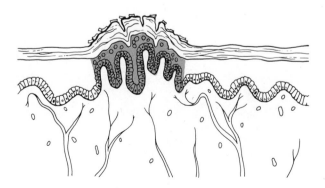

FIGURE 5 – 16. A cross-section through a wart. Note the thickened epidermis and hyperkeratosis.

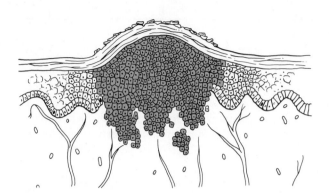

FIGURE 5–17. Cross-section through a squamous cell carcinoma. Note the invasion into the dermis.

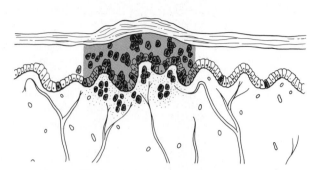

FIGURE 5–19. Cross-section through a melanoma. Note the nests of melanoma cells in the dermis.

with a squamous cell carcinoma in a surgical scar. Figure 5–17 shows a cross-section through a squamous cell carcinoma.

A *basal cell carcinoma* is a malignant neoplasm of the basal cells of the epidermis. The epidermis is thickened, and the dermis may be invaded by the malignant basal cells. It may appear as a papule with a ''pearly'' appearance having a central depression. If ulceration, bleeding, and crusting occur, a *rodent ulcer* is said to be present. Any nonhealing lesion should be carefully evaluated for the possibility of a basal cell carcinoma. Figure 5–18 and Plate II *B* illustrate the typical features of a basal cell carcinoma.

A *melanoma* is malignant neoplasm of the melanocytes of the epidermis. If untreated or unrecognized, a melanoma will cause fatal metastases. Most melanomas have a prolonged superficial, or horizontal, growth phase in which there is a progressive lateral expansion. With time, the melanoma enters the vertical, or deep, phase by penetrating into the dermis, and metastatic spread may occur. There are several types of melanomas: superficial spreading, nodular, lentigo, and acral-lentiginous.

Most melanomas have atypical pigmentation in the epidermis such as shades of red, white, gray, blue, brown, and black, all in a single lesion. Most melanomas (60–70%) are the superficial spreading variety. They occur in white individuals with a predilection for the backs of men and the legs of women. Less than 5% of all melanomas occur in the black population. The acral-lentiginous melanoma is the most common form in blacks and occurs on the palms, soles, and nail beds. These melanomas have a short superficial growth phase and an early vertical growth phase and, as such, are associated with a poor prognosis. A black patient with an acral-lentiginous melanoma on the sole of her foot is

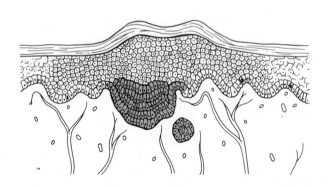

FIGURE 5–18. Cross-section through a basal cell carcinoma.

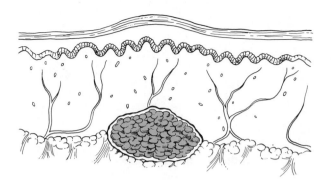

FIGURE 5–20. Cross-section through a lipoma.

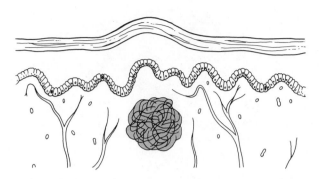

FIGURE 5–21. Cross-section through a neurofibroma. Notice that the tumor is a well-delimited mass of loosely packed neural elements.

shown in Plate II *C*. Figure 5–19 illustrates a cross-section through a melanoma.

A *lipoma* is a benign growth of subcutaneous fat that has a rubbery appearance. The epidermis is normal. Frequently, an encapsulated lipoma may grow to a very large size and elevate the overlying dermis and epidermis, as shown in Plate II *D* (see Fig. 5–20). Note that the examiner can easily push into the soft tissue tumor.

A *neurofibroma* is a tumor produced by a focal proliferation of neural tissue in the dermis. The epidermis is normal. Neurofibromas may appear as papules or nodules. Cutaneous neurofibromas are soft in consistency. Neurofibromatosis is a disorder in which multiple neurofibromas are present, sometimes as many as several hundred. Although the tumors themselves are benign, the occurrence of these space occupying lesions may produce severe disfigurement and/or neurologic disease. Other dermatologic features of neurofibromatosis include multiple café au lait patches and axillary freckling. Plate II *E* shows several neurofibromas in a patient with neurofibromatosis (see also Fig. 5–21).

Contact dermatitis is an inflammatory reaction of the skin that is precipitated by contact with an irritant or allergen such as detergents, acids, alkali, plants, medicines, and solvents. Vesicles in the epidermis as well as perivascular inflammation result. Plate II *F* shows a patient with contact dermatitis to poison ivy (see also Fig. 5–22). Note the characteristic linear distribution of papules, vesicles, and bullae on this patient's calf where the leaves of the plant touched the leg. The distribution of the bullous lesions together with their location is strongly suggestive of the diagnosis, which was confirmed by biopsy.

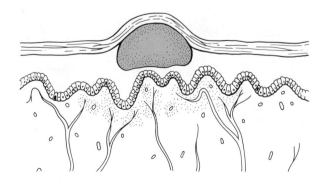

FIGURE 5–22. Cross-section through an area of contact dermatitis. Note the perivascular inflammation in the dermis as well as the vesicles and bullae in the epidermis.

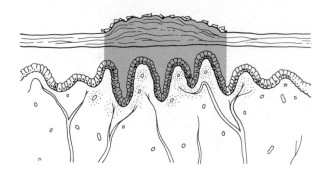

FIGURE 5–23. Cross-section through an area of psoriasis. Note the area of hyperkeratosis.

Psoriasis is an inflammatory rash resulting in hyperkeratosis of the epidermis. The stratum corneum thickens, and erythematous plaques with silvery scales result. Within the dermis, there is capillary proliferation with perivascular inflammation. The plaques are sharply demarcated. The lesions are characteristically located on the elbows, knees, scalp, and intergluteal cleft. Plate III *A* shows a patient with the classic scaling lesions of psoriasis at the intergluteal cleft. Figure 5–23 illustrates a cross-section through an area of psoriasis (see also Fig. 5–7).

Tinea corporis is "ringworm" infection. Fungal infections of the skin produce a scaling, erythematous patch, often with a reddened, raised, serpiginous border. The term *tinea* indicates the fungal etiology, whereas the second word denotes the area of the body involved: i.e., tinea corporis, body; tinea pedis, foot; tinea faciale, face; tinea cruris, groin; tinea capitis, head. In all cases, the epidermis is thickened, with the stratum corneum infiltrated with fungal hyphae. The underlying dermis shows mild inflammation. Figure 5–24 and Plate III *B* show the classic annular lesion of tinea corporis with its raised erythematous border and central clearing.

Pityriasis rosea is a common, acute, self-limiting inflammatory disease of unknown cause. Papulosquamous plaques appear over the trunk. The generalized eruption is preceded by a "herald patch," which is a single lesion resembling tinea corporis. In several days, the generalized eruption appears. Although the patient may complain of mild itching, he feels quite well. Slight hyperkeratosis of the epidermis with moderate dermal perivascular infiltration occurs. Plate III *C* shows a patient with a herald patch and the characteristic lesions of pityriasis rosea (see Fig. 5–25). Notice the delicate scale at the border of the

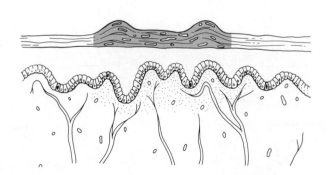

FIGURE 5–24. Tinea corporis. Cross-section through an area of tinea. Note the thickened stratum corneum, which is infiltrated by the fungus.

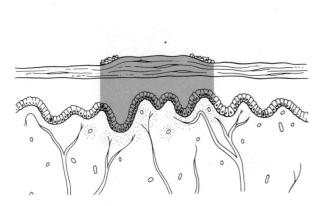

FIGURE 5–25. Pityriasis rosea. Cross-section through one of the lesions.

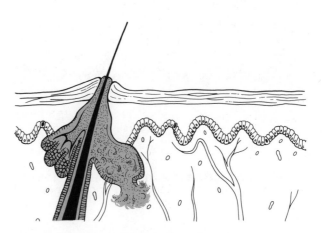

FIGURE 5–27. Cross-section through an area of acne. Note the rupturing of the sebaceous gland in the dermis as a result of a plugged hair follicle, which results in dermal inflammation.

annular lesion. Secondary syphilis may present with a similar eruption. It is therefore important to order a serologic test for syphilis in any individual with pityriasis rosea.

Herpes zoster, or shingles, is an intraepidermal vesicular eruption occurring in a dermatomal distribution. Bullae and multinucleated giant cells are present in the epidermis, with perivascular inflammation of the dermis. The condition is caused by activation of the zoster-varicella virus. Groups of vesicles and bullae on erythematous bases are present along the distribution of peripheral nerves. Severe pain often precedes the eruption. The distribution may occur along the spinal or cranial nerves. Plate III *D* shows a patient with herpes zoster along the T3 distribution (*see* Fig. 5–26 for cross-section).

Acne is a pustular disease affecting the hair follicles and sebaceous glands. In this condition, pustules, papules, and comedones are the primary lesions. There are collections of intradermal as well as intrafollicular neutrophils. Within the dermis, the hair follicle is occluded by a collection of keratin, sebum, and inflammatory cells. The hair follicle often ruptures into the dermis as a result of increasing pressure, leading to further dermal inflammation (Fig. 5–27; Plate III *E*).

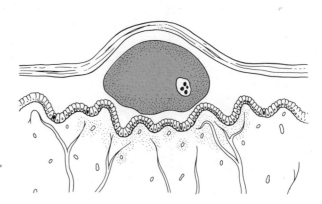

FIGURE 5–26. Herpes zoster. Cross-section through one of the vesicles. Note the large epidermal bullae with the classic multinuclear cells.

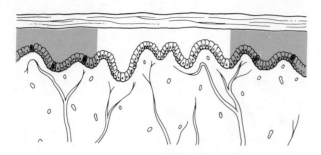

FIGURE 5–28. Cross-section through an area of vitiligo. Note the absence of melanocytes and skin pigment.

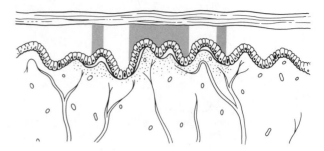

FIGURE 5–30. Cross-section through an area of erythema multiforme. Note the separation of the epidermis from the dermis.

Vitiligo consists of patches of lightened skin resulting from decreased melanin pigmentation. Vitiligo is essentially a large macule that is totally depigmented. The epidermis shows a complete absence of pigment, whereas the dermis is normal. Vitiligo can occur in any area, but it is most commonly found on the knees, elbows, and backs of the hands. Plate III *F* shows a woman with extensive vitiligo of her face and neck (see also Fig. 5–28).

Urticaria is a very common condition, the primary lesion of which is the wheal, or hive. In urticaria, the epidermis is normal. The dermis shows papillary edema. Inflammatory cells may be found surrounding dilated blood vessels. Itching is a common complaint. There are several mechanisms for the development of urticaria, which include both immunologic and nonimmunologic causes. Regardless of the cause, the common factor is the release of substances, such as histamine, that change the vascular permeability and produce dermal edema. Plate IV *A* shows a patient with giant urticaria (Fig. 5–29 depicts cross-section).

Erythema multiforme is an immunologic reaction in the skin triggered by infection or drugs. As the name implies, the condition includes a variety of lesions: papules, bullae, plaques, and "target lesions." Target lesions are the diagnostic lesions and have three zones of color. A central, tense bulla or dark area is surrounded by a zone of relative pallor that is rimmed by a thin area of erythema. Typically, target lesions are seen on the palms and soles. The epidermis is usually normal. In the dermis, there is a subepidermal separation with inflammatory cells in the papillary dermis. Penicillin and sulfonamides are the most common drugs implicated as the cause of this condition. The most severe form of erythema multiforme involves the mucous membranes and is called

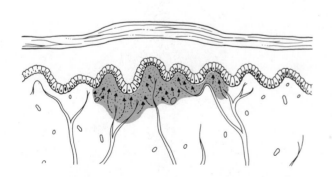

FIGURE 5–29. Cross-section through an area of urticaria.

TABLE 5–1. Common Maculopapular Diseases*

	Psoriasis	Pityriasis Rosea	Tinea Versicolor	Seborrheic Dermatitis	Lichen Planus
Color	Dull red, silvery	Pinkish yellow	Reddish brown	Pinkish yellow	Violaceous
Scale	Abundant	Fine, adherent	Fine	Greasy	Shiny, adherent
Induration	+	0	0	+	+
Face lesions	Rarely	Rarely	Occasionally	Common	Rarely
Oral lesions	0	0	0	0	2+
Nail lesions	4+	0	0	0	Rarely

* See Plates I *E*, III *A* and *C*, and VIII *C*.

Stevens-Johnson syndrome. A patient with the classic skin lesions of erythema multiforme is shown in Plate IV *B* (see also Fig. 5–30).

Kaposi's sarcoma is a neoplasm that is characterized by dark blue-purple macules, papules, nodules, and plaques on the legs, trunk, arms, neck, and head. The lesions start as lightish papules or nodules and coalesce into larger, darker lesions. Until recently, it was considered a rare disorder. Today, it is the most frequent neoplasm occurring in AIDS patients. Approximately 35% of gay patients with AIDS are affected, as opposed to about 5% of patients whose infection was acquired from intravenous drug abuse. Overall, 24% of all AIDS patients develop Kaposi's sarcoma. The average survival from the onset of the disease is less than 15 months. A patient with the classic skin lesions is shown in Plate IV *C*.

Scleroderma, also known as *progressive systemic sclerosis,* is an important rheumatic disease characterized by hardening of the skin. Vascular changes occur with visceral involvement and involve the microvessels and small arteries. The onset of the disease is often heralded by the development of Raynaud's phenomenon, which is discussed in Chapter 12, Peripheral Vascular System. The cutaneous manifestations of scleroderma involve tightening of the skin, especially on the face and hands. As a result of tendon contractures, flexion of the fingers results. Look at the fingers of the patient with scleroderma shown in Plate IV *D*. Notice that the skin is bound tightly and obscures the superficial vasculature. Skin lines are absent. Plate IV *E* shows the face of the same patient. Notice the tightening and wrinkling of the skin around her mouth and the fixed, expressionless countenance as a result of flattening of the nasolabial folds. The patient had great difficulty in opening her mouth. The skin around the mouth has many furrows radiating outward, giving a mouse-like appearance known as "mauskopf."

TABLE 5–2. Common Eczematous Diseases*

	Contact Dermatitis	Atopic Dermatitis	Neuro-Dermatitis	Stasis Dermatitis
History	Acute, localized to specific area	History in patient or family member of asthma, hayfever, or eczema	Chronic, in same areas, associated with anxiety	Varicosities, past history of thrombophlebitis or cellulitis
Location	Areas of exposure to allergen	Eyelids, groin, flexural areas	Head, lower legs, arms	Lower legs

* See Plates II *F*, X *D*, and XVI *C*.

TABLE 5–3. Vesiculobullous Diseases

	Pemphigus Vulgaris	Dermatitis Herpetiformis	Epidermolysis Bullosa*	Bullous Pemphigoid
Age of patient	40–60	Children or adults	Infants or children	60–70
Initial site	Oral mucosa	Scalp, trunk	Extremities	Extremities
Lesions	Normal skin at margins	Erythematous base	Bullae produced by trauma	Normal skin at margins
Sites	Mouth, abdomen, scalp, groin	Knees, sacrum, back, elbows	Hands, knees, elbows, mouth, toes	Trunk, extremities
Groupings	0	4+	1+	0
Weight loss	Marked	None	None	Minimal
Duration	1 or more years	Several years	Normal lifetime	Months to years
Pruritus	0	4+	0	±
Oral pain	4+	0	±	±
Palms/soles involved	No	No	Yes	Yes
Typical lesion	Flaccid bulla	Grouped vesicles	Flaccid vesicles	Tense bulla

* Refers not to a single disorder but to a group of inherited diseases.

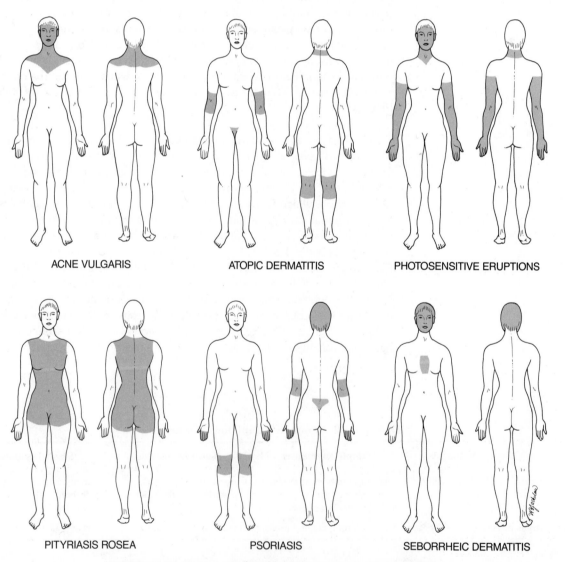

ACNE VULGARIS ATOPIC DERMATITIS PHOTOSENSITIVE ERUPTIONS

PITYRIASIS ROSEA PSORIASIS SEBORRHEIC DERMATITIS

FIGURE 5–31. Typical distribution of common skin conditions.

TABLE 5–4. Common Benign Tumors by Color

Color	Benign Tumor
Skin color	Warts (see Plate I F)
	Cysts
	Keloids
	Nevi
Pink or red	Hemangiomas (see Plate XV E)
	Keloids
Brown	Seborrheic keratoses
	Nevi
	Lentigines
	Dermatofibromas
Tannish yellow	Xanthomata (see Plate IX C)
	Xanthelasma (see Plate IX F)
	Warts
	Keloids
Dark blue or black	Seborrheic keratoses
	Hemangiomas
	Blue nevi
	Dermatofibromas

TABLE 5–5. Allergens Associated with Contact Dermatitis

Location	Possible Allergen
Scalp	Hair dyes
	Shampoos
	Tonics
Eyelids	Eye makeup
	Hair sprays
Neck	After shave lotions
	Perfumes
	Soaps
	Washing agents
	Nickel jewelry
Trunk	Clothing
	Washing agents
Axillae	Deodorants
	Soaps
Genitalia	Soaps
	Contraceptives
	Deodorants
	Washing agents
Feet	Shoes
	Sneakers
	Deodorants
	Socks
	Washing agents
Hands	Nickel jewelry
	Soaps
	Dyes
	Plants

Erythema nodosum is a common reaction associated with streptococcal infections, sarcoidosis, tuberculosis, inflammatory bowel diseases, and fungal diseases. It is infrequently associated with rheumatic disorders. The patient, primarily a young adult woman, seeks medical attention after the appearance of tender, erythematous nodules on her legs, especially over the anterior tibia. The lesions range in size from 1 to several centimeters in diameter. The lesions then coalesce and spread over the entire leg. The lesions of erythema nodosum begin to regress after 1–2 weeks. As they disappear, they undergo a series of characteristic color changes: bright erythema to shades of purple, yellow, and green. Plate IV F shows the early lesions of erythema nodosum in a 33 year old woman in whom sarcoidosis was diagnosed 3 months later.

Lichen planus is a common skin condition of unknown cause. The primary lesion is a polygonal, shiny, flat-topped papule with a violaceous hue. The lesions range in size from 2 mm to more than 1 cm. The sites of predilection are the flexural surfaces of the wrist, the legs, the genitalia, and the mucous membranes. Oral lesions are seen in 50% of all patients and consist of a white, lacy network on the buccal mucosa. A patient with the classic oral lesions is shown in Plate VIII C.

The typical distribution of lesions in six common skin disorders is shown in Figure 5–31.

Table 5–1 describes the differential diagnosis of common maculopapular diseases. Table 5–2 lists the differentiation of some common eczematous disorders and gives some special hints about their causes derived from the history. Table 5–3 provides a differential diagnosis of the vesiculobullous diseases. Table 5–4 classifies some of the common benign tumors by color. Table 5–5 lists some of the common allergens associated with contact dermatitis.

WRITING UP THE PHYSICAL EXAMINATION

Listed here are examples of the write-up for the examination of the skin.

There are oval plaques with well-defined borders and silvery scale symmetrically present on the elbows, knees, scalp, and gluteal cleft. The plaques in the scalp are along the hair line. The scales are large. Examination of the nails reveals pitting of the nail plates. The hair is of normal texture.

There is an annular lesion 3–4 cm in diameter on the right forearm. Scale is present on the narrow (1–2 mm), raised, erythematous border. The central area is slightly hypopigmented. The hair and nails are unremarkable.

There is a linear bullous eruption along the lateral aspect of the left leg. The eruption consists of bright red, edematous papules and bullae. There are no lesions on the palms or soles or in the mouth.

A wide variety of lesions are seen on the face, shoulders, and back. The predominant lesions are pustules on an inflammatory base. Many pustules are present, and several have become confluent over the chin and forehead. Open and closed comedones are present on the face, especially along the nasolabial folds. Inflammatory papules are present on the lower cheeks and chin. Large abscesses and ulcerated cysts are present over the upper shoulder areas. Numerous scars are present over the face and upper back.

A diffuse erythematous maculopapular rash is present on the trunk. Some excoriations are present over the shoulders and chest. Examination of the hair and nails is unremarkable.

Examination of the skin reveals several types of lesions. The main lesions seen are small papules in the antecubital and popliteal fossae. The papules in some areas have become confluent, and plaques are present. On the dorsum of the feet, there is eczema present with erythema, weeping, crusting, and scaling. Lichenification of the anogenital area, especially the scrotum, is present.

The skin is slightly cool and dry. Scattered lentigines are present over the trunk. The hair is very fine and soft. There is loss of the lateral one third of the eyebrows. No nail abnormalities are present.

BIBLIOGRAPHY

Braverman IM: Skin Signs of Systemic Disease. Philadelphia, WB Saunders Co, 1970.

Cage GW, Dobson RL: Sodium secretion and reabsorption in the human eccrine sweat gland. J Clin Invest 44:1270, 1965.

Ellis RA: Eccrine, sebaceous and apocrine glands. *In* Zelickson AS (ed): Ultrastructure of Normal and Abnormal Skin. Philadelphia, Lea and Febiger, 1967.

Flowers FP, Krusinski PA: Dermatology in Ambulatory and Emergency Medicine. Chicago, Year Book Medical Publishers, Inc, 1984.

Habif TP: Clinical Dermatology. St. Louis, CV Mosby Co, 1985.

Lever WF, Shaumburg-Lever G: Histology of the Skin. Philadelphia, JB Lippincott Co, 1975.

Lookingbill DP, Marks JG Jr.: Principles of Dermatology. Philadelphia, WB Saunders Co, 1986.

McMeekin TO, Moschella SL: Iatrogenic complications of dermatologic therapy. Med Clin North Am 63(2):441, 1979.

Montagna W: The Structure and Function of Skin. New York, Academic Press, 1962.

Rothman S: Physiology and Biochemistry of Skin. Chicago, University of Chicago Press, 1954.

Safai B, Johnson KG, Myskowski PL, Koziner B, Yang SY, Cunningham-Rundles S, Godbold JH, Dupont B: The natural history of Kaposi's sarcoma in the acquired immunodeficiency syndrome. Ann Intern Med 103:744, 1985.

Tragear RT: Physical Functions of Skin. New York, Academic Press, 1966.

THE HEAD AND NECK

A lady, aged twenty, became affected with some symptoms which were supposed to be hysterical...After she had been in this nervous state about three months it was observed that her pulse had become singularly rapid...She next complained of weakness on exertion and began to look pale and thin...It was observed that the eyes assumed a singular appearance, for the eyeballs were apparently enlarged. In a few months...a tumour, of a horseshoe shape, appeared on the front of the throat and exactly in the situation of the thyroid gland.

**Robert James Graves
1796 – 1853**

GENERAL CONSIDERATIONS

The appearance of the head and face, its contours and texture, often provides the first insight into the nature of illness. Sunken cheeks, wasting of the temporal muscles, and flushing of the face are important visible clues of systemic illness. Some facial appearances are pathognomonic of disease. The pale, puffy face of nephritis, the startled expression of hyperthyroidism, and the immobile stare of parkinsonism are examples of classic facies.

The appearance of the patient's face may also provide information regarding his psychological makeup: Is he happy, sad, angry, or anxious?

Thyroid disease takes many forms. The World Health Organization estimates that over 200 million people in the world have the condition of an enlarged thyroid, known as a *goiter*. The Asians first described the goiter around 1500 BC. Even at that time, they recognized that seaweed in the diet tended to make the goiter smaller. Iodine was not discovered until the nineteenth century, but it is now believed that these goiters were related to an iodine deficiency that was partially corrected by the iodine that was present in the seaweed.

The ancient Greeks and Romans recognized that when a thin thread tied around the neck of a newly married woman broke, she was pregnant. This was caused by an increase in the size of the thyroid during pregnancy.

In the United States, cancer of the head and neck composes about 5% of all malignancies in men and 2% in women. There are over 28,000 new cases a year. It has been estimated that nearly 90% of these cases are associated with poor dental hygiene, tobacco use, exposure to nickel, and alcohol. Tobacco, whether chewed, smoked, or simply kept in the buccal pouch, predisposes an individual to tumors of the upper aerodigestive tract (Vaughan et al, 1980). Pipe smokers and tobacco chewers are at risk for tumors of the oral cavity, and the Chinese are at risk for nasopharyngeal carcinomas.

STRUCTURE AND PHYSIOLOGY

The Head

The skull is composed of 22 bones, 14 in the face alone. This bony structure acts as a support and protection for the softer tissues within.

The *facial skeleton* is composed of the *mandible, maxilla, nasal, palatine, lacrimal,* and *vomer* bones. The unpaired *mandible* forms the lower jaw. The maxilla is an irregular bone and forms the upper jaw on each side. The nasal bones form the bridge of the nose. The other bones are not relevant to this discussion.

The main bones of the *cranial skeleton* include the *frontal, temporal, parietal,* and *occipital* bones. The frontal bones form the forehead. The temporal bones form the anterolateral walls of the brain. The *mastoid* process, which is part of the temporal bone, is particularly important in ear disease and is discussed in a subsequent chapter. The parietal bones form the top and posterolateral portions of the skull. The occipital bones form the posterior portion of the skull. The bones of the face and skull are shown in Figure 6–1.

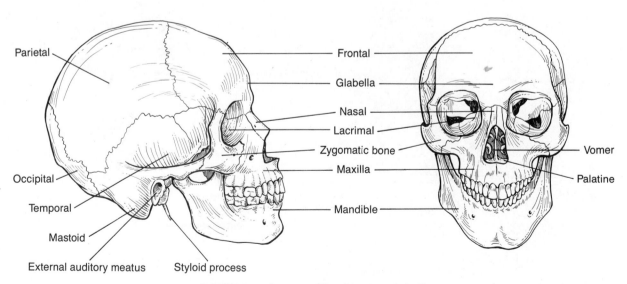

FIGURE 6–1. Bones of the face and skull.

The principal muscle of the mouth is the *orbicularis oris.* This single muscle surrounds the lips, with numerous other facial muscles inserting into it. The action of the orbicularis oris is to close the lips.

The *orbicularis oculi* muscle surrounds the eye. Its function is to close the eyelids. Chapter 7 further discusses this muscle and its action.

The *platysma* is a thin, superficial muscle of the neck, crossing the outer border of the mandible and extending over the lower anterior portion of the face. The main action of the platysma is to pull the mandible downward and backward, resulting in a mournful facial expression.

The muscles of mastication include the *masseter, pterygoid,* and *temporalis.* These muscles insert on the mandible and effect chewing. The masseter is a strong, thick muscle and is one of the most powerful muscles of the face. The action of the masseter is to close the jaw by elevating and drawing the mandible backward. Tension in the masseter may be felt by clenching the jaw. Although important in the functioning of the jaw, the other muscles of mastication are not clinically relevant to physical diagnosis and are not discussed in this text. The locations of these muscles are shown in Figure 6–2.

The muscles of the eye are discussed in Chapter 7, The Eye.

The *trigeminal,* or fifth cranial, nerve carries sensory fibers from the face, oral cavity, and teeth and carries efferent motor fibers to the muscles of mastication. The major divisions of this nerve are discussed in subsequent chapters.

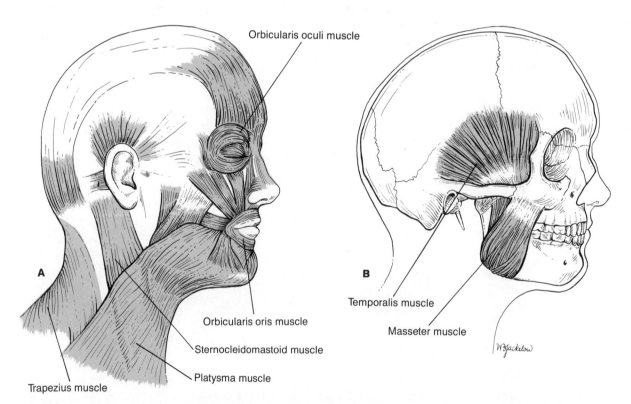

Orbicularis oculi muscle

A

Orbicularis oris muscle

Sternocleidomastoid muscle

Trapezius muscle

Platysma muscle

B

Temporalis muscle

Masseter muscle

FIGURE 6–2. Muscles of the face and skull. *A,* The more superficial muscles. *B,* The underlying muscles.

The Neck

The neck is divided by the sternocleidomastoid muscle into the anterior, or medial, triangle and the posterior, or lateral, triangle structures. This is illustrated in Figure 6–3.

The *sternocleidomastoid* is a strong muscle that serves to raise the sternum during respiration. The sternocleidomastoid has two heads: the *sternal* head arises from the manubrium sterni, whereas the *clavicular* head originates on the sternal end of the clavicle. The two heads unite and insert on the lateral aspect of the mastoid process. The sternocleidomastoid is innervated by the *spinal accessory,* or eleventh cranial, nerve.

Anterior to the sternocleidomastoid muscle is the *anterior triangle.* The other boundaries of the anterior triangle are the clavicle, inferiorly, and the midline, anteriorly. The anterior triangle contains the thyroid gland, the larynx, and the pharynx. The anterior triangle also contains lymph nodes, the submandibular salivary gland, and fat.

The *thyroid gland* envelops the upper trachea and consists of two lobes connected by an isthmus. It is the largest endocrine gland in the body. As seen from the front, the thyroid is butterfly shaped and wraps around the anterior and lateral portions of the larynx and trachea, as shown in Figure 6–4.

The thyroid isthmus lies across the trachea just below the cricoid cartilage of the larynx. The lateral lobes extend along either side of the larynx, reaching the level of the middle of the thyroid cartilage of the larynx. The function of the thyroid gland is to produce thyroid hormone in accordance with the needs of the body.

The pharynx and larynx are discussed in Chapter 9, The Oral Cavity and Pharynx.

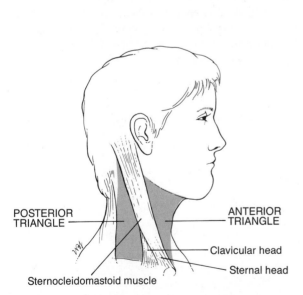

POSTERIOR TRIANGLE

ANTERIOR TRIANGLE

Clavicular head

Sternal head

Sternocleidomastoid muscle

FIGURE 6–3. The boundaries of the triangles of the neck.

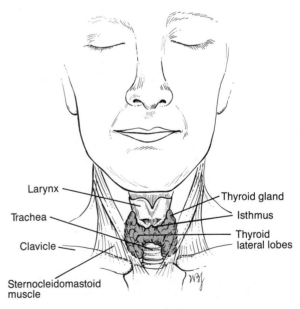

Larynx

Trachea

Clavicle

Sternocleidomastoid muscle

Thyroid gland

Isthmus

Thyroid lateral lobes

FIGURE 6–4. The thyroid gland.

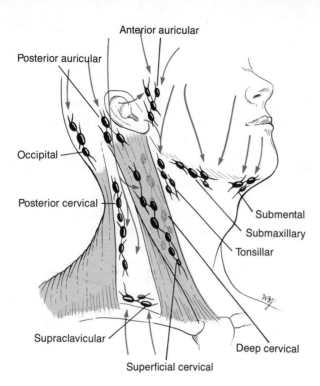

Anterior auricular

Posterior auricular

Occipital

Posterior cervical

Submental

Submaxillary

Tonsillar

Supraclavicular

Deep cervical

Superficial cervical

FIGURE 6-5. Lymph nodes of the neck and their drainage.

The sternocleidomastoid muscle overlies the *carotid sheath.* The carotid sheath lies lateral to the larynx. This sheath contains the common carotid artery, the internal jugular vein, and the vagus nerve.

Posterior to the sternocleidomastoid is the *posterior triangle.* This is bounded by the trapezius muscle, posteriorly, and by the clavicle, inferiorly. The posterior triangle also contains lymph nodes.

It has been estimated that the neck contains over 75 lymph nodes on each side. The chains of these lymph nodes are named for their location. Starting posteriorly, they are the *occipital, posterior auricular, posterior cervical, superficial* and *deep cervical* (adjacent to the sternocleidomastoid muscle), *tonsillar, submaxillary, submental* (at the tip of the jaw in the midline), *anterior auricular, and supraclavicular* (above the clavicle) chains. A knowledge of the lymphatic drainage is important, because the presence of an enlarged lymph node may signal disease in the area draining into it. The main groups of lymph nodes and their drainage areas are shown in Figure 6-5.

REVIEW OF SPECIFIC SYMPTOMS

The most common symptoms related to the neck include

- Neck mass
- Neck stiffness

Neck Mass

The most common symptom is a lump or swelling in the neck. Once a patient complains of a neck lump, ask the following questions:

"When did you first notice the lump?"
"Does it hurt?"
"Does the lump change in size?"
"Have you had any ear infections? . . . infections in your mouth?"
"Has there been hoarseness associated with the mass?"

If there is associated pain with a mass in the neck, an acute infection is likely. Masses that have been present for only a couple of days are commonly inflammatory, whereas those present for months are more likely to be neoplastic. A mass that has been present for months to years without any change in size will often turn out to be a benign or congenital lesion. Blockage of a salivary gland duct may produce a mass that fluctuates in size while the patient eats.

The *age of the patient* is relevant in the assessment of a neck mass. A lump in the neck of a patient under the age of 20 may be an enlarged tonsillar lymph node or a congenital mass. If the mass is in the midline, it is likely to be a thyroglossal cyst.* Between the ages of 20 and 40, thyroid disease is more common, although lymphoma must always be considered. Over the age of 40, a neck mass must always be considered malignant until proved otherwise.

The *location* of the mass is also important. Midline masses tend to be benign or congenital lesions such as thyroglossal cysts or dermoid cysts. Lateral masses are frequently neoplastic. Masses located in the lateral upper neck may be metastatic lesions from tumors of the head and neck, whereas masses in the lateral lower neck may be metastatic from tumors of the breast and stomach. One benign lateral neck mass is a branchial cleft cyst, which may present as a painless, lateral neck mass near the anterior upper third border of the sterno-cleidomastoid muscle.

Hoarseness in association with a thyroid nodule suggests vocal cord paralysis by impingement of the recurrent laryngeal nerve by tumor.

Neck Stiffness

Stiffness of the neck is usually caused by spasm of the cervical muscles and is commonly the cause of the tension headache. The sudden occurrence of a stiff neck, fever, and headache should alert suspicion of possible meningeal irritation. Neck pain may be associated with referred pain from the chest. Patients with angina or a myocardial infarction may complain of neck pain.

IMPACT OF HEAD AND NECK DISEASE ON THE PATIENT

The concept of body image is very important. The head and neck are the most visible portions of the body. The shape of our eyes, mouth, face, and nose is very important to all of us. There are many who dislike their body image and want to change it by cosmetic surgery. There are others who require cosmetic surgery to repair alterations that are due to trauma. There are still others who suffer from disfiguring head and neck cancer and need to undergo surgical

---

*A thyroglossal cyst may arise anywhere along the route of the thyroid gland's descent from the foramen cecum of the tongue to its adult location in the neck. It is a painless, mobile structure that moves on swallowing or with movement of the tongue. See Plate XVI *E*.

procedures for the removal of these lesions. Many of these procedures themselves are mutilating.

Distortion of the body image, especially on the head and neck, can produce a devastating effect on the patient. The most common reaction to head and neck disease is depression. Many of these patients suffer from feelings of sadness and hopelessness. They look in the mirror hoping someday they will see themselves with a more acceptable body image. Recurrent thoughts of suicide are common. Many of these depressed patients turn to alcohol or other drugs to try to escape from reality.

Occasionally, patients who have undergone cosmetic surgery are dissatisfied with the results. Many of these patients are trying to escape from feelings of inferiority and social maladjustment. They may have had only minor defects, but these defects are viewed as a major source of interpersonal problems. Cosmetic surgery is a way to change their image in the hope of improving their social maladjustment. Some individuals may even blame the physician for "destroying" their face. Even after further revisions, these patients may never be satisfied. One of the keys to success of cosmetic surgery is the proper selection of patients.

PHYSICAL EXAMINATION

> There is no special equipment needed for the examination of the head and neck.

The examination of the head and neck is performed with the patient seated, facing the examiner. The examination consists of

- Inspection
- Palpation

Inspection

Inspect the position of the head. Does the patient hold his head erect? Is there any asymmetry of the facial structure? Is the head proportioned to the rest of the body?

Inspect the scalp for lesions. Describe the hair.

Are any masses present? If so, describe the size, consistency, and symmetry.

Inspect the eyes for proptosis (a forward displacement, or bulging, of the eyeball). Proptosis may be caused by thyroid dysfunction or by a mass in the orbit.

Inspect the neck for areas of asymmetry. Ask the patient to extend his neck. Inspect the neck for scars, asymmetry, or masses. The normal thyroid is barely visible. You should ask the patient to swallow while you observe any upward motion of the thyroid with swallowing. A diffusely enlarged thyroid gland will often cause generalized enlargement of the neck. Look at the patient with diffuse thyromegaly shown in Plate V A. This patient has Graves' disease with bilateral proptosis.

Is nodularity of the neck seen? A patient with nodular neck masses that are due to a multinodular goiter is seen in Plate V B.

Is superficial venous distention present? Venous distention in the neck is important to evaluate, as this finding may be associated with a goiter.

Palpation

Palpate the Head and Neck

Palpation confirms the information obtained by inspection. The head should be slightly flexed and should be cradled in the examiner's hands, as shown in Figure 6–6.

All areas of the cranium should be palpated for tenderness or masses. The pads of the examiner's fingers should roll the underlying skin over the cranium in circular motions to assess its contour and to feel for the presence of lymph nodes or masses. Starting from the occipital region, the hands are moved into the posterior auricular region, which is superficial to the mastoid process; down into the posterior triangle to feel for the posterior cervical chain; along the sternocleidomastoid muscle to feel for the superficial cervical chain; hooking around the sternocleidomastoid muscle to feel for the deep cervical chain deep to the muscle; into the anterior triangle region; up to the jaw margin to feel for the tonsillar group; along the jaw to feel the submaxillary chain; to the tip of the jaw for the submental nodes; and up to the anterior auricular chain in front of the ear. This motion is shown in Figure 6–7.

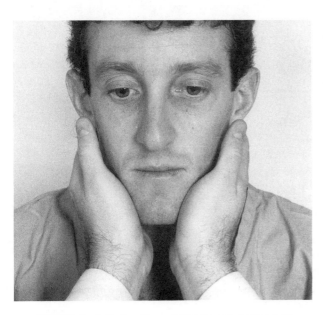

FIGURE 6–6. Palpation of the head and neck.

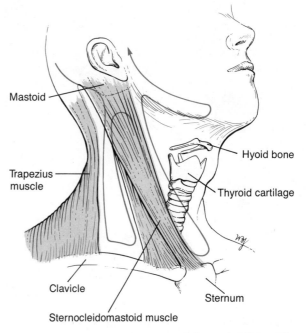

Mastoid

Trapezius muscle

Clavicle

Sternocleidomastoid muscle

Hyoid bone

Thyroid cartilage

Sternum

FIGURE 6–7. Suggested approach for palpation of the lymph nodes of the neck.

A patient with enlarged posterior auricular and posterior cervical nodes is shown in Plate V C.

Any nodes that are felt should be observed for mobility, consistency, and tenderness. Tender lymph nodes are suggestive of inflammation, whereas fixed, firm nodes are consistent with a malignancy.

Palpate the Thyroid Gland

There are two approaches to palpating the thyroid gland. The *anterior* approach is carried out with the patient and examiner sitting face to face. By flexing the patient's neck or turning the chin slightly to the right, the examiner can relax the sternocleidomastoid muscle on that side, making the examination easier to perform. The examiner's right hand should displace the larynx to the right, and, during swallowing, the displaced right thyroid lobe is palpated between the examiner's left thumb and index fingers. This is demonstrated in Figure 6–8. After the right lobe has been evaluated, the larynx is displaced to the left and the left lobe is evaluated by reversing the hand positions.

At this point in the examination, the examiner should stand behind the patient to palpate the thyroid by the posterior approach. The *posterior* approach involves placing the examiner's two hands around the neck of the patient, whose neck is slightly extended. The examiner uses his left hand to push the trachea to the right. The patient is asked to swallow while the examiner's right hand rolls over the thyroid cartilage. As the patient swallows, the examiner's right hand feels for the thyroid gland against the right sternocleidomastoid muscle. The patient is again asked to swallow as the trachea is pushed to the left, and the examiner uses his left hand to feel for the thyroid gland against the left sternocleidomastoid muscle. A drink of water given to the patient will facilitate swallowing. The posterior approach is shown in Figure 6–9.

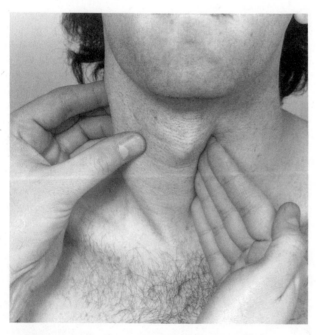

FIGURE 6–8. Anterior approach for palpation of the thyroid gland.

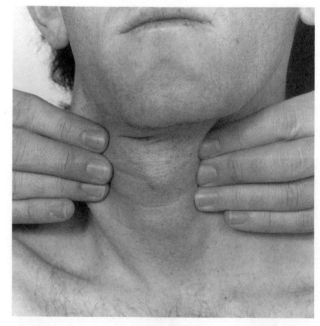

FIGURE 6–9. Posterior approach for palpation of the thyroid gland.

Although both the anterior and the posterior approaches of palpation are usually performed, the examiner rarely feels the thyroid gland in its normal state.

The *consistency* of the gland should be evaluated. The normal thyroid gland has a consistency of muscle tissue. Unusual hardness is associated with cancer or scarring. Softness, or sponginess, is often seen with a toxic goiter. *Tenderness* of the thyroid gland is associated with acute infections or with hemorrhage into the gland.

If the thyroid is enlarged, it should also be examined by auscultation. The bell of the stethoscope is placed over the lobes of the thyroid while the examiner listens for the presence of a bruit (a murmur heard when there is increased turbulence in a vessel). The finding of a systolic or a to-and-fro* *thyroid bruit*, particularly if heard over the superior pole, indicates an abnormally large blood flow and is highly suggestive of a *toxic goiter*.

Palpate for Supraclavicular Nodes

The palpation for supraclavicular nodes concludes the examination of the head and neck. The examiner stands behind the patient and places his fingers into the medial supraclavicular fossae, deep to the clavicle and adjacent to the sternocleidomastoid muscles. The patient is instructed to take a deep breath while the examiner presses deeply in and behind the clavicles. Any supraclavicular nodes that are enlarged will be felt as the patient inspires. This technique is shown in Figure 6–10.

The examination of the trachea is discussed in Chapter 10, The Chest. The examination of the carotid arterial and jugular venous pulsations is discussed in Chapter 11, The Heart.

---

* Refers to two separate murmurs, systolic and diastolic.

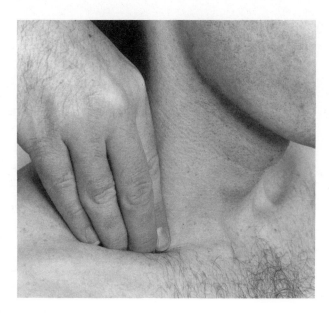

FIGURE 6–10. Technique for palpation of supraclavicular lymph nodes.

CLINICOPATHOLOGIC CORRELATIONS

Although iodine deficiency is still a worldwide cause of thyroid enlargement, infection, autoimmune disease, cancer, and isolated nodules are other important causes of goiter. An enlarged thyroid may be associated with *hyperthyroidism*, *hypothyroidism*, or a *simple* or *multinodular* goiter of normal function.

As indicated in the quote at the beginning of this chapter, hyperthyroidism may present with a variety of generalized symptoms and signs. It has been said, "To know thyroid disease is to know medicine," since there are so many generalized effects of thyroid hormone excess. Table 6–1 indicates the wide variety of clinical symptoms related to thyroid hormone excess.

Occasionally Graves' disease may present with unilateral proptosis, as shown in the patient in Plate V *D*. This patient presented with proptosis and was treated for Graves' disease 20 years before this photograph was taken. As is common, the proptosis never disappeared.

The nervous, perspiring patient with a stare and bulging eyes offers an unmistakable combination of physical signs associated with hyperthyroidism. The most common type of hyperthyroidism is the diffuse toxic goiter, known as Graves' disease. Graves' disease is viewed as an autoimmune disorder provoked by the elaboration of a thyroid stimulating immunoglobulin. There are many cutaneous signs of hyperthyroidism, including the following (p. 119):

TABLE 6–1. Symptoms of Hyperthyroidism

Organ System	Symptom
General	Preference for the cold Weight loss with good appetite
Eyes	Prominence of eyeballs* Puffiness of eyelids Double vision Decreased motility
Neck	Goiter
Cardiac	Palpitations Peripheral edema†
Gastrointestinal	Increased bowel movements
Genitourinary	Polyuria Decreased fertility
Neuromuscular	Fatigue Weakness Tremulousness
Emotional	Nervousness Irritability
Dermatologic	Hair thinning Increased perspiration Change in skin texture Change in pigmentation

* Appears to be due to mucopolysaccharide deposition behind the orbit.
† Appears to be due to excessive mucopolysaccharide deposition under the skin, especially in the legs.

TABLE 6–2. Distinctive Features of Graves' Disease and Plummer's Disease

Feature	Graves' Disease Toxic Diffuse Goiter*	Plummer's Disease Toxic Adenomatous Goiter†
Age of onset	40 years	40 years
Onset	Acute	Insidious
Goiter	Diffuse	Nodular
Signs/symptoms	Clear cut	Vague
Myopathy (muscle disease)	Present	Absent
Heart involvement	Sinus tachycardia Occasionally atrial fibrillation	Frequently atrial fibrillation Congestive heart failure
Ophthalmopathy	Exophthalmos Vision changes Motility abnormalities Chemosis (conjunctival edema)	Lid lag Lid retraction

* See Plate V A.
† See Plate V B.

- Warm skin
- Erythema
- Hyperhidrosis (increased sweating)
- Alopecia (hair loss)
- Hyperpigmentation
- Nail growth changes

Sometimes hyperthyroidism is caused by a single "hot" nodule.* Toxic adenomatous goiter, also known as *Plummer's disease,* accounts for less than 10% of all hyperthyroid patients. Hyperthyroidism may be caused by a single autonomously functioning thyroid adenoma. The adenoma is usually papillary

---

* The terms "hot" or "cold" are descriptions of nodules seen on a thyroid scan and are used to indicate whether a nodule accumulates more or less radioactive iodine than the surrounding thyroid tissue. A "hot" nodule is functioning thyroid tissue and has a greater uptake than the surrounding tissue. A "cold" nodule is nonfunctioning and will fail to take up the radioactive tracer.

TABLE 6–3. Characteristics of Benign and Malignant Thyroid Nodules

Characteristic	Benign Nodule	Malignant Nodule
Age of onset	Adult	Adult
Sex	Female	Male
Patient history	Symptoms present	Previous x-ray treatment to head or neck
Family history	Benign thyroid diseases	None
Speed of enlargement	Slow	Rapid
Change in voice	Absent	Present
Number of nodules	More than 1	1
Lymph nodes	Absent	Present
Remainder of thyroid	Abnormal	Normal

TABLE 6–4. Characteristics of Thyroid Nodules Suspicious for Cancer*

Characteristic	Sensitivity (%)	Specificity (%)
Palpable, hard nodule	42	89
Fixed mass	31	94
Local symptoms	3	97
Dysphagia	10	93
Unilateral adenopathy	5	96
Nodule found on routine examination	50	56
Family history of goiter	17	79

* Data from Hoffman, 1972; Kendall, 1976; and Haff, 1976.

and is unrelated to any autoimmune process. Hyperfunction may also occur in multiple nodules. The distinctive features of hyperthyroidism caused by Graves' and Plummer's diseases are summarized in Table 6–2.

Approximately 5% of the population have a single thyroid nodule larger than 1 cm. Though most of these nodules are benign and require no therapy, they should all be investigated for malignancy. The history and physical examination can provide some clues as to the nature of the "lump." Table 6–3 summarizes some of the important characteristics of benign and malignant nodules.

Many symptoms and signs of thyroid disease have been evaluated for their sensitivity and specificity. Most of these findings are specific but are too insensitive to make them useful. Table 6–4 summarizes the operating characteristics of certain findings in the evaluation of a thyroid nodule for malignancy. As can be seen, the most useful signs are a palpable, hard nodule and a fixed mass.

TABLE 6–5. Symptoms and Signs of Hypothyroidism

System	Symptom	Sign
General	Weight gain with regular diet Chilly while others are warm	Obesity
Gastrointestinal	Constipation	Enlarged tongue
Cardiovascular	Fatigue	Hypotension Bradycardia
Nervous	Speech disorders Short attention span Tremor	Hyporeflexia Defective abstract reasoning Spasticity Tremor Depressed affect
Musculoskeletal	Lethargy Thickened, dry skin Hair loss Brittle nails Leg cramps Puffy eyelids Puffy cheeks	Hypotonia Puffy facies
Reproductive	Heavier menses Decreased fertility	

The heavy, puffy-faced, lethargic patient with dry skin, sparse hair, and a hoarse voice provides the classic picture of hypothyroidism. Hypothyroidism develops insidiously. Often the only complaint is a tired or "run down" feeling. The careful interviewer and examiner must be on the alert for any patient, especially over the age of 60, with these symptoms. Patients with hypothyroidism commonly have *hung*, or delayed, reflexes. The measurement of the relaxation time of the Achilles tendon reflex has long been used to follow the effect of treatment in patients with hypothyroidism. However, it is useless as a screening technique because there may be many false negative or false positive results. Table 6–5 lists some of the major symptoms and signs of hypothyroidism.

USEFUL VOCABULARY

Listed here are the specific roots that are important in order to understand the terminology related to diseases of the head and neck.

ROOT	PERTAINING TO	EXAMPLE	DEFINITION
capit-	head	*capit*ate	Head shaped
cleido-	clavicle	*cleido*mastoid	Pertaining to the clavicle and mastoid process
cranio-	skull	*cranio*malacia	Abnormal softening of the skull
occipito-	back portion of the skull	*occipito*parietal	Pertaining to the occipital and parietal bones
odont(o)-	tooth; teeth	*odont*orrhagia	Hemorrhage following tooth extraction
thyro-	thyroid gland	*thyro*megaly	Enlargement of the thyroid gland

WRITING UP THE PHYSICAL EXAMINATION

Listed here are examples of the write-up for the examination of the head, neck, and thyroid.

The head is normocephalic without evidence of trauma. The neck is supple, with full range of motion. No adenopathy is present in the neck. The thyroid is nontender and is not enlarged. There are no thyroid nodules felt.

The head is normocephalic and atraumatic. There is a 2 cm, rubbery, nontender mass in the superficial cervical chain on the left side. The mass is freely mobile and is not fixed to the skin or underlying muscle. Another 4 cm, rubbery, nontender mass is felt in the right supraclavicular fossa. The thyroid is unremarkable.

There is frontal bossing of the head with prominence of the cheek bones. There is no evidence of trauma. The neck is supple, with no adenopathy present. There is a 2 cm, soft, painless thyroid nodule felt 3 cm from the midline in the upper portion of the right lobe (approximately at 10 o'clock). The nodule is not fixed to the overlying skin or muscles.

BIBLIOGRAPHY

Haff RC, Schecter BC, Armstrong RG, Evans WE: Factors increasing the probability of malignancy in thyroid nodules. Am J Surg *131*:707, 1976.

Hoffman GL, Thompson NW, Heffron C: The solitary thyroid nodule: A reassessment. Arch Surg *105*:379, 1972.

Kendall LW, Condon RE: Prediction of malignancy in solitary thyroid nodules. Lancet *1*:1019, 1976.

Shapiro HH: Applied Anatomy of the Head and Neck. Philadelphia, JB Lippincott Co, 1947.

Vaughan CW, Homburger F, Shapshay SM, Soto E, Bernfeld P: Carcinogenesis in the upper aerodigestive tract. Otolaryngol Clin North Am *13*(3):403, 1980.

Werner SC, Ingbar SH (eds): The Thyroid: A Fundamental and Clinical Text. New York, Harper and Row, 1971.

THE EYE

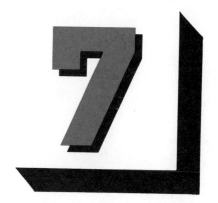

Who would believe that so small a space could contain the images of all the universe? O mighty process!

Leonardo da Vinci
1452–1519

HISTORICAL CONSIDERATIONS

The eyes are our windows to the world. Most of the sensory input to our brain is through our eyes. For centuries, the eye has been considered the essence of the person, representing the "I." When we review mythology and the writings of ancient times, we find many references to the eye as an organ associated with mystical powers.

The eye has long been associated with mythical gods. In ancient Egypt, the eye was always the symbol of the Great Goddess. The Eye of Horus was believed to protect against all evil and to ensure success. The "evil eye" from the myth of Medusa was an expression of envy and greed. Even today, many believe in the powers of an "evil eye."

Another interesting association is the subconscious linking of "eyeball" with genitalia. Blindness can symbolize castration, since both testicles and eyeballs have the same shape and are important in the development of the sense of identity. This linking goes back to the legend of Oedipus, who pierced his eyeballs when he discovered that he had been married to his mother and had killed his father. This can be thought of as an act of self-castration as well as a means of cutting oneself off from all worldly relationships. Throughout literature, the blinding of an individual was frequently a form of punishment for lust. The age-old notion that masturbation will cause blindness serves to further reinforce this close association of organs.

123

STRUCTURE AND PHYSIOLOGY

The external landmarks of the eye are shown in Figure 7–1, and the cross-sectional anatomy of the eye is shown in Figure 7–2.

The *eyelids* and *eyelashes* serve to protect the eyes. The eyelids cover the globe and lubricate its surface. The *meibomian glands* secrete an oily lubricating substance to retard evaporation. These glands have their openings at the lid margins.

The *orbicularis oculi* muscle encircles the lids and is responsible for their closure. This muscle is supplied by the facial, or seventh cranial, nerve. The *levator palpebrae* muscle serves to elevate the lids and is innervated by the oculomotor, or third cranial, nerve. *Müller's muscle* is a small part of the levator muscle, having sympathetic innervation.

The globe has six *extraocular muscles* that control its motion. There are four rectus and two oblique muscles. They are the medial rectus, the lateral rectus, the superior rectus, the inferior rectus, the superior oblique, and the inferior oblique muscles. The six extraocular muscles are shown in Figure 7–3.

The extraocular muscles work in a parallel, conjugate fashion to maintain single, binocular vision. When we turn our gaze to the left, for example, the *left lateral rectus* and the *right medial rectus* contract to turn our eyes to the *left*. The actions and innervations of the extraocular muscles are demonstrated in Table 7–1, and the extraocular movements are illustrated in Figure 7–4.

It is helpful to remember that the *lateral rectus* muscle, which is innervated by the *abducens* nerve, *abd*ucts the eye (turns it laterally), as do both oblique muscles.

The *conjunctiva* is a thin, vascular, transparent mucous membrane that lines the lids and the anterior portion of the globe continuously. The *palpebral* portion

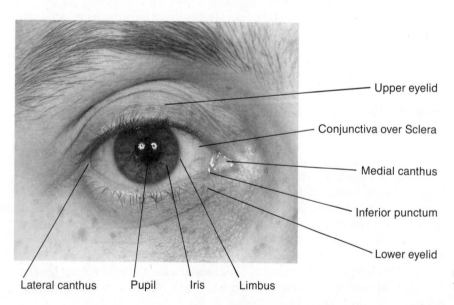

Upper eyelid

Conjunctiva over Sclera

Medial canthus

Inferior punctum

Lower eyelid

Lateral canthus   Pupil   Iris   Limbus

FIGURE 7–1. External landmarks of the eye.

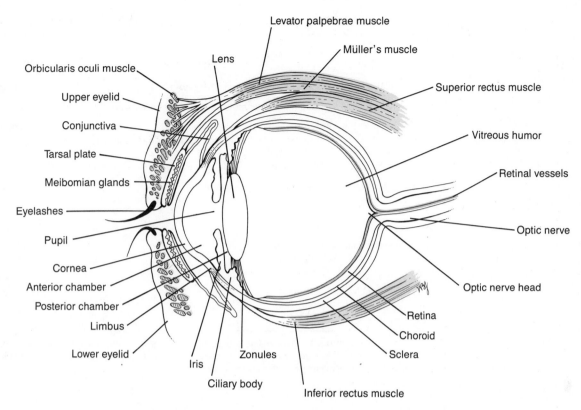

FIGURE 7–2. Cross-sectional anatomy of the eye.

covers the inner surface of the lids, whereas the *bulbar* portion covers the sclera up to the *limbus*, which is the corneal-scleral junction. The conjunctiva contains many small blood vessels, which when dilated can produce a "red" eye. There is little nervous innervation to the conjunctiva.

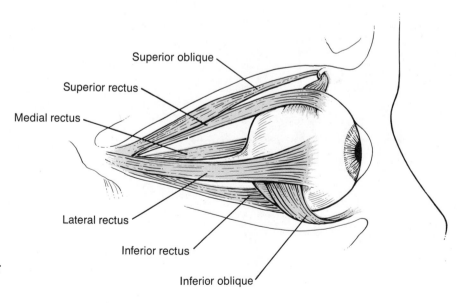

FIGURE 7–3. The extraocular muscles.

TABLE 7–1. Actions and Innervations of the Extraocular Muscles*

Muscle	Primary Action	Cranial Nerve Innervation
Medial rectus	Adduction (eye moves nasally)	Oculomotor (III)
Lateral rectus	Abduction (eye moves temporally [away from the nose])	Abducens (VI)
Inferior rectus	Depression (eye moves down) Extorsion (the 12 o'clock position on the cornea rotates temporally) Adduction	Oculomotor (III)
Superior rectus	Elevation (eye moves up) Intorsion (the 12 o'clock position on the cornea rotates nasally) Adduction	Oculomotor (III)
Superior oblique	Depression Intorsion Abduction	Trochlear (IV)
Inferior oblique	Elevation Extorsion Abduction	Oculomotor (III)

* Remember "LR$_6$SO$_4$." This mnemonic states that the lateral rectus (LR) muscle is innervated by the sixth cranial nerve and the superior oblique (SO) muscle is innervated by the fourth cranial nerve. All the other muscles are innervated by the third cranial nerve.

The *lacrimal apparatus* consists of the lacrimal gland, accessory tear glands, canaliculi, tear sac, and nasolacrimal duct. These are shown in Figure 7–5.

The *lacrimal gland* produces watery tears and is located above and slightly lateral to the globe. Secretion occurs mostly as reflex tearing or crying. Tears drain through the *puncta* on the lids and into the superior and inferior *canaliculi*. These canaliculi join and enter the *tear sac*, located at the medial *canthus* of the eye. The *nasolacrimal duct* drains the sac to the nose. Of the lacrimal apparatus, only the puncta are visible on routine examination.

The *sclera* is the white, fibrous, outer coat of the globe visible just beneath the conjunctiva. The extraocular muscles insert into the sclera.

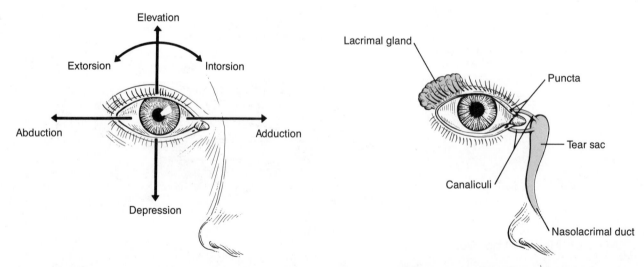

FIGURE 7–4. Extraocular movements.

FIGURE 7–5. The lacrimal apparatus.

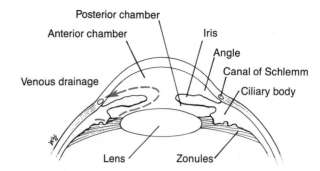

FIGURE 7–6. Cross-section of the normal angle structures, showing the flow of aqueous humor.

The *cornea* is a smooth, transparent, avascular tissue that covers the iris and joins with the sclera and conjunctival reflection at the limbus. The cornea functions as a protective window allowing light to pass into the eye. The cornea is richly innervated by the trigeminal, or fifth cranial, nerve and is therefore exquisitely sensitive to touch.

The *anterior chamber*, or space between the cornea anteriorly and the iris posteriorly, is filled with clear *aqueous humor*. Aqueous humor is produced by the *ciliary body* in the *posterior chamber*, the area behind the iris and in front of the lens. Aqueous humor circulates from the posterior chamber, through the pupil, into the anterior chamber, and is removed through the *canal of Schlemm*, from where it eventually enters the venous system. Pressure within the eye is regulated by this filtration. The *angle* is that formed by the juncture of the cornea and the iris at the limbus. A section through the eye at this level is shown in Figure 7–6.

The *iris* is the circular, colored portion of the eye. The small, round aperture in the middle of the iris is called the *pupil*. The pupil functions much as the aperture of a camera, controlling the amount of light that enters the eye.

When a light is shined on one eye, both pupils will constrict consensually. This is termed the *pupillary light reflex*. In order to understand this reflex, a brief review of the neuroanatomy is in order. Figure 7–7 illustrates the pathways of the pupillary light reflex.

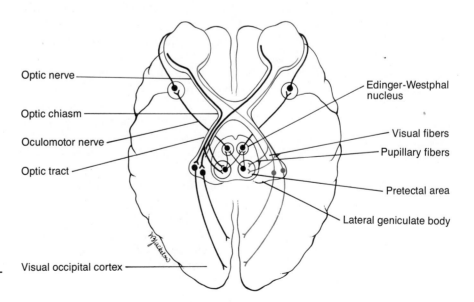

FIGURE 7–7. The pupillary light reflex.

The optic, or second cranial, nerves are composed of 80% *visual* and 20% afferent *pupillary* fibers. The optic nerves leave both retinae and travel a short course to where they join each other. This is the *optic chiasm*. At the optic chiasm, the nasal fibers cross and join the uncrossed fibers of the other side, forming the *optic tract*. The *visual* fibers continue in the optic tract to the *lateral geniculate body*, where synapses occur, the axons of which terminate in the primary visual cortex of the occipital lobe. The afferent pupillary fibers bypass the geniculate body and end in the *superior colliculus* and *pretectal* area of the midbrain.

Light impulses to the eye will cause the retina to transmit nerve impulses to the optic nerve, the optic tract, the midbrain, and the visual cortex of the occipital lobes. This is the *afferent limb* of the light reflex. In the midbrain, the pupillary fibers diverge and are relayed by crossed fibers to the opposite *Edinger-Westphal* nucleus of the oculomotor, or third cranial, nerve. Some fibers remain on the same side. The third cranial nerve is the *efferent limb*, which goes via the ciliary body to the sphincter muscle of the iris to cause it to contract. The *direct effect* is the constriction of the pupil of the eye upon which the light is shined (the *ipsilateral eye*). The *consensual effect* is the simultaneous constriction of the opposite pupil (the *contralateral eye*).

The *near reflex* occurs when the subject looks at a near target. The three parts of the near reflex are *accommodation, convergence*, and *pupillary constriction*. Accommodation is defined as the near focusing of the eye, which is effected by increasing the power of the lens by contraction of the ciliary muscle, innervated by the third cranial nerve.

There is also autonomic innervation of the eyes. The iris is supplied by both sympathetic and parasympathetic fibers. When the sympathetic fibers are stimulated, pupillary dilatation occurs as well as elevation of the eyelid. Think of the nervous cat stalking its prey, pupils dilated, ready to pounce in the dark. It needs all the light it can get. It is purely sympathetic. When the parasympathetic fibers in the oculomotor nerve are stimulated, pupillary constriction occurs.

The *choroid* is the middle, vascular layer of the globe. It acts as a source of nourishment as well as a heat sink, serving to remove the extreme heat produced by the light energy entering the eye.

The *lens* sits directly behind the iris. It is a biconvex, avascular, colorless structure that changes its shape to focus the image upon the retina. The shape is changed by the *ciliary body muscles*.

The *vitreous humor* is the transparent, avascular gel that is located behind the lens and in front of the retina.

The *retina* is the innermost layer, or "camera film," of the eye. Within the retina are several important structures: the optic disc, the retinal vessels, and the macula. Figure 7–8 illustrates the retina.

The *optic disc* is located at the nasal aspect of the posterior pole of the retina. This is the head of the optic nerve, from where the nerve fibers of the retina exit the eye. The optic disc is 1.5 mm in diameter and is ovoid in shape. It is lighter than the surrounding retina and appears yellowish-pink. The disc margins are sharp with some normal blurring of the nasal portion. Black patients may have pigmentation at the margins. The *physiologic cup* is the center of the disc, where the retinal vessels penetrate. This small depression occupies about 30% of the disc diameter.

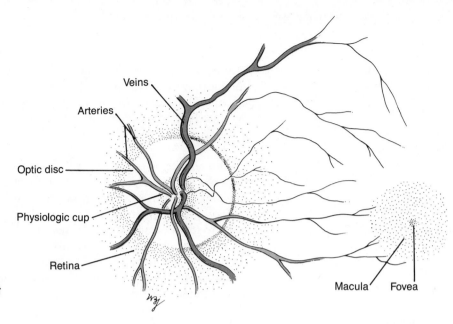

FIGURE 7-8. The retina of the left eye.

The *retinal vessels* emerge from the disc and arborize on the retinal surface. The arteries are brighter red and are thinner than the veins. An artery-to-vein ratio of 2:3 is normal.

The *macula* is a small, round area, approximately the size of the disc, located 3.5 mm temporal to and 0.5 mm inferior to the disc. The macula is easily seen, as it is devoid of retinal vessels. In the center of the macula is the *fovea*, a depressed area composed only of *cones*. Cones provide detailed vision and color perception.

The remaining areas of the retina contain mostly *rods*, which compose the other neurosensory element of the retina. The rods are responsible for motion detection and night vision. It should be remembered that the image on the retina is upside down and reversed left to right. The right world is projected on the left half of the retina. The left world is projected on the right half of the retina. An image in the superior world will strike the inferior part of the retina, and vice versa. This concept is shown in Figure 7-9.

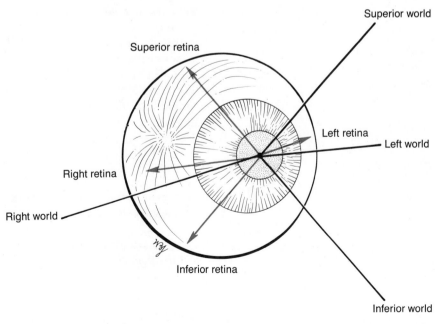

FIGURE 7-9. The images on the retina.

At birth, there is little pigment in the iris, which is why all babies are born with blue eyes. By 6 months, the pigmentation is completed. The lens is more spherical at birth than in later life. Most infants are born hyperopic (farsighted). By 3 months after birth, the medullation process of the optic nerve is completed. As the child grows, hyperopia increases until the age of 8 years and then gradually decreases. After age 8, myopia (nearsightedness) appears to increase.

With advancing age, there is the gradual loss of elasticity of the skin around the eyes. The cornea may show an infiltration of degenerative material around the limbus, which is known as an *arcus senilis*. The lens consistency changes from plastic to rigid, making it progressively more difficult to change its shape in order to focus on near objects. This condition is known as *presbyopia*. The lens may undergo changes that are due to metabolic disorders resulting in its opacification; this condition is called a *cataract*. The vitreous humor may develop condensations, called *floaters*. The retinal arteries may develop *atherosclerosis*, with resultant retinal ischemia or infarction.

REVIEW OF SPECIFIC SYMPTOMS

The major symptoms of *eye* disease are the following:

- Loss of vision
- Eye pain
- Diplopia (double vision)
- Tearing or dryness of the *eyes*
- Discharge
- Eye redness

Loss of Vision

When a patient complains of loss of vision, two questions must be asked:

"Did the loss of vision occur suddenly?"
"Is the eye painful?"

It is extremely important to ascertain the acuteness of the loss of vision and the presence or absence of pain. Sudden painless loss of vision may result from a retinal vascular occlusion or a retinal detachment. Sudden painful loss of vision is seen in attacks of acute narrow angle glaucoma. Gradual painless loss of vision is commonly seen in chronic simple glaucoma.

Eye Pain

Eye pain may result from a wide variety of causes. Ask the patient who has eye pain the following questions:

"Can you describe the pain?"
"Did the pain come on suddenly?"
"Does the light bother your eye?"
"Do you have pain when you blink?"

"Do you have the sensation of something in the eye?"
"Do you have headaches?"
"Do you have pain on movement of the eye?"
"Do you have pain over the brow on the same side?"

Pain may be experienced as "burning," "throbbing," "tenderness," or a "drawing sensation." Each of these descriptions may have a wide variety of etiologies. It is important to determine whether the patient has the sensation of a foreign body in the eye. Pain in the eye while blinking is seen in corneal abrasions and with foreign bodies in the eye. *Photophobia* is eye pain associated with light, as seen in inflammations of the iris and the middle layer of the eye. Inflammations of the conjunctiva, *conjunctivitis*, produce a gritty sensation. Diseases of the cornea are associated with significant pain because the cornea is so richly innervated. Headaches and eye pain are commonly seen in acute narrow angle glaucoma. Pain on motion of the eye is seen in optic neuritis. Eye pain associated with brow or temporal pain may be an indication of temporal arteritis.

Diplopia

Diplopia, or double vision, is a common complaint. Diplopia results from a faulty alignment of the eyes. Normally when the eyes fixate on a subject, the object is clearly seen despite the fact that the two retinal images are not exactly superimposed. These slightly different images, however, are fused by the brain; it is this fusion that produces *binocular vision*, or the perception of depth. When the eyes are misaligned, the two images fall on different parts of the retinae, only one falling normally on the fovea. The field of vision of the deviated eye is different, so that its image is not projected on its fovea; therefore, this second image will be different and not superimposable. The patient may close one eye to relieve this distressing situation. A compensatory head posture may be used by the patient to relieve the double vision. Elevation or depression of the patient's chin will be used to overcome a vertical deviation. Tilting of the head is often used to counteract the torsional and vertical deviation. Suggested questions for the patient with diplopia are found in Chapter 18, The Nervous System.

Tearing or Dryness

Excessive tearing or dryness of the eyes is a common complaint. Abnormal tearing may be caused either by overproduction of tears or by an obstruction of outflow. Dryness results from faulty secretion by the lacrimal or accessory tear glands. A common cause is *Sjögren's syndrome*, which is generalized failure of the secretory glands. This syndrome is associated with a wide variety of disease states.

Discharge

Discharge from the eye can be watery, mucoid, or purulent. A watery or mucoid discharge is often associated with allergic or viral conditions, whereas a purulent discharge is seen in association with bacterial infections.

Redness

The symptom of the red eye is very common. The interviewer should ask the following questions:

"Have you had any injury to the eye?"
"Does anyone else in the family have a red eye?"
"Have you had any recent coughing spells? . . . vomiting?"
"Have you had any associated eye pain?"
"Is there any associated discharge?"

The eye may appear bloodshot. Redness may result from trauma, infection, allergy, or increased pressure in the eye. Severe coughing spells or recurrent vomiting may cause a patient to have a conjunctival hemorrhage. A family member with viral conjunctivitis may be the source of this patient's red eye. Eye pain and a red eye may indicate acute narrow angle glaucoma. (See Table 7–9 for a summarization of the differential diagnosis of the red eye.)

General Suggestions

It is important to determine the medications that a patient is taking, as many drugs have deleterious effects on the eye. Some antimalarial, antituberculous, antiglaucoma, and anti-inflammatory drugs can cause eye pathology. A thor-

TABLE 7–2. Common Visual Eye Symptoms and Disease States

Visual Symptom	Associated Causes
Loss of vision	Optic neuritis Detached retina Retinal hemorrhage Central retinal vascular occlusion
Spots	No pathologic significance*
Flashes	Migraine Retinal detachment Posterior vitreous detachment
Loss of visual field or presence of shadows or curtains	Retinal detachment Retinal hemorrhage
Glare, photophobia	Iritis (inflammation of the iris) Meningitis (inflammation of the meninges)
Distortion of vision	Retinal detachment Macular edema
Difficulty seeing in dim light	Myopia Vitamin A deficiency Retinal degeneration
Colored haloes around lights	Acute narrow angle glaucoma Opacities in lens or cornea
Colored vision changes	Cataracts Drugs (digitalis increases yellow vision)
Double vision	Extraocular muscle paresis or paralysis

* May precede a retinal detachment or may be associated with fertility drugs.

TABLE 7–3. Common Nonvisual, Painful Eye Symptoms and Disease States

Nonvisual, Painful Symptom	Associated Causes
Foreign body sensation	Foreign body Corneal abrasion
Burning	Uncorrected refractive error Conjunctivitis Sjögren's syndrome
Throbbing, aching	Acute iritis (inflammation of the iris) Sinusitis (inflammation of the sinuses)
Tenderness	Lid inflammations Conjunctivitis Iritis
Headache	Refractive errors Migraine Sinusitis
Drawing sensation	Uncorrected refractive errors

ough family history will reveal familial disease tendencies such as glaucoma, cataracts, retinal degeneration, strabismus, or corneal dystrophies.

There are many specific symptoms related to eye disease. The common visual, nonvisual but painful, and nonvisual and painless symptoms and the associated causes are listed in Tables 7–2, 7–3, and 7–4, respectively.

TABLE 7–4. Common Nonvisual, Painless Eye Symptoms and Disease States

Nonvisual, Painless Symptom	Associated Causes
Itching	Dry eyes Eye fatigue Allergies
Tearing	Emotional states Hypersecretion of tears Blockage of drainage
Dryness	Sjögren's syndrome Decreased secretion as a result of aging
Sandiness, grittiness	Conjunctivitis
Fullness of eyes	Proptosis (bulging of the eyeball) Aging changes in the lids
Twitching	Fibrillation of orbicularis oculi
Eyelid heaviness	Fatigue Lid edema
Dizziness	Refractive error Cerebellar disease
Blinking	Local irritation Facial tic
Lids sticking together	Inflammatory disease of lids or conjunctivae

IMPACT OF BLINDNESS ON THE PATIENT

It is no wonder that the loss of sight is a terrifying experience. The sighted person lives mostly in a visual and auditory world illuminated by brilliant lights and colors. When blindness occurs, the patient loses not only his ability to see but also the perceptual center of his world. This center must now be replaced by hearing and touch. Because light is often equated with love and life, the inability to see light is associated with hate and death. If blindness occurs together with the actual loss of an eye, a patient may experience guilt feelings because the loss may be interpreted as punishment for sins. Whatever the cause, the newly blinded patient must take a new place in society. He can no longer read ordinary books; he can no longer receive visual stimuli; he is unable to appreciate the world of visual communication. This can result in a reactive depression. The physician must show genuine care for the blind patient and try to understand his feelings of discouragement and despair.

The person who is blind from birth or early childhood has little or no conception of the visual world. Having never been able to see, this patient has no frame of reference.

Occasionally, a blind individual recovers his sight as a result of a surgical procedure later in life. Many difficulties may arise, owing to the reorganization of his perception. His frame of reference has been shifted from touch to sight. Surprisingly, many of these patients become quite depressed after attaining vision. Facial expressions mean nothing, because only with experience can one understand them. The following quote from a case history illustrates the response of such an individual (Gregory and Wallace, 1963):

He suffered one of the greatest hardships (blindness) and yet he lived with energy and enthusiasm. When his handicap was apparently swept away, as by a miracle, he lost his peace and self-respect.

Not only does eye disease have an emotional impact on the patient, but also the patient with normal vision may conversely develop psychosomatic eye problems as a result of anxiety. The loss of vision that can accompany panic disorders should be mentioned. These individuals can lose either partial or complete vision in one or both eyes. Supportive care of the primary problem will usually result in the return of vision.

PHYSICAL EXAMINATION

The equipment necessary for the examination of the eye is as follows: an ophthalmoscope, a penlight, a pocket visual acuity card, and a 3×5 card.

The physical examination of the eye includes the following:

- Visual acuity
- Visual fields
- Ocular movements
- External and internal eye structures
- Ophthalmoscopic examination

Visual Acuity

Visual acuity is expressed as a ratio, such as 20/20. The first number is the distance at which the patient reads the chart. The second number is the distance at which a person with normal vision can read the same line of the chart. The term OD refers to the right eye; OS refers to the left eye; OU refers to both eyes.*

Using the Standard Snellen Chart

If a standard Snellen eye chart is available, the patient should stand 20 feet from the chart. If the patient wears glasses, have him wear them for the examination. The patient is asked to cover one eye with his palm† and read the smallest line possible. If the best he can see is the 20/200 line, the patient's vision in that eye is 20/200; this means that at 20 feet the patient can see what a person with normal vision can see at 200 feet. If a patient at 20 feet cannot see the 20/200 line, he is moved closer until the letters are recognized. If the patient can read these letters at 5 feet, the patient's visual acuity in that eye is 5/200.

Using a Pocket Visual Acuity Card

If the standard Snellen chart is not available, a pocket visual acuity card is helpful. This is viewed at 14 inches. The patient is again asked to read the smallest line possible. If neither eye chart is available, any printed material may be used. The examiner should remember that most patients over the age of 40 require reading glasses. Although the examiner will not be able to quantify the visual acuity, he can certainly determine if the patient has any vision. In such a case, the patient is asked to cover an eye and read the smallest line possible on a given printed page.

Evaluation of Patients with Low Vision

Patients with very poor vision who are unable to read any lines of print should be tested for finger counting ability. This crude measurement of visual acuity is obtained by holding up fingers in front of the patient's eye while his other eye is closed. The patient is then asked how many fingers are seen. If the patient is still unable to see, it is important to evaluate if he has any light perception. This is performed by covering one eye and directing a light at the other eye. The examiner asks the patient if he can see when the light is on and off. No light perception (NLP) is the term used when a person cannot perceive light.

Evaluation of Patients Who Cannot Read

For those individuals who cannot read, such as young children or the illiterate, the use of the letter "E" in different sizes and directions is helpful. The examiner asks the patient to point in the direction of the letter: up, down, right, left.

---

* Abbreviations are from the Latin: OD = oculus dexter; OS = oculus sinister; OU = oculi unitas.

† Always ask a patient to cover his eye with his palm. When fingers are used to cover the eye, a patient may peek between the fingers.

Visual Fields

Visual field testing is useful for determining lesions of the visual pathway. There are many techniques used for this purpose. It is important for the examiner to learn to perform the technique known as *confrontation visual field testing*. In this technique, the examiner will be comparing his peripheral vision with that of the patient's.

Assess Fields by Confrontation Testing

The examiner stands or sits 3 feet in front of and at eye level with the patient. The patient is asked to close his right eye while the examiner closes his left eye, each fixating on the other's nose. The examiner holds up his fists with his palms facing him. The examiner then shows one or two fingers on each hand simultaneously and asks the patient how many fingers he sees. The hands are moved from the upper to the lower quadrants, and the examination is repeated. The examination is then repeated, using the other eye of the patient and examiner. The fingers should be seen by both patient and examiner simultaneously. To position the patient to better advantage, the hands are held up slightly closer to the examiner. This provides a wider field for the patient. If the examiner can see the fingers, surely the patient can see them unless he has a field deficit. This technique for examining the patient's right eye is shown in Figure 7–10.

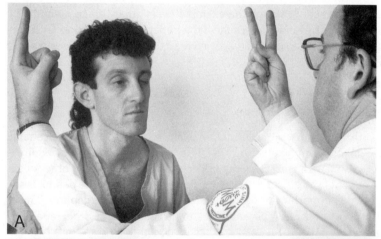

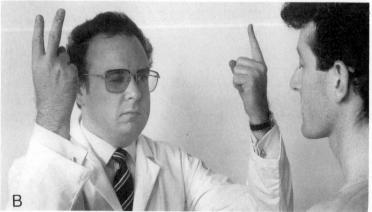

FIGURE 7–10. Confrontation visual field testing. *A,* View of the patient when examining the upper fields of the right eye. *B,* Position of the examiner when examining the upper fields of the patient's right eye.

Because lesions along the visual pathway develop insidiously, the patient may not be aware of any changes in visual fields until very late in the course of the disease. Confrontation fields, performed by the internist, may provide the first objective evidence that the patient has a lesion involving the visual pathway. An area of depressed vision is called a *scotoma*.

The normal central vision extends approximately 30° in all directions of central fixation. The *blind spot* is the physiologic scotoma located about 15–20° temporal to central fixation, corresponding to the optic nerve head. There are no sensory elements such as the rods or cones located on the nerve head.

Visual Field Abnormalities

There are pathologic scotomata that may be appreciated on visual field testing. Scotomata may result from primary ocular disease, such as glaucoma; or from lesions in the central nervous system, such as tumors. Figure 7–11 illustrates some of the common defects.

Total loss of vision in one eye is a *blind eye*, resulting from a disease of the eye, a lesion of its optic nerve, or a lesion of the corresponding occipital cortex.

Hemianopsia refers to absence of half of a visual field. A bilateral field defect in both temporal fields is termed *bitemporal hemianopsia*. It results from a lesion

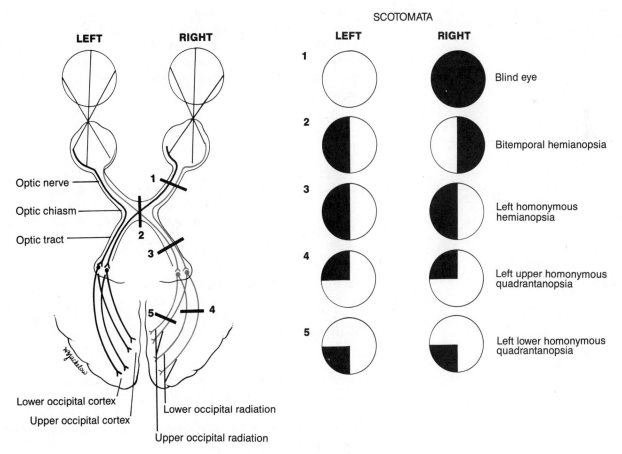

FIGURE 7–11. Visual field defects.

involving the optic nerves at the level of the optic chiasm. Pituitary tumors are common causes.

An *homonymous hemianopsia* results from damage to the optic tract, optic radiation, or occipital cortex. The term "homonymous" indicates that the visual loss is in similar fields. A patient with a left homonymous hemianopsia is unable to see the left half of the fields of both eyes. This defect occurs with damage to the right optic tract. Homonymous hemianopsia is the most common form of field loss and is seen frequently in patients with strokes.

A *quadrantanopsia* is a field loss in one quadrant. A patient with a left upper homonymous quadrantanopsia has damage to the right lower optic radiations or the right lower occipital region.

Patients with *tunnel vision* have visual fields that remain the same at all distances, a physiologically impossible phenomenon. This type of visual field abnormality is characteristic of hysteria.

Assess Optokinetic Nystagmus

Occasionally, a patient with psychiatric problems may feign blindness. A useful test to rule out such malingering involves *optokinetic nystagmus* (OKN). Optokinetic nystagmus is the rapid alternating motion of the eyes that occurs when the eyes try to fixate on a moving target. For example, observe the eyes of a person riding a train as it enters the station. The eyes move rapidly back and forth as the person tries to fixate on a station sign. The presence of optokinetic nystagmus indicates physiologic continuity of the optic pathways from the retina to the occipital cortex. Optokinetic nystagmus may be elicited in the examining room by having the patient fixate on the numbers on a tape measure while you rapidly pull out the tape. Because optokinetic nystagmus is involuntary, a positive response provides excellent verification that the patient is feigning blindness.

Ocular Movements

Ocular movements are effected by the contraction and relaxation of the extraocular muscles. This results in simultaneous movement of the eyes in tandem up or down or from side to side as well as in convergence.

Assess Eye Alignment

Alignment of the eyes is readily seen by observing the location of reflected light on the cornea. The penlight should be held directly in front of the patient. If the patient is looking straight ahead in the distance, the light reflex should be in the center of each cornea. If the light falls in the corneal center of one eye and is displaced away from the corneal center in the other eye, a *deviated* eye exists.

The condition of a deviated eye, or crossed eye, is called *strabismus*, or *tropia*. Strabismus is the nonalignment of the eyes such that the object being observed is not projected simultaneously on the fovea of each eye. *Esotropia* is defined as deviation of an eye nasally; *exotropia* is deviation of an eye temporally; *heterotropia* is deviation upward. An *alternating tropia* is the term used to describe the condition in which either eye is seen to deviate. Plate V *E* shows a patient with a left exotropia.

Perform the Cover Test

The cover test is useful to determine whether the eyes are straight or a deviated eye is present. The patient is instructed to look at a distant target. One eye is covered with a 3 × 5 card. The examiner should observe the uncovered eye. If the uncovered eye moves to take up fixation of the distant point, that eye was not straight before the other eye was covered. If the eye did not move, it was straight. The test is then repeated with the other eye.

Evaluate the Cardinal Positions of Gaze

An important cause of a deviated eye is a *paretic* (weak), or paralyzed, extraocular muscle. Paralysis of these muscles is detected by examination of the *six cardinal positions of gaze.* Hold the patient's chin steady with your right hand and ask him to follow your left hand as you trace a large "H" in the air. You should hold your left index finger about 10 inches from the patient's nose. From the midline, move the finger about a foot to the patient's right and pause; then up about 8 inches and pause, as shown in Figure 7–12; down about 16 inches and pause; and then slowly back to the midline. Cross the midline and repeat the finger movement on the other side. These are the six cardinal positions of gaze. You should observe the movement of both eyes, which should follow the finger smoothly. You should also observe for the parallel movements of the eyes in all directions.

Occasionally when looking to the extreme side, the eyes will develop a rhythmic motion called *endpoint nystagmus.* There is a quick motion in the direction of gaze, which is followed by a slow return. This test differentiates endpoint nystagmus from pathologic nystagmus, in which the quick movement is always in the same direction, regardless of gaze.

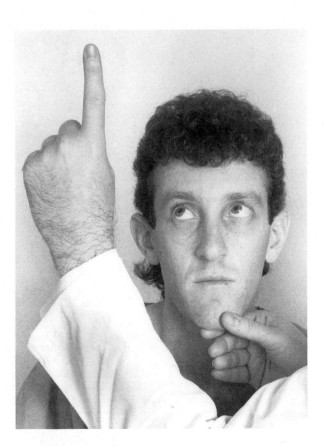

FIGURE 7–12. Technique for testing ocular motility.

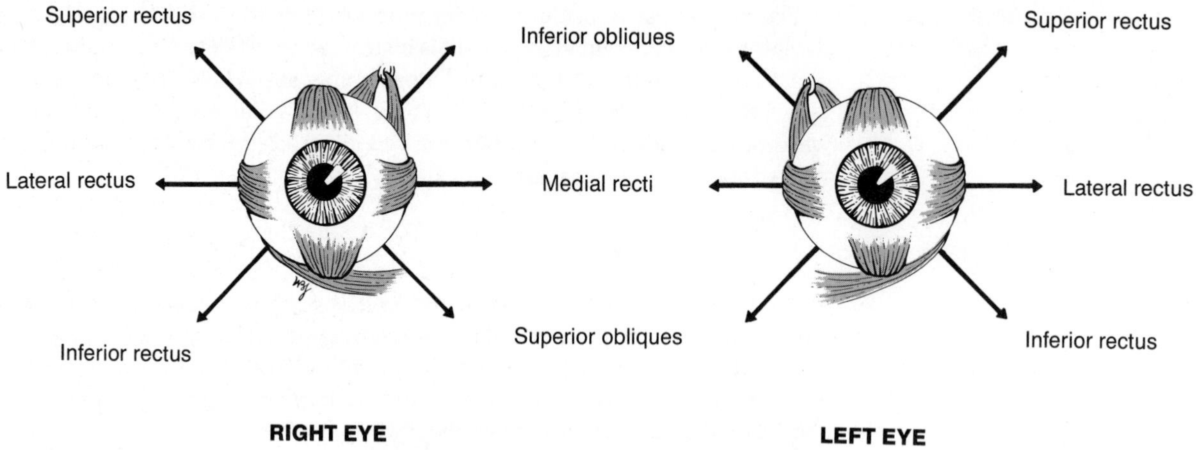

Superior rectus

Inferior obliques

Superior rectus

Lateral rectus

Medial recti

Lateral rectus

Inferior rectus

Superior obliques

Inferior rectus

RIGHT EYE

LEFT EYE

FIGURE 7–13. Cardinal positions of gaze.

If the eye and eyelid do not move together, *lid lag* is present.

The six cardinal positions of gaze are shown in Figure 7–13, and Table 7–5 summarizes the abnormal ocular motility that is due to paretic muscles.

The images projected on the retinae may be interpreted by the brain in one of three ways: fusion, diplopia, or suppression. Fusion and diplopia have already been discussed. In children, strabismus leads to diplopia, which leads to confusion, then *suppression* of the image, and finally *amblyopia*. Amblyopia is the loss of visual acuity secondary to suppression. Amblyopia is reversible until the retinae are fully developed, at about the age of 7 years. Amblyopia is a phenomenon that occurs only in children. An adult who acquires strabismus secondary to whatever cause cannot suppress the deviated eye's image and will have diplopia.

Evaluate the Pupillary Light Reflex

The examiner should ask the patient to look in the distance while he shines a bright light in the patient's eye. The light source should come from the side, using the nose as a barrier to light to the other eye. The examiner should observe the direct and consensual pupillary responses. The examiner then repeats the test on the other eye.

TABLE 7–5. Paretic Muscles Causing Abnormal Ocular Motility

Paretic Muscle	Position to Which Eye Will Not Turn
Medial rectus	Nasal
Inferior oblique	Up and nasal
Superior oblique	Down and nasal
Lateral rectus	Temporal
Superior rectus	Up and temporal
Inferior rectus	Down and temporal

The *swinging light test* is a modification for testing the pupillary light reflex. This test serves to reveal differences in the response to afferent stimuli between the eyes. In this test, the patient fixates on a distant target while the examiner rapidly swings a light from one eye to the other, observing for constriction of the pupils. In some conditions, there is a parodoxical dilatation of the pupil on which the light is shined. This condition, referred to as a *Marcus Gunn pupil,* is associated with an afferent limb defect in the eye being illuminated.

The most extreme example of an eye displaying the Marcus Gunn phenomenon is a blind eye. When light is shined into the blind eye, there is neither a direct nor a consensual response. When the light is moved to the other eye, there will be both a direct and a consensual response because both afferent and efferent pathways are normal. When the light is swung back to the blind eye, no impulses will be received by the retina (afferent), and the pupil of the blind eye will no longer remain constricted; it will dilate. There are different degrees of severity of Marcus Gunn pupils, depending upon the involvement of the optic nerve.

Evaluate the Near Reflex

The near reflex is tested by having the patient look alternately first at some distant target and then at a target placed about 5 inches away from his nose. When focusing on the near target, the eyes should converge and the pupils should constrict.

External and Internal Eye Structures

The examination of the external and internal eye structures includes the following:

- Lids
- Conjunctiva
- Sclera
- Cornea
- Pupils
- Iris
- Anterior chamber
- Lacrimal apparatus

Inspect the Lids

Examine the lids for evidence of drooping, infection, tumors, or other abnormalities. No edema or crusting should be present.

Have the patient open and close his eyelids. The motion should be smooth and symmetrical.

Inspect the eyelids for *xanthelasma.* Although not specific for hypercholesterolemia, these yellowish appearing plaques are commonly associated with lipid abnormalities. A patient with xanthelasma is seen in Plate IX *F.*

Notice the distribution of the eyelashes.

When the *eye* is open, the upper lid normally covers only the upper margin of the iris. When the *eye* is closed, the eyelids should approximate each other completely. The distance between the upper and lower lids is called the *palpebral fissure*. Plate V *F* shows a patient with marked bilateral ptosis and a narrowed palpebral fissure that are due to a muscle weakening disorder known as myasthenia gravis.

Inspect the Conjunctiva

The conjunctiva should be examined for signs of inflammation (i.e., injection, or dilatation of its blood vessels), unusual pigmentation, nodes, swelling, or hemorrhage. Both conjunctivae should be evaluated.

The tarsal conjunctiva may be seen by everting the lid. Ask the patient to keep his eyes open and look downward. You should grasp some of the eyelashes of the upper lid. The eyelid is then pulled away from the globe, and the tip of an applicator stick is pressed against the upper border of the tarsal plate. The tarsal plate is then quickly turned over the applicator stick, using it as a fulcrum. The thumb can now be used for holding the everted lid, and the applicator stick can be removed. After inspection of the tarsal conjunctiva, have the patient look up to return the lid to its normal position.

The normal conjunctiva should be pink. Note the number of blood vessels. Normally only a small number of vessels are seen. Ask the patient to look up, and pull down on the lower lids. Compare the vascularity.

Inspect the Sclera

The sclera is examined for nodules, hyperemia, and discoloration. The normal sclera should be white. In dark-skinned individuals, the sclera may be slightly "muddy" in color.

Inspect the Cornea

The cornea should be clear and without cloudiness or opacities. A whitish ring at the perimeter of the cornea is probably an arcus senilis. In patients over the age of 40 years, this finding is usually a normal aging phenomenon. Although there are many false positive findings, patients under the age of 40 may have hypercholesterolemia. An arcus senilis is seen in the patient shown in Plate VI *A*.

An abnormal greenish-yellow ring near the limbus, most evident superiorly and inferiorly, is a *Kayser-Fleischer ring*. This ring is a very specific and very sensitive sign of *Wilson's disease*, which is hepatolenticular degeneration as a result of an inherited disorder of copper metabolism. The Kayser-Fleischer ring is due to deposition of copper in the cornea.

Inspect the Pupils

The pupils should be equal in size, round, and reactive to light and accommodation. In about 5% of normal individuals, pupillary size is not equal; this is called *anisocoria*. Anisocoria may be an indication of neurologic disease. Pupillary enlargement, or *mydriasis*, is associated with sympathomimetic agents, glaucoma, or dilating drops. Pupillary constriction, or *miosis*, is seen with parasympathomimetic drugs, inflammation of the iris, and drug treatment for

TABLE 7–6. Pupillary Abnormalities

	Adie's Myotonic Pupil	Argyll Robertson Pupil	Horner's Syndrome
Laterality	Often unilateral	Bilateral	Unilateral
Reaction to light	Sluggishly reactive	Nonreactive	Reactive
Accommodation	Minimally reactive	Reactive	Reactive
Pupillary size	Mydriatic	Miotic	Miotic
Other signs	Absent or diminished tendon reflexes	Absent knee jerk reflexes	Slight ptosis* Anhidrosis

* The ptosis is *slight,* owing to interruption of the sympathetic chain innervating only the Müller's muscle portion of the levator palpebrae. The rest of the levator palpebrae functions normally; thus, ptosis is not *severe.*

glaucoma. Many medications can cause anisocoria. It is therefore very important to ascertain if the patient has used any *eye* drops or is on any medications.

Pupillary abnormalities are often markers of neurologic disease. A condition known as *Adie's myotonic pupil* is a dilated pupil 3–6 mm that constricts little to light and accommodation. This pupil is often associated with diminished to absent deep tendon reflexes in the extremities. It occurs more commonly in women 25–45 years of age, and the cause is unknown. There are no serious clinical implications. The *Argyll Robertson pupil* is a constricted pupil 1–2 mm that reacts to accommodation but is nonreactive to light. It is seen in association with neurosyphilis. *Horner's syndrome* is sympathetic paralysis of the eye that is due to interruption of the cervical sympathetic chain. In addition to the miosis and ptosis, anhidrosis* is also present. Table 7–6 indicates some of the more important pupillary abnormalities.

Inspect the Iris

The iris is evaluated for color, nodules, and vascularity. Normally, iris blood vessels cannot be seen with the naked eye.

Inspect the Depth of the Anterior Chamber

By shining a light obliquely across the eye, a rough estimation of the depth of the chamber can be made. If a crescentic shadow on the far portion of the iris is seen, the anterior chamber may be shallow. Shallowing of the anterior chamber refers to the decreased space between the iris and the cornea. The technique for estimating the depth of the anterior chamber is illustrated in Figure 7–14.

The presence of a shallow chamber predisposes an individual to a condition called *narrow angle glaucoma.* The term *glaucoma* refers to a symptom complex that occurs in a variety of disease states. The characteristic finding in all types of glaucoma is an increased intraocular pressure. This can be measured with the *Schiøtz tonometer,* which is a small, portable instrument used for the quantitative assessment of intraocular pressure. Palpation of the globe in order to determine intraocular pressure is a technique of very low sensitivity. Palpation,

* Absence of sweating in this syndrome is related to interruption of the sympathetic chain. The amount of sweating is assessed by examination of the forehead or the axilla of the affected side.

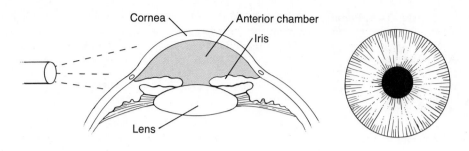

NORMAL ANGLE

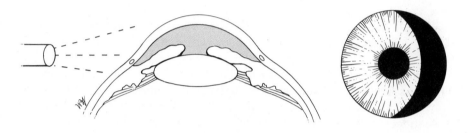

NARROW ANGLE

FIGURE 7–14. Assessing the depth of the anterior chamber.

if performed incorrectly, may also be deleterious because a retinal detachment may result. Therefore, palpation of the eye should *not* be performed.

Inspect the Lacrimal Apparatus

Generally, there is little to be seen of the lacrimal apparatus, with the exception of the punctum. If tearing, also known as *epiphora*, is present, there may be some obstruction to flow through the punctum. If excessive moisture is present, check for a blockage of the nasolacrimal duct by pressing the lacrimal sac gently against the inner orbital ring. If a blockage is present, material may be expressed through the punctum. Plate VI *B* shows a patient with massive lacrimal gland enlargement as a result of sarcoidosis.

OPHTHALMOSCOPIC EXAMINATION

The Ophthalmoscope

Before the examination of the retina is discussed, a few words about the ophthalmoscope are in order. The ophthalmoscope is an instrument with a mirror optical system for viewing the interior anatomy of the eye. There are two dials on the ophthalmoscope: one adjusts the light apertures (and filters), and the other changes the lenses to correct for the refractive errors of both the examiner and the patient.

The most important apertures and filters are the *small* aperture, the *large* aperture, and the *red-free* filter. The small aperture is for an undilated pupil; the large aperture is for a dilated pupil; and the red-free filter excludes rays of red light and is designed for visualization of blood vessels and hemorrhages. With this filter, the retina appears gray, the disc is white, the macula is yellow, and blood appears black.

Using the Ophthalmoscope

The ophthalmoscope is held in the *right* hand in front of the *right eye* of the examiner in order to examine the *right eye* of the patient. The patient is asked to look straight ahead and fixate on a distant target. If the examiner wears glasses, they should be removed for better visualization of the retina. The ophthalmoscope light is turned on, and the aperture is switched to the small aperture. The examiner should start with the lens diopter* dial set to "0" if he does not use glasses. The myopic examiner should start with "minus" lenses, which are indicated by red numbers; the hyperopic examiner will need "plus" lenses, which are indicated by black numbers. The index finger remains on the dial to permit easy focusing.

The ophthalmoscope is placed against the forehead of the examiner while the examiner's left thumb elevates the patient's right upper eyelid. The ophthalmoscope and the head of the examiner should function as one unit. The examiner looking through the ophthalmoscope should approach the patient at eye level from about 15 inches away at an angle of about 20° lateral from center as shown in Figure 7 – 15. The light should shine on the pupil. A red glow, the *red reflex*, can be seen in the pupil. The examiner should note any opacities in the cornea or lens.

By moving in toward the patient along the same 20° line, the examiner will begin to see the blood vessels of the retina. The examiner should move in close to the patient, bringing the hand holding the ophthalmoscope against the patient's cheek. As contact is made with the patient, the optic disc or vessels will be seen. By rotating the diopter wheel with the index finger, the examiner will bring these structures into sharp focus. Figure 7 – 16 shows the correct position of the examiner and patient; Figure 7 – 17 and Plate VI *C* show a normal retina.

---

* A unit of optical power of a lens to diverge or converge light rays.

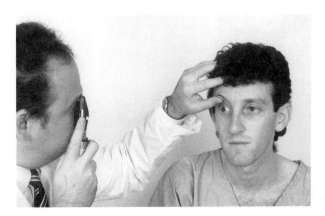

FIGURE 7 – 15. Correct position for holding the ophthalmoscope and patient's eye.

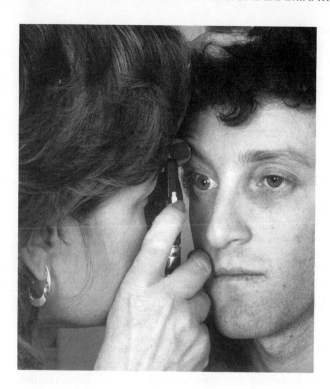

FIGURE 7–16. Correct position for examining the retina.

After the right *eye* is examined, the ophthalmoscope is held by the examiner's *left* hand with the examiner using his *left* eye to examine the patient's *left* eye.

Inspect the Optic Disc

A systematic approach to the retina is useful. The most conspicuous landmark of the retina is the optic disc. Its *margins, color,* and *cup-to-disc ratio* should be determined. The disc should be round, with sharp borders. The nasal border is normally slightly blurred. The color of the disc is pinkish in light-skinned individuals and yellowish-orange in darker-skinned individuals. The *cup*

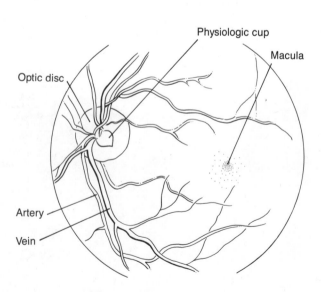

FIGURE 7–17. Schematic showing the landmarks of the retina.

is the portion of the disc that is central, lighter in color, and penetrated by the retinal vessels. The normal ratio of the cup-to-disc ratio varies from 0.1 to 0.5. The examiner should check the cup-to-disc ratio in both eyes for symmetry.

Inspect the Retinal Vessels

The vessels are evaluated as they arborize over the retina. The arteries are two thirds to four fifths the size of the veins in diameter and have a prominent *light reflex*. This light reflex is a reflection of the ophthalmoscope's light on the arterial wall and is normally about one quarter the diameter of the column of blood. The veins exhibit spontaneous pulsations in 85% of patients. This can best be demonstrated as the retinal vein enters the optic nerve, where it can be seen on end.

As all the vessels course away from the disc, they appear to narrow. The crossing of the arteries and veins occurs within 2 disc diameters from the disc.

The normal vessel wall is invisible, with its thin light reflex. In hypertension, the vessel may have focal or generalized areas of narrowing or spasm, causing the light reflex to be narrowed. With time, the vessel wall becomes thickened and sclerotic and there is a widening of the light reflex to greater than half of the diameter of the column of blood. The light reflex develops an orange metallic appearance, which is termed *copper wiring*. When such an artery crosses over a vein, there appears to be a discontinuity of the venous column as a result of the widened, but invisible, arterial wall. This is termed *arteriovenous (AV) nicking*.

Follow the vessels in all four directions: superior temporal, superior nasal, inferior nasal, and inferior temporal. Remember to move your head and the ophthalmoscope as one unit.

Inspect the Macula

When the ophthalmoscope is kept level with the disc and moved temporally about 2 disc diameters, the macula will be seen. This appears as an avascular area with a pinpoint reflective center, the fovea. If the examiner has difficulty in seeing the macula, the patient can be instructed to look directly into the light; the fovea will then be seen. The red-free filter is also helpful in locating the macula.

Describe Any Retinal Lesions

In scanning the fundus, the examiner may detect abnormalities. When a lesion is seen, its color and shape are important in determining its cause. Is it red, black, gray, or whitish? Red lesions are usually hemorrhages. They can be located best by using the green filter of the ophthalmoscope. Linear, or *flame-shaped*, hemorrhages occur in the nerve fiber layer of the retina, whereas round hemorrhages are located in deeper intraretinal layers.

Black lesions that are shaped like bone spicules are associated with retinitis pigmentosa. In this condition, melanin tends to ensheath the retinal vessels. A "doughnut" shaped lesion is often found in old chorioretinitis. A pigmented, raised, disc-shaped lesion suggests a melanoma. Diffuse spotting of the retina is often a degenerative state. Flat, *gray* lesions are usually benign nevi.

White lesions may appear as soft, cotton-wool areas or may be dense. White lesions are very common and are frequently associated with hypertension or

TABLE 7 – 7. Differentiation of Whitish-Colored Lesions of the Fundus

	Cotton-wool Spots*	Fatty Exudates†	Drusen‡	Chorioretinitis
Etiology§	Hypertension Diabetic retinopathy AIDS Lupus erythematosis Dermatomyositis Papilledema	Diabetes mellitus Retinal venous occlusion Hypertensive retinopathy	Normal with aging	Toxoplasmosis Sarcoidosis
Border	Fuzzy	Well defined	Well defined, nonpigmented	Often large with ragged edge, heavily pigmented
Shape	Irregular	Small, irregular	Round, well circumscribed	Very variable
Patterns	Variable	Often clustered in circles or stars	Variable. Symmetrical in both eyes.	Variable
Comments	Caused by an ischemic infarct of the nerve fiber layer of the retina. Obscures retinal blood vessels. Usually several in number.	In deep retinal layer	Often confused with fatty exudates. Deep to retinal blood vessels.	Acute with white exudate. Healed lesion with pigmented scar.

* See Figures 7 – 20 and 7 – 21 and Plate VII A.
† Also known as "edema residues."
‡ Also known as "colloid bodies."
§ The diseases noted do not compose a complete etiologic list. Only the most common causes are indicated.

diabetes. The differentiation of white lesions of the retina is summarized in Table 7 – 7.

Difficulties in Using the Ophthalmoscope

Frequently difficulties arise in the use of the ophthalmoscope. These include the following:

- A small pupil
- Extraneous light
- Improper use of the ophthalmoscope
- Myopia in the patient
- Cataract in the patient

The use of mydriatric drops in order to visualize the retina better is important. Many medical students fear that these drops will precipitate an attack of narrow angle glaucoma. It is clear from the data that more physicians miss retinal findings by not dilating the eyes than those who precipitate such an attack. Even if the 1 in 1000 persons should have an attack of glaucoma, he is in the best possible facility for treatment. The examiner should use one drop of tropicamide 1% in each eye. The mydriatic action is maximal in 15 minutes and lasts for 3 – 4 hours. The cycloplegic* action lasts for about 6 hours. These drops can be used in patients wearing contact lenses. Atropine should be avoided, because its effect lasts for up to 2 weeks. The large aperture of the ophthalmoscope is used when the eye is dilated. It is very important to record in the chart that the patient's eye(s) were dilated and the medications used.

The room should be darkened as much as possible for the easiest evaluation of the retina. Another common problem is corneal reflection. Often light is

---

* A drug that produces paralysis of accommodation.

reflected back from the cornea, which makes the examination more difficult. Use of the small aperture or a polarizing filter, which many ophthalmoscopes include, may be helpful.

The rules for the use of the ophthalmoscope are patient's *right eye*, examiner's *right eye*, and examiner's *right hand;* patient's *left eye*, examiner's *left eye*, and examiner's *left hand*. Practice will provide ease of use of the ophthalmoscope.

Patients with myopia provide the most problems for the novice examiner. In myopic eyes, the retinal image is enlarged, making it sometimes difficult to visualize the retina adequately. If the patient is severely myopic, it may be necessary to examine the patient while he wears his corrective lenses.

A cataract will not allow adequate visualization of the retina, especially if the cataract is central.

CLINICOPATHOLOGIC CORRELATIONS

There are many ophthalmoscopic conditions with which the examiner should be familiar. An image is normally focused directly on the retina. When the image is not focused on the retina, a refractive error is present. Lenses are used to correct refractive errors. The absence of a refractive error is called *emmetropia*. Refractive errors are extremely common. Listed here are the common refractive errors and their causes:

Hyperopia (farsightedness)	Light is focused posterior to the retina.
Myopia (nearsightedness)	Light is focused anterior to the retina.
Astigmatism	Light is not uniformly focused in all directions. This condition is commonly due to a cornea that is not perfectly spherical.
Presbyopia	Progressive decrease in near vision as a result of a decrease in the eye's ability to accommodate. Occurs after age 40.

Figure 7–18 illustrates emmetropic, hyperopic, myopic, and astigmatic eyes.

A *cataract* is the most common cause of blindness in the world. It is a type of degenerative eye disease. One of the first symptoms the cataract patient experiences is a "mistiness" of his vision or a sensation of a speck in front of his eye. He typically gives a history that his vision has become "like looking through a dirty window." As the lenticular opacity increases with time, there is a diminution of visual acuity associated with glare in bright light. This effect is due to the irregular refraction of the light rays through the lens. These patients may wear dark glasses and hold their heads down to avoid excess light.

Narrow angle glaucoma results from an obstruction to the drainage of aqueous humor at the canal of Schlemm. Patients with narrow angle glaucoma have periodic attacks of acute elevation of intraocular pressure caused by intermittent obstruction. This is associated with pain, halos, and poor vision.

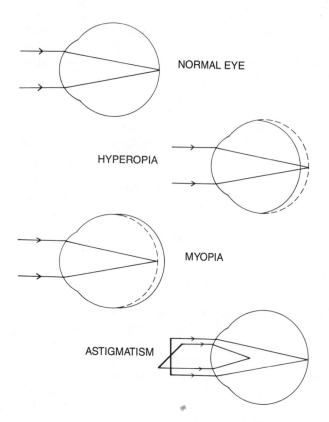

NORMAL EYE

HYPEROPIA

MYOPIA

ASTIGMATISM

FIGURE 7–18. Common refractive errors.

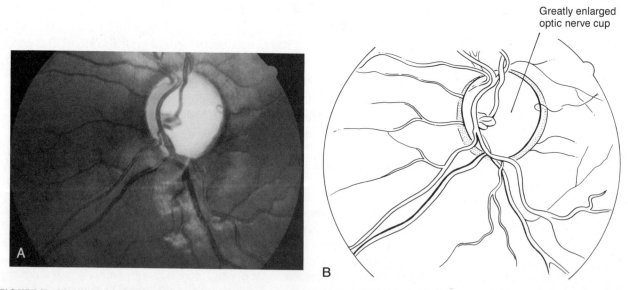

Greatly enlarged optic nerve cup

A

B

FIGURE 7–19. *A* and *B*, Black and white photograph and labeled schematic of Plate VI *D*, showing glaucomatous cupping of the optic nerve head. The cup-to-disc ratio is approximately 85%.

This type of glaucoma commonly occurs in a darkened room, when pupillary dilatation occurs. When the pupil is fully dilated in a person with a narrow angle, the redundant iris folds at its base cause the increased obstruction and decreased drainage.

Chronic simple glaucoma, in contrast, is associated with an open angle. There are many etiologies for simple glaucoma, which is a leading cause of slowly progressive blindness. The most important difference diagnostically between narrow angle glaucoma and chronic simple glaucoma is the absence of pain. Patients have reduced outflow of aqueous humor through the trabecular meshwork and into the canal of Schlemm, thus resulting in elevated intraocular pressure. As a result, progressive cupping of the optic nerve occurs (i.e., loss of nerve substance) and visual field changes are seen. The cup-to-disc ratio increases with loss of symmetry. Peripheral field defects, especially in the nasal aspect, are common early in the disease. As the disease progresses, vision is increasingly impaired. Late in the disease, only a small area on the nasal aspect of the nerve head may remain. Figure 7–19 and Plate VI *D* show marked glaucomatous cupping of the nerve head with an increased cup-to-disc ratio. Table 7–8 lists the major characteristics of both types of glaucoma.

TABLE 7–8. Characteristics of Glaucoma

	Narrow Angle Glaucoma	Chronic Simple Glaucoma
Occurrence	15% of all glaucoma cases	85% of all glaucoma cases
Cause	Closed angle prevents aqueous drainage	Unclear*
Age of onset	50–60	Variable
Type of patient	Type "A" personality	Not specific
Anterior chamber	Shallow	Usually normal
Chamber angle	Narrow	Normal
Symptoms	Headache Haloes around lights Sudden onset of severe eye pain Vomiting during attack	Generally none Decreased vision, late
Cupping of disc	After untreated attack(s)	Progressive if not treated (see Fig. 7–19 and Plate VI *D*)
Visual fields	Involvement is a late sign	Peripheral fields involved early Central involvement a very late sign
Ocular pressure	Early: with provocative tests only Late: high	Progressively higher if not medically controlled
Other signs	Fixed, mid-dilated pupil Conjunctival injection "Steamy" cornea†	
Treatment	Surgical	Medical Laser surgery
Prognosis	Good	Good, if recognized early Very dependent upon patient compliance

* Thought to be a defect in the trabecular network ultrastructure.
† Like looking through a steamy window.

TABLE 7-9. Differential Diagnosis of the Red Eye*

Presentation	Acute Conjunctivitis†	Acute Iritis	Narrow Angle Glaucoma	Corneal Abrasion
History	Sudden onset Exposure to pink eye	Fairly sudden onset Often recurrent	Very sudden onset Sometimes history of previous attack Highest incidence in Jews, Swedes, and the Inuit (Eskimos)	Trauma Pain
Vision	Normal	Impaired if untreated	Rapidly lost if untreated‡	Can be affected if central
Pain	Gritty feeling	Moderate	Severe	Exquisite
Bilaterality	Frequent	Occasional	Occasional	Usually unilateral
Vomiting	Absent	Absent	Common	Absent
Cornea	Clear (epidemic keratoconjunctivitis has corneal deposits)	Variable	"Steamy" (like looking through a steamy window)	Irregular light reflex
Pupil	Normal, reactive	Small, irregular, nonreactive	Mid-dilated, oval, nonreactive	Normal, reactive
Iris	Normal	Normal§	Difficult to see, owing to corneal edema	Shadow of corneal defect may be projected on the iris with penlight
Ocular discharge	Mucopurulent or watery	Watery	Watery	Watery or mucopurulent
Systemic effect	None	Few	Many	None
Prognosis	Self-limited	Poor if untreated	Poor if untreated	Good if not infected

* See Plate VI E.

† Can be viral, bacterial, or allergic.

‡ Seeing "rainbows" can be an early symptom during an acute attack.

§ The ophthalmologist can detect abnormalities with a slit lamp.

Acute eye inflammations are common. They may be associated with local or systemic diseases. The differential diagnosis of the red eye is important. The presence of pain, visual loss, and irregularities of the pupils are important signs signifying a serious, potentially blinding disorder. Plate VI E shows a patient with a red eye. Table 7-9 provides an approach to the diagnosis of the red eye.

Diabetes and hypertension are systemic illnesses with retinal manifestations. The retinal findings in a patient with diabetes are shown in Plate VI F. Plate VII A shows the retinal changes in a patient with hypertension (see Figs. 7-20 and 7-21). Increased pressure in the central nervous system produces a classic picture of papilledema in the retina. Blood dyscrasias are frequently first diagnosed from the examination of the retina. The retinal findings of these and other clinical states are summarized in Table 7-10.

Blurring of the disc margins may be the only sign of increased intracranial pressure. This finding, however, does occur with other conditions. Figure 7-22 and Plate VII B show the blurred disc margins of papilledema in a patient with increased intracranial pressure. Table 7-11 provides a differentiation of blurred disc margins.

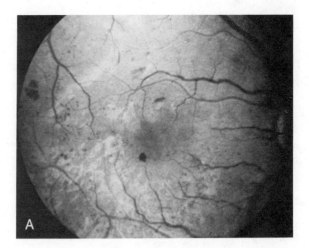

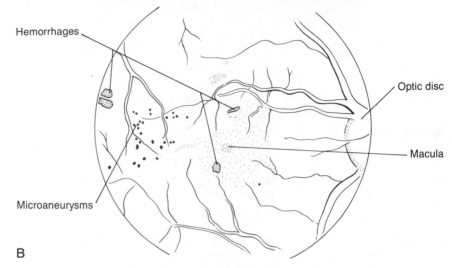

FIGURE 7-20. *A* and *B*, Black and white photograph and labeled schematic of Plate VI *F*, showing the retinal findings in the right eye in a patient with diabetes. Note the microaneurysms at the macula.

Hemorrhages

Optic disc

Macula

Microaneurysms

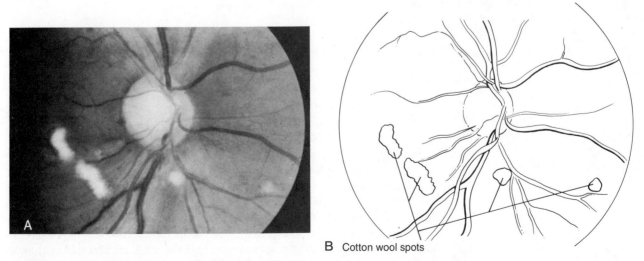

B Cotton wool spots

FIGURE 7-21. *A* and *B*, Black and white photograph and labeled schematic of Plate VII *A*, showing the retinal changes in a patient with long-standing hypertension. Note the "cotton-wool spots."

TABLE 7–10. Retinal Characteristics of Common Diseases

Condition	Primary Findings	Distribution	Secondary Findings
Diabetes (see Fig. 7–23 and Plates VI *F*, VII *C*)	Microaneurysms Neovascularization Retinitis proliferans*	Posterior pole	Hard exudates† Deep hemorrhages Retinal venous occlusions Vitreous hemorrhages
Hypertension (see Plate VII *A*)	Anteriolar narrowing "Copper wiring" Flame hemorrhages Arteriovenous nicking	Throughout retina	Hard and soft exudates Retinal venous occlusions Macular stars
Papilledema (see Fig. 7–22 and Plate VII *B*)	Hyperemia of the disc Venous engorgement Retinal hemorrhages Disc elevation Loss of spontaneous venous pulsations Cotton-wool spots	On or near disc	Hard exudates Optic atrophy, late
Retinal venous occlusion	Hemorrhages Neovascularization	Confined to area drained by affected vein	Exudates
Retinal arterial occlusion	Pallor of retina Decreased width of artery Embolus possibly visible	Confined to area supplied	Optic atrophy, late
Arteriolar sclerosis	Widening of light reflex "Copper wiring" Arteriovenous nicking	Throughout retina	Decrease in retinal pigment
Blood dyscrasias	Diffuse hemorrhages Venous dilatation, common Roth spots (hemorrhagic lesions with white centers)		
Sickle cell disease	Sharp cutoff of arterioles Arteriovenous anastomoses Neovascularization in "sea fan" formations (resemble the marine organism with a similar pattern)	Peripheral retina	Vitreous hemorrhages Retinal detachments

* A growth of a light-colored sheet of opaque connective tissue over the inner surface of the retina. Neovascularization of this tissue with tortuous vessels is seen. These vessels bleed easily.

† Exudate is the term used for small intraretinal lesions caused by retinal disturbances in a variety of disorders.

Many common diseases display their pathology at the macula of the retina. Table 7–12 provides a differentiation of some of these lesion types. Figure 7–23 and Plate VII *C* show circinate retinopathy in a diabetic patient.

Abnormalities of gaze are not uncommon. An *ophthalmoplegia* is a paralysis of the eye muscles. Lesions causing this paralysis may be acute, chronic, or progressive. Note the patient shown in Figure 7–24. When asked to look straight ahead, the patient has ptosis of the right eyelid and the right eye is abducted. When the patient is asked to look to the far right, both eyes move normally, although the right ptosis is well seen. When the patient is asked to look to the far left, the right eye cannot cross the midline. This patient has an acute oculomotor paralysis secondary to a fungal lesion near the nucleus of the third cranial nerve.

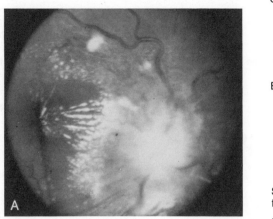

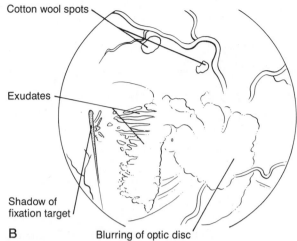

FIGURE 7–22. A and B, Black and white photograph and labeled schematic of Plate VII B, showing the retinal changes in chronic papilledema. Note the marked blurring of the right optic disc, the cotton-wool spots, and the exudates. The dark line at the macula is a shadow of the target at which the patient was asked to look.

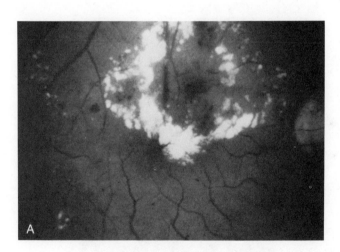

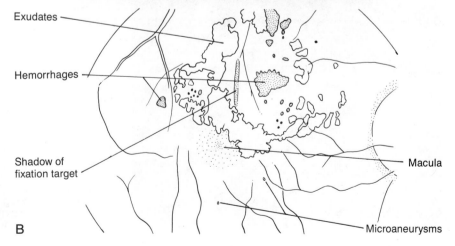

FIGURE 7–23. A and B, Black and white photograph and labeled schematic of Plate VII C, showing the retinal changes of severe diabetes called circinate retinopathy, which is a ring of exudates around the macula. This is the retina of the right eye.

TABLE 7–11. Differentiation of Blurred Disc Margins

Presentation	Papilledema*	Papillitis†	Drusen	Myelinated Nerve Fibers‡	Central Retinal Vein Occlusion
Visual acuity	Normal	Decreased	Normal	Normal	Decreased
Venous pulsations	Absent	Variable	Present	Present	Generally absent
Pain	Headache	Eye movement pain	No	No	No
Light reaction	Present	Marcus Gunn (see text)	Present	Present	Present
Hemorrhage	Present	Present	Uncommon	No	Marked
Visual fields	Enlarged blind spot	Central scotoma	Enlarged blind spot	Scotomata correspond to areas of myelination	Variable
Laterality	Bilateral	Unilateral	Bilateral	Often bilateral	Unilateral

* Edema of the optic disc resulting from increased intracranial pressure. See Figure 7–22 and Plate VII B.
† Inflammation of the optic disc.
‡ Myelination of the optic nerve ends at the optic disc. When it continues into the retina, white, flamed-shaped areas obscure the disc margins.

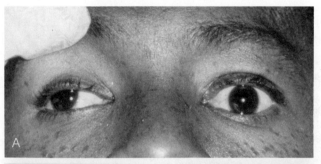

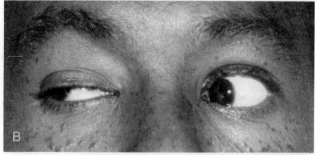

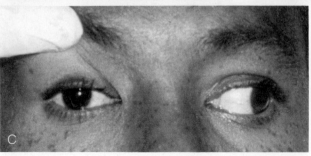

FIGURE 7–24. Acute oculomotor nerve paralysis. *A,* Notice that when the patient is asked to look straight ahead, the right eye is turned laterally (note the position of the corneal light reflexes). Also notice that the right palpebral fissure is markedly narrowed, requiring the lid to be elevated in order to visualize the position of the eye. *B,* When the patient is asked to look to the far right, both eyes are able to move in that direction. Note again the marked ptosis of the right lid. *C,* When the patient is asked to look to the far left, the right eye cannot cross the midline.

TABLE 7–12. Differentiation of Common Macular Lesions

	Macular Degeneration	Macular Star	Circinate Retinopathy*
Appearance	Pigmentary mottling, often with hemorrhage	Whitish exudate that radiates around macula	Broken ring–shaped whitish exudate around macula
Etiology	Often bilateral in the aged	Hypertension Papilledema Papillitis Central retinal vein occlusion	Diabetes Central retinal vein occlusion

* See Figure 7–23 and Plate VII C.

Note the patient shown in Figure 7–25. When the patient is asked to look straight ahead or to the right, both eyes move smoothly in the correct motion. However, when the patient is asked to look to the left, the left eye fails to cross the midline. Diplopia occurred as a result of a left abducens palsy secondary to carcinomatous meningitis.

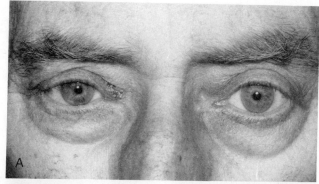

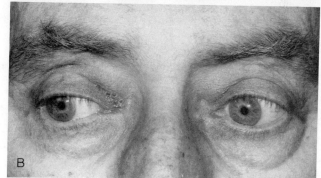

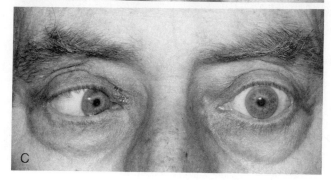

FIGURE 7–25. Acute left abducens paralysis. *A,* When the patient is asked to look straight ahead, both eyes are straight. *B,* When the patient is asked to look to the right, both eyes turn normally. *C,* When the patient is asked to look to the left, the left eye cannot cross the midline, indicating left abducens palsy.

Listed here are the specific roots that are important in order to understand the terminology related to diseases of the eye.

ROOT	PERTAINING TO	EXAMPLE	DEFINITION
blepharo-	eyelid	*blepharo*plasty	Surgical repair of eyelid
choroi-	choroid	*choroi*ditis	Inflammation of the choroid
-cor-	pupil	aniso*cor*ia	Unequal pupils
cyclo-	ciliary body	*cyclo*plegia	Paralysis of accommodation
dacryo-	tear	*dacryo*cystitis	Inflammation of the lacrimal gland
-duction	to lead	ab*duction*	Turning outward
irid-	iris	*irid*ectomy	Surgical excision of the iris
kerato-	cornea	*kerato*pathy	Disease of the cornea
lacri-	tears	*lacri*mal	Pertaining to the tears
nyct-	night	*nyct*alopia	Night blindness
-ocul-	eye	intra*ocul*ar	Within the eye
ophthalm-	eye	*ophthalm*oscope	Instrument for visualizing the eye
-opsia	vision	hemian*opsia*	Blindness in half of the visual field
-phak(os)-	lens	a*phak*ia	Without a lens
photo-	light	*photo*sensitive	Sensitive to light
presby-	old	*presby*opia	Impairment of vision as a result of increasing age
tars-	eyelid structure	*tars*orrhaphy	Surgical suturing of the lid
-trop-	turn	eso*trop*ia	Eye turning inward

WRITING UP THE PHYSICAL EXAMINATION

Listed here are examples of the write-up for the examination of the eye.

Visual acuity is OD 20/20 and OS 20/30 using the standard Snellen chart. The visual fields by confrontation are normal. Examination of the external structures of the eyes is normal. The pupils are equal, round, and reactive to light and to accommodation.* The extraocular movements† are normal. On ophthalmoscopic examination, the disc margins are sharp. A normal cup-to-disc ratio is present. The vasculature is normal.

Visual acuity is OD 20/60 and OS 20/20 using the pocket visual acuity card. Examination of the eyes reveals marked conjunctival injection on the right with a dilated pupil on the same side. The pupils are round and are reactive to light. Accommodation was not well seen. The visual fields by confrontation field testing are normal. The optic disc margins are sharp, and the vascularity of the retina appears normal.

The patient is able to read the newspaper without corrective lenses. The extraocular movements are normal. The left pupil is miotic and is 2 mm smaller than the right pupil. A mild ptosis of the left upper lid is present. Both pupils react to light directly and consensually. Confrontation fields are within normal limits. Funduscopic examination is within normal limits.

The visual acuity with corrected lenses appears normal. There is a paralysis of left lateral gaze, manifested by diplopia. The pupils are equal, round, and reactive to light. The optic disc margins are sharp. The vasculature is normal.

There is decreased visual acuity in both eyes. The patient has difficulty reading 1/4 inch print in the newspaper at about 6 inches with his right eye. There is OS NLP. The examination of the external eye is normal. The extraocular movements are intact. The left optic disc margin is slightly blurred on its nasal aspect. The cup-to-disc ratio is normal. There are multiple, soft, "cotton-wool" exudates seen bilaterally. A large, flame-shaped hemorrhage is seen in the right eye at 2 o'clock. Arterial-venous nicking is present bilaterally.

The visual acuity is OD 20/40 and OS 20/100 using the pocket visual acuity card. A bitemporal hemianopsia is present by confrontation field testing. EOMs are normal. Ophthalmoscopic examination reveals blurring of both optic discs with loss of spontaneous venous pulsations. A flame-shaped hemorrhage is present in the right eye 1 disc diameter at 10 o'clock.

* Often abbreviated as PERRLA.
† Often abbreviated as EOMs.

BIBLIOGRAPHY

Cassirer R: The Philosophy of Symbolic Forms. London, Oxford University Press, 1955.

Chevigny H, Braverman S: The Adjustment of the Blind. New Haven, CT, Yale University Press, 1950.

Diamond BL, Ross A: Emotional adjustments of newly blinded soldiers. Am J Psychiat 102:367, 1945.

Gregory RL, Wallace JG: Recovery from Early Blindness: A Case Study. Monograph 2, Experimental Psychology Society. Cambridge, Heffer, 1963.

Havener WH: Synopsis of Ophthalmology. St. Louis, CV Mosby, 1984.

Heaton JM: The Eye: Phenomenology and Psychology of Function and Disorder. Philadelphia, JB Lippincott, 1968.

Newell FW: Ophthalmology: Principles and Concepts. St Louis, CV Mosby, 1978.

Scheie HG, Albert DM: Textbook of Ophthalmology, 9th ed. Philadelphia, WB Saunders Co, 1977.

Steinmann WC, Millstein ME, Sinclair SH: Pupillary dilation with tropicamide 1% for fundoscopic screening: A study of duration of action. Ann Intern Med 107:181, 1987.

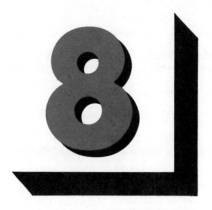

THE EAR AND NOSE

Yet it was not possible for me to say to people, "Speak louder, shout, for I am deaf" . . . Alas! how could I declare the weakness of a sense which in me ought to be more acute than in others — a sense which formerly I possessed in highest perfection, a perfection such as few in my profession enjoy, or ever have enjoyed.

**Ludwig van Beethoven
1770 – 1827**

GENERAL CONSIDERATIONS

Most of us are fortunate to hear the sounds of music, noise, and, above all, speech. Sometimes "silence is golden," but silence can only be golden when one can choose not to hear.

Though normal children are born with the apparatus necessary to produce speech, they are not born with speech. The ear and brain integrate and process sound, permitting the child to learn to imitate it. If sound cannot be heard, it cannot be imitated. Sounds will not become words; words will not become sentences; sentences will not become speech; speech will not become language.

Hearing is a perceptual process. To illustrate this concept, consider tinnitus as an example. *Tinnitus,* the name given to a sensation of sound in one or both ears, is a very common accompaniment to deafness. When tinnitus is present, there is nearly always some degree of hearing loss. Conversely, when there is no appreciable hearing loss, there is rarely tinnitus. However, children who are born deaf do *not* complain of tinnitus.

STRUCTURE AND PHYSIOLOGY
The Ear

The ear can be divided into the following four parts:

- External ear
- Middle ear
- Inner ear
- Nervous innervation

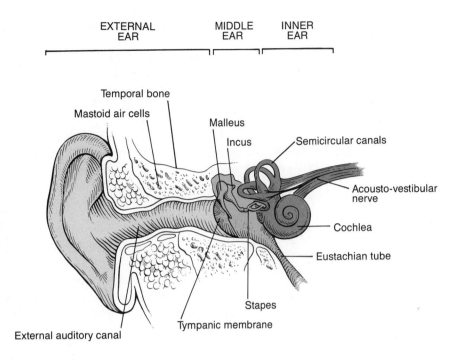

FIGURE 8-1. A cross-sectional view through the ear.

A cross-section through the ear is shown in Figure 8–1.

The *external ear* consists of the *pinna* and the *external auditory canal*. The pinna is composed of elastic cartilage and skin. Figure 8–2 illustrates the parts of the pinna.

The external auditory canal is about 1 inch in length. Its outer third is cartilaginous, whereas its inner two thirds are composed of bone. Within the

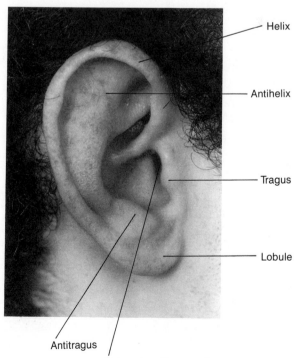

FIGURE 8-2. Landmarks of the pinna.

cartilaginous portion, there are hair follicles, pilosebaceous glands, and *ceruminous*, or wax producing, glands. The cartilaginous portion is continuous with the pinna. The canal curves slightly, being directed forward and downward. The innervation to most of the external canal is through the trigeminal nerve. The innermost portion of the canal is innervated by the vagus, or tenth cranial, nerve.*

The *middle ear*, or tympanic cavity, consists of connections to the *mastoid antrum* and to its connecting air cells and, through the *eustachian tube*, to the nasopharynx. The function of the eustachian tube is to provide an air passage from the nasopharynx to the ear to equalize pressure on both sides of the tympanic membrane. The eustachian tube is normally closed but opens during swallowing and yawning.

The *tympanic membrane* forms the lateral boundary of the middle ear. The medial boundary is formed by the *cochlea*. The tympanic membrane is gray in color with blood vessels at its periphery. It is composed of two parts: the *pars flaccida* and the *pars tensa*. The pars flaccida is the upper, smaller portion of the tympanic membrane. The pars tensa composes the remainder of the membrane. The handle of the malleus is a prominent landmark and divides the pars tensa into the *anterior and posterior folds*. The tympanic membrane is set slightly at an angle to the external canal. The inferior portion is more medial than the superior portion. Figure 8–3 illustrates the left tympanic membrane.

Sound is conducted from the tympanic membrane to the inner ear by way of three *auditory ossicles:* the *malleus,* the *incus,* and the *stapes.* The malleus is the largest ossicle. At its upper end is the *short process,* which appears as a tiny knob. The *handle* (long process) of the malleus, or *manubrium,* extends downward to its tip, called the *umbo.* Both the short process and the handle of the malleus attach directly to the tympanic membrane. At the other end of the malleus is its head, which articulates with the incus. The incus then articulates with the head of the stapes, the foot plate of which attaches to the *oval window* of the inner ear.

---

* Occasionally when the distal external canal is cleaned, coughing may result. This cough reflex is mediated through the vagus nerve.

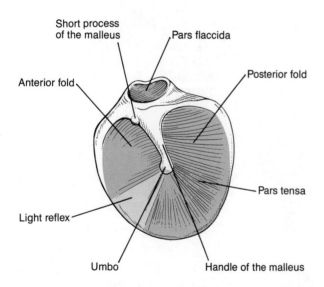

Short process of the malleus

Pars flaccida

Anterior fold

Posterior fold

Pars tensa

Light reflex

Umbo

Handle of the malleus

FIGURE 8–3. Landmarks of the left tympanic membrane.

The middle ear also contains two muscles: the *tensor tympani* and the *stapedius*. The tensor tympani muscle attaches to the malleus, whereas the stapedius muscle attaches to the neck of the stapes. The tensor tympani muscle is innervated by the trigeminal (fifth cranial) nerve, and the stapedius muscle is innervated by the facial, or seventh cranial, nerve. Both muscles contract in response to high intensity sound.

The facial nerve passes through the middle ear and provides, in addition to the nerve to the stapedius muscle, the *chorda tympani* nerve. The chorda tympani travels through the middle ear between the incus and the malleus and exits near the temporomandibular joint. It carries taste sensation from the anterior two thirds of the tongue.

The *inner ear* is the end organ for hearing and equilibrium. It is situated in the petrous portion of the temporal bone and consists of the three *semicircular canals,* the *vestibule,* and the *cochlea.* Each of these structures is made up of three parts: the *osseous labyrinth,* the *membranous labyrinth,* and the *space between.* The osseous labyrinth is the outer bone casing. The inner membranous labyrinth is within the osseous labyrinth and contains a fluid called *endolymph* and the sensory structures. The space between these two labyrinths is filled with another fluid, called *perilymph.* A section through this area is shown in Figure 8–4.

The three semicircular canals are directed posteriorly, superiorly, and horizontally. Each canal has a dilated end, the *ampulla,* which is the sensory end organ for balance.

The cochlea is a snail shell–shaped structure composed of two and three-quarter turns. Within its membranous labyrinth is the end organ for hearing. The *acoustic,* or eighth cranial, nerve consists of two parts: the *vestibular* and the *cochlear* divisions. These connect to the semicircular canals and cochlea, respectively. They join and pass through the internal auditory meatus to the brainstem.

Sound waves stimulate the afferent fibers either by *bone conduction* or by *air conduction.* Bone conduction is directly through the bones of the skull. Air conduction is through the external auditory canal, tympanic membrane, and ossicles to the oval window. Most hearing is mediated by air conduction.

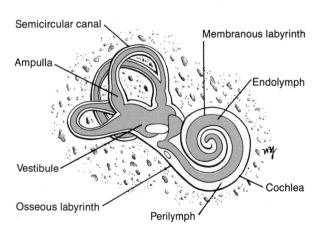

FIGURE 8–4. Cross-section through the cochlea.

Sound waves set up vibrations that enter the external canal and are transmitted to the ossicles, which vibrate. This vibration causes an inward motion of the footplate of the stapes and deforms the oval window. Waves are created in the perilymphatic fluid of the labyrinth. These fluid motion changes are transmitted in a wavelike fashion to the endolymphatic fluid, which causes distortion of the *hair cells* of the *organ of Corti.* These "hair" cells convert the mechanical force into an electrochemical signal that is propagated down the acoustic nerve and is ultimately interpreted as sound. It has been estimated that there are over 30,000 of these afferent hair fibers, which make up the auditory division. After many synapses, the impulse reaches the temporal cortex, where the appreciation of the sound occurs. A section through the cochlear duct is shown in Figure 8–5.

The sense of *balance* is achieved by visual, vestibular, and proprioceptive* senses. The loss of one of these senses will frequently go unnoticed. The vestibular apparatus appears to be the most important. Motion within the endolymphatic fluid stimulates the hair cells within the ampulla of the semicircular canals. Electrical impulses are transmitted to the vestibular portion of the eighth cranial nerve. Synapses occur in the vestibular and oculomotor nuclei, which send efferent fibers to the extraocular and skeletal muscles. This produces a deviation of the eyes with rapid compensatory motions to maintain gaze and increased tone in the skeletal muscles.

*Sensory stimulation from within the tissues of the body concerning their movement or position.

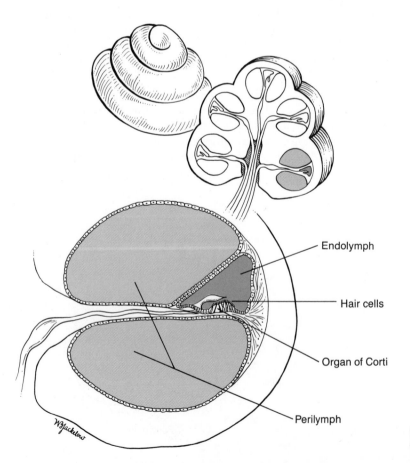

Endolymph

Hair cells

Organ of Corti

Perilymph

FIGURE 8–5. Cross-section through the cochlear duct.

Any alteration in the endolymphatic mechanism may affect the control of the eyes. *Nystagmus* is an involuntary rapid back and forth motion of the eyes, which can be horizontal, vertical, rotatory, or mixed. The direction of the nystagmus is determined by the direction of the quick component. Abnormalities of the labyrinth tend to produce *horizontal* nystagmus; brainstem disorders often produce *vertical* nystagmus; and retinal lesions may produce *ocular* nystagmus, which is slow and gives an irregular searching quality to the eyes.

The Nose

The external nasal skeleton consists of the *nasal bones,* part of the *maxilla,* and *cartilage.* The upper third of the skeleton is composed of nasal bones, which articulate with the maxilla and frontal bones. The lower two thirds are made of cartilage.

The internal portion of the nose consists of two cavities divided by the *nasal septum,* which forms the medial wall of the nasal cavity. Projecting from the lateral wall, there are three *turbinates,* or *chonchae.* The inferior turbinate is the largest and contains semierectile tissue. Inferior to each turbinate are openings to the *paranasal sinuses,* each opening known as a *meatus.* Each meatus is named for the turbinate above it. The *nasolacrimal duct* empties into the inferior meatus. The *middle meatus,* below the middle turbinate, contains the openings of the frontal, maxillary, and anterior ethmoid *sinuses.* The posterior ethmoid sinus drains into the superior meatus. The *olfactory region* is located high in the nose between the nasal septum and the superior turbinate. Figure 8–6 illustrates the lateral wall of the nose.

The blood supply to the nose is derived from the internal and external carotid arteries. The turbinates are very vascular and contain large vascular spaces. The blood vessels of the anterior nasal septum meet at an area about 1 inch from

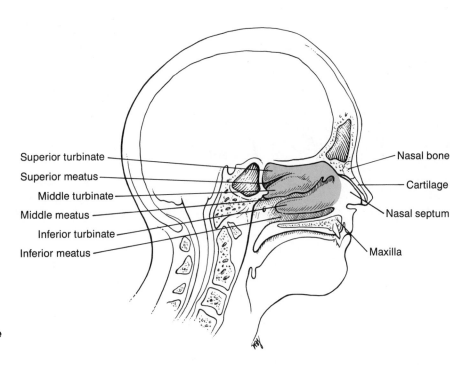

FIGURE 8–6. Lateral wall of the nose.

the mucocutaneous junction, known as *Little's area.* This is the area usually responsible for *epistaxis,* or nosebleeds. The blood vessels are under autonomic nervous system control. If there is an excess of *sympathetic* stimulation, the blood vessels constrict and the vascular spaces in the turbinates shrink. If there is an increase in *parasympathetic* tone, the blood pools in the turbinates, resulting in their swelling, obstruction to air flow, and elaboration of a watery discharge.

The nerve supply to the internal nose is from branches of the trigeminal nerve. The olfactory epithelium is supplied by the *olfactory,* or first cranial, nerve. Moist air with the dissolved odorous particles acts as a stimulus. The nerve fibers from this area pierce the *cribriform plate* to the olfactory bulb in the brain. The olfactory receptors in humans adapt rapidly to stimuli.

The main functions of the nose are to provide the following:

- An airway
- Olfaction
- Humidification of inspired air
- Warming of inspired air
- Filtering of inspired air

The inspired air flows above and below the middle turbinate. This produces eddy currents that serve to protect the olfactory epithelium in the superior portion of the nose. The nasal mucosa produces mucus, which increases the relative humidity to nearly 100%. This prevents drying out of the epithelium and possible infection. The air, by its circulation around the chonchae, is warmed to nearly body temperature by the time it enters the nasopharynx. The mucus and the nasal hairs, or *vibrissae,* prevent particulate matter from entering the distal respiratory tract. The mucous blanket is swept posteriorly by the *cilia* and is swallowed. The mucus also contains immunoglobulins and enzymes, which serve as a line of defense.

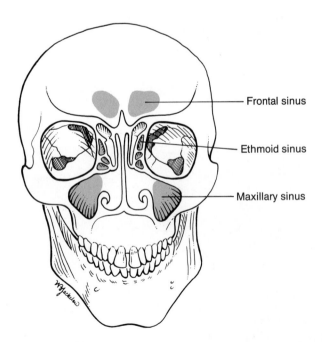

FIGURE 8–7. The nasal sinuses.

The four *paranasal sinuses* of the head are the *maxillary,* the *ethmoid,* the *frontal,* and the *sphenoid.* These are air-filled cavities lined with mucous membranes. The maxillary sinus is the largest and is bounded by the eye, the cheek, the nasal cavity, and the hard palate. The ethmoid sinuses are multiple and are present in the *ethmoid bone,* which lies medial to the orbit and extends to the pituitary fossa. The frontal sinus is located above the ethmoid sinuses and is bounded by the forehead, the orbit, and the anterior cranial fossa. Behind the ethmoid sinuses is the sphenoid sinus. There are no known functions for the paranasal sinuses. The maxillary, frontal, and ethmoid sinuses and their connections to the nose are illustrated in Figure 8–7.

REVIEW OF SPECIFIC SYMPTOMS

The Ear

The major symptoms of ear disease are the following:

- Hearing loss
- Dizziness or spinning sensation
- Hearing ringing or buzzing noises
- Discharge
- Ear pain
- Itching

Hearing Loss

Hearing loss may be unilateral or bilateral and may develop slowly or occur suddenly. In any patient with a hearing loss, ask the following questions:

"Is the hearing loss in one ear?"
"For how long have you known of a loss of hearing?"
"Was the loss sudden?"
"Is there a family history of hearing loss?"
"What type of work do you do?" "What have you done?"
"What types of hobbies do you have?"
"Have you noticed that you can hear better when it is noisy?"
"What kind of medications are you presently taking?"
"Do you know if you have ever been given an antibiotic called streptomycin or gentamicin?"

Occupational history is extremely important to ascertain. Patients with otosclerosis* can often hear better in a noisy environment. Drugs are well known to cause sudden bilateral hearing loss. Salicylates and diuretics such as furosemide and ethacrynic acid may produce transient loss of hearing when given in high doses. The aminoglycoside antibiotics such as streptomycin and gentamicin can destroy the hair cells of the organ of Corti and cause permanent hearing loss. An anti-cancer medication, cisplatin, is also associated with severe ototoxicity.

There are two main types of hearing loss: *conductive* and *sensorineural.* Any condition that interferes with or blocks the transmission of sound waves from

---

* Otosclerosis is the formation of new bone in the labyrinth causing progressive fixation of the footplate of the stapes to the oval window.

the external ear to the inner ear may result in a conductive hearing loss. Blockage may occur as a result of cerumen (earwax), foreign bodies, infection, or congenital abnormalities. Often the position of the cerumen is more important than the amount present. Not infrequently, a small amount of cerumen lying against the tympanic membrane can produce a significant hearing loss. Blockage by foreign bodies occurs in the 2 – 5 year old child. Once children discover the external canal, they may experiment and place beads or other objects inside. Effusions from infections in the middle ear represent one of the most common causes of conductive deafness in the 4 – 15 year old age group. The fluid impedes the transmission of the sound impulses by the tympanic membrane and the ossicles. Otosclerosis is the main cause of conductive hearing loss in individuals 15 – 50 years of age. With the exception of otosclerosis, conditions causing a conductive hearing loss cause alterations in the appearance of the tympanic membrane.

Sensorineural hearing loss is due to a disease process in the inner ear structures or auditory nerve. These conditions may be congenital or delayed-onset acquired. Congenital deafness accounts for 50% of all deaf children. In many cases of congenital sensorineural hearing loss, there may be no other congenital abnormality noted. At other times, deafness may accompany other defects, especially in the kidney. Infection with rubella in a woman during pregnancy accounts for most of the cases of sensorineural deafness that are due to anomalous development of the cochlea. The delayed-onset acquired types may, or may not, be genetic in origin. There are many syndromes, too numerous to mention, as well as viral infections and ototoxic drugs that may cause delayed-onset acquired sensorineural deafness. Systemic diseases, tumors, and noise are also associated with this type of hearing loss.

A patient's voice may give some ideas as to the nature of his deafness. One's speaking voice is regulated by the way he hears himself. A patient with a conductive hearing loss hears his own voice better by bone conduction than by air conduction. He will, therefore, think his voice is loud and will speak more softly. In contrast, the patient with a sensorineural hearing defect hears less by *both* air and bone conduction; therefore, he will tend to speak louder.

Vertigo

Vertigo is a sense of spinning or turning while in a resting position. It is frequently associated with a loss of vestibular function, such as unsteadiness of gait. In any patient with vertigo, ask the following questions:

> *"How long have you had this sensation?"*
> *"Have you had repeated attacks?"*
> *"How long does an attack last? . . . seconds? . . . minutes? . . . hours? . . . days?"*
> *"Is the onset of an attack abrupt?"*
> *"Was the sensation brought on by, or worsened by, changes in position?"*
> *"Does the spinning sensation progress during an attack?"*
> *"Are there any positions that make you feel better?"*
> *"During an attack have you had double vision? . . . loss of strength? . . . decreased hearing? . . . a disturbance of gait? . . . nausea? . . . vomiting? . . . ringing in your ears?"*
> *"What kind of medications are you presently taking?"*
> *"Do you know if you have ever been given an antibiotic called streptomycin or gentamicin?"*

Vertigo may result from otologic, neurologic, psychological, or iatrogenic causes. *Ménière's disease* causes severe paroxysmal vertigo as a result of labyrinthine lesions. The vertigo has an abrupt onset and may last several hours. It is often associated with nausea, vomiting, headache, a ringing sensation in the ear, and decreased hearing. The auditory abnormalities frequently antedate the vertigo. Vertigo associated with an acoustic neuroma is generally mild. Some antibiotics such as gentamicin, streptomycin, and kanamycin are vestibulotoxic and cause vertigo. The neurologic causes of vertigo are further discussed in Chapter 18, The Nervous System.

Tinnitus

Tinnitus is the sensation of hearing sound such as buzzing or ringing in the absence of environmental input. It is often associated with a conductive or sensorineural hearing loss. Usually the description of the type of tinnitus (e.g. "ringing" vs. "buzzing") is of little help in determining its cause. The most common causes result from inner ear disease such as from Ménière's disease, noise trauma, ototoxic drugs, and otosclerosis. Occasionally the patient may describe *pulsatile tinnitus*. This type of tinnitus beats at the same rate as the heart and may be a symptom of a vascular tumor of the head or neck. (See Table 8–6 for a list of some of the common causes of tinnitus.)

Otorrhea

Otorrhea, or discharge from the ear, generally indicates acute or chronic infection. Any patient complaining of an ear discharge should be asked the following:

"Can you describe the discharge?"
"Have you had similar episodes previously?"
"Do you experience 'dizziness'?"
"Do you have ear pain?"
"Have you had a recent ear or throat infection?"
"Have you had any change in your hearing?"
"Have you used ear drops?"
"Have you been swimming recently?"
"Have you had any recent head or ear injury?"

A bloody discharge may be associated with carcinoma or trauma. A clear, watery discharge may be associated with a leak of cerebrospinal fluid. It is important to determine the length of time the discharge has been present; its color, its smell; and its relationship to itching, pain, or trauma.

Otalgia

Otalgia, or ear pain, may be related to inflammatory conditions in or around the ear or may be referred* from distant anatomic sites in the head and neck. External otitis and otitis media are infections of the external and middle ear, respectively, and are very common causes of locally produced pain. Pain from the teeth, pharynx, or cervical spine is commonly referred to the ear. Inflamma-

---

* *Referred pain* is pain felt in an area that is separate from the area that is actually the source of the pain. For example, pain from gallbladder disease is frequently felt in the right shoulder. Chapter 14, The Abdomen, discusses further aspects of referred pain.

tion, trauma, or neoplasms anywhere along the course of the trigeminal, facial, glossopharyngeal, and vagus cranial nerves or cervical nerves C_2 or C_3 may be responsible for referred pain to the ipsilateral ear.

Itching

Pruritus (itching) of the ear may result from a primary disorder of the external ear or from a discharge from the middle ear. A systemic disease, such as diabetes, hepatitis, or lymphoma, may also be the cause.

The Nose

The specific symptoms related to the nose are the following:

- Obstruction
- Discharge
- Bleeding

Obstruction

The most common symptom of nasal disease is obstruction. If the symptom of nasal obstruction is present, ask these questions:

"Is the obstruction on one side?"
"Have you ever had an injury to your nose?"
"How long has the obstruction been present?"
"Do you have any allergies?"
"Does the obstruction worsen with stress?"
"Is there a history of nasal polyps?"
"Is the obstruction associated with other symptoms?"
"Is there a seasonal change in your symptoms?" If so, *"Which season is the worst?"*

Rhinitis, or the "stuffy nose," is a very common symptom and can be allergic or nonallergic in etiology. *Allergic rhinitis* is congestion of the nasal mucosa, triggered by an allergen such as pollen. The main symptoms include nasal obstruction; sneezing; and a clear, watery, nasal discharge. It is helpful to try to determine the allergen. Weeds pollinate in the spring and fall, trees in the spring, and grasses in the summer. Nonseasonal allergic rhinitis may be due to animal dander, mold, or dust. *Nonallergic rhinitis* produces the same symptoms but is nonseasonal and is not triggered by allergens. An example of nonallergic rhinitis is vasomotor rhinitis. Vasomotor rhinitis occurs at stressful times and results in venous engorgement of the chonchae causing obstruction. There are many other causes of vasomotor rhinitis, such as nasal spray abuse (also known as *rhinitis medicomentosa*), pregnancy, and hypothyroidism.

Nasal *polyps,* usually bilateral, also cause obstruction and are the most common cause of *anosmia,* or loss of smell. Nasal polyps are commonly seen in patients with allergic rhinitis.

Nasal obstruction may be responsible for symptoms referable to other organs. Eye tearing may result from obstruction of the nasolacrimal duct beneath the inferior turbinate. Sinus symptoms may result from obstruction to their drainage. Ear pain or a "clogged" sensation is commonly associated with eustachian tube obstruction.

Discharge

Nasal discharge can be unilateral or bilateral. It usually accompanies nasal obstruction. The discharge may be characterized as

- Thin and watery
- Thick and purulent
- Bloody
- Foul smelling

A *thin and watery* discharge is usually due to excess mucus production resulting from a viral infection or allergic condition. A *thick, purulent* nasal discharge results from bacterial infection. A *bloody* discharge can result from a neoplasm, trauma, or an opportunistic infection such as mucormycosis (fungal disease). A *foul smelling* discharge is often associated with foreign bodies in the nose, chronic sinusitis, or malignant disease. A clear, watery discharge that is increased by bending the head forward or by coughing suggests a cerebrospinal fluid leak.

Epistaxis

Epistaxis usually results from the traumatic or spontaneous rupture of the superficial mucosal vessels in Little's area. In order to exclude other causes, it is important to determine whether the epistaxis is related to trauma or a bleeding disorder. It may also result from chronic sinusitis or malignancy within the sinuses. The most common cause of epistaxis is nose picking. Another important etiologic factor is cocaine abuse.

Sinus Disease Symptoms

The symptoms of sinus disease are similar to the symptoms of nasal disease. Pain is an important symptom. Pain from localized sinus disease is generally present in the area overlying the involved sinus. The only exception is sphenoid sinus disease, which is felt diffusely. Maxillary sinus pain is felt behind the eye and near the second premolar and first and second molar teeth. Frontal sinus pain is localized to above the eye. Ethmoid sinus pain is usually periorbital. Sometimes sinus pain can be referred to another area.

In addition to pain, ocular abnormalities may also be present with diseases of the sinuses.

Table 8–1 summarizes the location of pain associated with sinus disease.

TABLE 8–1. Location of Pain Associated with Sinus Disease

Sinus Involved	Local Pain	Referred Pain
Maxillary	Behind eye Cheek Nose Upper teeth Upper lip	Teeth Retrobulbar
Ethmoid	Periorbital Retronasal Retrobulbar	Occipital Upper cervical
Frontal	Supraorbital Frontal	Bitemporal and occipital headache

**TABLE 8–2. Clinical Signs and Symptoms in
Sinus Disease**

Sinus Involved	Signs and Symptoms
Maxillary	Ocular abnormalities 　　Diplopia 　　Proptosis 　　Epiphora (tearing) Nasal obstruction and rhinorrhea Epistaxis Loosening of teeth
Ethmoid	Orbital swelling Nasal obstruction and purulent rhinorrhea Ocular abnormalities 　　Proptosis 　　Diplopia Tenderness over inner canthus of eye
Frontal	Nasal obstruction and rhinorrhea Tenderness over frontal sinus Pus in middle meatus Signs of meningitis

Table 8–2 lists the other clinical signs and symptoms associated with sinus disease.

IMPACT OF DEAFNESS ON THE PATIENT

The ear is the sensory organ of hearing. Audition is one of the main avenues of communication. Any disturbance in the reception of sound waves by the external ear to the transmission of the electrical impulses to the brain may result in an abnormal interpretation of language.

In 1977, it was estimated that there were over 14.2 million persons in the United States with some degree of hearing loss that interfered with their ability to understand speech (Ries, 1982). About half of these individuals, 7.2 million, had bilateral hearing problems. Although persons over the age of 70 years account for 30% of all deaf individuals, in 1971 there were over 202,000 deaf children under 3 years of age (Schein and Delk, 1974). In the past 10 years, the overall prevalence rate has increased substantially.

In order to understand the impact of deafness on an individual, it is necessary for us to consider the *age of onset,* the *severity* of the loss, the *rapidity* of the loss, and any *residual* hearing. Persons with insidious or sudden hearing loss experience grief and depression. Consider for example the grief expressed in the quote by Beethoven at the beginning of this chapter.

The psychological effects of deafness include *paranoia, depression, withdrawal, irritability,* and *anxiety.* Although it is not entirely resolved, it appears that the deaf person has an increased tendency toward paranoia. Most deaf individuals tend to be suspicious of others' conversations.

The most significant response to a severe hearing deficit is depression and withdrawal. The following quote by Beethoven dramatizes these responses:

Oh you men who think that I am malevolent, stubborn, or misanthropic, how greatly do you wrong me. You do not know the secret cause which makes me seem that way to you . . . For me there can be no relaxation with my fellow men, no refined conversations, no mutual exchange of ideas. I must live alone, like one who has been banished . . . What a humiliation for me when someone standing next to me heard a flute in the distance, and I heard nothing . . . a little more of that and I would have ended my life — it was only my art that held me back.

The hearing-impaired person has social identity problems as well. He is frequently set aside from his previous associations. If the person uses sign language, he can no longer enjoy the company of individuals who do not sign. His work or career may have to be altered. The stigma associated with wearing a hearing aid serves to reinforce his feeling of alienation from others. The patient may avoid wearing a hearing aid for fear of being stigmatized.

A deaf child presents even more severe problems. His lack of auditory input influences his character, early childhood experiences, attitudes, and interpersonal relationships. He is deprived of many of the reassuring, loving, and comforting sounds that facilitate the development of his personality. He is unable to obtain verbal cues of a parent's affection. He is also unable to be alerted by auditory signs of danger. As he grows older, he is denied his own language.

Psychological problems, social inadequacy, and educational retardation are very common in deaf children. The worse the handicap, the worse are the psychological and educational implications.

The young hearing-impaired child who shows a delay in language development may be diagnosed as *retarded*. Generally, children who are congenitally deaf or suffer from severe hearing impairment prior to 3 years of age suffer the most. As the type of lesion causing deafness progresses from the periphery inward, the deleterious effects increase.

PHYSICAL EXAMINATION

> The equipment necessary for the examination of the ear and nose is as follows: an otoscope, choice of specula, penlight, and a 512 Hz tuning fork. A nasal illuminator attachment for the otoscope and a nasal speculum are optional.

The physical examinations of the ear and the nose are performed with the examiner seated in front of the patient.

The Ear

If the patient has symptoms referable to one ear, examine the uninvolved ear first. The physical examination of the ear includes the following:

- External examination
- Auditory acuity
- Otoscopic examination

External Examination

Inspect the External Ear Structures

Inspect the pinna for size, position, and shape. The pinna should be positioned centrally and should be in proportion to the face and head.

A small dimple in front of the tragus is usually a remnant of the first branchial arch.

The external ear is inspected for deformities, nodules, inflammation, or lesions. The presence of *tophi* is a highly specific but nonsensitive sign of gout. Tophi are deposits of uric acid crystals. They appear as hard nodules in the helix or antihelix. Rarely, a white discharge may be seen in association with them. A "cauliflower ear" is a gnarled pinna as a result of repeated trauma.

Inspect for discharge. If discharge is present, note its characteristics, such as color, consistency, and clarity.

Palpate the External Ear Structures

The pinna is palpated for tenderness, swelling, or nodules. If pain is elicited by pulling up and down on the pinna or by pressing in on the tragus, an external ear infection is likely to be present.

The posterior auricular region should be inspected for scars or swelling. The examiner should apply pressure to the mastoid tip, which should be painless. Tenderness may indicate a suppurative process of the mastoid bone.

Auditory Acuity

Testing for auditory acuity is the next part of the physical examination. The easiest method for testing for a gross hearing loss is for the examiner to occlude one external canal by pressing inward on the tragus and speak softly into the other ear. The examiner should hide his mouth to prevent lip reading by the patient. The examiner should *whisper* words such as "park," "dark," or "daydream" in the nonoccluded ear and determine whether the patient can hear them. This procedure is then repeated using the other ear. Asking a patient if he hears a watch ticking when held to his ear is generally meaningless, since the patient knows what to expect.

The use of *tuning fork testing* for hearing loss is more accurate and should be performed regardless of the results of the whisper test. Although there are several tuning fork frequencies available, the best for evaluation of hearing is the 512 Hz fork.* A tuning fork is held by its stem, and its tip is briskly struck against the palm of the hand. It is *never* to be struck on a solid wooden or metal object. There are two tuning fork tests to assess hearing. They are

- The Rinne test
- The Weber test

The Rinne Test

The Rinne test compares air conduction with bone conduction. Each ear is tested separately. The examiner should strike a 512 Hz tuning fork and place its handle on the mastoid tip. The patient is then asked if he hears the sound and to indicate when he can no longer hear it. When the patient can no longer hear it, the tines of the vibrating tuning fork are placed in front of the external auditory

---

* Different examiners prefer different frequencies of tuning forks for determining auditory acuity. A tuning fork of too high a frequency will fade too quickly.

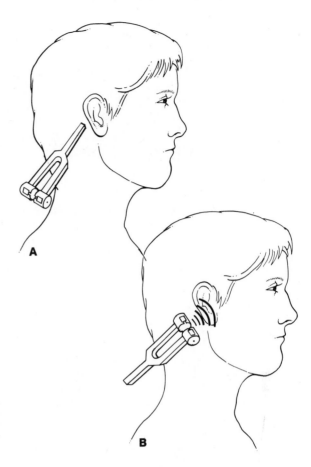

FIGURE 8–8. The Rinne test. The tuning fork is first placed on the mastoid process as shown in *A*. When the sound can no longer be heard, the tuning fork is placed in front of the external auditory meatus as shown in *B*. Normally, air conduction is better than bone conduction.

meatus of the same ear, and the patient is asked if he can still hear it. It is important that the tines of the vibrating tuning fork do not touch any hair, because the patient may have a hearing impairment but may still feel the vibration. The Rinne test is demonstrated in Figure 8–8.

Normally, air conduction (AC) is better than bone conduction (BC), and the patient will be able to hear the tuning fork at the external auditory meatus after he can no longer hear it on the mastoid tip; this is a *Rinne positive* test (AC > BC). Patients with a conductive hearing loss, however, have bone conduction that is better than air conduction: a *Rinne negative* test (BC > AC). Patients with sensorineural deafness will have impaired air *and* bone conduction but will maintain the normal AC > BC response. The middle ear will amplify the sound in both positions.

The Weber Test

The Weber test compares bone conduction in the two ears. Stand in front of the patient and place a vibrating 512 Hz tuning fork firmly against the center of the patient's forehead. Ask the patient to indicate whether he hears or feels the sound in his right ear, in his left ear, or in the middle of his forehead. Hearing the sound, or feeling the vibration, in the middle is the normal response. If the sound is not heard in the middle, the sound is said to be *lateralized,* and a hearing loss is present. Sound will be lateralized to the *affected* side in conductive deafness. Try it on yourself. Occlude your right ear and place a vibrating tuning fork in the center of your forehead. Where do you hear it? On the *right.* You have created a

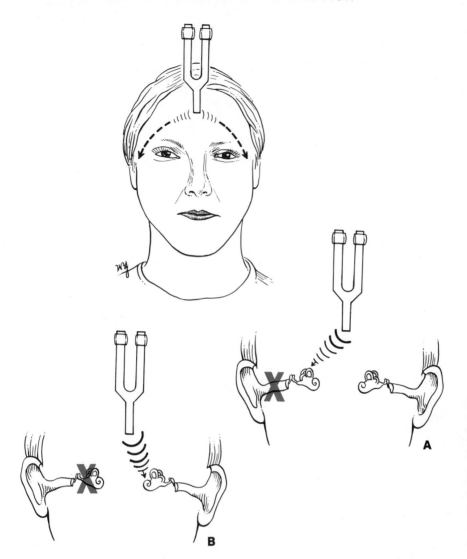

FIGURE 8–9. The Weber test. When a vibrating tuning fork is placed on the center of the forehead, the sound will be heard in the center without lateralization to either side (normal response). *A,* In the presence of a conductive hearing loss, the sound will be heard on the side of the conductive loss. *B,* In the presence of the sensorineural loss, the sound will be better heard on the opposite (unaffected) side.

conductive hearing loss on the right by blocking the right canal; the sound is lateralized to right side. The Weber test is illustrated in Figure 8–9.

The explanation for the Weber test is based on the masking effect of background noise. Under normal conditions, there is considerable background noise, which reaches the tympanic membrane by air conduction. This tends to mask the sound by the tuning fork heard by bone conduction. In an ear with a conductive hearing loss, the air conduction is decreased and the masking effect is, therefore, diminished. Thus, the affected ear will hear and feel the vibrating tuning fork better than the normal ear.

In patients with unilateral sensorineural deafness, the sound will not be heard on the affected side but will be heard by, or localized to, the *unaffected* ear.

In order to test the reliability of the patient's responses, it is useful to occasionally strike the tuning fork against the palm of the hand and hold it briefly to silence it. The two tests are then carried out as indicated, using the silent tuning fork. This serves as a good control.

Otoscopic Examination

The remainder of the examination of the ear is performed with the otoscope. You must take care in the use of the otoscope. The best visualization of the structures does *not* require the otoscope to be wedged into the canal! Be gentle, in order to achieve the best visualization of the anatomy.

Choose the correct speculum size: small enough to prevent discomfort to the patient, and large enough to provide an adequate beam of light.

The Techniques

To examine the patient's *right* ear, the examiner holds the otoscope in the *right* hand. The canal is straightened by the examiner's *left* hand, pulling the auricle *up, out, and back.* The straighter the canal, the easier the visualization and the more comfortable the examination will be for the patient.

In the child, the canal should be straightened by pulling the auricle *down and back.*

The patient is asked to turn his head to the side slightly so that the examiner can examine the ear more comfortably. The otoscope may be held in either of two positions. The first, and preferred, position involves holding the otoscope like a pencil, between the thumb and index fingers, in a *downward* position with the ulnar aspect of the examiner's hand braced against the side of the patient's face. This positioning provides a buffer against sudden movement of the patient. By holding the end of the otoscope's handle, the examiner then angles the speculum into the external canal. This technique at first feels more cumbersome than the alternate technique, but it is safer, especially for children. This technique is shown in Figure 8–10.

The second position involves holding the otoscope *upward* as the speculum is introduced into the canal. This technique feels more comfortable, but a sudden movement of the patient can cause pain and injury to the patient. This alternate technique is demonstrated in Figure 8–11.

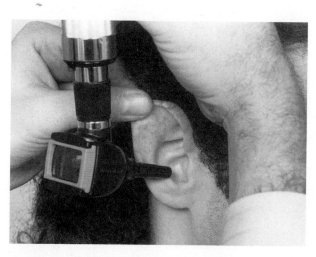

FIGURE 8–10. Technique for otoscopic examination. Notice that the ear is pulled up, out, and back.

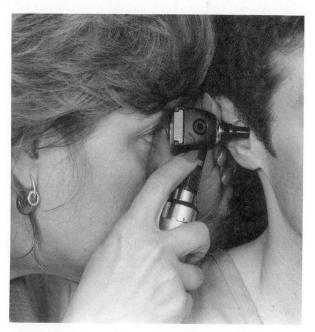

FIGURE 8–11. Alternate technique for otoscopic examination. The ear is again pulled up, out, and back.

Inspect the External Canal

Gently insert the speculum and inspect the external canal. There should be no evidence of redness, swelling, or tenderness, which indicates inflammation. The walls of the canal should be free of foreign bodies, scaliness, or discharge. If a foreign body is seen, pay particular attention to inspecting the opposite ear canal, nose, and other accessible body orifices carefully.

Any wax should be left as is, unless it interferes with the visualization of the rest of the canal and tympanic membrane. Removal of wax is best left to the experienced examiner, because any manipulation may result in trauma or abrasions.

If a discharge is present, look carefully for the site of origin.

Inspect the Tympanic Membrane

As the speculum is introduced further into the canal in a downward and forward direction, the tympanic membrane will be visualized. The tympanic membrane should appear as an intact, translucent, pearly gray membrane at the end of the canal. The handle of the malleus should be seen near the center of the tympanic membrane. From the lower end of the handle, there is frequently a bright triangular cone of light reflected from the pars tensa. This is called the *light reflex,* which is directed anteroinferiorly. The pars flaccida, the short process of the malleus, and the anterior and posterior folds should be identified. Figure 8–12 shows a normal tympanic membrane with the important landmarks identified (see also Plate VII *D*).

The presence or absence of the light reflex should not be considered indicative of normality or disease. The sensitivity of the presence of the light reflex indicating disease is low. There are as many normal tympanic membranes without a light reflex as abnormal membranes with a light reflex.

Describe the color, integrity, transparency, position, and landmarks of the tympanic membrane.

In health, the tympanic membrane is usually pearly gray. In disease, the tympanic membrane may be dull and become red or yellow. Is the drum injected? Injection refers to the dilatation of blood vessels, making them more

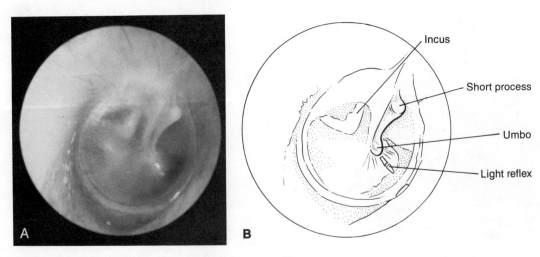

FIGURE 8–12. *A* and *B,* Black and white photograph and labeled schematic of Plate VII *D,* showing a normal right tympanic membrane.

apparent. The blood vessels should only be visible around the perimeter of the membrane. Dense, white plaques on the tympanic membrane may be due to tympanosclerosis.

Is the tympanic membrane bulging or retracted? Bulging of the membrane may indicate fluid or pus in the middle ear. There should be no bubbles or fluid seen behind the tympanic membrane in the middle ear. A retracted tympanic membrane occurs when intratympanic cavity pressures are reduced: for example, when the eustachian tube is obstructed.

If the tympanic membrane is perforated, describe the characteristics. Perforation of the tympanic membrane can occur after trauma or infection.

The normal position of the tympanic membrane is oblique to the external canal. The superior margin is closer to the examiner's eye. This is frequently better seen in infants than in adults.

In the normal ear, the handle of the malleus attached to the tympanic membrane is the primary landmark. Occasionally, the long process of the incus may be seen posterior to the malleus. Rarely, the chorda tympani nerve may be seen coursing behind the short process of the malleus. In the presence of a retracted tympanic membrane, the malleus is seen in sharp outline.

There are many differences in the color, shape, and contour of the tympanic membrane, which will be recognized only with experience.

After you have examined the right ear, examine the *left* ear by holding the otoscope in your *left* hand and straightening the canal with your *right* hand.

Determine the Mobility of the Tympanic Membrane

If there is a question of middle ear infection, pneumatic otoscopy should be performed. This technique can easily be accomplished by attaching a rubber squeeze bulb to the otoscope. By increasing and decreasing the pressure in the external canal, the normal tympanic membrane should move in and out, respectively. In patients with middle ear infections, this motion is diminished or absent despite the possible existence of a light reflex. The reduction of movement of the tympanic membrane increases the probability of middle ear infection by as much as 40%.

The Nose

The examination of the nose consists of

- External examination
- Internal examination

External Examination
Inspect the Nose

The external examination consists of inspection of the nose for any *swelling, trauma,* or *congenital anomalies.* Is the nose straight? Does a deviation involve the upper, bony portion or the lower, cartilaginous portion?

Inspect the external nares. Are they symmetrical?

Test the patency of each nostril. Occlude one nostril by *gently* placing your finger across the opening of the nostril. Ask the patient to sniff. It is important not to compress the contralateral nostril by aggressive pressure.

Any swelling or deformity should be palpated for pain and firmness.

Palpate the Sinuses

Palpation over the frontal and maxillary sinuses may reveal tenderness indicative of sinusitis.

Internal Examination

The key to the internal examination is the proper positioning of the head. Ask the patient to hold his head back. Place your left hand firmly on top of the patient's head, and use your left thumb to elevate the tip of the patient's nose. In this manner, you can change the position of the patient's head in order to visualize intranasal structures. Use a light source to illuminate the internal structures. This technique is demonstrated in Figure 8–13.

Inspect the position of the septum to the lateral cartilages on each side. Examine the vestibule for inflammation and the anterior septum for deviation or perforation. The *color* of the nasal mucous membrane should be evaluated. Normal nasal mucous membranes are dull red and moist and have a smooth, clean surface. Nasal mucosae are usually darker in color than oral mucosae. You should inspect for exudate, swelling, bleeding, or trauma. If epistaxis has occurred, careful examination of Little's area for vascular engorgement or crusting is important.

Is a discharge present? If present, it should be described as purulent, watery, cloudy, or bloody. Is crusting present? Are any masses or polyps present?

By tipping the head back further, check the posterior septum for deviation or perforation. The size and color of the inferior turbinates should be noted. The two inferior turbinates are rarely symmetrical.

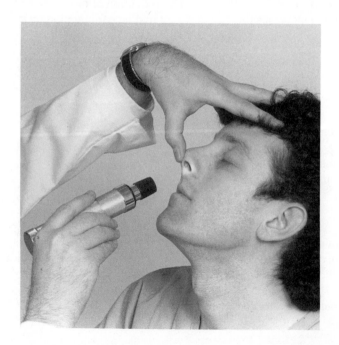

FIGURE 8–13. Inspection of the internal structures of the nose.

Inspect the size, color, and mucosal condition of the middle turbinates. Are polyps present? Most polyps are found in the middle meatus.

Using a Nasal Illuminator

If a nasal illuminator is used, the examiner places his left thumb on the tip of the patient's nose while the palm of his hand steadies the head. The patient's neck is slightly extended as the tip of the speculum of the illuminator is inserted into the nostril. After one nostril is evaluated, the illuminator is placed in the other nostril. The technique of using a nasal illuminator is shown in Figure 8–14.

Using a Nasal Speculum

If a nasal speculum is used, the instrument is held in the left hand and the speculum is introduced into the nostril in a vertical position (blades facing up and down). The speculum should not rest on the nasal septum. The blades are inserted about 1 cm into the vestibule, and the patient's neck should be slightly extended. The left index finger is placed on the ala of the nose to anchor the upper blade of the speculum while the right hand of the examiner steadies the patient's head. The right hand is used to change the head position for better visibility of the internal structures. After one nostril has been examined, the speculum, still being held in the left hand, is introduced into the other nostril. The technique of holding the speculum is shown in Figure 8–15. Although the nasal speculum provides the best method of inspection, the internist rarely uses this instrument.

Transillumination of the Sinuses

If a patient has symptoms referable to sinus problems, transillumination of the sinuses is performed. This examination is performed in a darkened room, where a bright light source is placed in the mouth of the patient on one side of the hard palate. The light is transmitted through the maxillary sinus cavity and is seen as a crescent-shaped dull glow under the eye. The other side is then examined.

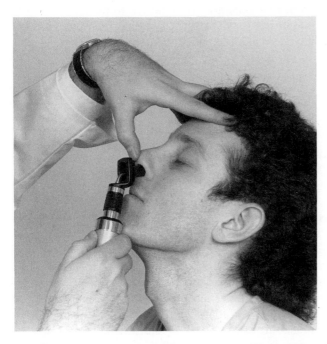

FIGURE 8–14. Using a nasal illuminator to inspect the internal structures of the nose.

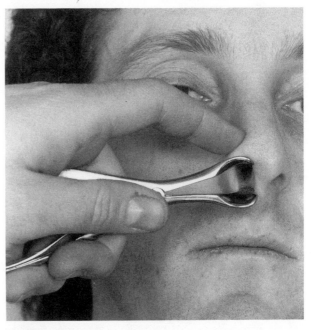

FIGURE 8–15. Using a nasal speculum to inspect the internal structures of the nose. Note the position of the left index finger.

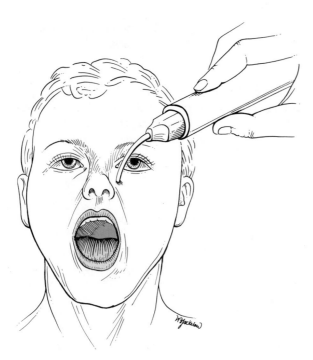

FIGURE 8-16. Transillumination of the maxillary sinus. Note the red glow seen on the hard palate.

Normally, the glow on each side should be equal. If one sinus contains fluid, a mass, or mucosal thickening, there will be a decrease in its glow, indicating loss of aeration on that side. An alternate method of examining the maxillary sinus is to direct a light downward from under the medial aspect of the eye. The patient is asked to open his mouth, and the glow is observed in the hard palate. This technique is illustrated in Figure 8-16. The frontal sinus can be examined in a similar fashion by directing the light upward under the medial aspect of the eyebrow and observing the glow above the eye.

The ethmoid and sphenoid sinuses cannot be examined by transillumination.

The variability of sinus transillumination from patient to patient is tremendous. It must be understood that in the absence of sinus symptoms, these differences in transillumination make the technique nonspecific.

CLINICOPATHOLOGIC CORRELATIONS

Infectious, inflammatory, traumatic, and neoplastic diseases are common in the organs of the ear and nose. Some of the more common ear infections are discussed in this section.

Acute otitis media is a bacterial infection of the middle ear, seen most commonly in children. Up to 50% of all children will experience an attack of acute otitis media before they reach 1 year of age, and 75% of children will be affected before the second birthday. After the age of 5 years, the incidence declines rapidly. The child suffers ear pain and has constitutional symptoms of fever and malaise, often associated with gastrointestinal problems and a conductive hearing loss. The tympanic membrane becomes injected, and the entire membrane becomes fiery red. A mucopurulent exudate in the middle ear causes the membrane to bulge outward. In most cases, antibiotic therapy will resolve the condition and restore normal hearing.

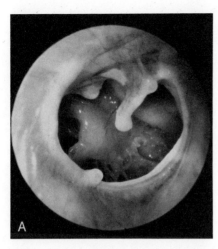

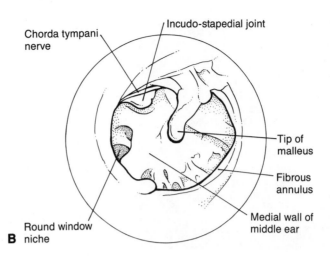

FIGURE 8–17. *A* and *B,* Black and white photograph and labeled schematic of Plate VII *E,* showing a central perforation of the right tympanic membrane.

If the tympanic membrane ruptures from the increased pressure, *advanced acute otitis media* is said to be present. The purulent exudate is then discharged into the external canal. Figure 8–17 and Plate VII *E* show a perforated tympanic membrane of a patient as a result of otitis media.

Perforations may be *central* or *marginal* and may result from either otitis or trauma. A central perforation does not involve the margin or annulus of the tympanic membrane; a marginal perforation involves the margin. Marginal perforations are more serious, as they predispose the patient to the development of a *cholesteatoma,* which is a chronic condition of the middle ear. A marginal perforation will allow squamous epithelium from the external canal to grow into the middle ear. As these cells invade, they desquamate and debris accumulates in the middle ear, forming a cholesteatoma. Slow enlargement of the cholesteatoma leads to erosion of the ossicles and expansion into the mastoid antrum. Plate VII *F* shows a patient with a cholesteatoma (see Fig. 8–18 for schematic).

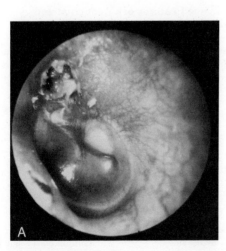

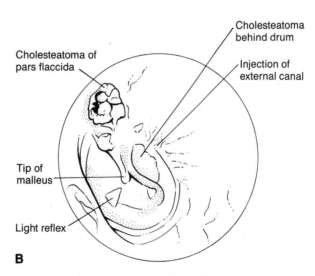

FIGURE 8–18. *A* and *B,* Black and white photograph and labeled schematic of Plate VII *F,* showing a cholesteatoma of the left ear that resulted from a marginal perforation of the tympanic membrane. Note the injection of the distal external canal.

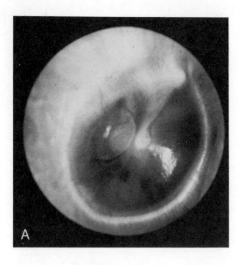

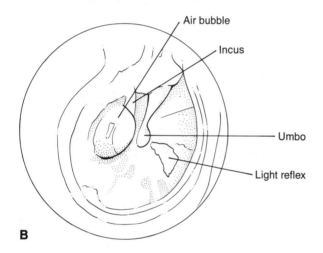

FIGURE 8 – 19. *A* and *B,* Black and white photograph and labeled schematic of Plate VIII *A,* showing serous otitis media of the right ear. Note the air bubble in the middle ear behind the tympanic membrane.

TABLE 8 – 3. Comparative Features of Conductive and Sensorineural Hearing Loss

	Conductive Hearing Loss	Sensorineural Hearing Loss
Pathology	External canal Middle ear	Cochlea Cochlear nerve Brainstem
Loudness of speech	Softer than normal	Louder than normal
External canal	May be abnormal	Normal
Tympanic membrane	Usually abnormal	Normal
Rinne test	Negative	Positive
Weber test	Heard on "deaf" side	Heard on better side (only in severe unilateral loss)

TABLE 8-4. Common Causes of Deafness

Patient	Conductive Deafness	Sensorineural Deafness
Child	Congenital	Congenital
	Acute otitis media	Mumps labyrinthitis
	Chronic otitis media	Maternal rubella during first trimester
	Cerumen	Birth trauma
	Trauma	Congenital syphilis
Adult	Serous otitis media	Delayed-onset congenital
	Chronic otitis media	Ménière's disease
	External otitis	Ototoxic drugs
	Cerumen	Viral labyrinthitis
	Eustachian tube blockage	Acoustic neuroma
	Viral myringitis	Presbycusis (age-related deafness)
	Cholesteatoma	
	Otosclerosis	

Serous otitis media occurs primarily in adults with a viral upper respiratory infection or during sudden atmospheric pressure changes. In the presence of a blocked eustachian tube, air becomes trapped within. The tiny blood vessels in the middle ear absorb much of the air, producing a vacuum that draws in or retracts the tympanic membrane. The sensation of "plugged ears" occurs. If the pressure is not relieved, this vacuum draws serous, nonpurulent fluid from the blood vessels into the middle ear. The tympanic membrane appears yellowish-orange as a result of the amber-colored fluid, and the landmarks are clearly seen as the membrane is retracted against these structures. Partial obstruction of the eustachian tube will produce air bubbles or an air-fluid level in the middle ear. Figure 8-19 and Plate VIII A show a tympanic membrane of a patient with serous otitis media.

Recurrent middle ear infections and tympanic membrane rupture may lead to *chronic otitis media*. Chronic infection may produce a foul smelling discharge, which is the main symptom of chronic otitis media; pain is usually not present. Erosion of the ossicles and scar tissue may develop, causing a conductive hearing loss.

TABLE 8-5. Differentiation of Acute External Otitis From Acute Otitis Media

Signs and Symptoms	Acute External Otitis	Acute Otitis Media
Pressure on tragus	Painful	No pain
Lymphadenopathy	Frequent	Absent
External canal	Edematous	Normal
Season	Summer	Winter
Tympanic membrane	Normal	Fluid behind drum, possibly perforated
Fever	Yes	Yes
Hearing loss	Slight or normal	Decreased

TABLE 8–6. Common Causes of Tinnitus

Location	Pulsatile/Clicking	Nonpulsatile
External ear	External otitis Bullous myringitis Foreign body	Cerumen Tympanic membrane perforation Foreign body
Middle ear	Otitis media Vascular anomalies Neoplasm Eustachian tube dysfunction	Otosclerosis Serous otitis
Inner ear	Vascular anomalies	Cochlear otosclerosis Ménière's disease Labyrinthitis Noise trauma Drug toxicity Presbycusis
Central nervous system	Vascular anomalies Hypertension	Syphilis Degenerative disease Cerebral atherosclerosis

Table 8–3 summarizes the comparative features of conductive and sensorineural deafness. Table 8–4 enumerates the common causes of deafness. Table 8–5 is a differentiation of acute external otitis from acute otitis media. Table 8–6 lists the multiple common causes of tinnitus.

WRITING UP THE PHYSICAL EXAMINATION

Listed here are examples of the write-up for the examinations of the ear and nose.

The external ear appears normal without evidence of inflammation or lesions. The patient has no difficulty hearing the whispered word. The Weber test result is midline. AC > BC. The external canals are normal, as are the tympanic membranes. There is no injection of the external canals or the tympanic membranes. No discharge is present.

A 1 cm, round, hard, painless mass is present on the right pinna. The patient has no problem with hearing. The Weber test result is midline. Air conduction is greater than bone conduction. The external canals and tympanic membranes are normal.

The external structures of the ears are within normal limits. There is a hearing loss in the left ear with bone conduction greater than air conduction. The Weber test lateralizes to the left ear. The left tympanic membrane appears opaque. The ossicles are not seen on the left. The right tympanic membrane appears normal. The ossicles appear normal on the right.

The nose is not deviated. There are no swellings seen. The anterior septum appears pink without discharge or vascular engorgement. The septum is midline. No sinus tenderness is present.

The nose appears deviated to the right. The nasal mucous membranes are bright red and moist. A whitish-yellow discharge is present on a deviated septum to the right. The sinuses are not tender.

USEFUL VOCABULARY

Listed here are the specific roots that are important in order to understand the terminology related to diseases of the ear and nose.

ROOT	PERTAINING TO	EXAMPLE	DEFINITION
audio-	to hear	*audio*meter	Device to measure hearing
aur-	ear	*aur*icle	Portion of the external ear not contained within the head
-cusis	hearing	presby*cusis*	Progressive decrease in hearing with age
-lalia	speech	echo*lalia*	Meaningless repetition by a patient of words addressed to him
myringo-	tympanic membrane	*myringo*tomy	Surgical incision of the tympanic membrane
ot(o)-	ear	*ot*itis	Inflammation of the ear
phon-	sound; often the sound of a voice	*phon*asthenia	Weakness of the voice
rhino-	nose	*rhino*plasty	Plastic surgery on the nose
tympan(o)-	middle ear	*tympan*otomy	Surgical puncture of the tympanic membrane

BIBLIOGRAPHY

Ballantyne J: Deafness. Edinburgh, Churchill Livingstone, 1977.

Dayal VS: Clinical Otolaryngology. Philadelphia, JB Lippincott Co, 1981.

DeWeese D, Saunders W: Textbook of Otolaryngology. St. Louis, CV Mosby, 1973.

English GM: Otolaryngology. New York, Harper and Row, 1976.

Furth HG: Thinking Without Language: Psychological Implications of Deafness. New York, Free Press, 1966.

Hawke M, Keene M, Alberti PW: Clinical Otoscopy: A Text and Colour Atlas. Edinburgh, Churchill Livingstone, 1984.

Hawke M, Kwok P: A mini-atlas of ear-drum pathology. Can Fam Physician 33:1501, 1987.

Lucente FE, Sobol SM: Essentials of Otolaryngology. New York, Raven Press, 1983.

Orlans H (ed): Adjustment to Adult Hearing Loss. San Diego, College-Hill Press, 1985.

Ries PW: Hearing ability of persons by sociodemographic and health characteristics: United States (Series 10, No. 140). Washington, DC, US Government Printing Office, 1982.

Schein J, Delk M Jr: The Deaf Population in the United States. Silver Springs, MD, National Association of the Deaf, 1974.

Zemlin WR: Speech and Hearing Science. Englewood Cliffs, NJ, Prentice-Hall, Inc, 1981.

THE ORAL CAVITY
AND PHARYNX

One should not converse at meals lest the windpipe acts before the gullet and his life will thereby be endangered.

The Talmud

GENERAL CONSIDERATIONS

The mouth and oral cavity are used by individuals to express a range of emotions from love to hate, from ecstasy to despair, from satisfaction to rage. As early as infancy, the mouth provides gratification and sensory pleasure.

Approximately 20% of all visits to the primary care physician are related to problems of the oral cavity and throat. The great majority of these patients present with throat pain, which may be acute and associated with fever or difficulty in swallowing. A sore throat may be the result of local disease or may be an early manifestation of a systemic problem.

Many visits are also associated with psychiatric disturbances. Often psychosomatic disease symptoms center themselves around the mouth. Patients with psychosomatic disease may complain of "burning" or "dryness" of the mouth or tongue. *Bruxism,* or grinding of one's teeth other than for chewing, occurs especially during sleep. This overuse of the muscles of mastication has often been interpreted as a manifestation of rage or aggression that is not overtly displayed. Bruxism may be an infantile response to reduce psychic tension. Bruxism may produce facial pain, which causes further spasm of the muscles and continued bruxism, all of which starts a vicious cycle. Individuals who habitually have something in their mouths, such as a pipe, a thumb, or a pencil, may actually cause damage to their oral cavities.

STRUCTURE AND PHYSIOLOGY

The Oral Cavity

The oral cavity consists of the following:

- Buccal mucosa
- Lips
- Tongue
- Hard and soft palate
- Teeth
- Salivary glands

The oral cavity extends from the inner surface of the teeth to the oral pharynx. Forming the roof of the mouth are the hard and soft palates. The soft palate terminates posteriorly at the *uvula.* The *tongue* forms the floor of the mouth. At the most posterior aspect of the oral cavity lie the *tonsils* between the anterior and posterior *pillars.* The oral cavity is shown in Figure 9–1.

The *buccal mucosa* is a mucous membrane that is continuous with the gingivae and lines the inside of the cheeks.

Lips are red as a result of the increased number of vascular dermal papillae and the thinness of the epidermis in this area. An increase in desaturated hemoglobin, *cyanosis,* is therefore apparent as blue lips. We are all familiar with the common blue discoloration of the lips in a cold environment, which is related to the decreased blood supply and increased extraction of oxygen under these conditions.

The tongue lies at the floor of the mouth and is attached to the *hyoid bone.* It is the main organ of taste, aids in speech, and serves an important function in mastication. The body of the tongue contains intrinsic and extrinsic muscles and is the strongest muscle of the body. The tongue is supplied by the *hypoglossal,* or twelfth cranial, nerve.

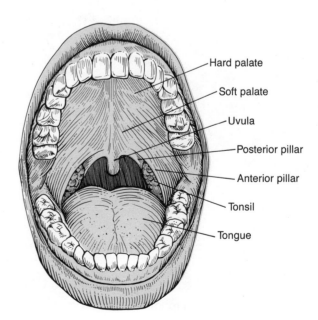

FIGURE 9–1. The oral cavity.

The dorsum of the tongue has a convex surface with a median sulcus. At the posterior portion of the sulcus is the *foramen cecum,* which marks the area of the origin of the *thyroid gland.* Behind the foramen cecum are mucin secreting glands and an aggregate of lymphatic tissue called the *lingual tonsils.* The rough texture of the tongue is due to the presence of papillae, the largest of which are the *circumvallate* papillae. There are approximately ten of these round papillae, which are located just in front of the foramen cecum and divide the tongue into the anterior two thirds and the posterior one third. *Filiform* papillae are the most common papillae, being present over the surface of the anterior portion of the tongue. The *fungiform* papillae are located at the tip and the sides of the tongue. These papillae can be recognized by their red color and broad surface. Figure 9–2 shows the tongue viewed from above.

The *taste buds* are located on the sides of the circumvallate and fungiform papillae. Taste is perceived from the anterior two thirds of the tongue by the *chorda tympani* nerve, a division of the facial nerve. The *glossopharyngeal,* or ninth cranial, nerve perceives taste sensation from the posterior third of the tongue. There are four basic taste sensations: sweet, salty, sour, and bitter. Sweetness is detected at the tip of the tongue. Saltiness is sensed at the lateral margins of the tongue. Sourness and bitterness are perceived at the posterior aspect of the tongue and are carried by the glossopharyngeal nerve.

When the tongue is elevated, a mucosal attachment, the *frenulum,* may be seen underneath the tongue in the midline connecting the tongue to the floor of the mouth.

The *hard palate* is a concave bone structure. The anterior portion has raised folds, or *rugae.* The *soft palate* is a muscular flexible area posterior to the hard palate. The posterior margin ends at the *uvula.* The uvula aids in closing off the nasopharynx during swallowing.

Teeth are composed of several tissues: *enamel, dentine, pulp,* and *cementum.* Enamel covers the tooth and is the most highly calcified tissue in the body. The bulk of the tooth is the dentine. Under the dentine is the pulp, which contains branches of the trigeminal nerve and blood vessels. The cementum covers the

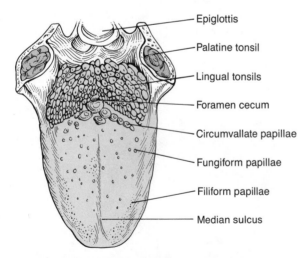

— Epiglottis

— Palatine tonsil

— Lingual tonsils

— Foramen cecum

— Circumvallate papillae

— Fungiform papillae

— Filiform papillae

— Median sulcus

FIGURE 9–2. The tongue viewed from above.

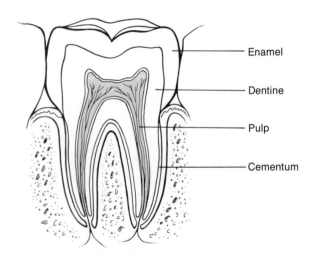

— Enamel

— Dentine

— Pulp

— Cementum

FIGURE 9–3. Cross-section through a molar tooth.

root of the tooth and attaches it to the bone. Figure 9–3 shows a section through a molar tooth.

The *primary dentition,* or the deciduous teeth, consists of 20 teeth that erupt between the ages of 6 and 30 months of age. The primary dentition per quadrant of jaw consists of two incisors, one canine, and two premolars. These teeth are then shed between the ages of 6 and 13 years. The *secondary dentition,* or the permanent teeth, consists of 32 teeth that erupt between the ages of 6 and 22 years. The secondary dentition per quadrant of jaw consists of two incisors, one canine, two premolars, and three molars. Figure 9–4 illustrates the primary and secondary dentition, and Table 20–6 summarizes the chronology of dentition.

Although not part of the oral cavity proper, the *salivary glands* are considered to be part of the mouth. There are three major salivary glands: the *parotid,* the *submandibular,* and the *sublingual* glands. The parotid gland is the largest of the salivary glands. It lies anterior to the ear on the side of the face. The facial nerve courses through the gland. The duct of the parotid gland is called *Stensen's duct* and enters the oral cavity through a small papilla opposite the upper first or second molar tooth. The submandibular gland is the second largest salivary gland. It is located below and in front of the angle of the mandible. The duct of the submandibular gland is called *Wharton's duct* and terminates in a papilla on either side of the frenulum at the base of the tongue. The sublingual gland is the smallest of the major salivary glands. It is located in the floor of the mouth beneath the tongue. There are numerous ducts of the sublingual gland, some of which open into Wharton's duct. In addition to these major salivary glands, there are hundreds of very small salivary glands located throughout the oral cavity.

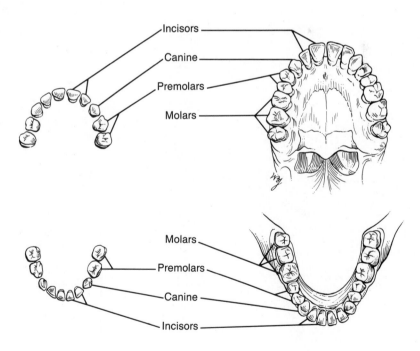

FIGURE 9–4. Primary and secondary dentition.

PRIMARY DENTITION

SECONDARY DENTITION

The Pharynx

The pharynx is divided into the *nasopharynx,* the *oropharynx,* and the *hypopharynx,* which is also known as the *laryngopharynx.* The nasopharynx lies above the soft palate and is posterior to the nasal cavities. On its posterolateral wall is the opening of the *eustachian tube.* The *adenoids* are pharyngeal tonsils and hang from the posterosuperior wall near the opening of the eustachian tube. The oropharynx lies below the soft palate, behind the mouth, and superior to the hyoid bone. Posteriorly it is bounded by the superior constrictor muscle and the cervical vertebrae. Below the oropharynx is the area known as the hypopharynx. The hypopharynx is surrounded by three constrictor muscles, which are innervated by the glossopharyngeal and vagus nerves. The hypopharynx ends at the level of the cricoid cartilage, where it communicates with the esophagus through the upper esophageal sphincter. Figure 9–5 illustrates the functional parts of the pharynx.

The muscular walls of the pharynx are formed by the constrictor muscles, which function during the act of swallowing. The blood supply is derived from the external carotid artery.

Lymphatic tissue is abundant in the pharynx. The lymphoid tissue consists of the *palatine tonsils,* the *adenoids,* and the *lingual tonsils.* These tissues form a ring known as *Waldeyer's ring.* The palatine tonsils lie in the tonsillar fossa, between the anterior and posterior pillars. The palatine tonsils are almond shaped and vary considerably in size. The adenoids lie on the posterior wall of the nasopharynx, and the lingual tonsils are located at the base of the tongue. The upper portion of the pharynx drains to the retropharyngeal nodes, whereas the lower part drains to the deep cervical lymph nodes.

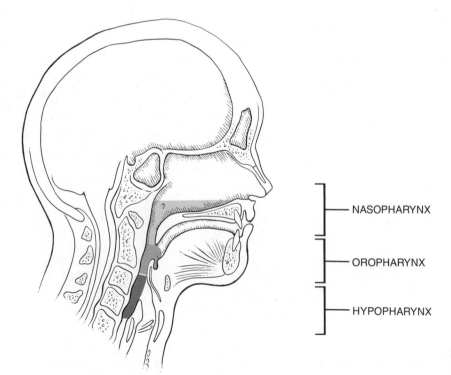

NASOPHARYNX

OROPHARYNX

HYPOPHARYNX

FIGURE 9–5. Functional parts of the pharynx.

The functions of the pharynx are

- Swallowing
- Speech
- An airway

Swallowing, or *deglutition,* is divided into three stages. The voluntary stage occurs when a bolus of food is forced by the tongue past the tonsils to the posterior pharyngeal wall. The second stage is involuntary constriction by the pharyngeal muscles propelling the bolus from the pharynx to the esophagus. The third stage is also involuntary, in which the esophageal muscles push the bolus down into the stomach. The larynx is first raised and then closed during the first two stages of swallowing. The eustachian tubes open during swallowing when the nasopharynx closes.

The pharynx also acts as a structure of resonation and articulation. *Resonation* refers to the vibration of a structure. *Articulation* is the change of shape of a structure to produce speech. By contracting the pharyngeal muscles, a change in the acoustical quality of speech results. Changes in the size and shape of the pharynx affect resonance. The soft palate affects resonance by opening and closing the partition between the oral and nasal cavities. If closure is incomplete, nasal speech will result.

The pharynx is part of the airway from the nose and mouth to the trachea.

The Larynx

The larynx is located at the superior margin of the trachea and below the hyoid bone, which is located at the base of the tongue. It is at the level of the fourth to sixth cervical vertebrae. The larynx functions dually as a guard against the entrance of solids and liquids into the trachea as well as the organ of voice production.

The *epiglottis* is attached above the larynx. Its function in humans is questionable.

The body of the larynx consists of a series of cartilaginous structures: the *cricoid,* the *thyroid,* and the *arytenoid* cartilages. The thyroid cartilage forms the bulk of the structure of the larynx and produces the prominence in the neck known as the "Adam's apple." Moving to the top of the thyroid cartilage is the *thyroid notch.* If one moves down on the thyroid cartilage, a space, the *cricothyroid space and membrane,* will be felt. This separates the thyroid cartilage from the cricoid cartilage. The cricoid cartilage articulates with the cricothyroid membrane superiorly and the trachea inferiorly. It is the only complete ring of cartilage in the larynx. The paired arytenoid cartilages provide an important area for attachment of the vocal cords. A projection of the thyroid and cricoid cartilages onto the neck is shown in Figure 9–6, and the laryngeal skeleton is shown in Figure 9–7.

The *vocal cords* vibrate in order to generate speech. Sound is produced by the rapid vibration of the vocal cords excited by the exhaled stream of air. The vocal cords are approximated, and their tension is changed by the action of various laryngeal muscles. The nerve supply to the larynx is derived from the superior

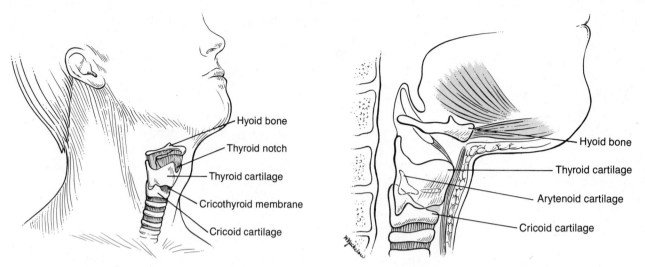

FIGURE 9–6. Laryngeal cartilages.
FIGURE 9–7. Laryngeal skeleton.

and recurrent laryngeal branches of the *vagus* nerve. Voice produced at the larynx is then modified by the pharynx and oronasal cavity.

REVIEW OF SPECIFIC SYMPTOMS

The Oral Cavity

The most important symptoms of disease of the oral cavity are the following:

- Pain
- Ulceration
- Bleeding
- A mass
- Halitosis (bad breath)

Pain

When a patient complains of oral pain, it is important to ask the following:

"Where is the pain?"
"Describe the pain."
"Do you feel the pain anywhere else?"
"How long has the pain been present?"
"What brings the pain on?"
"What makes it better? . . . worse?"
"When you have the pain, do you have any other symptoms?"

Tooth pain may be a symptom of underlying gingival disease. A careful history should be taken of dental procedures and recent dental work.

It must not be forgotten that pain in the teeth may sometimes be referred from the chest. Patients with angina may actually complain of pain in their teeth associated with exertion. Careful and thoughtful questioning is indicated.

Ulceration

Frequently, pain is related to ulceration of the lips or tongue. Cancer is *not* the most common cause of oral cavity ulceration, but it must always be considered. When a patient complains of ulceration, ask these questions:

"Do the lesions occur in groups?"
"Are the lesions painful?"
"Do the lesions recur?"
"Do you have other ulcerations, such as in the vagina? . . . in the urethra? . . . in the anus?"
"Do you smoke?" If so, *"How much?"*
"Do you have a history of venereal disease?"

It is very important to ask about a patient's sexual habits. These questions have already been discussed in Chapter 1. Smoking and drinking alcohol predispose an individual to precancerous lesions of the mouth.

Bleeding

Bleeding may result from a primary hematologic disorder or from a local inflammation or neoplasm. Many medications may also cause or predispose a patient to bleeding. Always ask if the patient is taking any medications.

Mass

If a patient complains of an intraoral mass or a mass in the region of a salivary gland, it is important to determine its duration and whether the mass is painful. Are there associated symptoms such as excessive salivation, known as *ptyalism,* or dryness of the mouth, known as *xerostomia?* Is dysphagia (difficulty in swallowing) present?

Halitosis

Most patients with halitosis have been told by others that they have bad breath. Bad breath may be a symptom or sign of gingival, tonsillar, sinus, or carious* disease. Uremia can also produce bad breath by the accumulations of waste products that are eliminated in the expired air.

The Pharynx

The most common symptoms of disease of the pharynx include the following:

- Nasal obstruction
- Pain
- Dysphagia
- Deafness
- Snoring

Obstruction

Nasal obstruction can result from enlarged adenoids or from tumor formation in the nasopharynx. It is important to determine whether the patient has any allergies or sinus trouble or has had nasal trauma.

* Affected with caries (tooth decay).

Pain

Pain can result from inflammation of the tonsils or posterior pharynx as well as from a tumor in this area. Is the pain acute? Acute throat pain may be caused by inflammatory processes or injury. Does the pain worsen upon swallowing? A foreign body in the pharynx often produces severe pain that is worsened by swallowing. Often throat pain may be referred to the ipsilateral ear. Chronic throat pain may be caused by inflammatory processes as well as by neoplasms. Enlarged thyroid lobes or diffuse thyroid enlargement may cause throat pain associated with dysphagia. Hysteria is another cause of chronic throat pain.

Dysphagia

Dysphagia is difficulty in swallowing. It is important to determine the site of obstruction. Does the dysphagia occur with liquids, solids, or tablets? Questions related to tonsillar infections are relevant, because enlarged tonsils may interfere with swallowing. It is prudent to ask if *regurgitation* of food occurs. This results from an abnormal pharyngeal pouch. The patient may describe that the "food gets stuck." This is often associated with significant disease.

Deafness

A tumor at the distal end of the eustachian tube in the nasopharynx can produce *conductive deafness*. Benign masses such as hypertrophied adenoids may be responsible. Nasopharyngeal malignancies may also be the cause of the conductive deafness. In many cases, serous effusions in the middle ear space cause eustachian tube dysfunction.

Snoring

Snoring is a very common complaint. The important problem often associated with heavy snoring is obstructive sleep apnea. These patients are frequently overweight and have a long history of excessive daytime sleepiness. A bed partner may describe the patient as sleeping quietly; then a transition occurs to louder snoring, followed by a period of cessation of snoring, during which time the patient becomes restless, has gasping motions, and appears to be struggling for breath. This period is then terminated by a loud snort, and the sequence may begin again. It is common for patients with sleep apnea to have many of these episodes each night.

The Larynx

Dysphonia

The major symptom of laryngeal disease is a change in the voice, especially the development of dysphonia, or hoarseness. Ask these questions:

> *"For how long have you had the hoarseness?"*
> *"What seems to make it better? . . . worse?"*
> *"Is there any time of day at which it is worse?"*
> *"Have you had any surgery requiring general anesthesia?"*
> *"Have you had any injury to your neck?"*

It is important to know whether the patient is (or was) a smoker. Recent onset of hoarseness may result from impingement upon the recurrent laryngeal nerve as it hooks around the left bronchus. This may be caused by a tumor, an enlarged left atrium, voice overuse, or a vocal cord neoplasm. General anesthesia requires the use of an endotracheal tube, which could potentially damage a vocal cord and cause hoarseness. It is also important to determine voice use, such as singing or public speaking.

IMPACT OF A VOICE DISORDER ON THE PATIENT

Phonation is the process of sound production by the interaction of airflow through the glottis and the opening and closing of the vocal cords of the larynx. Voice loudness is proportional to the air pressure below the glottis; pitch is related to this pressure and to the length of the vocal cords. Voice quality may change when there is interference with the vocal cords or pharyngeal cavity vibration, that is, resonance.

A voice disorder may be related to an increased size of the vocal cord, a laryngeal mass, or a neurologic or psychological problem. A voice disorder is defined as a voice that is different in pitch, quality, loudness, or flexibility as compared with other persons of similar age, sex, and ethnic group. An abnormal voice may be a symptom or sign of illness, and its cause should be determined.

In one study of a school-aged population, voice disorders were found in up to 23% of children (Silverman and Zimmer, 1975). Most of these disorders were related to voice abuse and not to organic problems. In another study, 7% of men and 5% of women between the ages of 18 and 82 years were found to have voice disorders (Laguaite, 1972). Most of these *were* related to organic problems.

The patient with an organic speech disorder is often rejected by other people. His speech may be high pitched or nasal, a cause for embarrassment. His self-image is low. He is rejected by others because his voice pattern is objectionable.

Just as a voice disorder has an impact on the person, so can a person *use* his voice to impact upon others. The manner in which a person speaks — the quality, pitch, loudness, stress patterns, rate — reflects his personality. The psychogenic voice disorders are those functional disorders that are manifestations of psychological imbalance. Voice is very useful as an indicator of *affective disorders*, such as depression, manic states, and mood swings, as well as *schizophrenia*. A voice disorder may also be an indication of a sexual identity problem.

PHYSICAL EXAMINATION

The equipment necessary for the examination of the oral cavity is the following: a penlight, gauze pads, gloves or finger cots, applicator sticks, and tongue depressors.

The Oral Cavity

The physical examination of the oral cavity includes inspection and palpation of the:

- Lips
- Buccal mucosa
- Teeth and gingivae
- Salivary glands
- Palate
- Floor of the mouth
- Tongue

The patient should be seated with the examiner seated or standing directly in front of him. The patient's face should be well illuminated. The examiner should work systematically from the front to the back so that no areas will be omitted. The examiner should put on a pair of gloves or finger cots when palpating any structure in the mouth. When any lesion is noted, its consistency and tenderness should be noted. If the patient is wearing dentures, he should be asked to remove them.

Inspect the Lips

The *color* of the lips should be assessed. Is cyanosis present? Are there any lesions on the lips? If a lesion is detected, careful palpation should be performed to characterize the lesion's texture and consistency. Plate VIII *B* shows a patient with multiple herpetic ulcers, commonly known as *cold sores,* on the lips and external nares. Plate XI *F* shows a patient with multiple telangiectatic lesions on her lips and tongue secondary to a condition known as Osler-Weber-Rendu syndrome.

Inspect the Buccal Mucosa

The patient should be asked to open his mouth widely. The mouth should be illuminated with a light source. The buccal mucosa must be evaluated for any lesions or color changes, and the buccal cavity is inspected for any evidence of asymmetry or areas of injection (dilated vessels usually indicative of inflammation). The buccal mucosa, teeth, and gingivae are easily evaluated by using a tongue depressor to pull the cheek away from the gums, as shown in Figure 9–8. Inspect for discolorations, evidence of trauma, and the condition of the parotid duct orifice. Are there any ulcerations of the buccal mucosa? Are there *white lesions* on the buccal mucosa? The most common painless white lesion in the mouth is *lichen planus,* which appears as a reticulated, or lace-like, eruption bilaterally on the buccal mucosa. An erosive variant is similar in appearance except for the presence of hemorrhagic and ulcerated lesions. A patient with nonerosive lichen planus is shown in Plate VIII *C.* Is *leukoplakia* present? Leukoplakia is a painless, precancerous white plaque on the mucous membranes of the cheeks, gums, and tongue.

Inspect the Gingivae

The gums are inspected. Are the gums swollen? Is there evidence of bleeding gums? Is gingival inflammation present? Is abnormal coloration present? Gingival hypertrophy is commonly seen in patients taking phenytoin (Dilantin), an anti-epilepsy medication. Another important cause of gingival hypertrophy is leukemia.

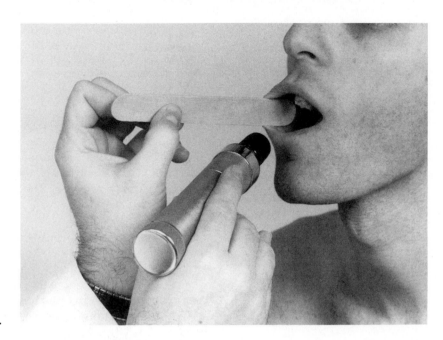

FIGURE 9–8. Inspection of the mouth.

Inspect the Teeth

The adult has 32 teeth in full dentition. The teeth should be inspected for caries and malocclusion. Is there any discoloration of the teeth? Is there tooth loss? Is bad breath present? Inspection of the teeth will often provide insight into the patient's attitude to general hygiene.

Evaluate the Salivary Glands

The ductal orifices of the parotid gland and the submandibular gland should be visualized. Inspect the condition of the papillae. Is there a flow of saliva? This is best evaluated by drying the papilla with a cotton applicator and observing the flow of saliva produced by exerting external pressure on the gland itself.

The salivary glands are usually not visible. Careful observation of the face will determine any asymmetry that is due to unilateral salivary gland enlargement. Obstruction to flow or infiltration of the gland will result in glandular enlargement. Plate VIII *D* illustrates a patient with parotid enlargement as a result of obstruction to flow.

Palpate the parotid and submandibular glands. Determine the consistency of each gland. Is tenderness present?

Inspect the Hard and Soft Palates

The palate should be inspected for ulceration or masses. Are there any white plaques present? Is the soft palate edematous? Is the uvula in the midline?

Are *petechiae* present? Petechiae (see Plate X *A*) are embolic phenomena commonly seen in association with subacute bacterial endocarditis or leukemia.

A common finding is a *torus palatinus*, which is an exostosis (a benign bony growth) in the midline of the hard palate. It is painless and asymptomatic.

Inspect the Floor of the Mouth

The flcor of the mouth is inspected by asking the patient to lift up his tongue to the roof of the mouth. Is there edema of the floor of the mouth? The opening of the submandibular gland, Wharton's duct, should be observed.

Examine the Tongue

Inspect the mucosa and note any masses. Is the tongue moist? Are there any mass lesions on the sides or undersurface of the tongue? Ask the patient to lift his tongue to the roof of the mouth so that the inferior aspect of the tongue may be inspected. In older individuals, the large veins on the ventral aspect of the tongue may become tortuous. These varicosities never bleed and have no clinical significance.

Is *candidiasis* present? Candidiasis, also known as moniliasis or *thrush,* is an opportunistic mycotic infection commonly associated with the use of broad spectrum antibiotics. It frequently involves the oral cavity, gastrointestinal tract, perineum, or vagina. The lesions appear as white, loosely adherent membranes, beneath which the mucosa is fiery red. Oral candidiasis is uncommon in healthy individuals who have not been on antibiotic therapy. The presence of thrush in such a patient may be an initial manifestation of AIDS. Candidiasis is the most common oral infection in AIDS patients. A patient with AIDS and oral candidiasis is shown in Plate VIII *E.*

Is leukoplakia present? A new form of leukoplakia termed *oral hairy leukoplakia* seems to be associated with the subsequent development of AIDS. The raised, white lesions appear corrugated or ''hairy'' and range in size from a few millimeters to 2 – 3 cm. They are most commonly found on the lateral margins of the tongue but may also be seen on the buccal mucosa. Plate VIII *F* shows an AIDS patient with hairy leukoplakia of the tongue.

Test Cranial Nerve XII

Ask the patient to stick out his tongue. Does the tongue deviate to one side? A *hypoglossal,* or twelfth cranial, nerve palsy does not allow the lingual muscles

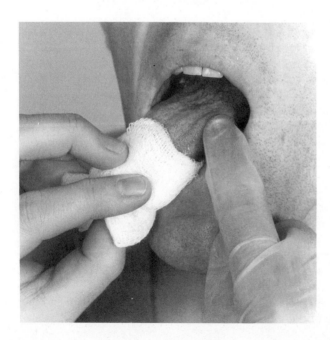

FIGURE 9–9. Palpation of the tongue.

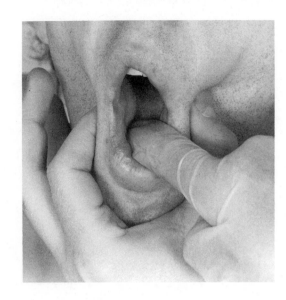

FIGURE 9-10. Technique for palpating oral structures.

on the affected side to contract normally. Consequently, the contralateral side "pushes" the tongue to the side of the lesion.

Palpate the Tongue

After a thorough inspection of the tongue, the examination proceeds with careful palpation. Palpation of the tongue is carried out by asking the patient to stick out his tongue onto a piece of gauze. The tongue is then held by the examiner's left hand as the sides of the tongue are inspected and palpated with the right hand. This is illustrated in Figure 9-9.

The anterior two thirds and the lateral margins of the tongue can be evaluated without causing a gag reflex. It is very important to palpate the lateral margins of the tongue, because over 85% of all lingual cancers arise in this area. All white lesions should be palpated. Is there evidence of induration (hardness)? Induration or ulceration strongly suggests carcinoma. After palpating the tongue, the tongue is unwrapped and the gauze is discarded.

Whenever palpating in a patient's mouth, the examiner should hold the patient's cheeks, as shown in Figure 9-10. This is a means of precaution in case the patient suddenly tries to speak or bite down on the examiner's finger.

Palpate the Floor of the Mouth

The floor of the mouth should be examined by bimanual palpation. This is performed by placing one finger under the tongue and another finger under the chin to assess any thickening or masses.

The Pharynx

Inspect the Pharynx

Examination of the pharynx is limited to inspection. In order to visualize the palate and oropharynx adequately, the examiner must usually depress the tongue with a tongue depressor stick. The patient is asked to open his mouth widely, stick out his tongue, and breathe slowly through his mouth. Occasion-

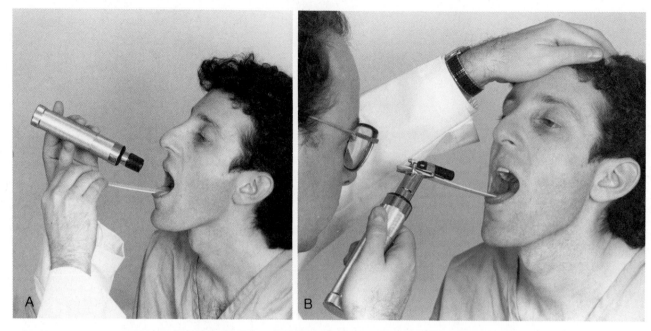

FIGURE 9–11. *A,* Use of the tongue depressor in inspecting the pharynx. *B,* Use of the tongue depressor attachment for inspecting the oral pharynx. Notice that the tongue blade is placed on the middle third of the tongue.

ally, leaving the tongue in the floor of the mouth will provide better visibility. The examiner should hold the tongue depressor in his right hand and a light source in his left. The tongue blade should be placed on the middle third of the tongue. The tongue is depressed and scooped forward. The examiner should be careful not to press the lower lip or tongue against the teeth with the tongue depressor. If the tongue depressor is placed too anteriorly, the posterior portion of the tongue will mound up, making inspection of the pharynx difficult; if placed too posteriorly, a gag reflex may result.

Is injection present? Is candidiasis present?

An accessory for the oto-ophthalmoscope handle is a light source that holds the tongue blade and makes the examination easier. Both techniques of holding the tongue depressor are shown in Figure 9–11.

Inspect the Tonsils

Evaluate tonsillar size. Tonsillar enlargement results from infection or tumor. In chronic tonsillar infection, the deep tonsillar crypts may contain cheese-like debris. Is there a *membrane* over the tonsils? A membrane is associated with acute tonsillitis, infectious mononucleosis, or diphtheria.

Inspect the Posterior Pharyngeal Wall

Is there a discharge, mass, ulceration, or injection present? Ask the patient to say "aahhh" as you observe for soft palate elevation.

Test Gag Reflex

At the end of the inspection, tell the patient that you are now going to test his gag reflex. The tip of the tongue depressor should gently touch the posterior

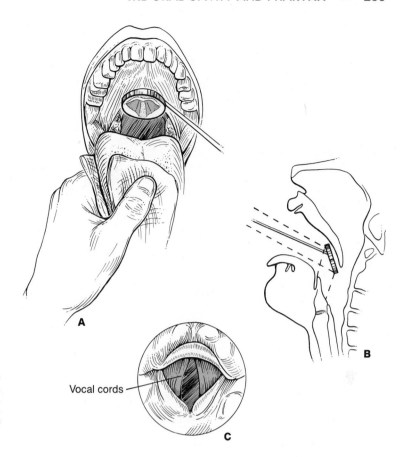

Vocal cords

FIGURE 9–12. Mirror laryngoscopy. *A* illustrates how the tongue is held and the placement of the mirror. *B* shows a cross-section through the pharynx, illustrating placement of the mirror. *C* shows the mirror reflection of the vocal cords.

surface of the tongue or the posterior pharyngeal wall. A rapid gag reflex should follow.

The Larynx

Using the Laryngeal Mirror

The tongue is held while a small, slightly warmed mirror is introduced into the mouth. The examiner should be careful that the mirror is not excessively warm and should avoid contact with the tongue. The patient is asked to breathe normally through his mouth. The mirror should be pushed upward against the uvula and positioned in the oropharynx. A beam of light can then be reflected off the mirror onto the internal laryngeal structures. This technique is shown in Figure 9–12.

Although the examination of the larynx is important, indirect laryngoscopy as just indicated is generally only performed by the specialist. Certainly, any patient having symptoms of laryngeal disease should be evaluated further.

CLINICOPATHOLOGIC CORRELATIONS

Lesions of the oral cavity are very common. Table 9–1 summarizes the important symptoms and signs of some of the most common etiologies. Table 20–6 lists the chronology of dentition.

TABLE 9–1. Symptoms and Signs of Oral Lesions

Lesion	Symptoms	Signs	Other Information
Aphthous ulcer (canker sore)	Painful, recurrent white sore with red border on lips, inner side of cheeks, tip and sides of tongue, or palate.	Single lesion 0.5–2 cm in diameter that first is maculopapular, but then ulcerates and has an area of erythema at its border. Lesions usually only on movable mucosal areas.	60% of population have periodic canker sores lasting up to 2 weeks. Etiology is unknown.
Herpetic ulcer (cold sore; fever blister) (see Plate VIII *B*)	Painful, recurrent sores on the lips.	Multiple papules, vesicles, or ulcers on the mucocutaneous junction, hard palate, or gingivae. As the bullae break, crusting occurs.	*Primary* herpetic infection in children under 16 months of age. Multiple lesions in clusters on fixed mucous membranes. Small, discrete, whitish vesicles prior to ulceration. Ulcers about 1 mm in diameter, which may coalesce. Tender lymphadenopathy, fever, and malaise present. Lip lesions represent the *recurrent* form, common in the adult. Self-limited illness, 1–2 weeks, in both the primary and recurrent forms.
Chancre	Painful sore on lips or tongue lasting for period of 2 weeks to 3 months.	Single ulcerated lesion with indurated border. Lesion without central necrotic material. Tender lymphadenitis may be present.	
Squamous cell carcinoma	Ulcerated sore of the lips, floor of the mouth, or tongue (especially lateral borders).	Single indurated lesion with indurated and raised border. Often in an area of leukoplakia. Absence of necrotic material in crater. Base often erythematous. Speech alterations may result if lesion is large. Painless lymphadenopathy may be present in neck. Evidence of distant metastasis may be present.	Frequently in alcoholics or smokers.
Erythema multiforme	Sudden onset of multiple burning ulcers in mouth or lips.	Hemorrhagic areas of ulceration with erythematous bases often with pseudomembrane. Lesions start as bullae. Skin involvement common (target lesions).	Many precipitating factors include drug reactions, viruses, endocrine changes, and an underlying malignancy. Most common in winter and spring in young adults. Frequently recurring.
Denture hyperplasia	Painless excess tissue at border of denture.	Spongy, redundant, often erythematous tissue with impression of edge of denture. Frequently seen on anterior maxillary mucosa.	

TABLE 9–1. Symptoms and Signs of Oral Lesions *(Continued)*

Lesion	Symptoms	Signs	Other Information
Candidiasis (moniliasis; thrush) (see Plate VIII *E*)	Burning areas of tongue, inside of cheek, or throat.	Whitish pseudomembrane, resembling milk curd, that can be peeled off, leaving a raw, erythematous area that may bleed.	Often seen in individuals who are chronically debilitated, patients who are immunosuppressed, or patients on long-term antibiotic therapy. Commonly seen in AIDS victims.
Leukoplakia (see Plate VIII *F*)	Painless white area on inside of cheek, tongue, lower lip, or floor of mouth.	Hyperkeratinized, whitish lesion that cannot be scraped off. Looks similar to flaking white paint. Often speckled with reddish areas. Associated adenopathy may indicate malignant changes of lesion.	Patients are usually men over the age of 40. Associated with smoking, AIDS, alcoholism, and chewing tobacco.
Lipoma	Slow growing, painless mass on inner surface of cheek.	Yellowish, nontender, soft mass. Freely mobile.	
Lichen planus (see Plate VIII *C*)	Usually no symptoms. Erosive form causes painful, burning sores of inner side of cheeks or tongue.	White lesions on buccal mucosa bilaterally in the form of reticulated papules in lace-like pattern. Erosive form appears as hemorrhagic, ulcerated lesion with possible white areas or bullae. Pseudomembrane may be present over lesion.	Non-erosive form is the most common cause of white lesions in the mouth. Skin involvement in 10–35% of patients. More frequently seen in patients with emotional stress.
Traumatic ulcer	Pain in an area of a sore. Short duration (1–2 weeks).	Single lesion with raised erythema at its border. Center often with necrotic debris. Occasionally purulent. Mild lymphadenitis may be present.	Patient can frequently relate the cause (e.g., biting cheek while eating).
Mucocele	Intermittent, painless swelling of the lower lip or inside of cheek. Slightly bluish. Occasionally ruptures.	Dome-shaped, 1–2 cm in diameter, freely mobile cystic lesion.	May be related to trauma or inflammation.
Hairy tongue	Gagging sensation associated with "hairy" sensation of tongue. Large, blackish, painless lesion on top of tongue.	Elongation of filiform papillae on the dorsum of tongue with a change in their color to almost black.	History of excessive antibiotic use, excessive use of mouthwash, poor oral hygiene, smoking, or alcohol is common.
Fordyce's spots	None	Clusters of small, yellowish, raised lesions best seen on the buccal mucosa opposite the molar teeth.	Common in older individuals. They are normal, hyperplastic sebaceous glands.

USEFUL VOCABULARY

Listed here are the specific roots that are important in order to understand the terminology related to diseases of the mouth and pharynx.

ROOT	PERTAINING TO	EXAMPLE	DEFINITION
arytenoid-	pitcher-shaped	*arytenoid*itis	Inflammation of the arytenoid cartilage
bucco-	cheek	*bucco*pharyngeal	Pertaining to the cheek and pharynx
dent-	tooth	*dent*al	Pertaining to the teeth
gingiv-	gums	*gingiv*ectomy	Surgical excision of diseased gum
gloss(o)-	tongue	*glosso*plegia	Paralysis of the tongue
-labi-	lips	naso*labi*al	Pertaining to the nose and lip
linguo-	tongue	*linguo*papillitis	Painful ulcers around the papillae of the tongue
ptyal-	saliva	*ptyal*ism	Excessive salivation
stoma-	mouth; opening	*stoma*titis	Inflammation of the mouth

WRITING UP THE PHYSICAL EXAMINATION

Listed here are examples of the write-up for the examinations of the oral cavity and pharynx.

The lips appear normal. The mucosa of the oral cavity is red and without masses, leukoplakia, or other lesions. There is good dentition and good dental hygiene. The tongue is midline and does not deviate to either side. The tonsils are absent. The pharynx appears normal.

There is a 1 – 2 cm, painful vesicular lesion at the mucocutaneous junction on the right side of the mouth. There is tonsillar hypertrophy with a purulent discharge in the crypts of both tonsils. There is bilateral anterior triangle lymphadenopathy, greater on the right. The remainder of the examination of the oral cavity is unremarkable.

There is a whitish pseudomembrane over the hard and soft palate, as well as over the tongue. When lifted, its erythematous base is friable and bleeds. The rest of the examination of the mouth and throat appears normal.

BIBLIOGRAPHY

Aronson AE: Clinical Voice Disorders: An Interdisciplinary Approach. New York, Thieme-Stratton, Inc, 1980.

Dayal VS: Clinical Otolaryngology. Philadelphia, JB Lippincott Co, 1981.

DeWeese D, Saunders W: Textbook of Otolaryngology. St. Louis, CV Mosby, 1973.

English GM: Otolaryngology. New York, Harper and Row, 1976.

Laguaite JK: Adult voice screening. J Speech Hear Disord 37:147, 1972.

Silverman EM, Zimmer CH: Incidence of chronic hoarseness among school-age children. J Speech Hear Disord 40:211, 1975.

Silverman S Jr, Migliorati CA, Lozada-Nur F, Greenspan D, Conant MA: Oral findings in people with or at high risk for AIDS: A study of 375 homosexual males. JADA 112:187, 1986.

Wood RP II, Northern JL: Manual of Otolaryngology. A Symptom-Oriented Text. Baltimore, Williams and Wilkins, 1979.

Zemlin WR: Speech and Hearing Science. Englewood Cliffs, NJ, Prentice-Hall, Inc, 1981.

THE CHEST

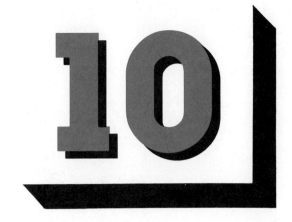

In the beginning the malady (tuberculosis) is easier to cure but difficult to detect, but later it becomes easy to detect but difficult to cure.

Niccolò Machiavelli
1469 – 1527

GENERAL CONSIDERATIONS

Oxygen is our breath of life, and without adequate lung function our lives cannot be sustained. Patients with pulmonary disease must work harder for adequate oxygenation. These patients complain of ''air hunger'' or ''too little air.'' Anyone who has traveled to areas of high altitude, where the oxygen concentration is reduced, has experienced shortness of breath.

The magnitude of pulmonary disease is enormous. It is estimated that over 80,000 individuals in the United States die yearly of chronic lung disease, over 5 million have some degree of pulmonary disability, and over 20 million have pulmonary symptoms (NIH Task Force Report, 1980). In 1967, the estimated cost of morbidity and mortality from lung disease was 1.8 billion dollars (National Heart and Lung Institute, 1972). By 1990, it is estimated that this figure will skyrocket to over 40 billion dollars.

Cancer of the lung is the leading cause of death from cancer in the United States. In 1986, there were nearly 150,000 new cases of lung cancer diagnosed, with over 130,000 deaths. In 1985, cancer of the lung was equal to cancer of the breast as the leading causes of death from cancer in women.

Pulmonary diseases arise when the lungs are unable to provide adequate oxygenation or to eliminate carbon dioxide. Any derangement of these functions indicates abnormal respiratory function.

During a 24 hour period, the lungs oxygenate over 6000 quarts of blood with over 12,000 quarts of air in the lungs. The total surface area of the alveoli of the lungs comprise an area larger than a tennis court.

STRUCTURE AND PHYSIOLOGY

The chest forms the bony case that houses and protects the lungs, the heart, and the esophagus as it passes into the stomach. The bony chest skeleton consists of 12 thoracic vertebrae, 12 pairs of ribs, the clavicle, and the sternum. The bony structure is shown in Figure 10–1.

The lungs continuously provide oxygen to and remove carbon dioxide from the circulatory system. The power required for breathing comes from the intercostal muscles and the diaphragm. The integrated action of these muscles acts as a bellows to suck air into the lungs. Expiration is passive. The control of breathing is complex and is controlled by the *breathing center* in the medulla of the brain.

Inspired air is warmed, filtered, and humidified by the upper respiratory passages. After passing through the cricoid cartilage of the larynx, air travels through a system of flexible tubes, the *trachea.* At the level of the fourth or fifth thoracic vertebrae, the trachea bifurcates into the *left* and *right bronchi.* The right bronchus is shorter, wider, and straighter than the left bronchus. The bronchi continue to subdivide into smaller bronchi, then into *bronchioles* within the lungs. Each respiratory bronchiole terminates in an *alveolar duct,* from which many *alveolar sacs* branch off. It is estimated that there are over 500 million alveoli in the lungs. Each alveolar wall contains elastin fibers that allow

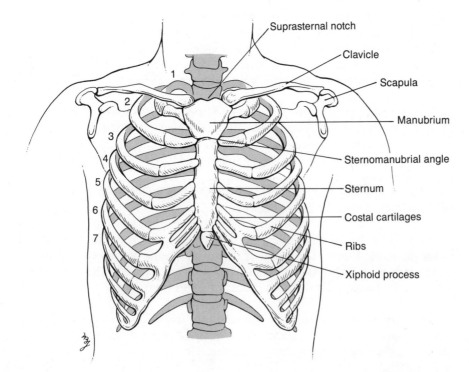

FIGURE 10–1. Bony chest skeleton.

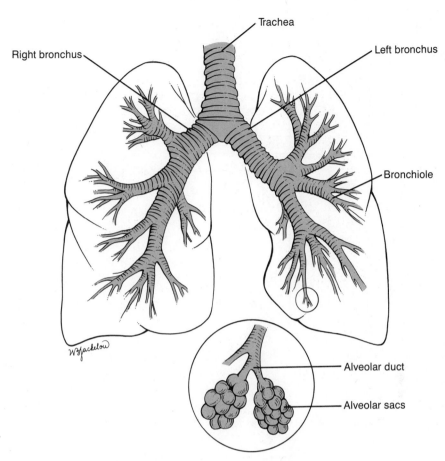

Figure 10-2. System of air conducting passages.

the sac to expand with inspiration and to contract with expiration by *elastic recoil*. This system of air conducting passages is shown in Figure 10-2.

The lungs are subdivided into lobes: the *upper, middle,* and *lower* on the *right,* and the *upper* and *lower* on the left. The lungs are enveloped in a thin sac, the *pleura.* The *visceral* pleura overlies the lung parenchyma, whereas the *parietal* pleura lines the chest wall. The two pleural surfaces glide over each other during inspiration and expiration. The space between the pleura is the pleural cavity.

In order to describe physical signs within the chest accurately, the examiner must understand the topographic landmarks of the chest wall. The landmarks of clinical importance are as follows:

- Sternum
- Clavicle
- Suprasternal notch
- Sternomanubrial angle
- Midsternal line
- Midclavicular lines
- Anterior axillary lines
- Midaxillary lines
- Posterior axillary lines
- Scapular lines
- Midspinal line

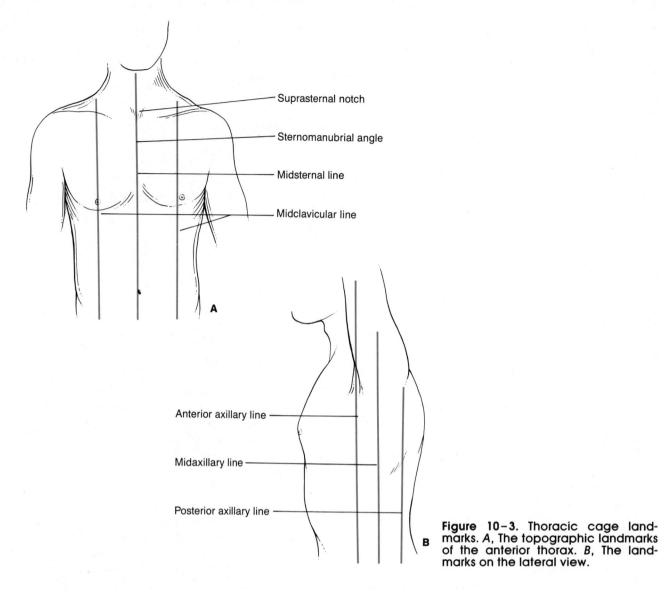

Figure 10-3. Thoracic cage landmarks. *A,* The topographic landmarks of the anterior thorax. *B,* The landmarks on the lateral view.

Figure 10-3 shows the anterior thorax and lateral views, and Figure 10-4 shows the posterior thorax.

The *suprasternal notch* is located at the top of the sternum and can be felt as a depression at the base of the neck. The *sternomanubrial angle* is often referred to as the *angle of Louis.* This bony ridge lies approximately 5 cm below the suprasternal notch. When you move your fingers off the ridge laterally, the adjacent rib is the second rib. The interspace below the second rib is the *second intercostal space.* Using this as a reference point, you should be able to identify the ribs and interspaces anteriorly. Try it on yourself.

In order to identify areas, several imaginary lines are drawn on the anterior and posterior chest. The *midsternal line* is drawn through the middle of the sternum. The *midclavicular lines* are those drawn through the middle points of the clavicles and parallel to the midsternal line. The *anterior axillary lines* are vertical lines drawn along the anterior axillary folds parallel to the midsternal line. The *midaxillary lines* are drawn from each vertex of the axillae parallel to

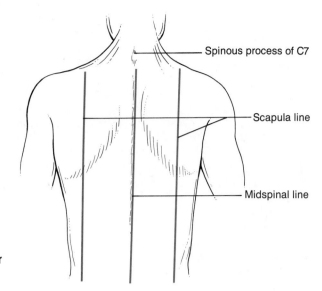

Spinous process of C7

Scapula line

Midspinal line

Figure 10–4. The topographic landmarks of the posterior thorax.

the midsternal line. The *posterior axillary lines* are parallel to the midsternal line and travel vertically along the posterior axillary folds. The *scapular lines* are parallel to the midspinal line and pass through the inferior angles of the scapulae. The *midspinal line* is a vertical line that passes through the posterior spinous processes of the vertebrae.

Rib counting from the posterior chest is slightly more complicated. The inferior wing of the *scapula* lies at the level of the seventh rib or interspace. Another useful landmark can be found by having the patient flex his neck; the most prominent cervical spinous process, the *vertebra prominens*, protrudes from the seventh cervical vertebra.

It is important to remember that only the first seven ribs articulate with the sternum. The eighth through tenth ribs articulate with the cartilage above. The eleventh and twelfth ribs are *floating* ribs and have a free anterior portion.

The *interlobar fissures*, shown in Figure 10–5, are situated between the lobes of the lungs. Both the right and left lungs have an *oblique fissure*, which begins on the anterior chest at the level of the sixth rib at the midclavicular line and extends laterally upward to the fifth rib in the midaxillary line, ending at the posterior chest at the spinous process of T3. The right lower lobe is located below the right oblique fissure; the right upper and middle lobes are superior to the right oblique fissure. The left lower lobe is below the left oblique fissure; the left upper lobe is superior to the left oblique fissure. The *horizontal fissure* is present only on the right and divides the right upper lobe from the right middle lobe. It extends from the fourth rib at the sternal border to the fifth rib at the midaxillary line.

The lungs extend superiorly about 3–4 cm above the medial end of the clavicles. The inferior margins of the lungs extend to the sixth rib at the midclavicular line, the eighth rib at the midaxillary line, and between T9 and T12 posteriorly. This variation is related to respiration. The bifurcation of the trachea, the *carina*, is located behind the angle of Louis at approximately level T4 on the posterior chest. The *right hemidiaphragm* at the end of expiration is located at the level of the fifth rib anteriorly and T9 posteriorly. The presence of

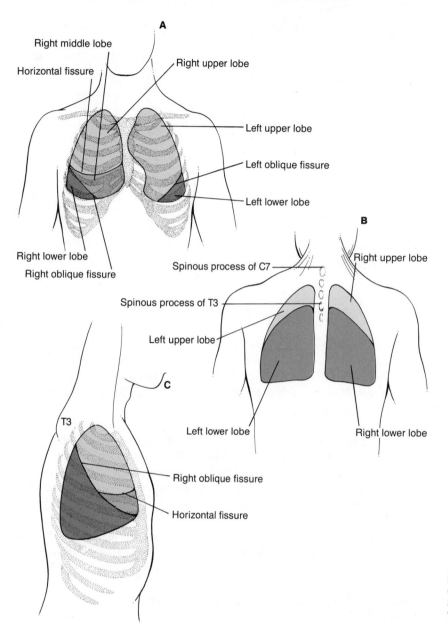

Figure 10–5. Surface topography and the underlying interlobar fissures. *A*, Anterior view. *B*, Posterior view. *C*, Lateral view.

the liver on the right side makes the right hemidiaphragm slightly higher than the left.

During quiet breathing, muscle contraction occurs only during inspiration. Expiration is passive, resulting from the elastic recoil of the lungs and chest.

REVIEW OF SPECIFIC SYMPTOMS

The main symptoms of pulmonary disease are the following:

- Cough
- Sputum production

- Hemoptysis (coughing up blood)
- Dyspnea (shortness of breath)
- Wheezing
- Cyanosis (bluish discoloration of the skin)
- Chest pain

Cough

The most common symptom of lung disease is the cough. Coughing is so common that it is frequently regarded as a trivial complaint. The cough reflex is a normal defense mechanism of the lungs that serves to protect the lungs from foreign bodies and excessive secretions. Infections of the upper respiratory tract are associated with coughing that usually improves in 2–3 weeks. A persistent cough deserves further investigation.

Coughing is a coordinated, forced expiration, interrupted by repeated closure of the glottis. The expiratory muscles contract against the partially closed glottis, creating high pressure within the lungs. When the glottis suddenly opens, there is an explosive rush of air that clears the air passages. When a patient complains of coughing, it is important to ask these questions:

"Can you describe your cough?"
"How long have you had a cough?"
"Was there a sudden onset of coughing?"
"Do you smoke?" If so, *"How much, and for how long?"*
"Does your cough produce sputum?" If so, *"Can you estimate the amount of your expectorations? What is the color of the sputum? Does the sputum have a foul order?"*
"Does the cough occur for prolonged periods?"
"Does the cough occur after eating?"
"Is the coughing worse in any position?"
"What relieves the cough?"
"Are there any other symptoms associated with the cough? . . . fever? . . . headaches? . . . night sweats? . . . chest pain? . . . a runny nose? . . . shortness of breath? . . . weight loss? . . . hoarseness? . . . loss of consciousness?"
"Do you have any birds as pets? Do you feed pigeons?"
"Have you ever been exposed to anyone with tuberculosis?"

Coughing may be voluntary or involuntary, productive or nonproductive. A *productive* cough is one in which mucus or other materials are expelled. A *dry* cough is one that does not produce any secretions.

Smoking is probably the most common cause of the chronic cough. Smoker's cough results from inhalation of irritants in tobacco and is most marked in the morning. Coughing is normally decreased during sleep. When the smoker awakens in the morning, productive coughing tends to clear the respiratory passages. Coughing decreases and may disappear in patients who stop smoking.

Coughing may also be *psychogenic*. This nonproductive cough occurs in individuals with emotional stress. When attention is drawn to it, the cough increases. During sleep, or when the patient is distracted, the coughing stops. Psychogenic coughing is a *diagnosis of exclusion:* only after all other causes of coughing have been eliminated can this diagnosis be made.

TABLE 10–1. Descriptors of Coughing

Description	Possible Causes
Dry, hacking	Viral infections, interstitial lung disease, tumor, allergies, anxiety
Chronic productive	Bronchiectasis, chronic bronchitis, abscess, bacterial pneumonia, tuberculosis
Wheezing	Bronchospasm, asthma, allergies
Barking	Epiglottal disease (e.g., croup)
Stridor	Tracheal obstruction
Morning	Smoking
Nocturnal	Postnasal drip, congestive heart failure
Associated with eating or drinking	Neuromuscular disease of the upper esophagus
Inadequate	Debility, weakness

There are many terms used by patients and physicians to describe a cough. Table 10–1 provides a list of some of the more common descriptors and their possible causes.

Sputum Production

Sputum is the substance expelled by coughing. Approximately 75–100 ml of sputum is secreted daily by the bronchi. By ciliary action, it is brought up to the throat and then swallowed unconsciously with the saliva. An increase in the quantity of sputum production is the earliest manifestation of bronchitis. Sputum may contain cellular debris, mucus, blood, pus, or microorganisms.

Sputum should be described according to color, consistency, quantity, occurrences during the day, and the presence or absence of blood. An adequate description may provide a cause of the disease process. Uninfected sputum is odorless, transparent, and whitish-gray, resembling mucus; it is termed *mucoid.* Infected sputum contains pus and is termed *purulent;* the sputum may be yellow, greenish, or red. Table 10–2 lists the appearances of sputum and their possible causes.

TABLE 10–2. Appearances of Sputum

Appearance	Possible Causes
Mucoid	Asthma, tumors, tuberculosis, emphysema
Mucopurulent	As above, pneumonia
Yellow-green purulent	Bronchiectasis, chronic bronchitis
Rusty purulent	Pneumococcal pneumonia
Red currant jelly	*Klebsiella pneumoniae*
Foul odor	Lung abscess
Pink, blood tinged	Streptococcal or staphylococcal pneumonia
Gravel	Broncholithiasis
Pink, frothy	Pulmonary edema
Profuse, colorless (also known as bronchorrhea)	Alveolar cell carcinoma
Bloody	Pulmonary emboli, bronchiectasis, abscess, tuberculosis, tumor, cardiac causes, bleeding disorders

Hemoptysis

Hemoptysis is the coughing up of blood. Few symptoms produce as much alarm in patients as does hemoptysis. The careful description of the hemoptysis is crucial, because the term "hemoptysis" includes both clots of blood as well as blood-tinged sputum. The implications of each are very different. Coughing up clots of blood is a symptom of extreme importance, because it often heralds a serious illness. Clots of blood are generally associated with a cavitary lung lesion, a tumor of the lung, certain cardiac diseases, or pulmonary embolism. Blood-tinged sputum is usually associated with smoking or minor infections *but* can be seen with tumors or more serious diseases as well. When a patient complains of hemoptysis, it is important to ask the following questions:

"Do you smoke?"
"Did the coughing up of blood occur suddenly?"
"Have there been recurrent episodes of coughing up blood?"
"Is the sputum blood tinged, or are there actual clots of blood?"
"For how long have you noticed the blood?"
"What seems to bring on the coughing up of blood? . . . vomiting? . . . coughing? . . . nausea?"
"Have you ever had tuberculosis?"
"Is there a family history of coughing up blood?"
"Have you had recent surgery?"
"Do you take any 'blood thinners'?"
"Are you aware of any bleeding tendency?"
"Have you had night sweats? . . . shortness of breath? . . . palpitations? . . . irregular heartbeats? . . . hoarseness? . . . weight loss? . . . swelling or pain in your legs?"
"Have you felt any unusual sensation in your chest after coughing up blood?" If so, *"Where?"*
For the woman with hemoptysis, *"Do you use oral contraceptives?"*

Any suppurative (associated with the production of pus) process of the airways or lungs can produce hemoptysis. Bronchitis is probably the most common cause of hemoptysis. Bronchiectasis and bronchogenic carcinoma are also major causes. Hemoptysis results from mucosal invasion, tumor necrosis, or pneumonia distal to bronchial obstruction by tumor. Pneumococcal pneumonia characteristically produces "rusty" colored sputum. Pink and frothy sputum can result from pulmonary edema.

Occasionally, patients have a warm sensation within their chest at the location from which the hemoptysis has originated. Therefore, it is useful to ask a patient who has had recent hemoptysis whether he has experienced such a sensation. This information may direct you to a more careful review of the physical examination and x-ray in that area.

Patients who have had recent surgery are at risk for deep vein thrombophlebitis with pulmonary embolism. Women taking oral contraceptives are likewise at risk for pulmonary embolic disease. Hemoptysis occurs when pulmonary emboli result in infarction with necrosis of the pulmonary parenchyma.

Recurrent episodes of hemoptysis may result from bronchiectasis, tuberculosis, or mitral stenosis. Atrial fibrillation is a common cause of "irregular heartbeats" and embolic phenomena.

TABLE 10–3. Characteristics Distinguishing Hemoptysis from Hematemesis

Features	Hemoptysis	Hematemesis
Prodrome	Coughing	Nausea and vomiting
Past history	Possible history of cardiopulmonary disease	Possible history of gastrointestinal disease
Appearance	Frothy	Not frothy
Color	Bright red	Dark red, brown, or "coffee grounds"
Mixed with	Pus	Food
Associated symptoms	Dyspnea	Nausea

At times, it may be difficult to ascertain whether the patient coughed up or vomited blood. Most patients can provide a sufficiently clear history. Table 10–3 lists characteristics that help distinguish hemoptysis from hematemesis (vomiting blood).

Dyspnea

The *subjective* sensation of "shortness of breath" is termed *dyspnea.* Dyspnea is an important manifestation of cardiopulmonary disease, although it is found in other states such as neurologic, metabolic, and psychological conditions. It is important to differentiate dyspnea from the *objective* finding of *tachypnea,* or rapid breathing. A patient may be observed to be breathing rapidly, while stating that he is not short of breath. The converse is also true: a patient may be breathing slowly but may have dyspnea. Never assume that a patient with a rapid respiratory rate is dyspneic.

It is important for the examiner to inquire when dyspnea occurs and in which position. *Paroxysmal nocturnal dyspnea* (PND) is the sudden onset of shortness of breath occurring at night while a patient sleeps. The patient suddenly is seized with an intense strangling sensation. He frantically sits up and, classically, runs to the window for "air." As soon as the patient assumes an upright position, his dyspnea usually improves. *Orthopnea* is difficulty in breathing while lying flat. The patient requires two or more pillows to breathe comfortably. *Platypnea* is a rare symptom of difficulty in breathing while sitting up and is relieved by a recumbent position. *Trepopnea* is a condition in which the patient is more comfortable breathing while lying on his side. (Some of the more common causes of positional dyspnea are listed in Table 10–4.) It is important to ask all patients complaining of dyspnea the following questions:

> *"For how long have you had shortness of breath?"*
> *"Did the shortness of breath occur suddenly?"*
> *"Is the shortness of breath constant?"*
> *"Does the shortness of breath occur with exertion? . . . at rest? . . . lying flat? . . . sitting up?"*
> *"What makes the shortness of breath worse? What relieves it?"*
> *"How many level blocks can you walk without becoming short of breath? How many could you walk 6 months ago?"*
> *"Is the shortness of breath accompanied by wheezing? . . . fever? . . . cough? . . . coughing up blood? . . . chest pain? . . . palpitations? . . . hoarseness?"*

TABLE 10-4. Positional Dyspnea

Type	Possible Causes
Orthopnea	Congestive heart failure
	Mitral valvular disease
	Severe asthma, rarely
	Emphysema, rarely
	Chronic bronchitis, rarely
	Neurologic diseases, rarely
Trepopnea	Congestive heart failure
Platypnea	Status post-pneumonectomy
	Neurologic diseases
	Cirrhosis (intrapulmonary shunts)
	Hypovolemia

"Do you smoke?" If so, *"How much? For how long?"*
"Have you had any exposure to asbestos? . . . sandblasting?
. . . pigeon breeding?"
"Have you had any exposure to individuals with tuberculosis?"
"Have you ever lived near the San Joaquin valley? . . . midwestern or
southeastern United States?"

It is essential to try to quantify the dyspnea. Questions such as *"How many level blocks can you walk?"* provide a framework for *exercise tolerance.* For example, if the patient answers, *"2 blocks,"* he is said to have *2 block dyspnea on exertion* (DOE). The interviewer can then ask, *"How many level blocks were you able to walk 6 months ago?"* The interviewer can now make a rough assessment of the progression of the disease or the efficacy of therapy.

Careful questioning regarding *industrial exposure* is paramount in any patient with unexplained dyspnea. Examples of further questions regarding occupational and environmental history are discussed in Chapter 1. Exposure to pigeons may result in psittacosis. Outbreaks of coccidioidomycosis have occurred in individuals living in the southwestern United States. Living in the midwestern and southeastern United States has been associated with outbreaks of histoplasmosis.

Wheezing

Wheezing is an abnormally high-pitched noise resulting from a partially obstructed airway. It is usually present during expiration when slight bronchoconstriction occurs physiologically. Bronchospasm, mucosal edema, loss of elastic support, and tortuosity of the airways are the usual causes. Asthma causes bronchospasm, which is the cause of the wheezing associated with this condition. Obstruction by intraluminal material, such as aspirated foreign bodies or secretions, is another important cause of wheezing. A well-localized wheeze, unchanged by coughing, may indicate a partially obstructed bronchus by a foreign body or tumor. When a patient complains of wheezing, the examiner must determine the following:

"At what age did the wheezing begin?"
"How often does it occur?"
"Are there any precipitating factors, such as foods, odors, emotions, animals, etc.?"
"What usually stops the attack?"
"Have the symptoms worsened over the years?"
"Are there any associated symptoms?"
"Is there a history of nasal polyps?"
"What is the smoking history?"
"Is there a history of heart disease?"

An important axiom to remember is

> **Asthma is associated with wheezing, but not all wheezing is asthma!**

Do not equate wheezing with asthma. As will be indicated subsequently, congestive heart failure is usually associated with abnormal breath sounds called crackles. Sometimes there is such severe bronchospasm in heart failure that the main physical finding is a wheeze and not a crackle.

A decrease in wheezing may result from either an opening up of the airway or a progressive closing off of the air passage. A "silent" chest in a patient with an acute asthmatic attack is generally a bad sign: it indicates worsening of the obstruction.

Cyanosis

Cyanosis is commonly detected by a family member. The subtle bluish discoloration may go completely unnoticed by the patient. *Central* cyanosis occurs with inadequate gas exchange in the lungs resulting in a significant reduction in arterial oxygenation. Primary pulmonary problems or diseases that cause mixed venous blood to bypass the lungs (e.g., intracardiac shunt) are frequently the cause. The bluish discoloration is best seen in the mucous membranes of the mouth (e.g., the frenulum) and lips. *Peripheral* cyanosis results from an excessive extraction of oxygen at the periphery. It is limited to cyanosis of the extremities (e.g., the fingers, toes, nose). Ask the following questions:

"Where is the cyanosis present?"
"For how long has the cyanosis been present?"
"Are you aware of any lung problem? . . . heart problem? . . . blood problem?"
"What makes the cyanosis worse?"
"Is there associated shortness of breath? . . . cough? . . . bleeding?"
"What types of work have you performed?"
"Is there anyone else in your family who has cyanosis?"

Cyanosis from birth is associated with congenital heart lesions. The acute development of cyanosis can occur in severe respiratory disease, especially acute airway obstruction. Peripheral cyanosis is due to increased oxygen extraction in low cardiac states and is seen in cooler areas of the body such as the nail beds and the outer surfaces of the lips. Peripheral cyanosis disappears as the area is warmed. Cyanosis of the nails and warm hands are suggestive that the cyanosis is central. Central cyanosis occurs only after the oxygen saturation has fallen to below 80%. Central cyanosis diffusely involves the skin *and* mucous membranes and does not disappear with warming of the area. At least 5 gm unsaturated hemoglobin per 100 ml of blood must be present for the patient to manifest central cyanosis. Exercise worsens central cyanosis, because the exercising muscles require an increased extraction of oxygen from the blood. In patients with severe anemia, in whom hemoglobin levels are markedly decreased, cyanosis may not be seen. Clubbing is seen in association with central cyanosis and significant cardiopulmonary pathology.

Some workers, such as arc welders, inhale toxic levels of nitrous gases that can produce cyanosis by methemoglobinemia. Hereditary methemoglobinemia is a primary hemoglobin abnormality causing congenital cyanosis.

Chest Pain

Chest pain related to pulmonary disease generally results from involvement of the chest wall or parietal pleura. Nerve fibers are abundant in this area. *Pleuritic pain* is a common symptom of inflammation of the parietal pleura. It is described as a sharp, stabbing pain, which is usually felt in inspiration. It may be localized to one side, and the patient may *splint** to avoid the pain. Chapter 11, The Heart, summarizes the important questions to ask a patient complaining of chest pain.

Acute dilatation of the main pulmonary artery may also produce a dull pressure sensation, often indistinguishable from angina pectoris. This results from nerve endings responding to the stretch on the main pulmonary artery.

Although chest pain is seen in pulmonary disease, chest pain is the cardinal symptom of cardiac disease and is discussed more completely in the next chapter.

Other Symptoms

In addition to the just cited main symptoms of pulmonary disease, there are other, less common symptoms. These include the following:

- Stridor (noisy breathing)
- Voice changes
- Swelling of the ankles (dependent edema)

Stridor is a harsh type of noisy breathing and is generally associated with obstruction of a major bronchus that occurs with aspiration. Voice changes can occur with inflammation of the vocal cords or interference with the recurrent laryngeal nerve. Swelling of the ankles is a manifestation of dependent edema, which is associated with right heart failure, renal disease, liver disease, or obstruction of venous flow. As the condition worsens, abnormal accumulations of fluid produce generalized edema, known as *anasarca.*

---

* Splinting is making the muscles rigid to avoid motion of that part of the chest.

IMPACT OF LUNG DISEASE ON THE PATIENT

The impact of lung disease on the patient varies greatly with the nature of the ailment. The subjective sensation of air hunger varies considerably. Some patients with lung disease are hardly aware of their dyspnea. The decrease in exercise tolerance is so insidious that these patients may not be aware of any problem. Only when asked to try to quantify the dyspnea can these patients realize their deficiency. In other patients, dyspnea is so rapidly progressive that they can experience severe depression. They recognize that little can be done to improve their lung condition, thus markedly altering their lifestyle. They become incapacitated, and many are forced to retire from work. They can no longer experience the slightest exertion without becoming dyspneic.

Often patients develop chronic lung disease secondary to occupational hazards. These patients are embittered and hostile. Today there is much publicity about occupational exposure, but there are still industries that provide little protection for their employees.

Chronic obstructive pulmonary disease (COPD) is a form of lung disease that can be subdivided into two types: emphysema and chronic bronchitis. Both are characterized by a slowly progressive course, obstruction to airflow, and destruction of the lung parenchyma. Classically, the patient with emphysema is the "pink puffer." He is thin and weak, having severe dyspnea associated with little cough and sputum production. The classic "blue bloater" suffers primarily from bronchitis. He is cyanotic and has a productive cough but is less troubled by dyspnea. He is short and stocky. These classic descriptions are interesting, but most patients with COPD have characteristics of both types.

Since early times, clinicians have recognized that emotional factors play a role in the onset and maintenance of symptoms in bronchial asthma. Attacks of asthma can be provoked by a wide range of emotions: fear, anger, anxiety, depression, guilt, frustration, joy. It is the patient's attempt to suppress the emotion, rather than the emotion itself, that precipitates the asthmatic attack (Rees, 1956).

The patient having an asthmatic attack becomes anxious and fearful, producing a vicious cycle that tends to perpetuate the attack. Hyperventilation may contribute to the breathlessness of the frightened patient. Despite being given adequate medical therapy, these patients remain dyspneic. In such patients, it is the *anxiety* and its causes that require attention. They need continuing medical *and* psychological support after the acute attack. Even as early as in the twelfth century, Maimonides recognized that "mere diet and medical treatment cannot fully cure this disorder."

The child with asthma presents a special problem. Anxiety, underachievement, peer pressure, and noncompliance with medications all contribute to exacerbate episodes of asthma. The child is absent from school more than his nonasthmatic peers, causing his school work to suffer; this creates another vicious cycle. The incidence of emotional disorders is greater than twofold in asthmatic school-aged children compared with the general population (Mattson, 1975).

Asthma can affect a person's sexual function physiologically as well as psychologically. The asthmatic patient may become more dyspneic as a result of the increased physical demands of sexual intercourse. Bronchospasm may occur, owing to excitement, anxiety, or panic (Conine and Evans, 1981). Anxiety about precipitating an asthmatic attack during sexual intercourse worsens the patient's dyspnea and sexual performance; another vicious cycle is set into motion. Patients may then tend to avoid sexual intercourse.

PHYSICAL EXAMINATION

> The equipment necessary for the examination of the chest is a stethoscope.

After a general assessment of the patient, the examination of the posterior chest is performed while the patient is still seated. The patient's arms should be folded in his lap. After the completion of the examination of the posterior chest, the patient is asked to lie down and the examination of the anterior chest is begun. During the examination, it is important for the examiner to try to imagine the underlying lung areas.

If the patient is a man, his gown should be removed to his waist. If the patient is a woman, the gown should be positioned to prevent unnecessary or embarrassing exposure of the breasts. The examiner should stand facing the patient.

The examination of the anterior and posterior aspects of the chest includes the following:

- Inspection
- Palpation
- Percussion
- Auscultation

General Assessment

Inspect the Patient's Facial Expression

Is the patient in acute distress? Is there nasal flaring* or pursed lip breathing? Are there audible signs of breathing, such as stridor and wheezing? These are related to obstruction to air flow.

Is cyanosis present?

Inspect the Patient's Posture

Patients with airway obstructive disease tend to prefer a position in which they can support their arms and fix the muscles of the shoulder and neck to aid in respiration. A common technique used by patients with bronchial obstruction is to clasp the sides of the bed and use the latissimus dorsi muscle to help overcome the increased resistance to outflow during expiration. Patients with orthopnea are seated or are lying on several pillows.

---

* Nasal flaring is the outward motion of the nares during inhalation. This is seen in any condition causing an increase in the work of breathing.

Inspect the Neck

Is the patient's breathing aided by the action of the *accessory muscles?* Use of the accessory muscles is one of the earliest signs of airway obstruction. In respiratory distress, the trapezius and sternocleidomastoid muscles contract during inspiration. The accessory muscles assist in ventilation, as they raise the clavicle and anterior chest to increase the lung volume and produce an increased negative intrathoracic pressure. This results in retraction of the supraclavicular fossae and intercostal muscles. An upward motion of the clavicle of more than 5 mm during respiration has been associated with *severe obstructive lung disease* (Anderson et al, 1980).

Inspect the Configuration of the Chest

A variety of conditions may interfere with adequate ventilation, and the configuration of the chest may indicate lung disease. An increase in the *antero-posterior* (AP) *diameter* is seen in advanced COPD. The AP diameter tends to equal the lateral diameter, and a *barrel chest* results. The ribs lose their 45° angle and become more horizontal. A *flail chest* is a chest configuration in which one chest wall moves paradoxically inward during inspiration. This condition is seen with multiple rib fractures. *Kyphoscoliosis* is a spinal deformity in which there is an abnormal AP and lateral curvature of the spine producing a severe restriction of chest and lung expansion. A *pectus excavatum,* or funnel chest, is a depression of the sternum, which will produce a restrictive lung problem only if the depression is marked. *Pectus carinatum,* or pigeon breast, which results from an anterior protrusion of the sternum, is a common deformity but does not compromise ventilation. Figure 10–6 illustrates the various configurations of the chest.

Assess the Respiratory Rate and Pattern

Never ask the patient to breathe "normally" when you assess respiratory rate. Individuals will voluntarily change their breathing pattern and rate once they are aware of it. A better way is, after taking the radial pulse, to direct your

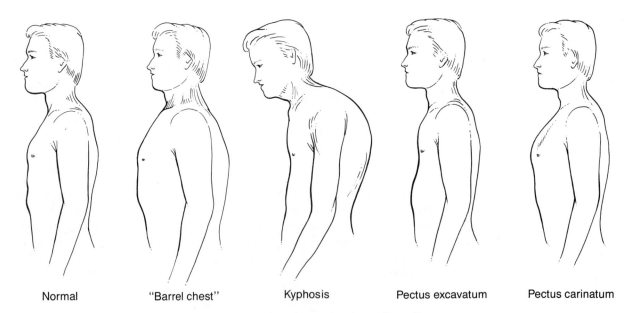

| Normal | "Barrel chest" | Kyphosis | Pectus excavatum | Pectus carinatum |

Figure 10–6. Common chest configurations.

eyes to the chest and evaluate the respirations while still holding the wrist. The patient is unaware that you are no longer taking the pulse, and voluntary changes in breathing will not occur. Counting the number of respirations in a 30 second period and multiplying this number by 2 will provide an accurate respiratory rate.

The normal adult takes about 10–14 breaths a minute. *Bradypnea* is an abnormal slowing of respiration; *tachypnea* is an abnormal increase. *Apnea* is the temporary cessation of breathing. The term *hyperpnea* is an increased depth of breathing, usually associated with metabolic acidosis. It is also known as *Kussmaul's breathing*. There are many types of abnormal breathing patterns. (Figure 10–22 illustrates and lists the more common types of abnormal breathing.)

Inspect the Hands

Is *clubbing* present? The technique for the evaluation of clubbing is described in Chapter 5, The Skin. The earliest finding of clubbing is the loss of the angle between the nail and the terminal phalanx. Look at Plate IX *A* comparing a normal index finger with a severely clubbed index finger of a patient with bronchogenic carcinoma.

Clubbing has been associated with a number of clinical disorders, such as the following:

- Intrathoracic tumors
- Mixed venous-to-arterial shunts
- Chronic pulmonary disease
- Chronic hepatic fibrosis

The pathogenesis of clubbing is unclear. In many of the first cited conditions, however, arterial desaturation occurs. This, in some way, may be the underlying problem.

Posterior Chest

You should now move to the back of the patient to examine the posterior chest.

Palpation is the "laying on of hands." Palpation is used in examination of the chest to assess the following:

- Areas of tenderness
- Symmetry of chest excursion
- Tactile fremitus

Palpate for Tenderness

All chest areas should be evaluated for areas of tenderness. Gently hit the patient's back with your fist. A complaint of "chest pain" may be related only to local musculoskeletal disease and not to disease of the heart or lungs. Be meticulous in assessing for areas of tenderness.

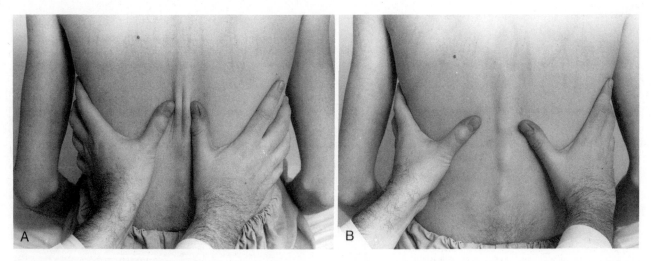

Figure 10-7. Technique for evaluating posterior chest excursion. *A,* Placement of the hands during normal expiration. *B,* Their location after normal inspiration.

Evaluate Posterior Chest Excursion

The degree of symmetry of chest excursion may be determined by placing your hands flat against the patient's back with the thumbs parallel to the midline at approximately the level of the tenth ribs and pulling the underlying skin slightly toward the midline. The patient is asked to inhale deeply, and the movement of the hands is noted. Symmetry of hand movement should be noted. Localized pulmonary disease may cause one side of the chest to move less than the opposite side. The placement of the hands is shown in Figure 10-7.

The Principle of Tactile Fremitus

The spoken word creates vibrations that can be heard when one listens to the chest and lungs. This is termed *vocal fremitus*. When one palpates the chest wall while an individual is speaking, these vibrations can be felt. This is *tactile fremitus*. Sound is conducted from the larynx through the bronchial tree to the lung parenchyma and the chest wall. Tactile fremitus provides useful information about the density of the underlying lung tissue and chest cavity. Conditions that increase the density of the lung and make it more solid, such as consolidation, increase the transmission of tactile fremitus. Clinical states that decrease the transmission of these sound waves will reduce tactile fremitus. If there is excess fat tissue on the chest, air or fluid in the chest cavity, or an overexpanded lung, tactile fremitus will be diminished.

Evaluate Tactile Fremitus

Tactile fremitus can be evaluated in one of two ways. The first technique involves the examiner placing the ulnar side of the right hand against the chest wall, as shown in Figure 10-8, and asking the patient to say "ninety-nine." Tactile fremitus is evaluated, and the examiner's hand is moved to the corresponding position on the other side. Tactile fremitus is then compared with the opposite side. By moving the hand from side to side and from top to bottom, the examiner can detect differences in the transmission of the sound to the chest wall. "Ninety-nine" is one of the phrases used because it causes good vibratory tones. Asking the patient to speak either louder or deeper will enhance the tactile sensation. Tactile fremitus should be evaluated in the five or six locations shown in Figure 10-9.

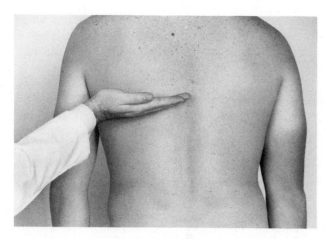

Figure 10–8. Technique for evaluating tactile fremitus.

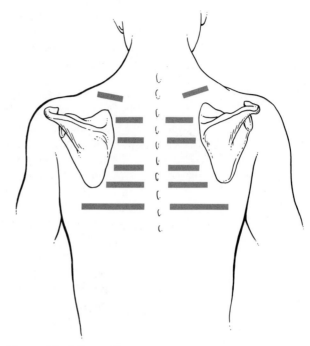

Figure 10–9. Locations on the posterior chest for evaluating tactile fremitus.

The other method of evaluating tactile fremitus uses the finger tips instead of the ulnar side of the hand. The same side to side and top to bottom positions as shown in Figure 10–9 are used. It is only necessary to perform one of these techniques. The examiner should try both methods initially to determine which one he prefers.

Table 10–5 provides a list of some of the important pathologic causes for changes in tactile fremitus.

The Principle of Percussion

Percussion refers to the tapping on a surface to determine the underlying structure. It is very similar to a radar or echo detection system. Tapping on the chest wall is transmitted to the underlying tissue, reflected back, and picked up by the examiner's tactile and auditory senses. The sound heard and the tactile

TABLE 10–5. Tactile Fremitus

Increased	Decreased
Pneumonia	Unilateral
Atelectasis (incomplete	Pneumothorax
expansion of lung tissue)	Pleural effusion
	Bronchial obstruction
	Bilateral
	Chronic obstructive lung disease
	Chest wall thickening (muscle, fat)

sensation felt are dependent upon the air-tissue ratio. The vibrations set up by the percussion of the chest can evaluate the lung tissue only to a depth of 5–6 cm, but percussion is valuable because many changes in the air-tissue ratio are readily apparent.

Percussion over a solid organ, such as the liver, produces a *dull,* low amplitude, short duration note without resonance. Percussion over a structure containing air and tissue, such as the lung, produces a *resonant,* higher amplitude, lower-pitched note. Percussion over a hollow air containing structure, such as the stomach, produces a *tympanic,* high-pitched, hollow quality note. Percussion over a large muscle mass, such as the thigh, produces a *flat,* high-pitched note.

Normally in the chest, dullness over the heart and resonance over the lung fields are heard and felt. As the lungs are filled with fluid and become more dense, as in pneumonia, resonance is replaced by dullness. The term *hyperresonance* has been applied to the percussion note obtained from a lung of decreased density, as is found in emphysema. Hyperresonance is a low-pitched, hollow quality, sustained resonant note bordering on tympany.

The Technique of Percussion

Percussion of the chest uses the middle finger of the left hand placed firmly against the chest wall parallel to the ribs in an interspace with the palm and other fingers held off the chest. The tip of the right middle finger strikes a quick, sharp blow to the terminal phalanx of the left finger on the chest wall. The motion of the striking finger should come from the wrist, and not from the elbow. Paddle ball players use this motion, whereas tennis players will now have to concentrate on using this wrist motion. The technique of percussion is diagrammed in Figure 10–10 and shown in Figure 10–11.

Try percussion on yourself. Percuss over your right lung (resonant), stomach (tympanic), liver (dull), and thigh (flat).

Percuss the Posterior Chest

The sites on the posterior chest for percussion are above, between, and below the scapulae in the intercostal spaces, as shown in Figure 10–12. The bony scapulae are not percussed. The examiner should start at the top and work downward, proceeding from side to side, comparing one side with the other.

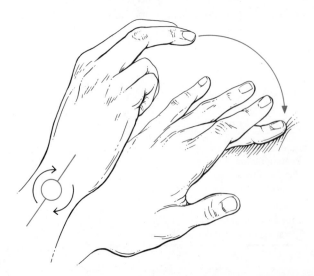

Figure 10–10. Technique of percussion.

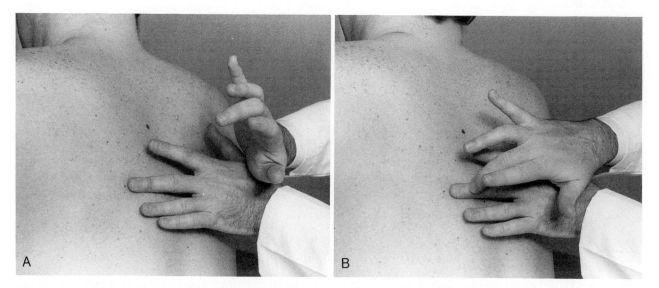

Figure 10–11. *A* shows the position of the right hand ready to percuss. *B* shows the location of the fingers after striking. Notice that the motion is from the wrist.

Evaluate Diaphragmatic Movement

Percussion is also used to detect diaphragmatic movement. The patient is asked to take a deep breath and hold it. Percussion at the right lung base determines the lowest area of resonance, which represents the lowest level of the diaphragm. Below this level is dullness from the liver. The patient is then instructed to exhale as much as possible, and the percussion is repeated. With expiration, the lung will contract, the liver will move up, and the same area will become dull. The level of dullness has moved upward. The difference between the inspiration and expiration levels represents diaphragmatic motion, which is normally 4–5 cm. Patients with emphysema have a reduced motion. Patients with a phrenic nerve palsy will have absent diaphragmatic motion. This test is illustrated in Figure 10–13.

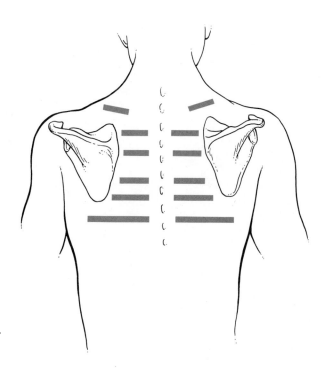

Figure 10–12. Locations on the posterior chest for percussion.

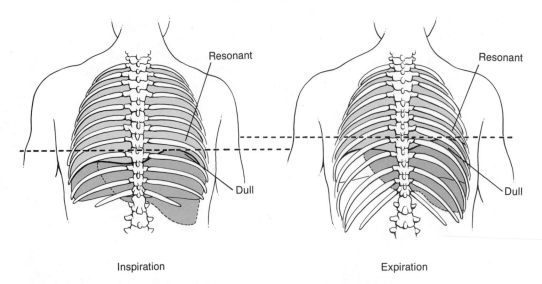

Figure 10-13. Technique for evaluating diaphragmatic motion. During inspiration, in the example on the left, percussion in the right seventh posterior interspace at the midscapular line would be resonant as a result of the presence of the underlying lung. During expiration, in the example on the right, the liver and diaphragm move up. Percussion in the same area would now be dull, owing to the presence of the underlying liver.

The Technique of Auscultation

Auscultation is the technique of listening for sounds produced in the body. Auscultation of the chest is used to identify lung sounds. The stethoscope usually has two heads: the bell and the diaphragm. The bell is used to detect low-pitched sounds, whereas the diaphragm is better at detecting higher-pitched sounds. The bell must be loosely applied to the skin; if it is pressed too tightly, the skin will act as a diaphragm and the lower-pitched sounds will be filtered out. In contrast, the diaphragm is applied firmly to the skin. In very cachectic individuals the bell may be more useful, as placement of the diaphragm is more difficult in these patients because of the protrusion of their ribs. The correct placement of the heads of the stethoscope is shown in Figure 10-14.

It is *never* acceptable to listen through clothing! The bell or the diaphragm of the stethoscope must always be in contact with the skin.

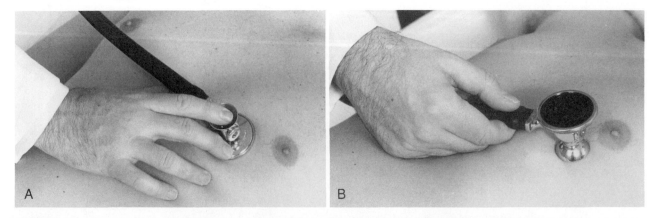

Figure 10-14. Placement of stethoscope heads. *A,* Correct placement of the diaphragm. Notice that the head is applied tightly to the skin. *B,* Placement of the bell. Notice that the bell is applied lightly to the skin.

Types of Breath Sounds

Breath sounds are heard over most of the lung fields. They consist of an inspiratory phase followed by an expiratory phase. There are four types of normal breath sounds. They are as follows:

- Tracheal
- Bronchial
- Bronchovesicular
- Vesicular

Tracheal breath sounds are very harsh, loud, and high-pitched sounds heard over the extrathoracic portion of the trachea. The two components are approximately equal in length. Although always present when one listens over the trachea, they are rarely evaluated because they do not represent any clinical lung problems.

Bronchial breath sounds are loud, high pitched, and sound like air rushing through a tube. The expiratory component is louder and longer than the inspiratory component. These sounds are present normally when one is listening over the manubrium. When one listens carefully, a definite pause is heard between the two phases.

Bronchovesicular breath sounds are a mixture of bronchial and vesicular sounds. The inspiratory and expiratory components are equal in length. They are normally heard only in the first and second interspaces anteriorly and between the scapulae posteriorly. This is near the carina and mainstem bronchi.

Vesicular breath sounds are the soft, low-pitched sounds heard over most of the lung fields. The inspiratory component is much longer than the expiratory component, which is also much softer and frequently inaudible.

The four types of breath sounds are shown and summarized in Figure 10–15.

CHARACTERISTICS OF BREATH SOUNDS

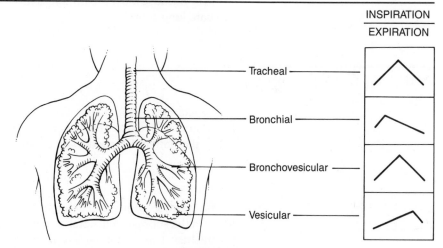

Figure 10–15.

Characteristic	Tracheal	Bronchial	Bronchovesicular	Vesicular
Intensity	Very loud	Loud	Moderate	Soft
Pitch	Very high	High	Moderate	Low
I:E Ratio*	1:1	1:3	1:1	3:1
Description	Harsh	Tubular	Rustling, but tubular	Gentle rustling
Normal locations	Extrathoracic trachea	Manubrium	Over mainstem bronchi	Most of peripheral lung

* Ratio of duration of inspiration to expiration.

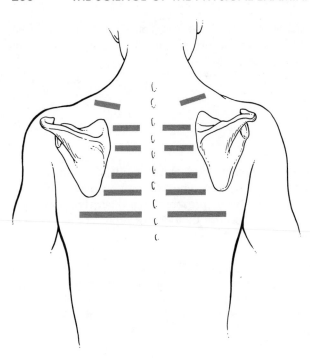

Figure 10-16. Locations on the posterior chest for auscultation.

Auscultate the Posterior Chest

Auscultation should be performed in a quiet environment. The patient is asked to breathe in and out through his mouth. The examiner should first concentrate on the length of inspiration and then on expiration. When the breath sounds are very soft, the term *distant* is used. Distant breath sounds are commonly found in patients with hyperinflated lungs, as in emphysema.

The examination should proceed from side to side and from top to bottom, comparing one side with the other. The positions are illustrated in Figure 10-16. Because most breath sounds are high pitched, the diaphragm is used to evaluate lung sounds.

Anterior Chest

The examiner should now move to the front of the patient. The first part of the examination of the anterior chest is performed with the patient seated, after which the patient is asked to lie down.

Evaluate Position of the Trachea

The position of the trachea can be determined by placing the right index finger in the suprasternal notch and moving slightly lateral to feel the location of the trachea. This technique is repeated, moving the finger from the suprasternal notch to the other side. The space between the trachea and the clavicle should be equal. A shift of the mediastinum can displace the trachea to one side. This technique is shown in Figure 10-17.

Look at the patient shown in Plate IX *B*. Notice that the trachea is markedly displaced to the right in this very cachectic woman. The diagnosis of a mass either pushing or pulling the trachea to the right is suggested.

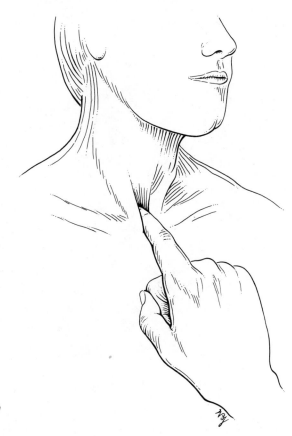

Figure 10–17. Technique for determining the position of the trachea.

Evaluate the Mobility of the Trachea

The upward motion of the trachea is used to ascertain whether the trachea is *fixed* in the mediastinum. The technique is called the *tracheal tug*. The patient's head should be slightly flexed, and your left hand should support the back of the patient's head. Your right hand should be placed parallel against the trachea with the palm facing out. The middle fingers should slide into the cricothyroid space, and the larynx is pushed upward. The larynx and trachea normally move about 1 – 2 cm. After moving the larynx upward, slowly lower it before removing your fingers. Do not suddenly release it from its superior position. A fixed trachea indicates mediastinal fixation, which can occur with neoplasm or tuberculosis. You must be careful not to place the examining fingers horizontally, push backward, or drop the trachea. These maneuvers can cause the patient much discomfort. The correct position is shown in Figure 10 – 18.

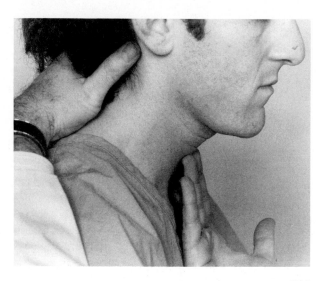

Figure 10–18. Technique for the tracheal tug.

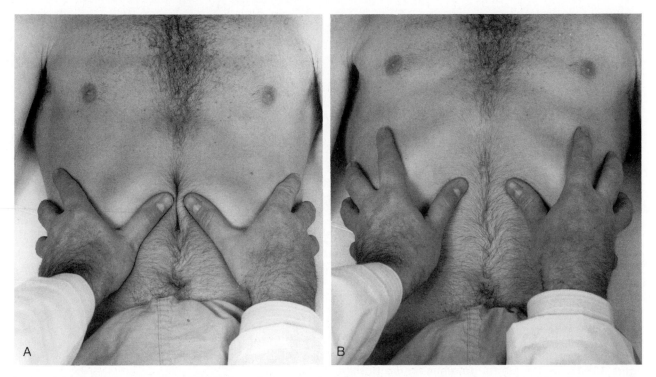

Figure 10–19. Technique for evaluating anterior chest excursion. *A* shows the placement of the hands during normal expiration. *B* shows their location after normal inspiration.

Now ask the patient to lie on his back for the rest of the examination of the anterior chest. The patient's arms are at his side. If the patient is a woman, either have her elevate her breasts or displace them yourself as necessary during palpation, percussion, and auscultation. These examinations should not be performed over breast tissue.

Evaluate Anterior Chest Excursion

The symmetry of anterior chest excursion is performed by placing your hands along the lateral rib margins, as shown in Figure 10–19. Instruct the patient to inhale deeply as you observe the motion of your hands.

Evaluate Tactile Fremitus

Tactile fremitus is assessed in the supraclavicular fossae and in alternate anterior interspaces, beginning at the clavicle. The techniques for evaluating tactile fremitus have already been discussed. The examiner should proceed from the supraclavicular fossae downward, comparing one side with the other.

Percuss the Anterior Chest

Percussion of the anterior chest includes the supraclavicular fossae, the axillae, and the anterior interspaces, as shown in Figure 10–20. The percussion note on one side is always compared with the corresponding position on the other side. Dullness may be elicited in the third to fifth intercostal spaces to the left of the sternum, which is related to the presence of the heart. It is important to percuss high in the axillae, because the upper lobes are best evaluated at these positions. Axillary percussion is sometimes easier to perform while the patient is in a sitting position.

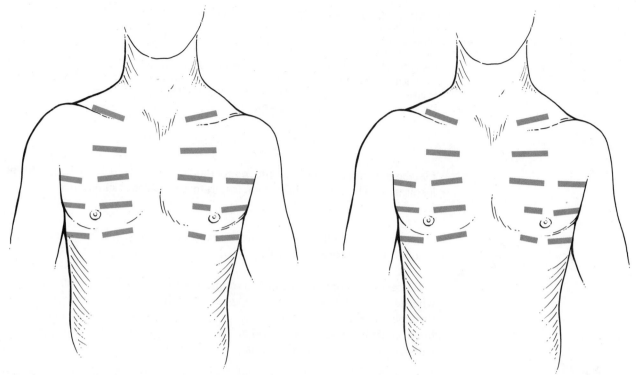

Figure 10–20. Locations on the anterior chest for percussion.

Figure 10–21. Locations on the anterior chest for auscultation.

Auscultate the Anterior Chest

Auscultation of the anterior chest is performed in the supraclavicular fossae, the axillae, and the anterior chest interspaces, as illustrated in Figure 10–21. The techniques of auscultation have already been discussed. The breath sounds of one side are compared with the breath sounds in the corresponding position on the other side.

CLINICOPATHOLOGIC CORRELATIONS

In addition to the normal breath sounds previously discussed, other lung sounds may be produced in abnormal clinical states. These abnormal sounds heard during auscultation are called *adventitious* sounds. Adventitious sounds include the following:

- Crackles
- Wheezes
- Pleural rubs

Crackles are short, discontinuous, nonmusical sounds heard mostly during inspiration. They have also been previously called *rales*. Since 1980, however, the correct terminology is *crackle*. It appears that crackles are produced when there is fluid inside a bronchus and there is a collapse of the distal airways and alveoli. A sudden equalization of pressure seems to result in a crackle. Coarser crackles are related to larger airways. Crackles are likened to the sound made by rubbing hair next to the ear, or the sound made when Velcro is opened. They

TABLE 10-6. Timing of Common Inspiratory Crackles

Disease	Early Crackle	Late Crackle
Congestive heart failure	Very common	Common
Obstructive lung disease	Present	Absent
Interstitial fibrosis	Absent	Present
Pneumonia	Absent	Present

may be described as early or late, depending upon when they are heard during inspiration. The timing of common inspiratory crackles is summarized in Table 10-6.

The most common causes of crackles are pulmonary edema, congestive heart failure, and pulmonary fibrosis.

Wheezes are continuous musical sounds heard mostly during expiration. The wheeze is also known as the *rhonchus*. The wheeze is produced by air flow through a narrowed bronchus. Thus narrowing may be due to swelling, secretions, spasm, a tumor, or a foreign body. Wheezes are commonly associated with the bronchospasm of asthma.

A *pleural rub* is a grating sound produced by motion of the pleura, which is impeded by frictional resistance. It is best heard at the end of inspiration and at the beginning of expiration. The sound of a pleural rub has been described as the sound made by creaking leather. Pleural rubs are heard when pleural surfaces are roughened or thickened by inflammatory or neoplastic cells or by fibrin deposits.

All of the adventitious sounds should be described as to their location, timing, and intensity.

There is much confusion regarding the terminology of adventitious sounds. Table 10-7 summarizes the adventitious sounds.

Occasionally, breath sounds are transmitted abnormally. This may result in auscultatory changes known as

- Egophony
- Whispered pectoriloquy
- Bronchophony

TABLE 10-7. Adventitious Sounds

Recommended Term	Older Term	Mechanism	Etiology
Crackle	Rale Crepitation	Excess airway secretions	Bronchitis, respiratory infections, pulmonary edema, atelectasis, fibrosis, congestive heart failure
Wheeze	Sibilant rale Sibilant rhonchus Musical rale Sonorous rale Low-pitched wheeze	Rapid airflow through obstructed airway	Asthma, pulmonary edema, bronchitis, congestive heart failure
Pleural rub		Inflammation of the pleura	Pneumonia, pulmonary infarction

PATTERNS OF ABNORMAL BREATHING

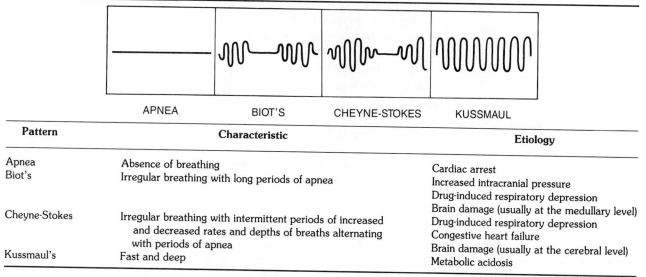

Pattern	Characteristic	Etiology
Apnea	Absence of breathing	Cardiac arrest
Biot's	Irregular breathing with long periods of apnea	Increased intracranial pressure
		Drug-induced respiratory depression
		Brain damage (usually at the medullary level)
Cheyne-Stokes	Irregular breathing with intermittent periods of increased and decreased rates and depths of breaths alternating with periods of apnea	Drug-induced respiratory depression
		Congestive heart failure
		Brain damage (usually at the cerebral level)
Kussmaul's	Fast and deep	Metabolic acidosis

Figure 10–22.

Egophony (egobronchophony) is said to be present when the spoken word heard through the lungs is increased in intensity and takes on a nasal or bleating quality. The patient is asked to say "eeee" while the examiner listens to an area in which consolidation is suspected. If egophony is present, the "eeee" will be heard as "aaaa." This "e to a" change is seen in consolidation of lung tissue. The area of compressed lung above a pleural effusion often produces egophony.

Whispered pectoriloquy is the term given to the intensification of the whispered word heard in consolidation of the lung. The patient is instructed to whisper "one-two-three" while the examiner listens to the area suspected of having consolidation. Normally, whispering produces high-pitched sounds that tend to be filtered out by the lungs. Little or nothing may be heard when one listens to a normal chest. However, if consolidation is present, the transmission of the spoken words will be increased and the words will be clearly heard.

TABLE 10–8. Common Conditions Associated with Dyspnea

Condition	Dyspnea	Other Symptoms
Asthma	Episodic, symptom-free between attacks	Wheezing, chest pain, productive cough
Pneumonia	Insidious dyspnea	Cough
Pulmonary fibrosis	Abrupt Gradual	Tachypnea, cough, orthopnea and PND* with chronic state.
Pulmonary fibrosis	Progressive	Tachypnea, dry cough, chest pain
Pneumonia	Exertional	Productive cough, pleuritic pain
Pneumothorax	Sudden, moderate to severe	Sudden pleuritic pain
Emphysema	Insidious onset, severe	Cough as disease progresses
Chronic bronchitis	As disease progresses and with infection	Chronic, productive cough
Obesity	Exertional	

* Paroxysmal nocturnal dyspnea.

Bronchophony is the increased transmission of spoken words heard in consolidation of the lungs. The patient is asked to say "ninety-nine" while the examiner listens to the chest. If bronchophony is present, the words will be transmitted louder than normally and will be heard as "NINETY-NINE."

One of the most important principles for the examination of the chest is to correlate percussion, palpation, and the auscultatory findings. Dullness, crackles, increased breath sounds, and increased tactile fremitus suggest consolidation. Dullness, decreased breath sounds, and decreased tactile fremitus suggest a pleural effusion.

Table 10–1 lists some of the common terms used by patients to describe their coughing and some possible causes. Table 10–2 describes the appear-

TABLE 10–9. Differentiation of Common Pulmonary Conditions

Condition	Vital Signs	Inspection	Palpation	Percussion	Auscultation
Asthma*	Tachypnea; tachycardia	Dyspnea; use of accessory muscles; possible cyanosis; hyperinflation	Often normal; decreased fremitus	Often normal; hyperresonant; low diaphragms	Prolonged expiration; wheezes; decreased lung sounds
Emphysema	Stable	Increased AP diameter; use of accessory muscles; thin individual	Decreased tactile fremitus	Increased resonance; decreased excursion of diaphragm	Decreased lung sounds; decreased vocal fremitus
Chronic bronchitis	Tachycardia	Possible cyanosis; short, stocky individual	Often normal	Often normal	Early crackles
Pneumonia	Tachycardia; fever; tachypnea	Possible cyanosis; possible splinting on affected side	Increased tactile fremitus	Dull	Late crackles; bronchial breath sounds†
Pulmonary embolism	Tachycardia; tachypnea	Often normal	Usually normal	Usually normal	Usually normal
Pulmonary edema	Tachycardia; tachypnea	Possible signs of elevated right heart pressures‡	Often normal	Often normal	Early crackles; wheezes
Pneumothorax	Tachypnea; tachycardia	Often normal lag on affected side	Absent fremitus; trachea may be shifted to other side	Hyperresonant	Absent breath sounds
Pleural effusion	Tachypnea; tachycardia	Often normal; lag on affected side	Decreased fremitus; trachea shifted to other side	Dullness	Absent breath sounds
Atelectasis	Tachypnea	Often normal; lag on affected side	Decreased fremitus; trachea shifted to same side	Dullness	Absent breath sounds
ARDS§	Tachycardia; tachypnea	Use of accessory muscles; cyanosis	Usually normal	Often normal	Normal initially; crackles and decreased lung sounds, late

* Often the physical findings in asthma are not reliable in predicting its severity.
† Bronchophony, pectoriloquy, and egophony are also often present.
‡ Elevated jugular venous distention, pedal edema, hepatomegaly.
§ Adult respiratory distress syndrome.

ances of classic types of sputum and their etiologies. Table 10–4 lists the types of positional dyspnea and their causes. Figure 10–22 illustrates and summarizes the major types of abnormal breathing patterns. Table 10–5 lists some of the etiologies for changes in tactile fremitus. Table 10–8 lists some of the common causes of dyspnea and their associated symptoms. Table 10–9 summarizes some important manifestations of common pulmonary conditions.

USEFUL VOCABULARY

Listed here are the specific roots that are important in order to understand the terminology related to diseases of the chest.

ROOT	PERTAINING TO	EXAMPLE	DEFINITION
broncho-	bronchus	**bronch**itis	Inflammation of the bronchus
chondro-	cartilage	**chrondr**oma	Hyperplastic growth of cartilage
costo-	ribs	**costo**chondritis	Inflammation of the rib cartilage
phren-	diaphragm	**phreno**hepatic	Pertaining to the diaphragm and liver
pleur(o)-	pleura	**pleur**itic	Pertaining to inflammation of the pleura
-pne(o)-	breath	dys**pne**a	"Bad" breathing; shortness of breath
pneumo-	lungs	**pneumo**nectomy	Surgical removal of lung tissue
spiro-	to breathe	**spiro**gram	A tracing of respiratory movements
-stern(o)-	sternum	costo**stern**al	Pertaining to the ribs and sternum

WRITING UP THE PHYSICAL EXAMINATION

Listed here are examples of the write-up for the examination of the chest.

The trachea is midline and is not fixed. The chest is normal in appearance. Palpation is normal. The chest is clear to percussion and auscultation.

The trachea is midline. There is a mild pectus excavatum present. There is increased tactile fremitus at the left posterior chest, up one third from the base. This area is also dull to percussion. Bronchial breath sounds and crackles are present in the area of dullness. Bronchophony and whispered pectoriloquy are also present in this area.

The trachea is deviated to the left. The chest structure is within normal limits. There is decreased tactile fremitus on the right chest posteriorly, up three quarters from the base. The percussion note is dull in the area of decreased fremitus. There are no breath sounds heard in this area. An area of egophony is present above the area of dullness.

The trachea is midline. Tactile fremitus is normal, as is percussion. Auscultation reveals normal breath sounds with bilateral basilar crackles present.

BIBLIOGRAPHY

Anderson CL, Shankar PS, Scott JH: Physiological significance of sternomastoid muscle contraction in chronic obstructive pulmonary disease. Respir Care 25:937, 1980.

Conine TA, Evans JH: Sexual adjustment in chronic obstructive pulmonary disease. Respir Care 26:871, 1981.

Forgacs P: Lung Sounds. London, Bailliere Tindall, 1978.

Forgacs P: The functional basis of pulmonary sounds. Chest 73:399, 1978.

Gershwin ME: Bronchial Asthma. New York, Grune and Stratton, 1981.

Glauser FL: Signs and Symptoms in Pulmonary Medicine. Philadelphia, JB Lippincott Co, 1983.

Hinshaw HC, Murray JF: Diseases of the Chest, 4th ed. Philadelphia, WB Saunders Co, 1980.

Mattson A: Psychologic aspects of childhood asthma. Pediatr Clin North Am 2:77, 1975.

National Institute of Health (NIH): Epidemiology of Respiratory Diseases — Task Force Report. NIH Publication No. 81-2019, Oct 1980.

Raffin TA: Separating cardiac from pulmonary dyspnea. JAMA 238:206, 1977.

Rees L: Physical and emotional factors in bronchial asthma. J Psychosomatic Res 1:98, 1956.

Stubbing DG, Mathur PN, Roberts RS: Some physical signs in patients with chronic airway obstruction. Am Rev Respir Dis 125:549, 1982.

THE HEART

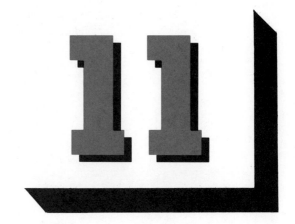

. . . For it is the heart by whose virtue and pulse the blood is moved, perfected, made apt to nourish and is preserved from corruption and coagulation. . . . It is indeed the fountain of life, the source of all action.

William Harvey
1578–1657

GENERAL CONSIDERATIONS

The heart does not rest for more than a fraction of a second at a time. During a lifetime, it contracts more than 4 billion times. In order to support this active state, the coronary arteries supply greater than 10 million liters of blood to the myocardium and more than 200 million liters to the systemic circulation. Cardiac output can vary under physiologic conditions from 3 to 30 liters per minute, and regional blood flow can vary by 200%. This wide range occurs without any loss of efficiency in the normal state.

Diseases of the heart are very common. The major disease categories are coronary artery disease, hypertension, rheumatic heart disease, bacterial endocarditis, and congenital heart disease. The clinical consequences of these conditions are generally very serious.

Coronary artery disease is the leading cause of death in the United States. By the age of 60, nearly one in five American males has symptomatic coronary artery disease caused by coronary atherosclerosis. Autopsy studies during the Korean War showed that 40% of all American soldiers who were killed in their early twenties had atheromatous involvement of one or more of their coronary arteries.

In the United States, over 1 million myocardial infarctions are suffered annually with greater than 650,000 deaths, half of which are sudden. An additional 200,000 individuals die from strokes and related vascular diseases. The cost of diseases related to the cardiovascular system exceeds 40 billion dollars. Unlike other forms of cardiac disease, coronary atherosclerotic disease may be severe and life-threatening despite a normal physical examination, electrocardiogram, and chest x-ray.

Systemic arterial hypertension affects approximately 20% of the American population. It is a major risk factor for coronary artery disease as well as being a prime cause of congestive heart failure and strokes. It has been well established that patients with higher systolic or diastolic pressures have a greater incidence of morbidity and mortality.

Since the implementation of antibiotic therapy, the incidence of rheumatic heart disease has been decreasing in the more affluent countries. In areas of overcrowding and in less affluent areas, rheumatic fever and valvular heart disease that results from it are still a major cause of cardiac morbidity and mortality.

Bacterial endocarditis remains a significant medical problem despite the wide use of antibiotics. The increasing number of cases is related to intravenous use of "street" drugs. The diagnosis of endocarditis is often not suspected until serious sequelae develop. In addition to valvular damage, the persistent bacteremia can spread the infection to the brain, myocardium, spleen, kidneys, and other sites in the body.

The incidence of congenital heart disease averages 5 in 1000 live births. If one includes other commonly found congenital conditions, such as bicuspid aortic valve and mitral valve prolapse, the incidence approaches 1 in 100 live births.

It is clear that the magnitude of cardiac disease is enormous, and the cost of the morbidity and mortality is directly proportional.

STRUCTURE AND PHYSIOLOGY

The principal function of the cardiovascular system is to deliver nutrients to and remove metabolites from *every* cell in the body. This metabolic exchange system is produced by a high pressure delivery system, an area of exchange, and a low pressure return system. The high pressure delivery system is the *left* heart and *arteries,* whereas the low pressure return system includes the *veins* and the *right* heart. The circulation of blood through the heart is illustrated in Figure 11 – 1.

The heart is enveloped by a thin *pericardial sac.* This sac is adherent to the diaphragm below and is loosely attached above to the upper portion of the sternum. The *visceral* pericardium is the epicardial, or outermost layer, of cells of the heart. The *parietal* pericardium is the outer sac. Between these two surfaces, a small amount of pericardial fluid in the pericardial sac provides a lubricating interface for the constantly moving heart. The parietal pericardium is innervated by the phrenic nerve, which contains pain fibers. The visceral pericardium is insensitive to pain.

The synchronous contraction of the heart results from the conduction of impulses generated by the *sino-atrial* (SA) *node* and propagated through the *conduction system.* The sino-atrial node is located at the juncture of the superior

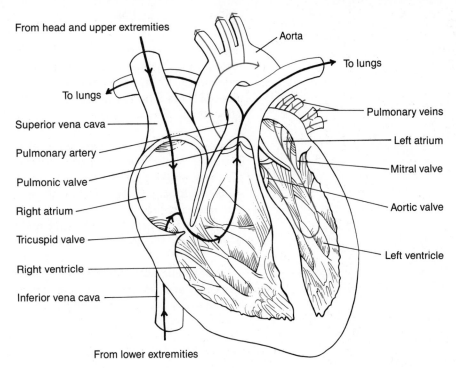

FIGURE 11-1. Circulation of blood through the heart.

From head and upper extremities

Aorta

To lungs

To lungs

Pulmonary veins

Superior vena cava

Left atrium

Pulmonary artery

Mitral valve

Pulmonic valve

Aortic valve

Right atrium

Tricuspid valve

Left ventricle

Right ventricle

Inferior vena cava

From lower extremities

vena cava and the right atrium. The sino-atrial impulse spreads from its point of origin concentrically. When the impulse reaches the *atrio-ventricular* (AV) *node,* in the interatrial septum near the entrance of the coronary sinus, the impulse is slowed. It is then transmitted to the specialized conducting tissue known as the *right and left bundle branches,* which conduct the impulse to the specialized conducting pathways within the ventricles, the *Purkinje fibers.* The impulse spreads from the endocardial to the epicardial surface of the heart. These conducting pathways are illustrated in Figure 11-2.

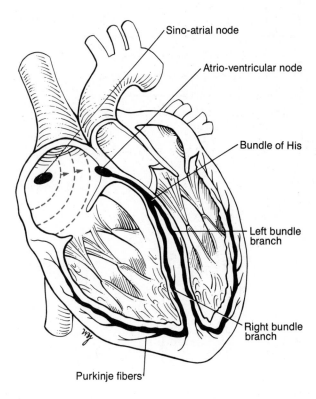

Sino-atrial node

Atrio-ventricular node

Bundle of His

Left bundle branch

Right bundle branch

Purkinje fibers

FIGURE 11-2. Conducting pathways in the heart.

The heart is innervated extensively by branches of the autonomic nervous system. Both sympathetic and parasympathetic fibers are present in the sinoatrial and atrioventricular nodes. The atrial muscle is also innervated by both types of fibers. The ventricular musculature is innervated predominantly by the sympathetic nervous system.

The *parasympathetic* fibers travel along the vagus, or tenth cranial, nerve. The *sympathetic* fibers descend in the spinal cord to the level of T1–T5, where they emerge through the ventral roots to synapse in the thoracic and cervical *sympathetic ganglia*. The postganglionic fibers travel through the cervical *cardiac nerves* to join the parasympathetic fibers in forming the *cardiac plexus,* which is located near the aortic arch and the tracheal bifurcation. These neural pathways are shown in Figure 11–3.

Sympathetic stimulation by *norepinephrine* produces marked increases in heart rate and contractility. Parasympathetic stimulation mediated by *acetylcholine* slows the heart rate and decreases contractility.

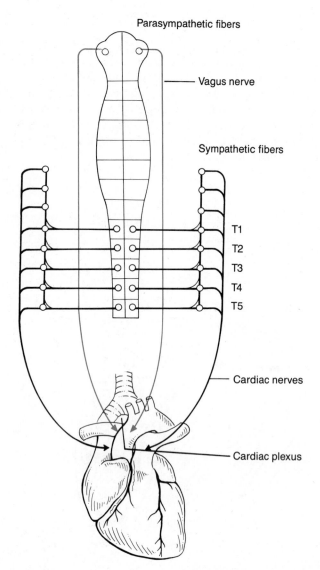

FIGURE 11–3. Autonomic neural pathways of the heart.

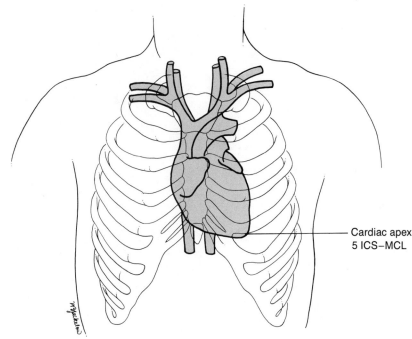

Cardiac apex
5 ICS–MCL

FIGURE 11–4. Surface topography of the heart.

In addition, there are several receptor sites that provide circulatory information to the *medullary cardiovascular center* in the brain. This center has cardioexcitatory and cardioinhibitory areas that regulate the neural output to the sympathetic and parasympathetic fibers. *Stretch* receptors in the aortic arch and in the carotid sinus monitor blood pressure. These *baroreceptors* respond to a decrease in blood pressure by decreasing their impulses to the medullary center. The center senses this decreased activity and increases its sympathetic efferent activity and decreases its parasympathetic efferent activity. The net result is to increase the heart rate and contractility. An increase in blood pressure causes an increase in afferent activity to the center, and the opposite changes occur.

In order to describe physical signs, the examiner must be able to identify the important surface topographic landmarks. Chapter 10, The Chest, describes the major areas. The reader should review these areas at this time.

The surface projection of the heart and great vessels is shown in Figure 11–4. Most of the anterior cardiac surface is the right ventricle. The right atrium forms a narrow border from the third to the fifth rib to the right of the sternum. The left ventricle lies to the left and behind the right ventricle. The left ventricular *apex* is normally in the *fifth* intercostal space at the *midclavicular line*. This location is commonly written as *5ICS-MCL*. This *apical impulse* is called the *point of maximum impulse,* or the *PMI*. The other chambers and vessels of the heart are usually not identifiable on examination.

The four classic *auscultatory areas* correspond to points over the precordium at which events originating at each valve are best heard. The areas are not necessarily related to the anatomic position of the valve, nor are all sounds heard in the area directly produced by the valve that names the area. The areas are as follows:

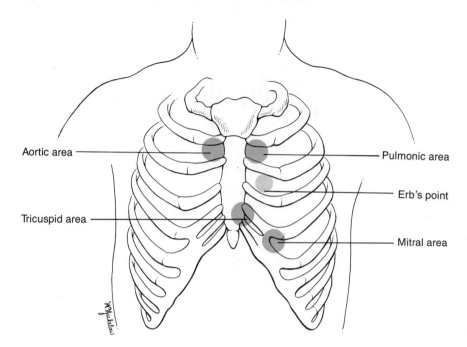

FIGURE 11–5. Auscultatory areas.

Aortic	Second intercostal space, right sternal border (2ICS-RSB)
Pulmonic	Second intercostal space, left sternal border (2ICS-LSB)
Tricuspid	Left lower sternal border (LLSB)
Mitral	Cardiac apex

In addition to these four areas, the third left interspace, known as *Erb's point,* is frequently the area to which pulmonic or aortic sounds radiate. The five areas are illustrated in Figure 11–5. The second intercostal space to the right and left of the sternum is commonly called the *base.*

It should be remembered that the left atrium is the most posterior portion of the heart. When the left atrium enlarges, it extends posteriorly and to the right.

The Cardiac Cycle

To understand the cardiac cycle, the reader should review the motion of the valves and the pressures within the chambers. The interrelationships of valve motion are critically important and must be understood before proceeding further. Only with the knowledge of these cycles can the reader fully comprehend the cardiac physical examination and heart sounds. The pressure tracings and valve motions are shown in Figure 11–6.

Normally, only the closing of the heart valves can be heard. The closure of the *atrioventricular valves,* the tricuspid and the mitral, produces the *first heart sound, S_1.* The closure of the *semilunar valves,* the aortic and the pulmonic, produces the *second heart sound, S_2.*

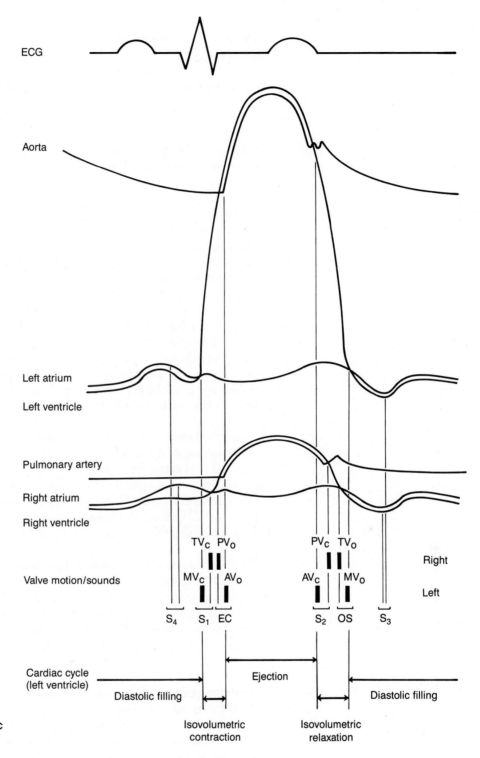

FIGURE 11-6 The cardiac cycle.

The opening of the valves can be heard only if they are damaged. When an atrioventricular valve is narrowed, or *stenotic,* the opening of the valve may be heard and is termed an *opening snap.* If a semilunar valve is stenotic, the opening may be heard and is termed an *ejection click.* It should be noted from Figure 11–6 that the term "opening snap" refers to the opening of a pathologically damaged atrioventricular valve that occurs during *diastole;* the term "ejection click" refers to the opening of a damaged semilunar valve that occurs during *systole.*

The sequence of the opening and closing of the four valves is as follows:

$$MV_c \ TV_c \ PV_o \ AV_o \ AV_c \ PV_c \ TV_o \ MV_o$$

in which MV = mitral valve, TV = tricuspid valve, PV = pulmonic valve, AV = aortic valve, $_c$ = closing, $_o$ = opening, EC = ejection click, and OS = opening snap.

The mitral component of S_1 occurs as a result of the closure of the mitral valve when the left ventricular pressure rises above left atrial pressure. It is commonly written as M_1. The tricuspid component of S_1 occurs as a result of closure of the tricuspid valve when right ventricular pressure rises above right atrial pressure. It is commonly written as T_1.

The time between the closure of the atrioventricular valves and the opening of the semilunar valves is the period of *isovolumetric contraction.* When the pressure in the right ventricle exceeds the diastolic pressure in the pulmonary artery, the pulmonic valve opens. A pulmonic ejection click will be heard at this time if the pulmonic valve is stenotic. When the pressure in the left ventricle exceeds the diastolic pressure in the aorta, the aortic valve opens. An aortic ejection click will be heard at this time if the aortic valve is stenotic.

The time between the opening and the closing of the semilunar valves is the systolic period of *ejection.* The point at which ejection is completed and the aortic and left ventricular curves separate is called the *incisura,* or *dicrotic notch,* and is simultaneous with the aortic component of S_2, or closure of the aortic valve. This is commonly written as A_2. The pulmonic valve closes at the point when the right ventricular pressure falls below the pulmonary diastolic pressure. This is the pulmonic component of S_2 and is commonly written as P_2.

The time between the closure of the semilunar valves and the opening of the atrioventricular valves is called *isovolumetric relaxation.* The tricuspid valve opens when the pressure in the right atrium exceeds right ventricular pressure. A tricuspid opening snap may be heard if the tricuspid valve is stenotic. The mitral valve opens when the pressure in the left atrium exceeds left ventricular pressure. A mitral opening snap may occur at this point if the mitral valve is stenotic.

With the opening of the atrioventricular valves, the period of rapid filling of the ventricles occurs. Approximately 80% of ventricular filling occurs at this point. It is at the end of the rapid filling period that a *third heart sound,* an S_3, may be heard. An S_3 occurs 120–170 msec after S_2. This period is approximately the same time as it takes to say "me too." The "me" is the S_2, whereas the "too" is the S_3. An S_3 is normal in children and young adults. When present in individuals over the age of 30, it signifies a volume overload to the ventricle. Regurgitant valvular lesions and congestive heart failure may be responsible.

At the end of diastole, *atrial contraction* and the additional 20% of ventricular filling occur. A *fourth heart sound,* an S_4, may be heard. The interval from the S_4 to the S_1 is approximately the time it takes to say "middle." The "mi" is the S_4, whereas the "ddle" is the S_1. It should also be noted that the "mi" is much softer than the "ddle," quite similar to the $S_4 - S_1$ cadence. An S_4 is normal in

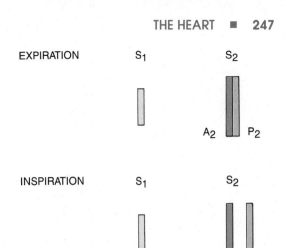

FIGURE 11-7. Physiologic splitting of the second heart sound.

children and young adults. When present in individuals over the age of 30, it indicates a *noncompliant,* or "stiff," ventricle. Pressure overload on a ventricle causes concentric hypertrophy, which produces a noncompliant ventricle. In addition, coronary artery disease is a major cause of a stiff ventricle.

The presence of an S_3 or an S_4 creates a cadence resembling the gallop of a horse. These sounds are, therefore, called *gallop* sounds or rhythms.

The first heart sound is loudest at the cardiac apex. *Splitting* of the first heart sound may be heard in the tricuspid area. The second heart sound is loudest at the base.

The terms A_2 and P_2 indicate the aortic component and the pulmonic component of S_2, respectively. A_2 normally precedes P_2, meaning that the aortic valve closes before the pulmonic valve. With inspiration, the intrathoracic pressure lowers. This draws more blood from the superior and inferior venae cavae into the right heart. The right ventricle enlarges, and it takes longer for all the blood to be ejected into the pulmonary artery: thus, the pulmonic valve stays open longer. P_2 occurs later in inspiration, and the split between A_2 and P_2 is widened during inspiration compared with expiration. This is the cause of *physiologic splitting* of S_2. Physiologic splitting of S_2 is diagrammed in Figure 11-7.

The blood in the right ventricle is then pumped into the large capacitance bed of the lungs. Therefore, the return of blood from the lungs to the left heart is decreased, and the left atrium and left ventricle become smaller. Atrial receptors trigger a reflex tachycardia that compensates for the decreased left ventricular volume. This increase in heart rate with inspiration is termed *sinus arrhythmia.* It is a misnomer, because it is really not an arrhythmia but a normal physiologic response to a decreased left ventricular volume during inspiration.

The Arterial Pulse

The arterial pulse is produced by the ejection of blood into the aorta. The normal configuration of the pulse consists of a smooth and rapid upstroke that begins about 80 msec after the first component of S_1. There is sometimes a slight notch in the arterial pulsation toward the end of the rapid ejection period. This is called the *anacrotic notch.* The peak of the pulse is smooth, dome shaped, and occurs about 100 msec after the onset of the pulse. The descending

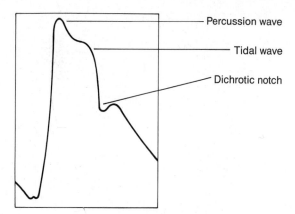

— Percussion wave

— Tidal wave

— Dichrotic notch

FIGURE 11–8. The arterial pulse.

limb from the peak is less steep. There is a gradual descent to the *dicrotic notch,* which represents the closure of the aortic valve. Figure 11–8 shows a characteristic arterial pulse.

As the arterial pulse travels to the periphery, there are several changes. The initial upstroke becomes steeper, the systolic peak is higher, and the anacrotic notch becomes less evident. In addition, the dicrotic notch occurs later in the peripheral pulse. This occurs approximately 300 msec after the onset of the pulse. The positive wave that follows the dicrotic notch is called the *dicrotic wave.*

Commonly there may be two waves present in the arterial pulse that precede the dicrotic notch. The *percussion wave* is the earlier wave and is associated with the rate of flow in the artery. The percussion wave occurs during peak velocity of flow. The *tidal wave* is the second wave and is related to pressure in the vessel. The tidal wave occurs during peak systolic pressure. The tidal wave is usually smaller than the percussion wave, but it may be increased in hypertensive or elderly patients.

Blood Pressure

Arterial blood pressure is the lateral pressure exerted by a column of blood against the arterial wall. It is the result of cardiac output and peripheral vascular resistance. Blood pressure is dependent upon the volume of blood ejected, its velocity, the distensibility of the arterial wall, the viscosity of the blood, and the pressure within the vessel after the last ejection.

Systolic blood pressure is the peak pressure in the arteries. It is regulated by the stroke volume and the compliance of the blood vessels. Diastolic blood pressure is the lowest pressure in the arteries and is dependent upon peripheral resistance. The difference in the systolic and diastolic pressure is the *pulse pressure.* The blood pressure in the right arm is usually 5–10 mm Hg higher than in the left arm. Systolic blood pressure in the legs is 15–20 mm Hg greater than in the arms, even while the individual is lying flat. This is in part related to Poiseuille's law, which in essence states that the total resistance of vessels connected in parallel is greater than the resistance of a single large vessel. The blood pressure in the aorta is less than the blood pressure in the branched arteries of the lower extremities.

Blood pressure varies greatly, according to the patient's degree of excitement, degree of activity, smoking habits, pain, bladder distention, or dietary pattern. There is normally an inspiratory decline of up to 10 mm Hg in systolic blood pressure during quiet respiration.

Jugular Venous Pulse

The jugular venous pulse provides direct information about the pressures in the right heart because the jugular system is in direct continuity with the right atrium. During diastole, when the tricuspid valve is open, the jugular veins are continuous with the right ventricle as well. Provided that there is no stenotic lesion at the pulmonic or mitral valves, the right ventricle will indirectly monitor the pressures in the left atrium and left ventricle. Remember that the most common cause of *right* heart failure is *left* heart failure. Examination of the neck veins also provides valuable information about the cardiac rhythm.

The understanding of the normal physiology is important in the consideration of the jugular venous pulsation. Figure 11–9 is an enlargement of the atrial and ventricular pressure curves shown in Figure 11–6.

The *a wave* of the jugular venous pulse is produced by right atrial contraction. When the "a" wave is timed with the electrocardiogram, it is found to occur about 90 msec after the onset of the P wave. This time delay is related to the time from electrical stimulation of the atria, to atrial contraction, and to the resultant wave propagated in the neck. The *x descent* is caused by atrial relaxation, which occurs just prior to ventricular contraction. This drop in right atrial pressure is terminated by the *c wave.* This increase in right atrial pressure is due to tricuspid valve closure secondary to right ventricular contraction. The descent of the atrioventricular valve rings produces the next change in right atrial pressure, called the *x prime descent.* As the free wall of the right ventricle approaches the septum during contraction, the atrioventricular valve rings descend toward the apex as contraction progresses. This increases the size of the atrium, causing a fall in its pressure: the "x prime" descent. During ventricular systole, the right atrium begins to fill with blood returning via the venae cavae. This increase in right atrial pressure as a result of its filling produces the ascending limb of the *v wave.* At the end of ventricular systole, right ventricular pressure falls rapidly. At the point at which it falls below the right atrial pressure,

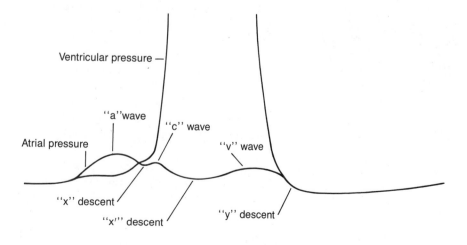

Ventricular pressure —

"a" wave

"c" wave

Atrial pressure

"v" wave

"x" descent

"x'" descent

"y" descent

FIGURE 11–9. The venous pulse.

the tricuspid valve opens. This drop in right atrial pressure produces the *y descent*.

Normally, only the "a" and "v" waves are visible on examination. Because the "c" wave is frequently not observed, the "x" and "x prime" descents are summated into a single "x" descent. Occasionally the later portion of the "c" wave may be enlarged by a carotid artery pulsation artifact.

REVIEW OF SPECIFIC SYMPTOMS

The important symptoms of cardiac disease include the following:

- Chest pain
- Irregularities of heart rhythm (palpitations)
- Dyspnea (shortness of breath)
- Syncope (fainting)
- Fatigue
- Dependent edema (swelling of legs)
- Hemoptysis (coughing up blood)
- Cyanosis (bluish discoloration of skin)

Chest Pain

Chest pain is probably the most important symptom of cardiac disease. It is, however, not pathognomonic for heart disease. It is well known that chest pain may result from pulmonary, intestinal, gallbladder, and musculoskeletal disorders. Ask the following questions of any patients with chest pain:

"Where is the pain?"
"For how long have you had the pain?"
"Do you have recurrent episodes of pain?"
"What is the duration of the pain?"
"How often do you get the pain?"
"What do you do to make it better?"
"What makes the pain worse? . . . breathing? . . . lying flat? . . . moving your arms or neck?"
"How would you describe the pain?* . . . burning? . . . pressing? . . . crushing? . . . dull? . . . aching? . . . throbbing? . . . knife-like? . . . sharp? . . . constricting? . . . sticking?"
"Does the pain occur at rest? . . . with exertion? . . . after eating? . . . when moving your arms? . . . with emotional strain? . . . while sleeping? . . . during sexual intercourse?"
"Is the pain associated with shortness of breath? . . . palpitations? . . . nausea or vomiting? . . . coughing? . . . fever? . . . coughing up blood? . . . leg pain?"

---

* Generally, it is best to allow the patient to describe the character of the pain. These descriptors are provided for the interviewer to use only when the patient is unable to characterize the pain.

TABLE 11–1. Characteristics of Chest Pain*

	Angina	Not Angina
Location	Retrosternal, diffuse	Left inframammary, localized
Radiation	Left arm, jaw, back	Right arm
Description	"Aching," "dull," "pressing," "squeezing," "vice-like"	"Sharp," "shooting," "cutting"
Intensity	Mild to severe	Excruciating
Duration	Minutes	Seconds, hours, days
Precipitated by	Effort, emotion, eating, cold	Respiration, posture, motion
Relieved by	Rest, nitroglycerin	Anything

*Angina and other chest pain may present in a variety of ways. The characteristics listed here are the common presentations. This list, however, is not absolute. This list should only be used as a guide.

Angina pectoris is the true symptom of coronary artery disease. Angina is commonly the consequence of hypoxia of the myocardium resulting from an imbalance of coronary supply and myocardial demand. Table 11–1 lists the characteristics that differentiate angina pectoris from the other types of chest pain.

Very commonly, a patient may describe his angina by clenching his fist and placing it over his sternum. This is a pathognomonic sign of angina commonly referred to as *Levine's sign*. Figure 11–10 demonstrates this body language.

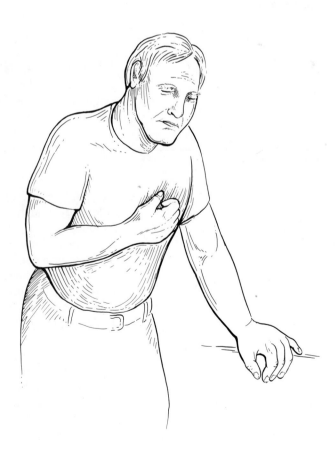

FIGURE 11–10. Levine's sign.

TABLE 11-2. Common Causes of Chest Pain

Organ System	Cause
Cardiac	Coronary artery disease
	Aortic valvular disease
	Pulmonary hypertension
	Mitral valve prolapse
	Pericarditis
	Idiopathic hypertrophic subaortic stenosis (IHSS)
Vascular	Dissection of the aorta
Pulmonary	Pulmonary embolism
	Pneumonia
	Pleuritis
	Pneumothorax
Musculoskeletal	Costochondritis*
	Arthritis
	Muscular spasm
	Bone tumor
Neural	Herpes zoster†
Gastrointestinal	Ulcer disease
	Bowel disease
	Hiatal hernia
	Pancreatitis
	Cholecystitis
Emotional	Anxiety
	Depression

* Tietze's syndrome, which is an inflammation of the costal cartilages.
† Shingles, which is a viral invasion of the peripheral nerves in a dermatomal distribution.

TABLE 11-3. Common Causes of Palpitations

Extrasystoles
  Atrial premature beats (APB)*
  Nodal premature beats
  Ventricular premature beats (VPB)†
Tachyarrhythmias
  Paroxysmal supraventricular tachycardia (PSVT)
  Atrial flutter (AFl)
  Atrial fibrillation (AF)
  Multifocal atrial tachycardia (MAT)
  Ventricular tachycardia (VT)
Bradyarrhythmias
  Heart block
  Sinus arrest
Drugs
  Bronchodilators
  Digitalis
  Antidepressants
Smoking
Caffeine
Thyrotoxicosis

* Also known as an atrial premature contraction (APC) or a premature atrial contraction (PAC).
† Also known as a ventricular premature contraction (VPC) or a premature ventricular contraction (PVC).

When chest pain is related to a cardiac etiology, coronary atherosclerosis and aortic valvular disease are the most common causes. Table 11-2 lists some common causes of chest pain.

Palpitations

Palpitations are the uncomfortable sensations in the chest associated with a wide range of arrhythmias. Patients may describe palpitations as "fluttering," "skipped beats," "pounding," "jumping," "stopping," or "irregularity." It is important to determine whether the patient has had similar episodes in the past and what was done to extinguish them. Palpitations are very common and do not necessarily indicate serious heart disease. Any condition in which there is an increased stroke volume, as in aortic regurgitation, may be associated with a sensation of "forceful contraction." When a patient complains of palpitations, it is important to ask the following questions:

"For how long have you had palpitations?"
"Do you have recurrent attacks?" If so, *"How frequently do they occur?"*
"When did the current attack begin?"
"How long did it last?"
"What did it feel like?"
"Did any maneuvers or positions stop it?"

"Did it stop abruptly?"
"Could you count your pulse during the attack?"
"Can you tap out on the table what the rhythm was like?"
"Have you noticed palpitations after strenuous exercise? . . . on exertion? . . . while lying on your left side? . . . after a meal? . . . when tired?"
"During the palpitations, have you ever fainted? . . . had chest pain?"
*"Was there an associated flush, headache, or sweating associated with the palpitations?"**
"Have you noticed an intolerance to heat? . . . cold?"
"What kind of medications are you taking?"
"Do you take any medications for your lungs?"
"Are you taking any thyroid medications?"
"Have you ever been told that you had a problem with your thyroid?"
"How much tea, coffee, or cola sodas do you consume a day?"
"Do you smoke?"
"Do you drink alcoholic beverages?"
"Did you notice that after the palpitations you had to urinate?"†

In addition to primary cardiovascular causes, thyrotoxicosis, hypoglycemia, fever, anemia, pheochromocytoma, and anxiety states are commonly associated with palpitations. Hyperthyroidism is an important cause of rhythm disturbances that originate outside the cardiovascular system. Caffeine, tobacco, and drugs are also important factors in arrhythmogenicity. Sympathomimetic amines used in the treatment of bronchoconstriction are potent stimuli for arrhythmia as well. In patients with panic disorders and other anxiety states, the sensation of palpitations may occur during periods of normal rate and rhythm.

Patients who have had previous attacks of palpitations should be asked the following:

"How was your previous attack terminated?"
"How often do you get the attacks?"
"Are you able to terminate them?" If so, *"How?"*
"Have you ever been told that you have Wolff-Parkinson-White syndrome?"‡

Table 11–3 outlines the common causes of palpitations.

Dyspnea

The complaint of dyspnea is very important. A patient will describe that he has "shortness of breath" or that he "can't get enough air." Dyspnea is commonly related to cardiac or pulmonary conditions. The questions relating to dyspnea are discussed in Chapter 10, The Chest. This section further delineates dyspnea as a *cardiac* symptom.

Paroxysmal nocturnal dyspnea (PND) occurs at night or when the patient is supine. This position increases the intrathoracic blood volume, and a weakened

---

* Symptoms associated with a pheochromocytoma.

† After an attack of paroxysmal atrial tachycardia (PAT), patients often have an urge to urinate. The pathophysiology is not well understood, but the association is present.

‡ The use of this technical term is appropriate, because a patient having this form of pre-excitation may have been told of this condition and may recognize the name.

TABLE 11–4. Common Causes of Dyspnea

Organ System or Condition	Cause
Cardiac	Left ventricular failure
	Mitral stenosis
Pulmonary	Obstructive lung disease
	Asthma
	Restrictive lung disease
	Pulmonary embolism
	Pulmonary hypertension
Emotional	Anxiety
High altitude exposure	Decreased oxygen pressure
Anemia	Decreased oxygen carrying capacity

heart may be unable to handle this increased load; congestive heart failure may result. The patient is awakened about 2 hours after having fallen asleep, is markedly dyspneic, is often coughing, and seeks relief by running to a window to "get more air." Episodes of PND are relatively specific for congestive heart failure.

The symptom of PND is often associated with the symptom of *orthopnea.* Orthopnea is the need for using more pillows on which to sleep. It is important to inquire of all patients, "How many pillows do you need in order to sleep?" To help quantify the orthopnea, one can state, for example, "3 pillow orthopnea for the past 4 months."

Dyspnea on exertion (DOE) is usually due to chronic congestive heart failure or severe pulmonary disease. It is important to quantify the severity of the dyspnea by asking, "How many level blocks can you walk now?" "How many level blocks could you walk 6 months ago?" The examiner can now attempt to quantify the dyspnea. For example, "The patient has had 1 block DOE for the past 6 months. Prior to 6 months ago, the patient was able to walk 4 blocks without becoming short of breath. In addition, over the past 3 months the patient has noted 4 pillow orthopnea."

Trepopnea is a rare form of positional dyspnea in which the dyspneic patient has less dyspnea while lying on his left or right side. The pathophysiology of trepopnea is not well understood.

Table 11–4 lists the common causes of dyspnea.

Syncope

Fainting, or syncope, is the transient loss of consciousness that is due to inadequate cerebral perfusion. It is very important to ask the patient what *he* means by "fainting" or "dizziness." Syncope may be related to cardiac as well as noncardiac causes. When a patient describes fainting, it is important to ask the following questions:

"What were you doing just before you fainted?"

"Have you had recurrent fainting spells?" If so, *"How often do you have these attacks?"*

"Was there an abrupt onset to the fainting?"

"Did you lose consciousness?"

"In what position were you when you fainted?"

"Was the fainting preceded by any other symptom? . . . nausea? . . . chest pain? . . . palpitations? . . . confusion? . . . numbness? . . . hunger?"

"Did you have any warning that you were going to faint?"

"Did you have any black, tarry bowel movements after the faint?"

The activity that preceded the syncope is important because some cardiac etiologies are associated with syncope during exercise, e.g., valvular aortic stenosis, idiopathic hypertrophic subaortic stenosis, and primary pulmonary hypertension. If a patient describes palpitations prior to the syncope, an arrhythmogenic cause may be present. Cardiac output may be reduced by arrhythmias or obstructive lesions.

The position of the patient just before fainting is important because this information may help determine the cause of the syncope. For example, if a patient fainted after rising suddenly from bed in the middle of the night to run to answer the telephone, *orthostatic hypotension* may be the cause. Orthostatic hypotension is a form of postural syncope and is the result of a peripheral autonomic limitation. There is a sudden fall in systemic blood pressure resulting from a failure of adaptive reflexes to compensate for an erect posture. *Micturition syncope* is that occurring usually during straining with nocturnal urination. It is usually seen after considerable alcohol consumption.

Vasovagal syncope is the most common type of fainting. Vasovagal syncope occurs during periods of emotional strain, such as donating blood, receiving bad

TABLE 11–5. Common Causes of Syncope

Organ System or Condition	Cause
Cardiac	Decreased cerebral perfusion secondary to cardiac rhythm disturbance Left ventricular output obstruction
Metabolic	Hypoglycemia Hyperventilation Hypoxia
Psychiatric	Hysteria
Neurologic	Epilepsy Cerebrovascular disease
Orthostatic hypotension	Volume depletion Antidepressant medications Antihypertensive medications
Vasovagal	Vasodepression
Micturition	Visceral reflex (vasodepressor)
Cough	Chronic lung disease
Carotid sinus	Vasodepressor response to carotid sinus sensitivity

news, or a stressful situation. It is often preceded by nausea, weakness, perspiration, epigastric discomfort, or a "sinking feeling." There is a sudden fall in systemic vascular resistance without a compensatory increase in cardiac output as a result of an increased vagotonia. *Carotid sinus syncope* is associated with a hypersensitive carotid sinus and is seen more commonly in the aged. Whenever a patient with carotid sinus syncope wears a tight shirt collar or turns his neck in a certain fashion, there is an increased stimulation of the carotid sinus. This causes a sudden fall in systemic pressure, and syncope results. Two types of carotid sinus hypersensitivity exist: a cardioinhibitory (bradycardia) type, and a vasodepressor (hypotension without bradycardia) type. *Post-tussive syncope* occurs generally in patients with chronic obstructive lung disease. Several mechanisms have been postulated to explain its occurrence. It is generally accepted that coughing produces an increase in intrathoracic pressure that decreases venous return and decreases cardiac output. There may also be a rise in cerebrospinal fluid pressure producing a decreased perfusion to the brain.

There are other suggested questions to ask a patient with syncope that direct one's attention to a neurologic etiology. These are summarized in Chapter 18, The Nervous System. Table 11 – 5 lists the common causes of syncope.

Fatigue

Fatigue is a common symptom of decreased cardiac output. Patients with congestive heart failure and mitral valvular disease frequently complain of fatigue. Fatigue, however, is not specific for cardiac problems. The most common causes of fatigue are anxiety and depression. Other conditions associated with fatigue include anemia and chronic diseases. The line of questioning must attempt to differentiate organic fatigue from psychogenic fatigue. Ask the following questions:

"For how long have you been tired?"
"Was the onset abrupt?"
"Do you feel tired all day? . . . in the morning? . . . in the evening?"
"When do you feel least tired?"
"Do you feel more tired at home than at work?"
"Is the fatigue relieved by rest?"

Patients with psychogenic fatigue are tired "all the time." They are often more tired at home than at work, but occasionally describe being more tired in the morning. They may feel their best at the *end* of the day, when most patients with organic causes feel the worst.

Edema

Swelling of the legs, a form of *dependent edema,* is a very frequent complaint of patients. The interviewer should ask:

"When was the swelling first noted?"
"Are both legs swollen equally?"
"Did the swelling appear suddenly?"
"Is the swelling worse at any time of the day?"
"Does it disappear after a night's sleep?"

"Does elevation of your feet make the swelling less?"
"What kind of medications are you taking?"
"Is there a history of kidney, heart, or liver disease?"
"Do you have shortness of breath?" If so, *"Which came first, the edema, or the shortness of breath?"*
"Do you have pain in the legs?"
"Do you have any ulcers on your legs?"
If the patient is a woman, *"Are you taking oral contraceptives?" "Is the edema associated with menstrual changes?"*

The patient with congestive heart failure has symmetric edema of the lower extremities that worsens as the day progresses. It is best in the morning after sleeping with elevation of the legs in bed. If the patient also complains of dyspnea, it is helpful to determine which symptom came first. In patients with dyspnea and edema secondary to cardiac causes, the dyspnea usually precedes the edema.

Hemoptysis

Hemoptysis is discussed in Chapter 10, The Chest. In addition to the pulmonary causes, mitral stenosis should not be forgotten as an important cause of hemoptysis. Rupture of the bronchial veins, which are under high back pressure, produces the hemoptysis.

Cyanosis

Cyanosis is discussed in Chapter 10. The important questions regarding cyanosis are indicated in that chapter.

One may occasionally note cyanosis of only the lower extremities. This is termed *differential cyanosis.* It is related to a right-to-left shunt through a patent ductus arteriosus (PDA). In a right-to-left shunt resulting from pulmonary hypertension, blood in the pulmonary artery crosses the PDA, which is located below the level of the carotid and left subclavian arteries; deoxygenated blood is pumped only to the lower extremity to produce cyanosis in only that location. Some blood does get to the lungs for oxygenation and is ultimately pumped out through the aorta to produce normal skin color in the upper extremity.

IMPACT OF CARDIAC DISEASE ON THE PATIENT

The cardiac patient is intensely fearful. Once a patient has been diagnosed as having cardiac disease, a series of reactions occur. Fear, depression, and anxiety are the end-points. The patient, who was totally asymptomatic until his episode of "sudden death" resulting from a coronary occlusion, is scared. He was resuscitated the first time; will it happen again? When? During his recovery in the hospital, he is afraid to leave the intensive care unit for fear that "no one will be watching." At the time of discharge from the hospital, he is filled with anxiety. Although he desperately wants to go home, he asks himself, "What will happen if I have chest pain at home? Who will provide medical assistance?" He now goes through a period of depression, recognizing what he has gone through. After his convalescence, he becomes fearful of daily situations that may provoke another attack. Can he go back to the daily "hassles" at work? Is it safe to have sexual intercourse? Despite appropriate reassurances from his physician, his anxiety level may remain high. The "cardiac cripple" has developed.

The cardiac patient who has witnessed a fatal cardiac arrest of another patient in his room will often refuse to admit how stressful this event really was. The patient will freely discuss the efficiency of the cardiac arrest team, or complain that the noise kept him from sleeping. He will refuse to identify with the deceased patient.

The cardiac patient approaching surgery has the same fears as all surgical patients; these fears are discussed in Chapter 2, The Patient's Responses. However, surgical procedures for the cardiac patient involve the "nucleus" of the body. The conscientious physician will take time to explain the nature of the problem and the surgical approach. Before the procedure, the physician should allow the patient, and especially the family, to visit the intensive care unit where the patient will be for a few days after surgery. The patient should be reassured that *everything* possible will be done in his behalf. *His* courage and determination and *the physician's* support are essential.

PHYSICAL EXAMINATION

> The equipment necessary for the examination of the heart is the following: a stethoscope, a penlight, and an applicator stick.

The physical examination of the heart includes the following:

- Inspection of the patient
- Blood pressure assessment
- Assessment of the arterial pulse
- Assessment of the jugular venous pulse
- Percussion of the heart
- Palpation of the heart
- Auscultation of the heart
- Evaluation for dependent edema

The patient should be lying supine, with the examiner standing on the right side of the bed. The head of the bed may be elevated slightly if the patient is more comfortable in this position.

Inspection

Evaluate General Appearance

The general inspection of the patient offers valuable clues to cardiac diagnosis. Is the patient in acute distress? What is the patient's breathing like? Is it labored? Are accessory muscles being used?

Inspect the Skin

The skin can reveal many changes associated with cardiac disease. Is cyanosis present? If so, does it appear central or peripheral?

The *temperature* of the skin may reflect cardiac disease. Severe anemia, beriberi, and thyrotoxicosis tend to make the skin warmer; intermittent claudication is associated with coolness of the lower extremity compared with the upper extremity.

Are *xanthomata* present? Tendon xanthomata are stony hard, slightly yellowish masses that are commonly bound on the extensor tendons of the fingers and are pathognomonic for familial hypercholesterolemia. The Achilles tendon and plantar tendons of the soles are also common locations for tendon xanthomata. A patient with a total cholesterol concentration of greater than 450 mg/dL* with tendon xanthomata on the extensor surfaces of his fingers is shown in Plate IX *C*.

Is a rash present? The presence of *erythema marginatum* (erythema in which the reddened areas are disc shaped with raised edges) in a febrile patient suggests acute rheumatic fever.

Inspect the Nails

Frequently, *splinter hemorrhages* may be visible as small reddish-brown lines in the nail bed. These hemorrhages run from the free margin proximally and are classically associated with subacute bacterial endocarditis. However, the finding is nonspecific because it is found in many other conditions, including even local trauma to the nail. A finger having splinter hemorrhages of a patient with endocarditis is shown in Plate IX *D*.

Inspect the Facies

Abnormalities of the heart may also be associated with peculiarities of the face and head. Supravalvular aortic stenosis, a congenital problem, is seen in association with widely set eyes, strabismus, low set ears, an upturned nose, and hypoplasia of the mandible. Moon facies and widely spaced eyes are suggestive of pulmonic stenosis. Expressionless facies with puffy eyelids and loss of the outer third of the eyebrow is seen in hypothyroidism. These individuals may have a cardiomyopathy. The *ear lobe crease,* or Lichtstein's sign, is an oblique crease, often bilateral, seen frequently in patients over the age of 50 with significant coronary artery disease. This is shown in Plate IX *E*. Although it is a useful sign, there are too many false positives and false negatives to make this finding very reliable.

Inspect the Eyes

The presence of yellowish appearing plaques on the eyelids, called *xanthelasma,* should raise the suspicion of an underlying hyperlipoproteinemia, even though this lesion is less specific than the xanthoma. A patient with xanthelasma and hypercholesterolemia is shown in Plate IX *F*.

Examination of the eyes may reveal an *arcus senilis.* An arcus (see Plate VI *A*) seen in a patient *under* the age of 40 years should raise the suspicion of *hypercholesterolemia.* Opacities in the cornea may be evidence for sarcoidosis,

---

* The total cholesterol concentration for an adult is normally less than 220 mg/dL.

which may be responsible for cor pulmonale or myocardial involvement. Displacement of the lens is frequently seen in patients with *Marfan's syndrome,* an important cause of aortic regurgitation. Conjunctival hemorrhages are commonly seen in infective endocarditis. *Hypertelorism,* or widely set eyes, is associated with congenital heart disease, especially pulmonic stenosis and supravalvular aortic stenosis. Retinal evaluation may furnish valuable information about diabetes, hypertension, and atherosclerosis.

Inspect the Mouth

Have the patient open his mouth widely. Inspect the palate. Is the palate high arched? A high-arched palate may be associated with congenital heart problems such as mitral valve prolapse.

Are there *petechiae* on the palate? Subacute bacterial endocarditis is often associated with palatal petechiae, as seen in the patient in Plate X *A.*

Inspect the Neck

Examination of the neck may reveal webbing. Webbing is seen in individuals with Turner's syndrome,* who may have coarctation of the aorta, or in Noonan's syndrome.† Pulmonic stenosis is the associated cardiac abnormality in this condition.

Inspect the Chest Configuration

Inspection of the chest often reveals information about the heart. Because the chest and the heart develop at about the same time during embryogenesis, it is not surprising that anything interfering with the development of the chest may interfere with the heart. A *pectus excavatum,* or caved-in chest, is seen in Marfan's syndrome and in mitral valve prolapse. *Pectus carinatum,* or pigeon breast, is also associated with Marfan's syndrome.

Are there any visible cardiac motions?

Inspect the Extremities

Some congenital abnormalities of the heart are associated with abnormalities of the extremities. Patients with atrial septal defects may have an extra phalanx, an extra finger, or an extra toe. Long, slender fingers suggest Marfan's syndrome and possible aortic regurgitation.

Blood Pressure Assessment

The Principles

Blood pressure can be measured directly with an intra-arterial catheter or indirectly with a sphygmomanometer. The sphygmomanometer consists of an inflatable rubber bladder within a cloth cover, a rubber bulb to inflate the bladder, and a manometer to measure the pressure in the bladder. Indirect measurement of blood pressure involves the auscultatory detection of the appearance and disappearance of the *Korotkoff sounds* over the compressed

---

* Short stature, retarded sexual development, and webbed neck in a female associated with an abnormality of the sex chromosomes (45 XO).
† Male Turner's syndrome (46 XY).

artery. Korotkoff sounds are low-pitched sounds originating in the vessel that are related to turbulence produced by partially occluding an artery with a blood pressure cuff. There are several phases that occur in sequence as the occluding pressure drops. Phase 1 occurs when the occluding pressure falls to the systolic blood pressure. The tapping sounds are clear and gradually increase in intensity as the occluding pressure falls. Phase 2 occurs at a pressure about 10–15 mm Hg lower than phase 1 and consists of tapping sounds followed by murmurs.* Phase 3 occurs when the occluding pressure falls enough to allow a large amount of volume to cross the partially occluded artery. The sounds are similar to the sounds of phase 2 except that only the tapping sounds are heard. Phase 4 is the abrupt muffling and decreased intensity of the sounds as the pressure approaches the diastolic blood pressure. Phase 5 is the complete disappearance of the sounds. The vessel is no longer compressed by the occluding cuff. Turbulent flow is no longer present.

The normal blood pressure for adults is up to 140 mm Hg systolic and up to 95 mm Hg diastolic. The point of disappearance of the Korotkoff sounds is probably more accurate than the point of muffling for the diastolic blood pressure reading (London and London, 1976). However, if the point of disappearance is more than 10 mm Hg lower than the point of muffling, the point of muffling is probably more accurate (Freis, 1968). Recording both the point of muffling and disappearance frequently helps in communication. A blood pressure might be recorded as *125/75–65*. The systolic blood pressure is 125; the point of muffling is 75; the point of disappearance is 65 (the diastolic blood pressure).

Blood pressure should be recorded only to the nearest 5 mm Hg, because there is a ±3 mm Hg limit of accuracy for all sphygmomanometers. In addition, normal blood pressure changes occur from moment to moment and measuring to less than 5 mm Hg provides a false sense of accuracy.

The size of the cuff is important for the accurate determination of blood pressure. It is recommended that the cuff be snugly applied around the arm with its lowest edge 1 inch above the antecubital fossa. The cuff should be approximately 20% wider than the diameter of the extremity. The bladder should overlie the artery. The use of a cuff that is too small for a large arm will result in an erroneously high blood pressure.

The *auscultatory gap* is the silence caused by the disappearance of the Korotkoff sounds after the initial appearance and the reappearance at a lower pressure. The auscultatory gap is present when there is a decreased blood flow to the extremities, as is found in hypertension and in aortic stenosis. The clinical importance lies in the fact that the systolic blood pressure may be mistaken for the lower blood pressure, the point of reappearance.

Determine Blood Pressure by Palpation

Blood pressure assessment is performed with the patient lying comfortably in the supine position. The cuff bladder is centered over the right brachial artery. If the arm is obese, a thigh cuff should be used. The arm should be slightly flexed, and it should be supported at approximately the level of the heart. In order to determine the systolic blood pressure adequately and to exclude an error as a result of an auscultatory gap, blood pressure is first assessed by palpation. In

---

* A murmur is a blowing auscultatory sign produced by turbulence in blood flow. These vibrations can originate in the heart or in blood vessels as a result of hemodynamic changes.

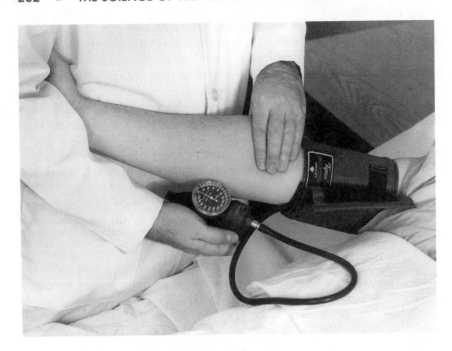

FIGURE 11–11. Technique for blood pressure assessment by palpation.

this procedure, the right brachial or right radial artery is palpated while the cuff is inflated above the pressure required to obliterate the pulse. The adjustable screw is opened slowly for slow deflation. The systolic pressure is identified by the reappearance of the brachial pulse. As soon as the pulse is felt, the adjustable screw is opened for rapid deflation. This is the systolic blood pressure. This is shown in Figure 11–11.

Determine Blood Pressure by Auscultation

Blood pressure by auscultation is assessed in the right arm by inflating the cuff to about 20 mm Hg above the systolic pressure that was determined by palpation. The diaphragm of the stethoscope should be placed over the artery as close to the *edge* of the cuff as possible, preferably just under the edge. The cuff is deflated *slowly,* while the Korotkoff sounds are evaluated. The systolic blood pressure, the point of muffling, and the point of disappearance are determined. The systolic blood pressure is the point at which the initial tapping sounds are heard. The technique of determining auscultatory blood pressure is shown in Figure 11–12. If the blood pressure is high, it is useful to retake the blood pressure at the end of the examination, when the patient may be more calm.

Rule Out Orthostatic Hypotension

Orthostatic hypotension is evaluated by having the patient sit up while the cuff pressure is raised. The blood pressure is then assessed for any drop related to the sitting posture. A fall of 15 mm Hg or more in the systolic blood pressure is a sign of orthostatic, or postural, hypotension. In most patients, there is also an increase in the heart rate when the patient sits up.

Rule Out Supravalvular Aortic Stenosis

If hypertension is detected in the right arm, perform the following test: Place the cuff on the left arm, and determine only the auscultatory pressure. It is not necessary to retake the palpatory pressure or reevaluate for orthostatic

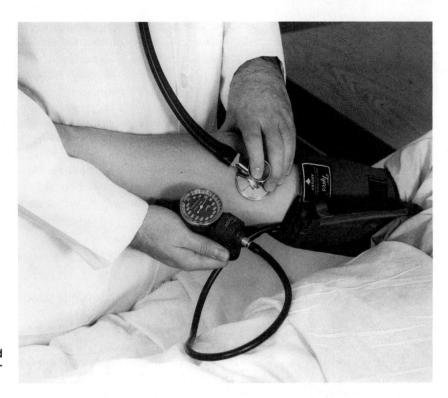

FIGURE 11-12. Technique for blood pressure assessment by auscultation.

changes. In supravalvular aortic stenosis, there is a difference in the blood pressures in the arms; hypertension may be detected in the right arm, whereas hypotension will be present in the left arm.

Rule Out Coarctation of the Aorta

If the blood pressure is elevated in the arms, determination of the blood pressure in the lower extremities is important to exclude coarctation of the aorta. The patient is asked to lie on his abdomen while the thigh cuff, which is 6 cm wider than the arm cuff, is placed around the posterior aspect of the midthigh. The stethoscope is placed over the artery in the popliteal fossa. The Korotkoff sounds are determined as in the upper extremity. If a thigh cuff is not available, the regular cuff can be applied to the lower leg with the distal border just at the malleoli. The stethoscope is placed over either the posterior tibial or the dorsalis pedis artery, and the auscultatory blood pressure is taken. A systolic blood pressure in the leg that is lower than in the arm is suspicious for coarctation of the aorta.

Rule Out Cardiac Tamponade

In the presence of low arterial blood pressure and a rapid and feeble pulse, it is necessary to rule out the presence of cardiac tamponade. A valuable clinical sign suggesting cardiac tamponade is the presence of a marked *paradoxical pulse,* which is characterized by an exaggeration of the normal inspiratory fall in systolic pressure. There is much confusion about the definition of a paradoxical pulse (also known as a *pulsus paradoxus*). A paradoxical pulse should be defined as the *normal* fall (about 5 mm Hg) in systolic arterial pressure during inspiration (Henkind et al, 1987). It is the *magnitude* of the phenomenon that should determine whether the pulsus paradoxus is normal or abnormal.

The technique for assessing the magnitude of a paradoxical pulse is as follows: Have the patient breathe as normally as possible. Inflate the blood pressure cuff until no sounds are heard. Gradually deflate the cuff until sounds are heard in expiration only. Note this pressure. Continue to deflate the cuff *slowly* until sounds are heard during inspiration. Note this pressure. If the difference in these two pressures exceeds 10 mm Hg, a marked pulsus paradoxus is said to be present; cardiac tamponade may be the cause. Cardiac tamponade results when there is an increase in intrapericardial pressure that interferes with normal diastolic filling. An exaggerated pulsus paradoxus is not a specific phenomenon for tamponade because it is also seen in large pericardial effusions; in constrictive pericarditis; and in conditions associated with increased ventilatory effort, such as asthma and emphysema.

The Arterial Pulse

The following information is gained from palpation of the arterial pulse:

- The rate and rhythm of the heart
- The contour of the pulse
- The amplitude of the pulse

Determine the Cardiac Rate

Cardiac rate is routinely assessed by the radial pulse. The examiner should stand in front of the patient and grasp both radial arteries. The second, third, and fourth fingers should overlie the radial artery, as shown in Figure 11–13. The examiner should count the pulse for a period of 30 seconds and multiply the number of beats by 2 to obtain the beats per minute. This method is accurate for most *regular* rhythms. If the patient has an irregularly irregular rhythm, as is found in atrial fibrillation, a *pulse deficit* may be present. In atrial fibrillation, many impulses bombard the atrioventricular node and ventricles. Owing to the varying lengths of diastolic filling periods, some of the contractions may be very weak and unable to produce an adequate pulse wave despite ventricular contraction. A pulse deficit, which is the difference between the apical (precordial) and radial pulses, will occur. In such cases, only auscultation of the heart will provide an accurate assessment of the cardiac rate, and *not* the radial pulse.

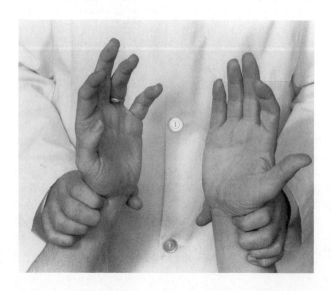

FIGURE 11–13. Technique for evaluating the radial artery pulses.

Determine the Cardiac Rhythm

When palpating the pulse, carefully evaluate the regularity of the rhythm. The slower the rate, the longer you should palpate. If the rhythm is irregular, is there a pattern to the irregularity?

Cardiac rhythm may be described as *regular, regularly irregular,* or *irregularly irregular.* A regularly irregular rhythm is a pulse having an irregularity that occurs in a definite pattern. An irregularly irregular pulse has no pattern.

The electrocardiogram is really the best way of diagnosing the rhythm, but the physical examination may provide some clues. *Premature beats* may be recognized by the presence of isolated extra beats during a regular rhythm. *Bigeminy* is a coupled rhythm of beats in pairs. The first beat is the sinus beat, which is followed by a premature, usually ventricular, beat. If the premature beat is very early in the diastolic period, the pulse from this beat may be missed if the examiner evaluates the rhythm by palpation alone. A rhythm that is grossly irregular with no pattern is termed "irregularly irregular" and is the pulse seen in patients with *atrial fibrillation.*

Palpate the Carotid Artery

Assess the carotid artery pulse by standing at the patient's right side with the patient lying on his back. Place your index and third fingers on the thyroid cartilage and slip them laterally between the trachea and the sternocleidomastoid muscle. You should be able to feel the carotid pulsations just medial to the sternocleidomastoid muscle. Palpation should be performed low in the neck to avoid pressure on the carotid sinus, which would cause a reflex drop in blood pressure and heart rate. Each carotid is evaluated separately. *Never* press on both carotids at the same time! After the right carotid is evaluated, stand in the same position and place the same fingers back on the trachea and slip them laterally to the left to feel the left carotid artery. This technique is demonstrated in Figure 11–14.

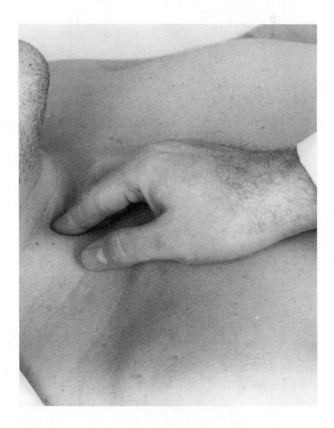

FIGURE 11–14. Technique for evaluating the carotid artery pulsations.

Evaluate the Characteristics of the Pulse

The carotid artery is used for the assessment of the contour and amplitude of the pulse. Contour is the shape of the wave. It is frequently described as the speed of the upslope, downslope, and duration of the wave. The examiner should place his hand firmly against the carotid artery until maximal force is felt. At this moment, the waveform should be discernible. The pulse may be described as *normal, diminished, increased,* or *double peaked.* The normal carotid pulse wave is smooth, with the upstroke steeper and more rapid than the downstroke. A diminished pulse is a small, weak pulse. The palpating finger feels a gentle pressure rise with a distinct peak. An increased pulse is a large, strong, hyperkinetic pulse. The palpating finger feels an increased rate of rise of the ascending limb of the pulse and a brisk tap at its peak. A double-peaked pulse has a prominent percussion and tidal wave with or without a dicrotic wave. (A summary of arterial pulse abnormalities may be found in Figure 11–29.)

The Jugular Venous Pulse

The *internal jugular vein* provides information about the wave forms and right atrial pressure. The pulsations of the internal jugular vein are beneath the sternocleidomastoid muscle and are visible as they are transmitted through the surrounding tissue. The vein itself is not visible. Because the right internal jugular vein is straighter than the left, only the right internal jugular vein is evaluated. The external jugular system, which is easier to visualize, is much less accurate and should not be used.

Determine the Jugular Wave Forms

In order to visualize the jugular wave forms, the examiner should have the patient lie flat without a pillow so that the neck will not be flexed and interfere with the pulsations. The patient's trunk should be at approximately 25° to the horizontal. The higher the venous pressure, the greater the elevation that will be required; the lower the pressure, the lower the elevation needed. The patient's head should be turned slightly to the right and slightly down to relax the right

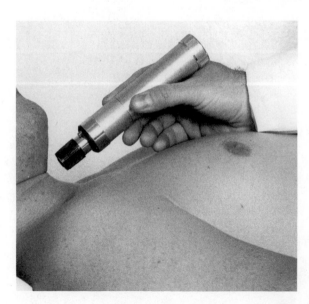

FIGURE 11–15. Technique for evaluating the jugular wave forms.

TABLE 11–6. Differentiation of Jugular and Carotid Wave Forms

	Internal Jugular Pulse	Carotid Pulse
Palpation	Not palpable	Palpable
Wave forms	Multiform: 2 or 3 components	Single
Quality	Soft, undulating	Vigorous
Pressure*	Wave forms obliterated	No effect
Inspiration	Decreased height of wave forms	No effect
Sitting up	Decreased height of wave forms	No effect
Valsalva maneuver	Increased height of wave forms	No effect

* Light pressure on the vessel above the sternal end of clavicle.

sternocleidomastoid muscle. Standing on the patient's right side, the examiner should place his right hand, holding a small pocket flashlight, on the patient's sternum and shine the light tangentially across the right side of the patient's neck. Shadows of the pulsations will be cast on the sheet behind the patient. The light and shadows serve to magnify the wave forms. This technique is shown in Figure 11–15. If no wave forms are seen, the angle of elevation of the head of the bed should be reduced. To help identify the wave forms, the examiner can time the cardiac cycle by palpating the cardiac impulse beneath his right hand or by feeling the left carotid impulse with his left hand. The descents, rather than the waves themselves, tend to be more obvious. If the neck veins are visible at the jaw margin while the patient is seated, the examiner should watch for the waveforms at the angle of the jaw with the patient seated upright.

The jugular pulse must be differentiated from the pulsation of the carotid artery. Table 11–6 lists the most important characteristic differences of these pulses.

Estimate the Jugular Venous Pressure

In order to assess the pressure in the right heart, it is necessary to establish a reference level. The standard reference is the manubriosternal angle. At any degree of elevation, one uses this position to measure the pressure in the internal jugular system. The examiner must first determine the height of the venous distention by noting the top of the wave forms in the internal jugular venous pulsations. An imaginary horizontal line is then drawn from this height to the sternal angle. The examiner should then measure the distance from the sternal angle to this imaginary line. The angle of elevation of the head of the bed is also estimated. It might be stated, "At 45° elevation, the jugular pulse is 7 cm above the sternal angle." At 45°, the upper limit of normal is 4–5 cm above the sternal angle; if the patient is at 30°, the upper limit of normal is 6 cm. When the height of the venous column is equal or lower than the sternal angle in the supine position, venous pressure is usually normal.

There is tremendous inaccuracy in attempting to determine the pressure in the right atrium by the jugular manometer as just indicated. It has been demonstrated numerous times that the sensitivity and specificity of this test are low, thus rendering this test inaccurate in predicting elevated pressures. The only accurate statement one can make is that right atrial pressure is high when there is neck vein distention up to the jaw margin while the patient is seated at 90°. At this time, the right atrial pressure generally exceeds 15 mm Hg. The patient shown in Plate X B has distended neck veins to the angle of the jaw while seated upright. His right atrial pressure was 21 mm Hg.

Evaluate the Hepatojugular Reflux

A useful test in assessing high jugular venous pressure is the hepatojugular reflux. This test is also known as abdominal compression. By applying pressure over the liver, one can grossly assess right ventricular function. The patient with right ventricular failure has a liver with dilated sinusoids. Pressure on the liver pushes blood out of these sinusoids and into the inferior vena cava and right heart, causing further distention of the neck veins. The procedure is performed with the patient lying in bed, his mouth open, breathing normally; this prevents a Valsalva maneuver. The examiner places his right hand over the liver in the right upper quadrant and applies a firm, progressive pressure. Compression is maintained for about 20–30 seconds. The normal response is for the internal and external jugular veins to show a transient increase in distention during the first few cardiac cycles, which is followed by a fall to baseline levels during the later part of the compression. In right ventricular failure, there is a maintenance of the distended neck veins during the entire period of compression, which falls rapidly upon sudden release of the compressing hand. If the examination is incorrectly performed with the patient's mouth closed, a Valsalva maneuver will result and will produce inaccurate results of the hepatojugular reflux test.

Several investigators feel that the hepatojugular reflux test is a technique of low sensitivity and specificity. This is usually related to incorrect technique. If performed correctly as indicated, the accuracy rate should be acceptable.

Percussion

Percuss the Heart's Borders

The technique of percussion has been discussed in the previous chapter. Percussion is performed at the third, fourth, and fifth intercostal spaces from the left anterior axillary line to the right anterior axillary line. Normally, there will be a change in the percussion note from resonance to dullness about 6 cm lateral to the left of the sternum. This dullness is due to the presence of the heart.

Most clinicians feel that percussion of the heart to estimate its size contributes little, because the sensitivity of the technique is low. In some clinical conditions, percussion may be useful. These include dextrocardia* and tension pneumothorax† of the left chest. In these conditions, abnormal dullness to the right of the sternum may be found.

Palpation

Palpation is performed in order to evaluate the apical impulse, the right ventricle, the pulmonary artery, and the left ventricular motions. The presence or absence of *thrills*‡ is also determined by palpation. The apical impulse, or the

---

* The heart is in the right chest with the apex directed to the right.
† Air in the pleural cavity.
‡ Low frequency cutaneous vibrations associated with loud heart murmurs.

point of maximum impulse (PMI), describes the outward motion of the cardiac apex as it rotates counterclockwise, as viewed from below, to strike the anterior chest wall during isovolumetric contraction.

Palpate the Point of Maximum Impulse

The examiner should stand on the right side of the patient, with the bed at a comfortable level for the examiner. Palpation for the point of maximum impulse is most easily performed with the patient in a sitting position. Only the fingertips should be applied to the chest in the fifth intercostal space, midclavicular line, because they are the most sensitive for assessing localized motion. The point of maximum impulse should be noted. This technique is demonstrated in Figure 11–16. If the apical impulse is not felt, the examiner should move the fingertips in the area of the cardiac apex. The point of maximum impulse is usually within 10 cm from the midsternal line and is no larger than 2–3 cm in diameter. A point of maximum impulse that is laterally displaced or is felt in two interspaces during the same phase of respiration suggests cardiomegaly.

The point of maximum impulse is felt in approximately 70% of normal individuals while sitting. If the point of maximum impulse cannot be felt in the sitting position, the patient should be re-evaluated while lying supine and in the left lateral decubitus position. The position of the point of maximum impulse in the left lateral decubitus position must be assessed with the understanding that the normal cardiac impulse will now be shifted slightly to the left. If in the left lateral decubitus position the point of maximum impulse is not laterally displaced, one can suspect that cardiomegaly is not present. If the apical impulse *is* laterally displaced, no definite appraisal can be made.

Although the point of maximum impulse usually corresponds to the *left* ventricular apex, in patients with an enlarged right ventricle, the heart rotates clockwise, as viewed from below, and the point of maximum impulse may actually be produced by the *right* ventricle. This rotation turns the left ventricle posteriorly and makes it difficult to palpate. The apical impulse by the right ventricle is more diffuse than that of the left ventricle, which tends to be more localized.

In patients with chronic obstructive lung disease, the overinflation of the lungs displaces the point of maximum impulse downward and to the right. The point of maximum impulse in such patients is felt in the *epigastric* area, at the lower end of the sternum. In patients with chronic obstructive lung disease, a point of maximum impulse in the normal location suggests cardiomegaly.

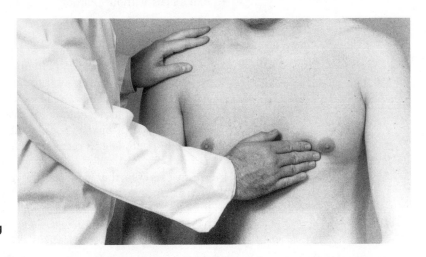

FIGURE 11–16. Technique for assessing the point of maximum impulse.

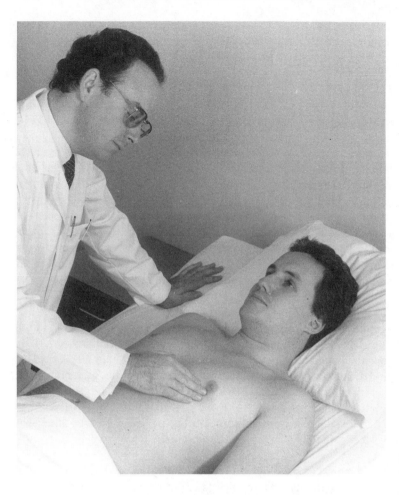

FIGURE 11–17. Technique for assessing localized cardiac movement.

Palpate for Localized Motion

The patient should be now instructed to lie down so that palpation of all four main cardiac areas can be performed. The examiner uses the fingertips to assess any localized motion. This technique is shown in Figure 11–17.

The presence of a systolic impulse in the second intercostal space to the left of the sternum is suspicious for pulmonary hypertension. This impulse is due to the closure of the pulmonic valve under increased pressure. The presence of this impulse suggests a dilated pulmonary artery, but it may also be felt in thin individuals without pulmonary hypertension.

Palpate for Generalized Motion

After the chest has been palpated with the fingertips, the examiner uses the proximal portion of the hand to feel for any large area of sustained outward motion, called a *heave* or *lift.* The examiner again palpates each of the four main cardiac areas. The technique for assessing heaves is shown in Figure 11–18. The presence of an *RV rock,* which is a sustained left parasternal impulse associated with lateral retraction, suggests a large right ventricle.

Any condition that increases the rate of ventricular filling during early diastole can produce a palpable impulse that occurs *after* the main left ventricular impulse. This second impulse in the area of the point of maximum impulse is usually felt in association with an S_3. Frequently an S_3 is easier felt than heard.

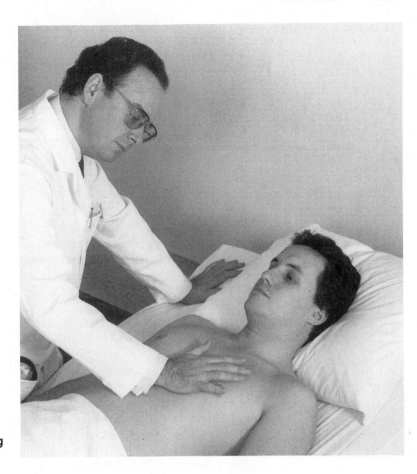

FIGURE 11-18. Technique for assessing generalized cardiac movement.

The use of a tongue blade or an applicator stick can be helpful to reinforce visually what has been palpated. The tip of the stick is placed directly over the area and held in place by the examiner's finger. This acts as a fulcrum, and the motions tend to be magnified by the movement of the stick. The technique is shown in Figure 11-19.

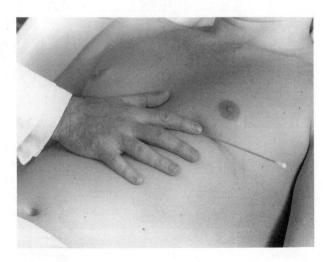

FIGURE 11-19. Technique for amplifying detection of cardiac movement.

Palpate for Thrills

Thrills are the superficial vibratory sensations felt on the skin overlying an area of turbulence. The presence of a thrill indicates a loud murmur. Thrills are best felt by using the heads of the metacarpal bones rather than the fingertips and applying very gentle pressure on the skin. If too much pressure is applied, thrills will not be appreciated. The palpation of thrills is generally of little importance, because auscultation will reveal the presence of the loud murmur that has produced the thrill. Therefore, the finding of a thrill adds little to the diagnosis, but it is an interesting physical sign to alert the examiner as to what will be heard.

Auscultation

The Technique

Proper auscultation requires a quiet area. Every attempt should be made to eliminate extraneous noise from radios, televisions, and so forth. The earpieces of the stethoscope are directed anteriorly, or parallel to the direction of the external auditory canal. If the earpieces are put in backward, the openings of the earpieces will impinge on the wall of the external canal and lower the intensity of the sounds. The earpieces should fit properly so as to be comfortable but tight enough to exclude external noises.

It is often useful for you to close your eyes when listening to the heart. Sounds that are more difficult to hear will actually sound louder. This is related to the fact that our brains are flooded with all types of sensory input. The input from our eyes appears to be the most important. The next important sensory input is auditory input, which is followed by tactile input. If you eliminate the distraction of visual stimuli, more concentration by the brain will be placed on the auditory input and the sounds will become more evident.

As indicated in the previous chapter, the bell of the stethoscope should be applied lightly to the skin, whereas the diaphragm should be pressed tightly to the skin. High-pitched sounds, such as valve closure, systolic events, and regurgitant murmurs, are better heard with the diaphragm. Low-pitched sounds, such as gallop rhythms or the murmur of atrioventricular stenosis, are better heard with the bell.

Never listen through *any* type of clothing!

Auscultate the Cardiac Areas

The examiner should be on the right side of the patient while the patient lies flat on his back. If not already at the proper height, the bed should be adjusted so that the examiner will be comfortable. The examiner should listen in the aortic, pulmonic, tricuspid, and mitral areas. However, the examiner should not limit his auscultation to these areas alone. The examiner should start at any area and "inch" the stethoscope over the precordium from area to area. The areas have been established to provide some degree of standardization.

While listening at the apex and left lower sternal border with the bell, the examiner should determine whether an S_3 or an S_4 is present.

Cardiac murmurs may radiate widely. The important observation is to determine where the sounds are loudest or best heard. There are no acoustic walls in the chest. A murmur typically heard at the apex with radiation to the axilla may be heard in the neck, if it is loud enough. The murmur in this example is probably loudest at the apex and axilla.

The Standard Auscultation Positions

The four standard positions for auscultation are shown in Figure 11–20. They are as follows:

- Supine
- Left lateral decubitus
- Upright
- Upright, leaning forward

All precordial areas are examined while the patient is supine. Using a systematic approach, the examiner starts at either the aortic area or the apex and carefully listens to the heart sounds. After all areas are examined, the patient is then instructed to turn on his left side. The examiner should now listen at the apex for the low-pitched diastolic murmur of *mitral stenosis,* which is best heard with the bell of the stethoscope. The examiner has the patient sit upright and examines all areas with the diaphragm of the stethoscope. Finally, the patient is asked to sit up and lean forward. The patient is asked to exhale and hold his breath while the examiner, using the diaphragm, listens for the high-pitched diastolic murmur of *aortic regurgitation* at the right and left second and third intercostal spaces.

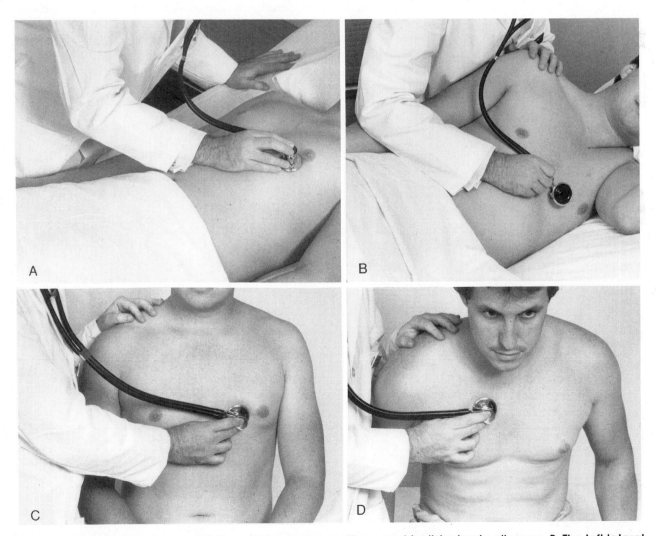

FIGURE 11–20. Positions for auscultation. *A,* The supine position, used for listening to all areas. *B,* The left lateral decubitus position, used for listening with the bell in the mitral area. *C,* The upright position, used for listening to all areas. *D,* The upright, leaning forward position, used for listening at the base positions.

The Influence of Breathing

The examiner should pay special attention to the influence of breathing on the intensity of heart sounds. Most murmurs or sounds originating in the right heart will be accentuated with inspiration. This is related to the increased return of blood that occurs with inspiration and the resultant increased right ventricular output. In addition, an S_3 or an S_4 originating in the right heart will likewise be accentuated during inspiration.

Time the Cardiac Events

In order to interpret heart sounds accurately, the examiner must be able to time the events of the cardiac cycle. The most reliable way of identifying S_1 and S_2 is to time the sounds by palpating the carotid artery. While the examiner's right hand is positioning the stethoscope, the left hand is placed on the patient's carotid artery. This technique is demonstrated in Figure 11–21. The sound that precedes the carotid pulse is the S_1. The S_2 follows the pulse. It is most important that the carotid and *not* the radial pulse be used. The time delay from S_1 to the radial pulse is significant, and errors in timing will result.

Approach to Careful Auscultation

Until the examiner gains expertise in cardiac examination, he should evaluate heart sounds in the manner suggested in Table 11–7. The examiner should take his time in each area before continuing on to the next area. He should listen to several cardiac cycles at each position in order to be certain of the observations made, which include respiratory effects.

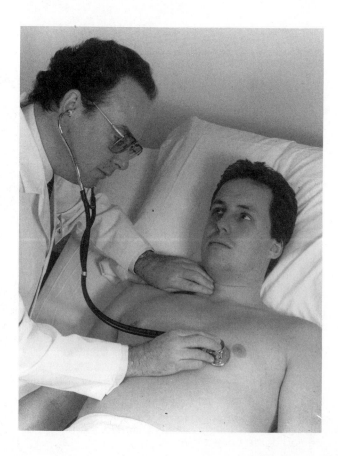

FIGURE 11–21. Technique for timing the heart sounds.

TABLE 11–7. Approach to Cardiac Auscultation

Position	Evaluate
Supine	S_1 in all areas
	S_2 in all areas
	Systolic murmurs or sounds in all areas
Left lateral decubitus	Diastolic events at apex with bell of stethoscope
Upright	S_1 in all areas
	S_2 in all areas
	Systolic murmurs or sounds in all areas
	Diastolic murmurs or sounds in all areas
Upright, leaning forward	Diastolic events at base with diaphragm of stethoscope

Describe Any Murmurs Present

If a murmur is present, attention should be directed to the following features:

- Timing in the cardiac cycle
- Location
- Radiation
- Duration
- Intensity
- Pitch
- Quality
- Relationship to respiration
- Relationship to body position

Timing of murmurs as to systole and diastole is paramount. Does the systolic murmur begin with, or after, S_1? Does it end before, with, or after S_2? Does the murmur occupy the entire systolic period? Murmurs occurring throughout systole are termed *holosystolic* or *pansystolic*. These murmurs begin with S_1 and end after S_2. A *systolic ejection* murmur begins after S_1 and ends before S_2. Does the murmur occur only in early systole, mid-systole, or late systole? Does the murmur persist throughout the entire diastolic period? Such murmurs are termed *holodiastolic*.

In which area is the murmur best heard?

The *radiation* of the murmur can provide a clue as to its cause. Does it radiate to the axilla? the neck? the back?

The intensity of a murmur is graded from I to VI, based on increasing loudness. The following grading system, though antiquated, serves as a means of communicating to others the intensity of the murmur.

I Lowest intensity, often not heard by inexperienced listeners

II Low intensity, usually audible by inexperienced listeners

III Medium intensity without a thrill

IV Medium intensity with a thrill

V Loudest murmur that is audible when the stethoscope is placed on the chest. Associated with a thrill.

VI Loudest intensity: audible when stethoscope is removed from chest. Associated with a thrill.

Murmurs can be described, for example, as "grade II/VI," "grade IV/VI," or "grade II–III/VI." Any murmur associated with a thrill must be at least a grade IV/VI. It is important to understand that a grade IV/VI murmur is louder than a grade II/VI murmur only because there is more turbulence; both or neither may be of clinical significance. The "/VI" is used because there is another less popular grading system using only four categories. An important axiom to remember is the following:

> **In general, the intensity of a murmur tells you nothing about the severity of the clinical state!**

The *quality* of a murmur can be described as "rumbling," "blowing," "harsh," "musical," "machinery," or "scratchy."

Describe Any Pericardial Rubs

Friction rubs are extracardiac sounds of short duration that have a unique quality similar to the sound of scratching on sandpaper. Rubs may result from irritation of the pleura (i.e., a pleural rub), or of the pericardium (i.e., a pericardial rub). Pericardial rubs typically have three components: one systolic and two diastolic. The systolic component occurs during ejection; the two diastolic components occur during rapid filling and atrial contraction. Pericardial rubs are best heard with the patient sitting while holding his breath in expiration. Patients with pericardial rubs commonly have chest pain that is lessened by sitting forward. A rub that disappears while the patient holds his breath originates from the pleura.

The Goals of Auscultation

The goals at the end of auscultation are to be able to describe the following:

- The intensity of S_1 in all areas
- The intensity of S_2 in all areas
- The characterization of any systolic sounds
- The characterization of any diastolic sounds

With experience, the examiner will be able to listen to all parts of the cardiac cycle in one area and compare the sounds and events with other areas. Normally, S_1 is loudest at the apex and S_2 is loudest at the base. Splitting of S_2 into A_2 and P_2 during inspiration is best heard at the pulmonic area with the patient lying on his back. As previously indicated, this increases venous return and widens the A_2-P_2 split.

Examination for Edema

When peripheral venous pressure is high, as in congestive heart failure, pressure within the veins is distributed retrograde to the smaller vessels. Transudation of fluid occurs, and edema of dependent areas results. This increase in tissue fluid produces edema that "pits."

Test for Edema

To test for pitting edema, the fingers are pressed into a dependent area, such as the shin, for 2 – 3 seconds. If pitting edema is present, the fingers will sink into the tissue, and when the fingers are removed, the impression of the fingers will remain. This technique is shown in Figure 11 – 22.

Pitting edema is usually quantified from 1 + to 4 +, depending upon how long the indentation persists. The most noticeable is 4 +. In patients who are bedridden, the dependent area is usually the sacrum and not the shins. The examiner should evaluate for edema at the sacrum in these patients. Figure 11 – 23 illustrates 4 + sacral edema in a bedridden patient.

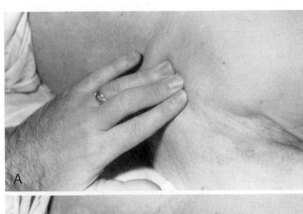

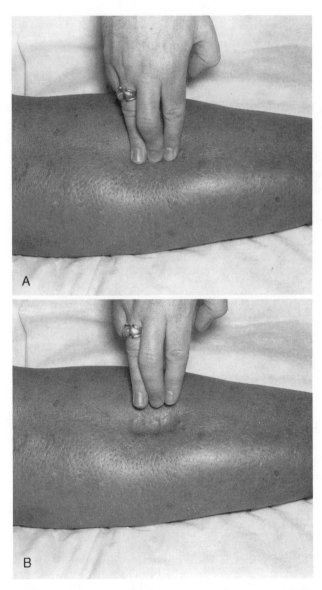

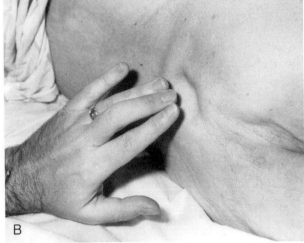

FIGURE 11 – 22. Technique for testing for pitting edema. *A* shows the examiner pressing into the shin area. *B* shows the indentation that occurs after the fingers are lifted when pitting edema is present.

FIGURE 11 – 23. Technique for testing for pitting edema of the sacrum. *A* shows the examiner pressing at the sacrum. *B* shows the pitting edema in this bedridden patient.

CLINICOPATHOLOGIC CORRELATIONS

Attention will now be focused on the pathologic changes, which result in the following:

- Abnormalities of the first heart sound
- Abnormalities of the second heart sound
- Systolic clicks
- Diastolic opening snaps
- Murmurs

Abnormalities of the First Heart Sound

Abnormalities of the Intensity of S_1

The factors that are responsible for the intensity of S_1 are as follows:

- The rate of rise of ventricular pressure
- The condition of the valve
- The position of the valve
- The distance of the heart from the chest wall

The faster the *rate of rise* of left ventricular pressure, the louder the mitral component of S_1 will be. Increased contractility will increase the intensity of S_1. Decreased contractility will soften S_1.

When the atrioventricular valve stiffens as a result of fibrosis or calcification, its closure will be louder. The pathologically deformed valve of mitral stenosis will produce an accentuated or louder S_1. After many years, as the valve becomes more and more calcified, it will be unable to move, causing S_1 to soften.

The *position of the valve* at the time of ventricular contraction affects the intensity of S_1. The *arc of coaptation* is the angle through which the valve closes. If the valve is in a midposition, it travels less than when it closes from a widely opened position. The more it is opened, the wider the arc of coaptation, and the louder is S_1. This is directly related to the pressure in the left atrium at the moment that the left ventricular pressure exceeds it and closes the valve. This can be seen in conditions in which there is a shortened PR interval on the electrocardiogram. The mitral valve is opened normally during diastole for ventricular filling. The P wave of the electrocardiogram corresponds to atrial contraction, which elevates left atrial pressure (the ''a'' wave of the left atrial tracing), further opening the mitral valve in late diastole. If the PR interval is short, ventricular contraction occurs so quickly after atrial contraction that the atrial pressure is still high when the left ventricular pressure exceeds it. The mitral valve stays open longer and closes later than normal, during the rapid rate of rise of the ventricle, which accentuates S_1.

In general, the longer the PR interval, the softer the S_1. Lengthening of the PR intervals, as is seen in Wenckebach's phenomenon,* produces an S_1 that softens until the dropped beat occurs.

---

* Gradually increasing PR intervals until a dropped beat occurs.

Whenever the heart is *further from the chest wall,* S_1 will be softer than normal. In patients who are very obese or have chronic obstructive lung disease, the intensity of S_1 will be softer than normal. In patients with a large pericardial effusion, S_1 will likewise be soft.

Abnormalities of the Second Heart Sound

Abnormalities of the Intensity of S_2

The conditions that change the intensity of S_2 are as follows:

- Changes in systolic pressure
- Condition of the valve

Any condition that produces an increase in the systolic pressure will increase the intensity of S_2. Conversely, conditions that lower the systolic pressure will soften S_2. Hypertension raises aortic systolic pressure and produces a loud A_2 component of S_2.

Calcification or *fibrosis* of the semilunar valves will produce a softening of their closure, S_2. Because the semilunar valves are a morphologically different type of valve, fibrosis does not cause an increased intensity, as in closure of a fibrotic atrioventricular valve.

Abnormalities of Splitting of S_2

Normal physiologic splitting of the second heart sound has already been discussed in the section on anatomy and physiology. The section will deal with abnormalities of splitting.

Any condition that delays right ventricular systole, either electrically or mechanically, will delay P_2 and produce a widened splitting of S_2. Right ventricular emptying will be delayed by a right bundle branch block or pulmonic stenosis. The pulmonic component of S_2 will be delayed during both inspiration and expiration, and *wide splitting* of S_2 will occur.

Any condition that shortens left ventricular systole will allow A_2 to occur earlier than normal, and wide splitting will likewise occur. Conditions such as mitral regurgitation, ventricular septal defect, or patent ductus arteriosus will shorten left ventricular systole, and the S_1 to A_2 interval will be shorter than normal. In these conditions, there is a "double outlet" to the left ventricle, and systole will therefore be shorter. In a ventricular septal defect with a left-to-right shunt, not only will left ventricular systole be shorter, but also right ventricular systole will be prolonged, both factors being key in producing the wide splitting of S_2.

Any condition, either electrical or mechanical, that delays left ventricular emptying will produce *paradoxical splitting* of S_2. Left bundle branch block or aortic stenosis will delay left ventricular emptying. These conditions delay the closure of the aortic valve *after* right ventricular systole and P_2 have occurred. The normal sequence of A_2-P_2 is reversed. During inspiration, P_2 moves normally away from S_1 toward A_2. The split is said to be *narrowed*. With expiration, P_2 moves normally and approaches S_1: the P_2-A_2 split widens. This widening during expiration is paradoxical. Other conditions, such as left ventric-

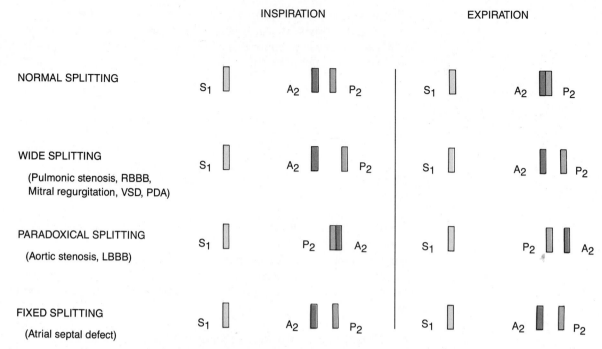

FIGURE 11–24. Abnormalities of splitting of the second heart sound. RBBB = right bundle branch block; VSD = ventricular septal defect; PDA = patent ductus arteriosus; LBBB = left bundle branch block.

ular failure and severe hypertension, delay left ventricular ejection and cause paradoxical splitting of S_2.

Fixed splitting of S_2 is the auscultatory hallmark of an atrial septal defect. In this situation, the split is wide and does not change with respiration. This is because inspiratory increases in venous return to the right atrium normally raise its pressure. During expiration, the right atrial pressure is lower, but the left-to-right atrial shunt keeps the volume in the right atrium constant during respiration; therefore, normal splitting does not occur.

Normal physiologic splitting of the second heart sound and abnormalities of splitting are illustrated in Figure 11–24.

Systolic Clicks

Ejection clicks are high-pitched sounds that occur early in systole at the onset of ejection and are produced by the opening of pathologically deformed semilunar valves. Pulmonic or aortic stenosis may produce ejection clicks. The sounds are short and have the quality of a "click." Pulmonic ejection clicks are best heard at the pulmonic area, whereas aortic ejection clicks are heard at the aortic area. As calcification progresses, the mobility of the valve decreases and the ejection click disappears.

Midsystolic clicks are not ejection clicks. They occur in the middle of systole. They may be single or multiple, and they may change in position during the cardiac cycle with various maneuvers that change ventricular geometry. The most common condition associated with a midsystolic click is prolapse of the mitral or tricuspid valve.

Diastolic Opening Snaps

The opening of an atrioventricular valve is normally silent and occurs about 100 msec after S_2. This is about as long as it takes to say "ma-ma" quickly. An *opening snap* is a diastolic event that is the sound of the opening of a pathologically deformed atrioventricular valve. The sound is sharp and high pitched. The mitral opening snap of mitral stenosis occurs after A_2; the tricuspid opening snap of tricuspid stenosis occurs after P_2.

The interval between S_2 and the opening snap is termed the $S_2 - OS$ *interval* and has specific significance as to the severity of the stenosis. As mitral stenosis worsens, the greater will be the resistance and obstruction to flow. Pressure in the left atrium will increase, and the gradient across the mitral valve will increase. The mitral valve will therefore open earlier than normal, when the left ventricular pressure falls below left atrial pressure. The $S_2 - OS$ time will shorten as the severity increases. Try saying "ma-da" as quickly as possible. This interval is about $50 - 60$ msec and approximates a very short $S_2 - OS$ interval, as heard in severe mitral stenosis.

Murmurs

Murmurs are produced when there is turbulent energy in the walls of the heart and blood vessels. Obstruction to flow or flowing from a narrow to a larger diameter vessel produces turbulence. Turbulence sets up eddies that strike the walls to produce vibrations that the examiner recognizes as a murmur. Murmurs can also be produced when there is a large volume of blood through a normal opening. In this circumstance, the normal opening is relatively stenotic for the increased volume. "Blowing" murmurs are produced by large gradients with variable flow volumes. "Rumbling" murmurs result from areas of small gradients that are dependent upon flow. "Harsh" murmurs result from large gradients and high flow.

The term *ejection murmur* refers to a murmur produced by turbulence across a semilunar valve during systole such as in aortic stenosis or pulmonic stenosis. Ejection murmurs are diamond shaped and are described as "crescendo-decrescendo." They begin slightly after S_1 and end before S_2. An ejection click from stenosis of the semilunar valve may precede the murmur. These murmurs are medium pitched and are best heard with the diaphragm of the stethoscope. Because they are based on flow, the intensity of these murmurs does not indicate the degree of severity. Increased flow across a minimally narrowed aortic valve produces a loud murmur; decreased flow across a severely stenotic aortic valve may produce a barely audible murmur. Any increase in flow or volume may produce an ejection murmur even in the presence of a normal valve. An ejection murmur as a sign of aortic stenosis is a finding of high sensitivity but low specificity. Figure $11 - 25$ illustrates an ejection murmur.

Regurgitant systolic murmurs are produced by retrograde flow from a higher pressure area to a lower pressure area during systole, such as in mitral or tricuspid regurgitation. These murmurs are termed *holosystolic* or *pansystolic*. They begin with S_1 and end after S_2. These murmurs extend past S_2 because ventricular pressure is higher than atrial pressure even after the closure of the semilunar valve. An S_3 indicative of volume overload to the ventricle is often heard. These murmurs are high pitched and are best heard with the diaphragm. The terms "regurgitation," "incompetence," and "insufficiency" are often

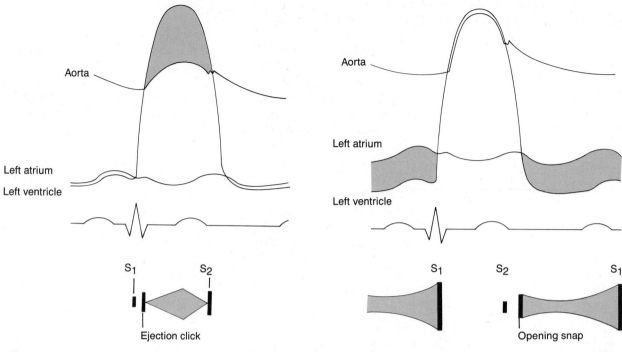

FIGURE 11–25. A systolic ejection murmur such as that of aortic stenosis.

FIGURE 11–27. A diastolic atrioventricular murmur such as that of mitral stenosis.

used synonymously for this type of murmur. The preferred term is "regurgitation," because it implies the retrograde direction of flow. The holosystolic murmur of atrioventricular valve regurgitation is a finding of high sensitivity. Figure 11–26 illustrates a regurgitant murmur.

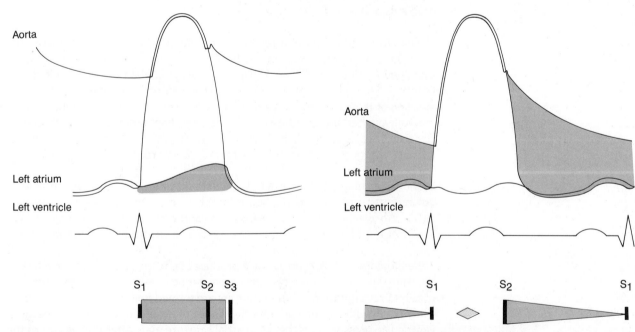

FIGURE 11–26. A systolic regurgitant murmur such as that of mitral regurgitation.

FIGURE 11–28. A diastolic semilunar murmur such as that of aortic regurgitation. Note the systolic ejection murmur, which is related to the increased volume and flow.

ARTERIAL PULSE ABNORMALITIES

Type	Description	Cause
Anacrotic*	Small, slow rising, delayed pulse with a notch or shoulder on the ascending limb	Aortic stenosis
Waterhammer	Rapid and sudden systolic expansion	Aortic regurgitation
Bisferiens	Double-peaked pulse with a midsystolic dip	Aortic regurgitation Combined aortic stenosis and aortic regurgitation Idiopathic hypertrophic subaortic stenosis (IHSS)
Alternans	Alternating amplitude of pulse pressure	Congestive heart failure
Paradoxical (marked)	Detected by blood pressure assessment. An exaggerated drop in systolic blood pressure during inspiration	Tamponade Constrictive pericarditis Chronic obstructive lung disease

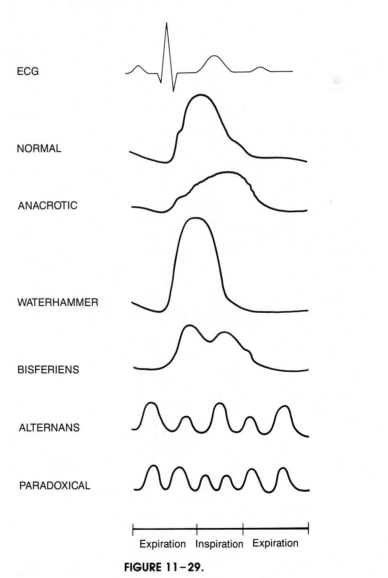

FIGURE 11–29.

* Also known as plateau pulse or *pulsus parvus et tardus*.

TABLE 11-8. Cardiac Sounds

Cardiac Cycle	Sound
Early systolic	Ejection click
	Aortic prosthetic valve opening sound*
Mid/late systolic	Midsystolic click
	Rub
Early diastolic	Opening snap
	S₃
	Mitral prosthetic valve opening sound†
	Tumor plop‡
Mid-diastolic	S₃
	Summation gallop§
Late diastolic (sometimes called *presystolic*)	S₄
	Pacemaker sound

* Opening and closure of the prosthetic aortic valve are heard with many prosthetic valves. The opening is comparable to an ejection click; the closing is a "prosthetic" S_2.

† Opening and closure of the prosthetic mitral valve are heard with many prosthetic valves. The opening is comparable to an opening snap; the closing is a "prosthetic" S_1.

‡ An atrial myxoma that is pedunculated may "plop" in and out of the mitral annulus, simulating the signs of mitral stenosis.

§ At fast heart rates, the diastolic period shortens. If an S_3 and S_4 are present, the sounds may be "summated" into a single sound called a summation gallop.

Diastolic atrioventricular murmurs begin a finite time after S_2 with the opening of the atrioventricular valve. Mitral stenosis and tricuspid stenosis are examples of this type of murmur. There is a pause between S_2 and the beginning of the murmur. Isovolumetric relaxation is occurring during this period. The murmur is decrescendo in shape, beginning with an opening snap, if the valve is mobile. These murmurs are low pitched and are best heard with the bell of the stethoscope with the patient lying in the left lateral decubitus position. Because the atrioventricular valve is stenotic, rapid filling does not occur and a gradient persists throughout diastole. If the patient is in normal sinus rhythm, atrial contraction will increase the gradient at the end of diastole, or presystole, and there will be an increase in the murmur at this time. The diastolic atrioventricular murmur is a sensitive and specific sign of atrioventricular valve stenosis. Figure 11-27 illustrates a diastolic atrioventricular murmur.

TABLE 11-9. Differentiation of Other Systolic Murmurs

	Pulmonic Stenosis	Tricuspid Regurgitation	Ventricular Septal Defect	Venous Hum	Innocent Murmur
Location	Pulmonic area	Tricuspid area	Tricuspid area	Above clavicle	Widespread*
Radiation	Neck	Right of sternum	Right of sternum	Right neck	Minimal
Shape	Diamond	Holosystolic	Holosystolic	Continuous	Diamond
Pitch	Medium	High	High	High	Medium
Quality	Harsh	Blowing	Harsh	Roaring; humming	Twanging; vibratory

* Usually between the apex and the left lower sternal border.

SYSTOLIC MURMURS

	Aortic Stenosis	Mitral Regurgitation
Location	Aortic area	Apex
Radiation	Neck	Axilla
Shape	Diamond	Holosystolic
Pitch	Medium	High
Quality	Harsh	Blowing
Associated signs	Decreased A_2	Decreased S_1
	Ejection click	S_3
	S_4	Laterally displaced diffuse PMI
	Narrow pulse pressure	
	Slow rising and delayed pulse	

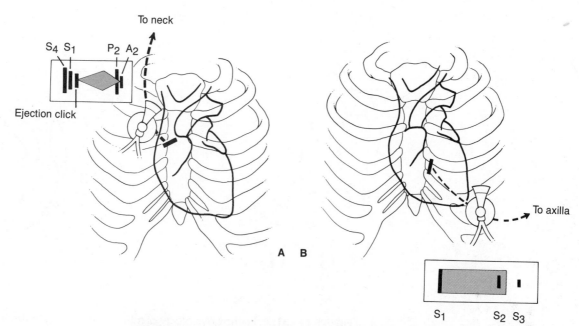

FIGURE 11–30. *A,* Pathophysiology of aortic stenosis. Note the paradoxical splitting of the second heart sound, the S_4, and the ejection click. *B,* Mitral regurgitation. Notice that the murmur ends after S_2, and note the presence of the S_3.

Diastolic semilunar murmurs begin immediately after S_2, as heard in aortic or pulmonic regurgitation. Unlike the diastolic atrioventricular murmurs, there is no delay after S_2 to the beginning of the murmur. The high-pitched murmur is decrescendo in shape and is best heard with the diaphragm of the stethoscope while the patient is sitting up, leaning forward. A diastolic semilunar murmur is a sign of low sensitivity but high specificity. Figure 11–28 illustrates the pressure curves responsible for the generation of a diastolic semilunar murmur.

Figure 11–29 describes and illustrates common arterial pulse abnormalities. Table 11–8 lists important cardiac sounds according to the cardiac cycle. Figure 11–30 lists important characteristics of the systolic murmurs of aortic stenosis and mitral regurgitation. Table 11–9 summarizes the differentiation of some additional systolic murmurs. Figure 11–31 lists important characteristics of the diastolic murmurs of mitral stenosis and aortic regurgitation.

DIASTOLIC MURMURS

	Mitral Stenosis	Aortic Regurgitation
Location	Apex	Aortic area
Radiation	No	No
Shape	Decrescendo	Decrescendo
Pitch	Low	High
Quality	Rumbling	Blowing
Associated signs	Increased S_1	S_3
	Opening snap	Laterally displaced PMI
	RV rock§	Wide pulse pressure*
	Presystolic accentuation	Bounding pulses
		Austin Flint murmur†
		Systolic ejection murmur‡

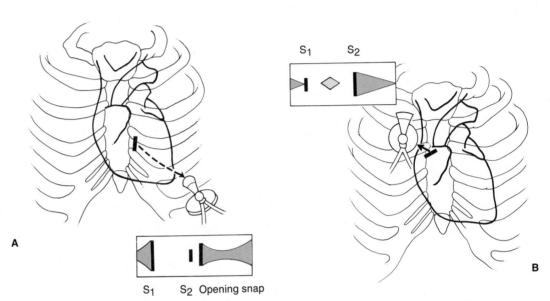

FIGURE 11–31. *A*, Pathophysiology of mitral stenosis. Note the intensity of S_1 and the accentuation of the diastolic murmur in late diastole. *B*, Aortic regurgitation. Note the systolic flow murmur.

* The wide pulse pressure is the cause of the many physical signs of aortic regurgitation: Quincke's pulse, de Musset's sign, Duroziez' sign, Corrigan's pulse, etc.

† An apical diastolic murmur heard in association with aortic regurgitation mimicking mitral stenosis.

‡ A flow murmur across a valve that is relatively narrow for the increased blood volume as a result of aortic regurgitation. It is relatively stenotic and need not be anatomically stenotic, as in true aortic stenosis.

§ Right ventricular impulse at lower left sternal border.

USEFUL VOCABULARY

Listed here are the specific roots that are important in order to understand the terminology related to cardiac disease.

ROOT	PERTAINING TO	EXAMPLE	DEFINITION
brady-	slow	**brady**cardia	Slow heart rate
-cardio-	heart	**cardio**megaly	Enlargement of the heart
sphygmo-	pulse	**sphygmo**manometer	Instrument for measuring blood pressure
supra-	above	**supra**ventricular	Above the level of the ventricles
tachy-	fast	**tachy**cardia	Rapid heart rate

WRITING UP THE PHYSICAL EXAMINATION

Listed here are examples of the write-up for the examination of the heart.

The PMI is in the fifth intercostal space, midclavicular line. S_1 and S_2 are normal.* Physiologic splitting is present. There are no murmurs, gallops, or rubs heard. There is no clubbing, cyanosis, or edema.

The PMI is in the sixth intercostal space, anterior axillary line. S_1 is soft. S_2 is widely split on inspiration and expiration. A grade III/VI, high-pitched, holosystolic murmur is heard at the apex with radiation to the axilla. A palpable S_3 is present at the apex. There is 2 + pitting edema on the shins bilaterally. No cyanosis or clubbing is present.

The PMI is in the fifth intercostal space, midclavicular line. S_1 is normal. S_2 is soft. An S_4 is present at the apex. A grade IV/VI, harsh, medium-pitched, crescendo-decrescendo murmur, beginning slightly after S_1 and ending before S_2, is present at the aortic area. This murmur radiates to both carotids. There is no clubbing, cyanosis, or edema present.

The PMI is in the fifth intercostal space, midclavicular line. S_1 is accentuated. S_2 is normal. An RV rock is present at the left lower sternal border. There is a grade II/VI, low-pitched, diastolic rumble heard at the apex, best heard in the left lateral decubitus position. A grade III/VI, high-pitched, holosystolic murmur is heard at the left lower sternal border, which increases in intensity with inspiration. A right ventricular S_3 may be present at the left lower sternal border.† There is 4 + pitting sacral edema. No cyanosis or clubbing is present.

* The descriptors for S_1 and S_2 are *normal, increased, decreased, widely split, narrowly split, fixed split,* or *paradoxically split.* Never indicate that S_1 and S_2 are present.

† Notice that in this example, the examiner stated that a finding *may* be present.

BIBLIOGRAPHY

Braunwald E: Heart Disease: A Textbook of Cardiovascular Medicine, 3rd ed. Philadelphia, WB Saunders Co, 1988.

Chung EK: Quick Reference to Cardiovascular Diseases. Philadelphia, JB Lippincott Co, 1983.

Constant J: Bedside Cardiology. Boston, Little, Brown and Co, 1985.

Elliott WJ: Ear lobe crease and coronary artery disease. Am J Med 75:1024, 1983.

Freis ED: Auscultatory indication of diastolic blood pressure. Cardiol Digest 3:13, 1968.

Henkind SJ, Benis AM, Teichholz LE: The paradox of pulsus paradoxus. Am Heart J 114:198, 1987.

Hurst JW: The Heart, Arteries and Veins. New York, McGraw-Hill, 1982.

Johnson R, Swartz MH: A Simplified Approach To Electrocardiography. Philadelphia, WB Saunders Co, 1986.

London SR, London RE: Critique of indirect diastolic end-point. Arch Intern Med 119:39, 1976.

Maisel AS, Atwood JE, Goldberger AL: Hepatojugular reflux: Useful in the bedside diagnosis of tricuspid regurgitation. Ann Intern Med 101:781, 1984.

Rothman A, Goldberger AL: Aids to cardiac auscultation. Ann Intern Med 99:346, 1983.

Thomas JE, Schirger A, Fealey RD, Sheps SG: Orthostatic hypotension. Mayo Clinic Proc 56:117, 1981.

12

THE PERIPHERAL VASCULAR SYSTEM

Veins which by the thickening of their tunicles in the old restrict the passage of blood, and by this lack of nourishment destroy their life without any fever, the old coming to fail little by little in slow death.

Leonardo da Vinci
1452–1519

GENERAL CONSIDERATIONS

Diseases of the peripheral vascular system are extremely common and may involve the arteries, veins, or lymphatics. The arterial conditions include cerebrovascular, aorto-iliac, femoral-popliteal, renal, and aortic occlusive and aneurysmal disease. The two most important diseases of the peripheral arteries are atherosclerosis of the larger arteries and microvascular disease.

The most common cause of peripheral arterial occlusive disease is atherosclerosis affecting the medium- and large-sized vessels of the extremities. The narrowing of the vessel results in a decreased blood supply resulting in ischemia. Atherosclerosis may in addition manifest itself by aneurysmal dilatation. The abdominal aorta is the artery most frequently involved. The aneurysm is commonly below the renal arteries and may extend to as far as the external iliac arteries. Often, these aneurysms produce few symptoms, if any. The examiner may discover a pulsatile mass as an incidental finding. Not infrequently, the first presentation may be the catastrophic rupture of the aneurysm. An abdominal aortic aneurysm greater than 5 cm in diameter carries a 20% risk of rupturing within the first year of discovery, and a 50% risk within 5 years. However, it was not until 1951 that the first abdominal aneurysm was surgically treated by resection and grafting. Since 1951, great strides have been made in understanding the natural history of vascular disease as well as in the institution of new technology to help diagnose and treat it.

Microvascular arterial disease occurs in patients with diabetes. Changes develop in the small arterioles that impair circulation to the skin or nerves, especially of the lower extremities, producing symptoms of ischemia. Peripheral neuropathy is a common sequela to microvascular disease. This neuropathy may be manifested as a defect in the sensory, motor, or autonomic system. Microvascular disease affects over 15 million individuals in the United States.

Peripheral venous disease often progresses to venous stasis and thrombotic disorders. One of the dread complications of thrombotic disease is pulmonary embolism. In the United States, more than 175,000 deaths per year are attributed to acute pulmonary embolism.

STRUCTURE AND PHYSIOLOGY

Diseases of the peripheral *arterial* system cause ischemia of the extremities. When the body is at rest, collateral blood vessels may be able to provide adequate circulation. During exercise, when oxygen demand increases, this circulation may not be sufficient for the actively contracting muscles, resulting in ischemia.

The *venous* system consists of a series of low pressure capacitance vessels. Nearly 70% of the blood volume is contained in this system. Though offering little resistance, the veins are controlled by a variety of neural and humoral stimuli that enhance venous return to the right heart. In addition, valves aid in the return of blood.

In the upright posture, the venous pressure in the lower extremity is the highest. Over a period of many years, dilatation of the veins occurs as a result of the weakening of their walls. As the walls dilate, the veins are unable to close adequately, and reflux of blood occurs. In addition, there is a loss of the efficiency of the venous pump in returning blood to the heart. Both of these factors are responsible for the venous stasis seen in patients with chronic venous insufficiency. Complications from venous stasis include pigmentation, dermatitis, cellulitis, ulceration, and thrombus formation.

The *lymphatic* system is responsible for returning tissue fluid back to the venous system. The extremities are richly supplied with lymphatic tissue. Lymph nodes, many of which are located between major proximal joints, aid in filtering the lymphatic fluid before it enters the blood. The most important clinical symptoms of lymphatic obstruction are *lymphedema* and lymphangitis.

REVIEW OF SPECIFIC SYMPTOMS

Many patients with peripheral vascular disease are asymptomatic. When symptomatic, vascular disease causes the following:

- Pain
- Changes in skin temperature and color
- Edema
- Ulceration
- Emboli
- Stroke
- Dizziness

Pain

Pain is the principal symptom of atherosclerosis. Whenever a patient complains of pain in the calf, arch, thighs, hips, or buttocks while walking, peripheral vascular disease of the arteries must be considered. The symptom of pain occurring during exercise is known as *intermittent claudication*. The site of the pain is always distal to the occlusive disease. As the disease progresses, pain at rest occurs. This is often severe and is aggravated by cool temperatures and elevation, especially during the night in bed. Pain may also occur with deep vein thrombosis.

If a male patient complains of buttock or thigh pain while walking, the interviewer should inquire about impotence. *Leriche's syndrome* is chronic aorto-iliac obstruction; the patient presents with intermittent claudication and impotence. In this condition, the terminal aorta and iliac arteries are involved by severe atherosclerosis at the aortic bifurcation.

Patients occasionally complain of bilateral leg pain or numbness occurring while walking as well as at rest. This is termed *pseudoclaudication* and is a symptom of musculoskeletal disease in the lumbar area.

Skin Changes

Color changes are common with vascular disease. Chronic *arterial* insufficiency produces a cool and pale extremity. Chronic *venous* insufficiency produces a warmer than normal extremity. The leg becomes erythematous, and erosions produced by excoriations result. With chronic insufficiency, stasis changes produce increased pigmentation, swelling, and an "aching" or "heaviness" in the legs. These changes are characteristically in the lower third of the extremity and are more prominent medially. When venous insufficiency occurs, edema of dependent areas result.

Patients with acute deep vein thrombosis have secondary inflammation of the tissue surrounding the vein. This produces signs of inflammation: warmth, redness, and fever. Swelling is the most reliable symptom and sign associated with venous obstruction. This finding is indicative of severe deep venous obstruction because the superficial veins of the lower extremity carry only 20% of the total drainage and are not associated with swelling. The extremities should be compared, and a difference in circumference of 2 cm at the ankle or midcalf should be considered significant.

Edema

Lymphedema results from either a primary abnormality in the development of the lymphatic system or an acquired obstruction to flow. Whether one is dealing with the congenital or the acquired form, the net result is stasis of lymph fluid in the tissues producing a *firm, nonpitting edema*. Over several years, the skin takes on a rough consistency similar to pigskin. Because lymphedema is usually painless, the only symptom is "heaviness" of the extremity.

Ulceration

Persistent ischemia of a limb is associated with ischemic ulceration and gangrene. Ulceration is almost inevitable once skin has become thickened and the circulation is compromised. Ulceration related to arterial insufficiency occurs as a result of trauma to the toes and heel. These ulcers are painful, have discrete edges producing a "punched out" appearance, and are often covered with crust. When infected, the tissue is erythematous.

In contrast to arterial insufficiency ulceration, venous insufficiency leads to stasis ulceration, which is painless and occurs in the ankle area or lower leg just above the medial malleolus. The classic presentation is a diffusely reddened, thickened area over the medial malleolus. The skin has a cobblestone appearance, which has resulted from fibrosis and venous stasis. Ulceration occurs with the slightest trauma. Rapidly developing ulcers are commonly arterial, whereas slowly developing ulceration is usually venous.

Emboli

A history of emboli is important. Thrombus formation results from stasis and hypercoagulability. It appears, however, that venous stasis is the most important cause of thrombus formation. Bed rest, congestive heart failure, obesity, pregnancy, and oral contraceptives have been associated with thrombus formation and emboli. Patients with leg ulcers should be asked the following:

"What did the ulcer look like when it first appeared?"
"What do you think started the ulcer?"
"How quickly did it develop?"
"How painful is the ulcer?"
"What kind of medication(s) have you been taking?"
"Is there a history of any generalized diseases? . . . such as anemia? . . . rheumatoid arthritis?"
"Is there a family history of leg ulcers?"

Symptoms secondary to emboli can include shortness of breath from pulmonary emboli; abdominal pain from splenic, intestinal, or renal artery emboli; neurologic symptoms from carotid or vertebral-basilar artery emboli; and pain and paresthesias from peripheral artery emboli.

Neurologic Symptoms

Cerebrovascular occlusive disease causes many neurologic symptoms, including strokes,* dizziness, and changes in consciousness. Occlusion of the internal carotid artery produces a syndrome of contralateral hemiplegia, contralateral sensory deficits, and dysphasia. Vertebrobasilar disease is associated with diplopia, cerebellar dysfunction, changes in consciousness, and facial paresis.

---

* A stroke is also known as a cerebrovascular accident (CVA).

IMPACT OF VASCULAR DISEASE ON THE PATIENT

The patient with chronic arterial insufficiency has progressive pain while walking. As the condition progresses, ulceration of the toes, feet, and areas susceptible to trauma, such as the shin, develops. Pain may become excruciating. Gangrene of a toe may develop, and amputation of it is frequently followed by amputation of the foot and leg. The patient becomes more and more depressed as ongoing mutilation of his body occurs.

PHYSICAL EXAMINATION

> The equipment necessary for the examination of the peripheral vascular system is the following: a stethoscope, a tourniquet, and a tape measure.

The physical examination of the peripheral vascular system consists of inspection, palpation of the arterial pulses, and some additional tests if disease is felt to be present. All of these techniques are usually integrated with the rest of the physical examination.

The patient lies supine, with the examiner standing to the right of the bed. The evaluation of the peripheral vascular system includes the following:

- Inspection
- Palpation of the arterial pulses
- Examination of the lymphatic system
- Other special techniques

Inspection

Inspect for Symmetry of the Extremities

The extremities should be compared for symmetrical differences in size, color, temperature, and venous patterns. Look at the patient in Plate X C. This patient has massive lymphedema of her right upper extremity secondary to a right mastectomy 18 years earlier.

Inspect the Lower Extremities

The lower extremities should be inspected for pigmentary abnormalities, ulcers, edema, and venous patterns. Is cyanosis present? Is edema present? If edema is present, does it pit? Look at the bilateral color changes and swelling of the legs of the patient shown in Plate X D. This patient had chronic venous insufficiency. She died of a massive pulmonary embolus 1 day after this photograph was taken.

Assess the Skin Temperature

Evaluate the temperature by using the back of your hand. Compare comparable areas of each extremity. A cool extremity is commonly found with arterial insufficiency.

| Inspect for Varicosities | Ask the patient to stand, and inspect the lower extremities for varicosities. Look at the area of the proximal femoral ring as well as in the distal portion of the legs. Varicose veins in these locations may not have been visible when the patient was lying. |

Examination of the Arterial Pulses

The most important finding when one is examining the peripheral arterial tree is a decreased or absent pulse. The peripheral arterial pulses routinely evaluated are the radial, brachial, femoral, popliteal, dorsalis pedis, and the posterior tibial.

| Palpate the Radial Pulse | The examiner should stand in front of the patient. The radial pulses are evaluated by the examiner grasping both of the patient's wrists and palpating the pulses with the index, middle, and fourth fingers. The examiner holds the patient's right wrist with his left fingers and the patient's left wrist with his right fingers, as shown in Figure 11–13. The symmetry of the pulses is then evaluated for timing and strength. |

| Palpate the Brachial Pulse | Because the brachial pulse is stronger than the digital pulses, the examiner may use his thumbs to palpate the patient's brachial pulses. The brachial artery may be felt medially just under the belly or tendon of the biceps muscle. With the examiner still standing in front of the patient, both brachial arteries may be felt simultaneously. The examiner's left hand holds the patient's right arm while the right hand holds the patient's left arm. Once the examiner feels the brachial pulsation with his thumbs, he should apply progressive pressure to it until the maximal systolic force is felt. This is demonstrated in Figure 12–1. The examiner should now be able to assess its waveform. |

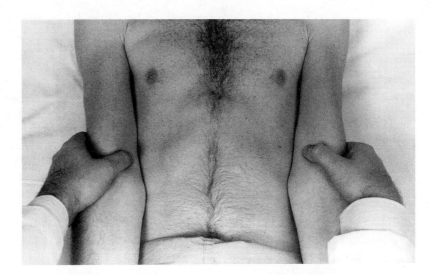

FIGURE 12–1. Technique for brachial artery palpation.

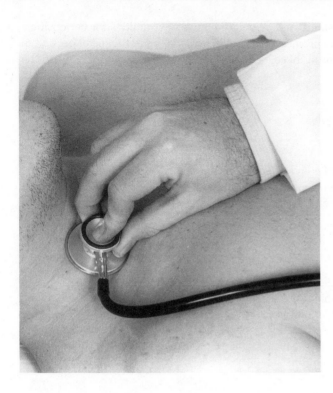

FIGURE 12-2. Technique for auscultation of the carotid artery.

Rule Out Carotid Bruits

Auscultation for carotid bruits* is performed by having the examiner place the diaphragm of the stethoscope over the carotid artery while the patient is lying supine. This is illustrated in Figure 12-2. The head of the patient should be slightly elevated on a pillow and turned away slightly from the carotid artery being evaluated. It is often helpful for the examiner to ask the patient to hold his breath during the auscultation. Normally, either nothing or transmitted heart sounds will be heard. After one carotid artery is evaluated, the other carotid artery is examined.

The presence of a murmur is to be noted. This may be a bruit resulting from atherosclerotic disease of the carotid artery. Occasionally, loud murmurs originating from the heart can be transmitted to the neck. With experience, the examiner will be able to determine whether the pathology is local in the neck or distal in the heart.

Rule Out an Abdominal Aneurysm

Palpate deeply in the midabdomen. The presence of a mass with laterally expansile pulsation suggests an abdominal aortic aneurysm. Caution is urged in making this diagnosis in a thin individual in whom the normal pulsatile aorta may be commonly palpated. In less than 10% of patients with an abdominal aneurysm, a bruit may be present. Acute rupture of an abdominal aortic aneurysm is suggested when this finding is associated with severe pain the abdomen or back and an absent or diminished distal pulse that later returns.

---

* A bruit is a sound or murmur heard in a vessel as a result of increased turbulence.

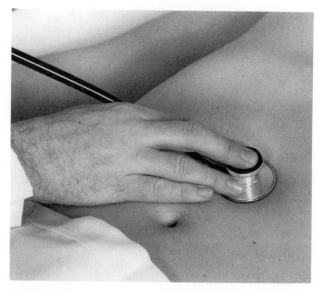

FIGURE 12–3. Technique for auscultation of the abdominal aorta.

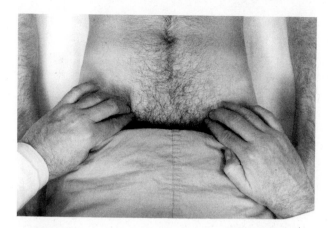

FIGURE 12–4. Technique for palpation of the femoral arteries.

Exclude Abdominal Bruits

The patient should be lying supine. The examiner should place the diaphragm of the stethoscope in the midline of the abdomen about 2 inches above the umbilicus and listen carefully for the presence of an *aortic* bruit. This technique is shown in Figure 12–3.

A *renal* bruit may be the only clue to renal artery stenosis. Auscultation should be performed about 2 inches above the umbilicus and 1–2 inches laterally to the right and to the left of midposition. The presence of a bruit in these positions suggests renal artery stenosis.

Palpate the Femoral Pulse

The femoral pulse is evaluated with the patient lying on his back and the examiner at the patient's right side. The lateral corners of the pubic hair triangle are observed and palpated. The femoral artery should run obliquely through the corner of the pubic hair triangle below the inguinal ligament and midway between the pubic symphysis and the anterior superior iliac spine. Both femoral pulses may be compared simultaneously. The technique is shown in Figure 12–4.

If one of the femoral pulses is diminished or absent, auscultation for a bruit is necessary. The diaphragm of the stethoscope is placed over the femoral artery. The presence of a bruit may indicate obstructive aorto-ilio-femoral disease.

Rule Out Coarctation of the Aorta

The timing of the femoral and radial pulses is important. Normally, these pulses peak either at the same time or with the femoral pulse preceding the radial pulse. By placing one hand on the femoral artery and the other on the radial artery, the examiner can determine the peaking of these pulses. The technique need only be performed on one side. Any delay in the femoral pulse is

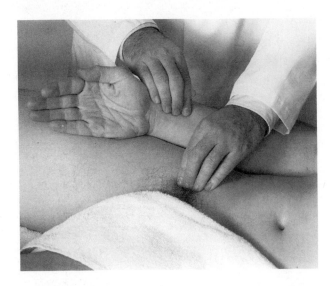

FIGURE 12-5. Technique for timing the femoral and radial arteries.

suspicious for coarctation of the aorta, especially in the hypertensive individual. This technique is shown in Figure 12-5.

Palpate the Popliteal Pulse

The popliteal artery is often difficult to assess. Each artery is evaluated separately. While the patient is lying on his back, the examiner places his thumbs on the patella and his remaining fingers of both hands in the popliteal space behind, as shown in Figure 12-6. The examiner should hold the leg in a mild degree of flexion. The patient should not be asked to elevate his leg, as this will only tighten the muscles and make it more difficult to feel the pulse. Both hands should squeeze in the popliteal fossa. Firm pressure is required to feel the pulsation.

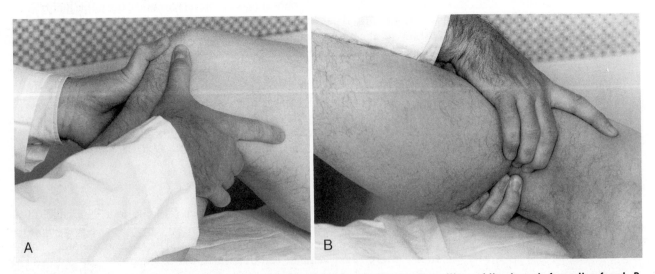

FIGURE 12-6. Technique for palpation of the popliteal artery. *A,* Correct position of the hands from the front. *B,* View from behind the popliteal fossa.

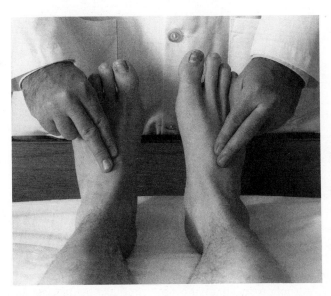

FIGURE 12–7. Technique for palpation of the dorsalis pedis arteries.

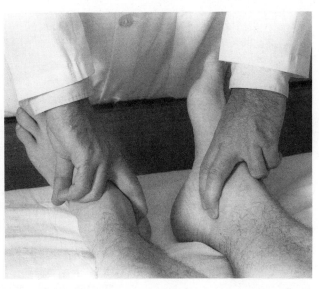

FIGURE 12–8. Technique for palpation of the posterior tibial arteries.

Palpate the Dorsalis Pedis Pulse	The dorsalis pedis pulse is best felt by dorsiflexion of the foot. The dorsalis pedis artery passes along a line from the extensor retinaculum of the ankle to a point just lateral to the extensor tendon of the great toe. The dorsalis pedis pulses may be felt simultaneously, as shown in Figure 12–7.
Palpate the Posterior Tibial Pulse	The posterior tibial artery can be felt as it wraps around the medial malleolus during plantar flexion. Both arteries may be evaluated simultaneously. Figure 12–8 illustrates this procedure. Although 15% of normal young subjects have absent posterior tibial pulses, the most sensitive sign of occlusive peripheral arterial disease in patients over the age of 60 years is the absence of the posterior tibial pulse.
Grading of Pulses	The description of the amplitude of the pulse is most important. The following is the most accepted grading system:

0   Absent
1   Diminished
2   Normal
3   Increased
4   Bounding

It is important that the patient's socks or stockings be removed in order for the examiner to assess the peripheral pulses of the lower extremities. If there is confusion about whether the examiner is feeling the patient's pulse or his own, the examiner may wish to palpate the patient's pulse with his right hand and use his left hand to palpate his own right radial pulse. If they are different, the examiner is feeling the patient's pulse with his right hand.

Examination of the Lymphatic System

Physical signs of lymphatic system disease include the following:

- Palpable lymph nodes
- Lymphangitis
- Lymphedema

Lymph nodes should be described as painless or tender, and single or matted. Generalized lymphadenopathy suggests different diagnoses then localized adenopathy. *Generalized* lymphadenopathy is the presence of palpable lymph nodes in three or more lymph node chains. Lymphoma; leukemia; collagen vascular disorders; and systemic bacterial, viral, or protozoal infections may be responsible. *Localized* lymphadenopathy is usually the result of localized infection or neoplasm. *Lymphangitis* is lymphatic spread manifested by thin red streaks on the skin. Obstruction to lymphatic flow produces *lymphedema,* which is usually indistinguishable from other types of edema.

The examinations for lymphadenopathy of the head, neck, and supraclavicular areas are described in Chapters 6 and 10. Chapter 13, The Breast, describes the examination for palpating axillary adenopathy. Chapter 15, The Male Genitalia, describes the technique for palpating inguinal lymph nodes. The only other important lymph node chain are the epitrochlear nodes, which are discussed in the following section.

Palpate for Epitrochlear Nodes

Epitrochlear nodes are palpated by having the patient flex his elbow about 90°. The examiner should feel for the nodes in the fossa about 3 cm proximal to the medial epicondyle of the humerus, in the groove between the biceps and the triceps muscles. Epitrochlear nodes are rarely palpable but, if present, should be described as to their size, consistency, and tenderness. Acute infections of the ulnar aspect of the forearm and hand may be responsible for epitrochlear adenopathy. Epitrochlear nodes are also seen in non-Hodgkin's lymphomas.

Other Special Techniques

Evaluate Arterial Supply in the Lower Extremity

The most important sign of arterial insufficiency is a decreased pulse. In patients in whom chronic arterial insufficiency of the lower extremity is suspected, another test may be useful. The degree of pallor that develops after elevation and dependency of the ischemic extremity provides a rough guide to the degree of decreased circulation. The patient is asked to lie on his back, while the examiner elevates the patient's legs at about 45° above the bed. The patient is asked to move his ankles in order to help drain the blood from the venous system, making the color changes more obvious. After about 30 seconds, the feet are inspected for pallor. Mild pallor is normal. At this point, the patient is asked to sit dangling his feet off the side of the bed and the examiner quickly assesses the time for color return. Normally, it takes 10 seconds for color to return and 15 seconds for the superficial veins to fill. A prolongation is related to arterial insufficiency, as is the development of a dusky or cyanotic color. This test is useful only if the superficial veins are competent.

Evaluate Arterial Supply in the Upper Extremity

Chronic arterial insufficiency of the upper extremity is much less common than that of the lower extremity. The *Allen test* may be used to determine whether arterial insufficiency exists in the upper extremity. This test takes advantage of the radial-ulnar loop. The ulnar artery is normally not palpable. Allen's test determines the patency of the radial and ulnar arteries. The radial artery is first occluded by the examiner applying firm pressure over it. The patient is then asked to clench his fist tightly. The patient is asked to open his fist, and the color of the palm is observed. The test is repeated with occlusion of the ulnar artery. Pallor of the palm during compression of one artery indicates occlusion of the other.

Test for Incompetent Saphenous Veins

The diagnosis of incompetent saphenous veins valves is easy to demonstrate on examination. The patient is asked to stand, and the dilated varicose vein will become obvious. The examiner compresses the proximal end of the varicose vein with one hand while placing the other hand about 15–20 cm below it at the distal end of the vein. Incompetent saphenous valves present between the portion of the vein examined will produce a transmission of an impulse to the distal fingers.

Test for Retrograde Filling

Another test, called the *Trendelenburg maneuver,* tests for retrograde filling of the superficial venous system. A tourniquet is placed around the upper thigh of a patient's leg after it has been elevated 90° for 15 seconds. The tourniquet should not occlude the arterial pulse. The patient is then instructed to stand, while the examiner watches for venous filling. The saphenous vein should fill slowly from below in about 30 seconds. Filling from above indicates retrograde flow. After 30 seconds, the tourniquet is released. Any sudden filling also indicates incompetent saphenous vein valves.

All of the described tests are to be used in conjunction with other forms of testing. Each of these special vascular techniques has been associated with many false positive and false negative findings. The results, therefore, must be considered in the light of the total evaluation.

CLINICOPATHOLOGIC CORRELATIONS

The signs of an acute arterial occlusion are the *five Ps: pain, pallor, paresthesia, paralysis,* and *pulselessness.*

Chronic progressive small vessel disease is characteristic of diabetes mellitus. It is commonly observed that arterial pulses are present despite a gangrenous extremity. Look at the diabetic patient shown in Plate X E. This patient had dry gangrene of his toes.

Diabetes has been associated with many skin disorders. The cutaneous hallmark of diabetes is a waxy, yellow, reddish-brown, sharply demarcated, plaque-like lesion known as *necrobiosis lipoidica diabeticorum.* These lesions are classically found on the anterior surface of the lower legs. They are shiny and atrophic with marked telangiectasia over their surface. The lesions have a tendency to ulcerate, and, once present, the ulcers heal very slowly. Necrobiosis

TABLE 12–1. Precipitating Factors in Thromboembolism

Factor	Etiology
Stasis	Arrhythmias Heart failure Immobilization Obesity Varicose veins Dehydration
Blood vessel injury	Trauma Fracture
Increased coagulability	Neoplasm Oral contraceptives Pregnancy Polycythemia Previous thromboembolism

lipoidica diabeticorum often predates the frank development of diabetes. The severity of the cutaneous lesion is not related to the severity of the diabetes. Plate X *F* shows a patient with such a lesion.

Deep vein thrombosis of a lower extremity is diagnosed when there is unilateral marked swelling, venous distention, erythema, pain, increased warmth, and tenderness. There is often resistance to dorsiflexion of the ankle. Calf swelling is present in most patients with femoral or popliteal venous involvement, whereas thigh swelling occurs with iliofemoral thrombosis.

Gentle squeezing of the affected calf or slow dorsiflexion of the ankle may produce calf pain in approximately 50% of patients with femoral vein thrombosis. Pain elicited in this technique is referred to as a *positive Homans sign.* Unfortunately, owing to the low sensitivity of Homans sign, this finding should not be used as single criterion for deep vein thrombophlebitis. There are also a wide variety of unrelated conditions that may elicit a false positive response.

As a result of the venous thrombosis, a secondary inflammation around the vein may result. Erythema, warmth, and fever will then occur, and *thrombophlebitis* is present. Not infrequently, the examiner can palpate this tender, indurated vein in the groin or medial thigh. This is commonly referred to as a *cord.*

TABLE 12–2. Differential Diagnosis of Raynaud's Disease from Raynaud's Phenomenon

Feature	Raynaud's Disease	Raynaud's Phenomenon
Sex	Female	Male
Bilaterality	Present (often symmetrical)	±(asymmetric)
Ischemic changes	Rare	Common
Precipitated by cold	Common	Uncommon
Gangrene	Rare	Common
Underlying condition*	No	Yes

* Such as scleroderma, systemic lupus erythematosus, dermatomyositis, or rheumatoid arthritis.

TABLE 12–3. Differential Diagnosis of the Main Vascular Diseases Causing Gangrene

Feature	Diabetes	Atherosclerosis	Thromboangiitis Obliterans	Raynaud's Disease	Arterial Embolism
Age	Any	Over 60 years	Under 40 years	Under 40 years	Any
Sex	Either	Either	Male	Female	Either
Onset	Gradual	Gradual	Gradual	Gradual	Sudden
Pain	Moderate	Moderate	Severe	Moderate	Often severe
Distal pulses	May be absent	May be absent	May be absent	Present	Absent*

* Affected artery does not have pulsation.

Deep venous thrombophlebitis (DVT) is associated with symptomatic *pulmonary embolism* in approximately 10% of patients. If the embolus is large, main pulmonary artery obstruction may occur, which can result in death. It is estimated that an additional 45% of patients with thrombophlebitis suffer asymptomatic pulmonary emboli.

There are several factors that are important in precipitating thromboembolism. These are outlined in Table 12–1.

A very important and common peripheral vascular condition is *Raynaud's disease or phenomenon.* Classically, this condition is associated with three color changes of the distal fingers or toes: white *(pallor),* blue *(cyanosis),* and red *(rubor).* These color changes are related to arteriospasm and decreased blood supply (pallor); increased peripheral extraction of oxygen (cyanosis); and return of blood supply (rubor). The patient may experience pain or numbness of the involved area as a result of the pallor and cyanosis. During the hyperemic or rubor stage, the patient may complain of burning paresthesias. Between episodes, there may be no symptoms or signs of the condition.

Primary or idiopathic Raynaud's *disease* must be differentiated from secondary Raynaud's *phenomenon.* Table 12–2 lists some of the differential characteristics of these conditions. *Gangrene* is necrosis of the deep tissues resulting from a decreased blood supply. A summary of the major features of the main vascular diseases causing gangrene of the lower extremities is shown in Table 12–3.

USEFUL VOCABULARY

Listed here are the specific roots that are important in order to understand the terminology related to vascular disease.

ROOT	PERTAINING TO	EXAMPLE	DEFINITION
angi(o)-	blood vessel	*angio*graphy	X-ray visualization of blood vessels
embolo-	wedge; stopper	*embol*ism	Sudden blocking of a vessel by a clot
phleb(o)-	veins	*phlebo*tomy	Incision into a vein for blood removal
thrombo-	clot	*thrombo*embolism	Obstruction of a blood vessel by a clot that has broken loose from its site of formation
varico-	twisted; swollen	*varico*se	Unnaturally swollen and twisted

WRITING UP THE PHYSICAL EXAMINATION

Listed here are examples of the write-up for the examination of the vascular system.

The extremities are normal in color, size, and temperature. All pulses in the upper and lower extremities are grade 2 and are equal. No bruits are present. There is no clubbing, cyanosis, or edema present.

There are bilateral, yellow appearing, waxy, sharply demarcated lesions on both anterior shins. Both legs appear slightly cool, the left greater than the right. There is a punched out ulceration on the lateral aspect of the left ankle. The left big toe is blackened, with a sharp demarcation. The femoral pulses are grade 2 bilaterally. There are no distal pulses felt. There is 1 + pretibial edema present bilaterally. No clubbing or cyanosis is present.

The right lower extremity is 3 cm larger than the left, measured 4 cm below the inferior aspect of the patella. The right calf is tender, warm, and erythematous. A cord is palpated in the right groin. Both lower extremities are edematous and hyperpigmented. There is 3 + pretibial edema on the right and 2 + pretibial edema on the left. A small ulceration is present above the left medial malleolus. The arterial pulses are grade 2 at the femorals and grade 1 at the popliteals. No pulses are palpated distal to the popliteals. No clubbing or cyanosis is present.

BIBLIOGRAPHY

Juergens JL, Spittell JA Jr, Fairbairn JF II: Allen-Barker-Hines Peripheral Vascular Diseases, 5th ed. Philadelphia, WB Saunders Co, 1980.
Kurtz KJ: Dynamic vascular auscultation. Am J Med 76:1066, 1984.

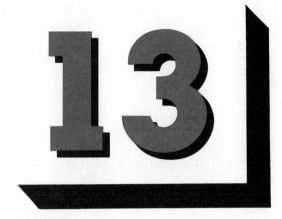

THE BREAST

The shape of the breast is like a gourd. They are round for holding blood to be changed into milk . . . They have teats, that the new born child may suck therefrom.

**Mondino De' Luzzi
1275 – 1326**

GENERAL CONSIDERATIONS

In the United States, 1 woman out of 11 will develop breast cancer at some time during her life. Among the malignant diseases, breast cancer is the most common cause of death in women. It accounts for 26% of new cancers in American women and 18% of cancer deaths. In 1986 in the United States, there were over 120,000 new cases with over 40,000 deaths. The incidence of cancer of the breast is higher in the United States than in European or Asian countries. It has been well established that women in underdeveloped nations have lower rates of breast cancer than those from more affluent societies.

Once breast cancer has occurred in a family, the risk of other women in the same family developing breast cancer is significantly higher. First degree relatives, such as sisters or daughters, are at more than twice the risk of developing breast cancer if the original patient developed cancer in one breast post-menopause. Women with a family history of pre-menopausal breast cancer in one breast have a three times greater risk. If the original patient had post-menopausal cancer in both breasts, the first degree relatives are at more than four times the risk. First degree relatives of patients with cancer in both breasts prior to menopause have nearly a *nine* times greater risk.

The age of onset of menarche and the reproductive cycle seems to play some role in the development of breast cancer. Women with menarche before the age of 12 appear to have an increased incidence of breast cancer. Women who had

303

their first child at the age of 30 or older have a three times greater risk than those having their first child at a younger age.

Most breast cancers are detected as painless masses detected by either the patient or the examiner during a routine physical examination. The earlier the diagnosis, the better the prognosis.

STRUCTURE AND PHYSIOLOGY

The *mammary glands* are the distinguishing feature of all mammals. Human breasts are conical in form but are often unequal in size. The breast extends from the second or third rib to the sixth or seventh rib, from the sternal edge to the anterior axillary line. The "tail" of the breast extends into the axilla and tends to be thicker than the other breast areas. This upper outer quadrant contains the greater bulk of mammary tissue and is frequently the site of neoplasia. Figure 13–1 illustrates the normal breast.

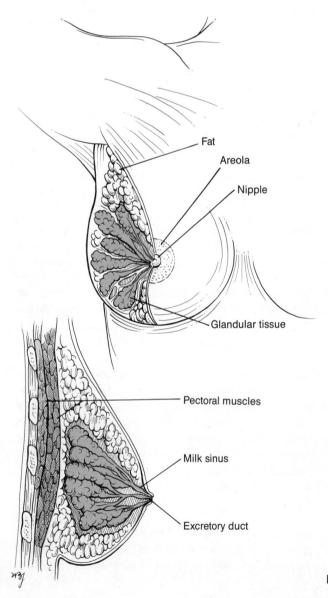

Fat

Areola

Nipple

Glandular tissue

Pectoral muscles

Milk sinus

Excretory duct

FIGURE 13–1. Anatomy of a normal breast.

The normal breast consists of glandular tissue, ducts, supporting muscular tissue, fat, blood vessels, nerves, and lymphatics. The glandular tissue consists of 15–25 lobes, each of which drains into a separate excretory duct that terminates in the nipple. Each duct dilates as it enters the base of the nipple to form a *milk sinus*. This serves as a reservoir for milk during lactation. Each lobe is subdivided into 50–75 lobules, which drain into a duct that empties into the excretory duct of the lobe.

Both the nipple and areola contain smooth muscle that serves to contract the areola and compress the nipple. Contraction of the smooth muscle makes the nipple erect and firm, thereby facilitating the emptying of the milk sinuses.

The skin of the nipple is deeply pigmented and hairless. The dermal papillae contain many sebaceous glands, which are grouped near the openings of the milk sinuses. The skin of the areola is also deeply pigmented but unlike the skin of the nipple contains occasional hair follicles. Its sebaceous glands are commonly seen as small nodules on the areolar surface and are termed *Montgomery's tubercles*.

Cooper's ligaments are projections of the breast tissue that fuse with the outer layers of the superficial fascia and serve as suspensory structures.

The blood supply to the breast consists of the internal mammary artery. The breast has an extensive network of venous and lymphatic drainage. Most of the lymphatic drainage empties into the nodes in the axilla. Other nodes lie beneath the lateral margin of the pectoralis major muscle, along the medial side of the axilla, and in the subclavicular region. The main lymph node chains and lymphatic drainage of the breast are shown in Figure 13–2.

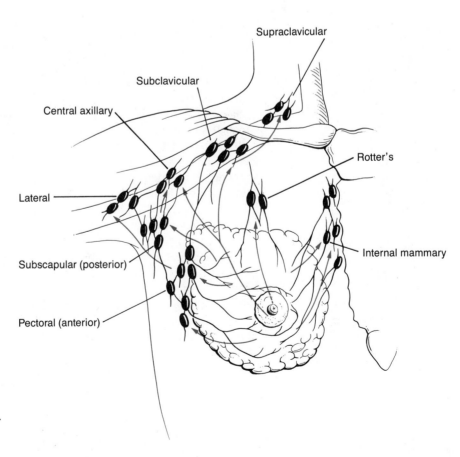

FIGURE 13–2. Lymphatic drainage of the breast.

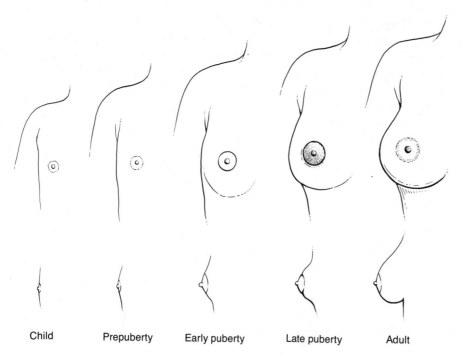

Child   Prepuberty   Early puberty   Late puberty   Adult

FIGURE 13-3. Stages of breast development.

There are several physiologic changes that occur in the breast. These changes are a result of the following factors:

- Growth and aging
- The menstrual cycle
- Pregnancy

At birth, the breasts contain a branching system of ducts emptying into a developed nipple. There is elevation of only the nipple at this stage. Shortly after birth, there is a slight secretion of milky material. After 5-7 days, this secretory activity stops. Prior to puberty, there is elevation of the breast and nipple, called the "breast bud" stage. The areola has increased in size. At the onset of puberty, the areola enlarges further and darkens in color. A distinct mass of glandular tissue begins to develop beneath the areola. By the onset of menstruation, the breasts are well developed and there is forward projection of the areola and nipple at the apex of the breast. One to two years later, when the breast has reached maturity, only the nipple projects forward, whereas the areola has receded to the general contour of the breast. The stages of breast development from birth to adulthood are illustrated in Figure 13-3. Figure 20-13 (Chapter 20, The Pediatric Patient) further illustrates and describes the breast developmental stages.

The nodularity, density, and fullness of the adult breast are dependent upon several factors. Most important is the presence of excess adipose tissue. Because the mammary gland consists mainly of adipose tissue, women who are overweight have larger breasts. Pregnancy and nursing will also alter the character of the breasts. Women who have nursed often have softer, less nodular breasts. However, because the glandular tissue is approximately equal in all women, the size of the breast is unrelated to nursing. With menopause, the breasts decrease in size and become less dense. There is an associated increase in elastic tissue as the woman ages.

The major physiologic change related to the menstrual cycle is engorgement, occurring 3-5 days prior to menstruation. This occurs as a result of an increase

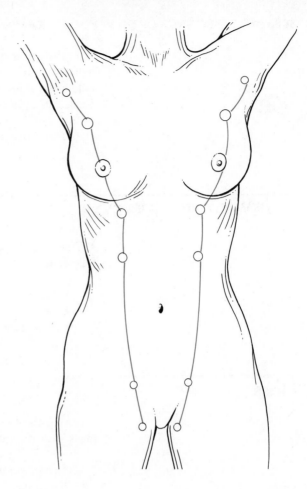

FIGURE 13–4. The milk line.

in the size, density, and nodularity of the breasts. There is also an increased sensitivity of the breasts at this time. Because there is an increase in the nodularity of the breasts during this period, the examiner should not attempt to diagnose a breast mass at this time. The patient should be re-evaluated during the mid-period of the next cycle.

With pregnancy, the breasts become fuller and more firm. The areola darkens, and the nipples become erect as they enlarge. As the woman approaches the third trimester, a thin, yellowish secretion, called *colostrum,* may occur. After the birth of the child, if the mother begins nursing within 24 hours, the secretion of colostrum will stop and the secretion of milk will begin. During nursing, the breasts become markedly engorged. After the woman has stopped nursing, lactation will continue for a short period.

The neuroendocrine control of the breasts can be outlined as follows: Suckling produces nerve impulses that travel to the hypothalamus. The hypothalamus stimulates the anterior pituitary to secrete *prolactin,* which acts on the glandular tissue of the breast to produce milk. The hypothalamus also stimulates the posterior pituitary to produce *oxytocin,* which stimulates the muscle cells surrounding the glandular tissue to contract and force the milk into the ductular system.

Many abnormalities of the breast are related to its embryology. It should be remembered that an epithelial ridge called the *milk line* forms along each side of the body from the axilla to the inguinal region. Along this milk line are multiple rudiments for future breast development. In humans, only one rudimentary pair in the pectoral region persists and eventually develops into normal breasts. Accessory breasts or nipples do occur in as many as 2% of white women.

Accessory breasts may exist as glandular tissue, nipple, or only the areola. The axilla is the most common site for these anomalous structures, followed by just below the normal breast. In over 50% of all patients with accessory breast tissue, the anomalies are bilateral. Generally, accessory breast tissue is of little clinical significance. It usually has no physiologic function and is rarely associated with disease. Figure 13–4 illustrates the milk line.

REVIEW OF SPECIFIC SYMPTOMS

The most important symptoms of breast disease are the presence of the following:

- Mass
- Pain
- Nipple discharge

Mass

During the technique of self-examination, a patient may discover a breast mass. Ask the following questions:

"When did you first notice the lump?"
"Have you noticed that the mass changes in size during your menstrual periods?"
"Is the mass tender?"
"Have you ever noticed a mass in your breast before?"
"Have you noticed any skin changes on the breast?"
"Have you had any recent injury to the breast?"
"Is there any nipple discharge? . . . nipple retraction?"

If the lump enlarges during the premenstrual and menstrual stages of the cycle, it is likely that the woman is detecting only physiologic nodularity. The association of nipple discharge, nipple inversion, or skin changes overlying the mass is strongly suggestive of neoplasm.

Pain

Breast pain or tenderness is a common symptom. Most often, these symptoms are due to the normal physiologic cycle. Ask the following questions of any patient with breast pain:

"Can you describe the pain?"
"When did you first experience the pain?"
"Are there any changes in the pain with your menstrual cycle?"
"Do you have pain in both breasts?"
"Have you had any injury to the breast?"
"Is the pain associated with a mass in the breast? . . . nipple discharge? . . . nipple retraction?"
"Has there been a change in your brassiere size?"

Rapidly enlarging cysts may be painful. Cystic disease of the breasts as well as breast cancer is usually painless.

Nipple Discharge

The symptom of nipple discharge is not common, but it should always raise the suspicion of breast disease, especially if the discharge occurs spontaneously. Any patient who describes a nipple discharge should be asked the following questions:

"What is the color of the discharge?"
"Do you have a discharge from both breasts?"
"When did you first notice the discharge?"
"Is the discharge related to your menstrual cycle?"
"When was your last menstrual cycle?"
"Is the discharge associated with nipple retraction? . . . a breast mass? . . . breast tenderness?"
"Do you have headaches?"
"Are you taking any medications?"
"Are you using oral contraceptives?"
If the woman has recently delivered a child, ask, *"Were there any problems during the delivery of your last child?"*

The most common types of discharge are serous or bloody. A *serous* discharge is thin and watery and may appear as a yellowish stain on the patient's garments. This commonly results from an intraductal papilloma in one of the larger subareolar ducts. Women taking oral contraceptives may complain of bilateral serous discharge. A serous discharge can also occur in women with breast carcinoma.

A *bloody* discharge is associated with an intraductal papilloma occurring frequently during pregnancy or menstruation. It may, however, be associated with a malignant intraductal papillary carcinoma. The presence of any nipple discharge is more important than its character, because both types of discharges are associated with benign or malignant disease.

A "milky" discharge is usually milk. It is common for women to continue to secrete milk for a few months even after they stopped nursing. Rarely, the secretion may continue for a year. Persistent lactation, also known as *galactorrhea*, can be a result of massive hemorrhage occurring during childbirth and producing pituitary necrosis. Abnormal lactation may also result from a pituitary tumor that interferes with the normal hypothalamic-pituitary feedback loop or from the use of certain tranquilizing medications. Mechanical stimulation or suckling may produce physiologic stimulation.

General Suggestions

The interviewer should pay special attention to the family history of any woman presenting with symptoms of breast disease. As indicated earlier, breast cancer is a familial disorder. The occurrence of breast disease in a close relative and the age at which it developed are relevant to the patient's disease.

IMPACT OF BREAST DISEASE ON THE PATIENT

The psychosocial problems resulting from breast cancer are far reaching. Although the loss of an extremity is far more disabling in everyday life, the loss of a breast produces intense feelings of loss of the feminine identity. Many of these women become depressed, as they feel their symbol of femininity has been removed. They are afraid that they will no longer be considered "whole" women because their bodies have been maimed. They fear that they can no longer be loved normally, and that they can no longer experience sexual satisfaction. They fear looking at themselves in a mirror and now perceive themselves as "ugly." The asymmetry is often described as "mutilation" or "a bomb crater." Often women after mastectomy suffer from sexual inhibition and sexual frustration.

Once a woman has discovered a mass in the breast, she becomes intensely fearful. The fear of breast cancer is twofold: it is a cancer, often with a bad prognosis, and it is associated with disfigurement. For these reasons, the patient commonly denies the presence of the mass and delays seeking medical attention. It is not uncommon for a patient to seek medical assistance for the first time with a large tumor mass the size of an orange that has eroded through the skin and has become infected. When asked how long the mass has been present, the woman might answer that she "discovered it yesterday"!

After a mastectomy, the patient will probably suffer from depression and low self-esteem. The patient should be supported and counseled if necessary. Open communication and sharing of feelings among the patient, husband, physician, and family are important factors in the psychologic rehabilitation of the woman.

Look at the woman shown in Plate XI A. She has inflammatory carcinoma of her left breast with massive lymphedema of the left arm. The patient had noticed that her arm had been swelling for the past few months, and she now needed support in order to raise it. She presented to the clinic complaining only about the heaviness of her arm. When examination revealed the breast lesion, she stated that she had noticed the breast changes "only a few days ago." This is the tragic story of denial.

PHYSICAL EXAMINATION

There is no special equipment necessary for the examination of the breast.

The examination of the breast consists of the following:

- Inspection
- Examination of the axilla
- Palpation

To facilitate communication, the breast is divided into four quadrants. Two imaginary lines are drawn through the nipple at right angles to each other. If one visualizes the breast as a face of a clock, one line is the "12 o'clock – 6 o'clock"

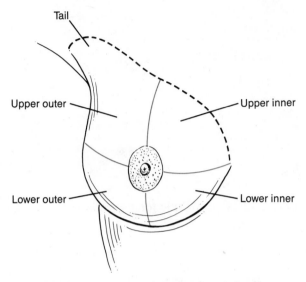

FIGURE 13–5. The four breast quadrants.

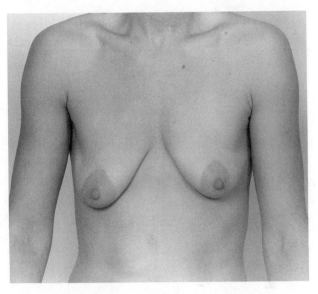

FIGURE 13–6. Inspection of the breasts.

line and the other is the "3 o'clock – 9 o'clock" line. The resulting four quadrants are the upper outer, upper inner, lower outer, and lower inner. The "tail" is an extension of the upper outer quadrant. This is illustrated in Figure 13–5.

Inspection

The woman should be seated facing the examiner. The examiner should ask the woman to remove her gown to her waist.

Inspect the Breasts

Inspection is first carried out with the patient's arms at her side, as shown in Figure 13–6. The breasts are inspected for size, shape, symmetry, contour, color, and edema. The nipples are inspected as to size, shape, inversion, eversion, or discharge. The nipples should be symmetrical. Is any abnormal bulging present?

The skin of the breast is observed for edema. Edema of the skin of the breast that overlies a malignancy may show *peau d'orange,* or an orange skin appearance. This is usually related to lymphatic obstruction resulting in tissue edema. The openings of the sweat glands are clearly visualized as small, deep pits surrounded by the edematous skin.

Is erythema present? Erythema is associated with infection as well as with inflammatory carcinoma of the breast.

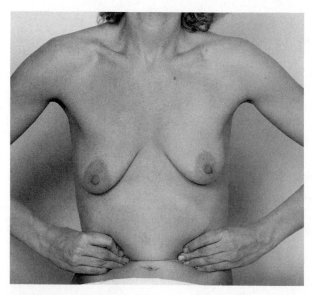

FIGURE 13–7. Technique for tensing the pectoralis muscles.

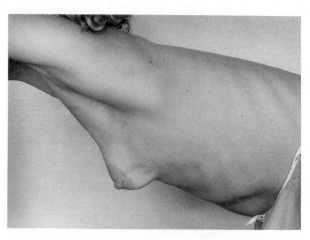

FIGURE 13–8. Technique for inspecting the breasts.

Is dimpling present? The examiner must inspect the breasts for the presence of *retraction phenomena*. Dimpling is a sign of retraction phenomena that are due to an underlying neoplasm and its fibrotic response. Skin retraction is commonly associated with malignancy that causes an abnormal traction on Cooper's ligaments. The shortening of the larger mammary ducts by cancer produces a flattened or inverted nipple. A change in the position of the nipple is important, because many women have a congenitally inverted nipple on one or both sides. The patient shown in Plate XI *B* has dimpling of the breast associated with a bloody nipple discharge, both secondary to carcinoma.

Inspect the Breasts in Various Postures

Inspection is next performed while the woman assumes several postures that may bring out signs of retraction that were previously less evident. Ask the woman to press her arms against her hips. This maneuver tenses the pectoralis muscles, which may bring out dimpling caused by fixation of the breast to the underlying muscles. This technique is shown in Figure 13–7. If a malignancy is present, the abnormal attachment of the tumor to the fascia and pectoralis muscle will draw on the skin and produce skin dimpling. Any bulging may also indicate an underlying mass.

Another maneuver, which is useful for the woman with pendulous breasts, involves asking her to bend at the waist and allow her breasts to hang free from the chest wall. This technique is shown in Figure 13–8. A carcinoma producing fibrosis in one breast will produce a change in the contour of that breast.

Axillary Examination

The axillary examination is performed with the patient seated facing the examiner.

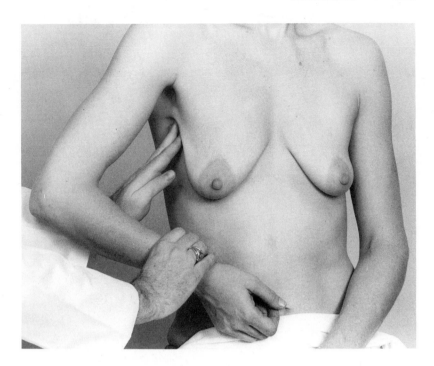

FIGURE 13–9. Technique for axillary examination.

Palpate Axillary Nodes

Examination of the axilla is best accomplished by relaxing the pectoral muscles. To examine the right axilla, the patient's right forearm is supported by the examiner's right hand. The tips of the fingers of the examiner's left hand start low in the axilla, and, as the patient's right arm is drawn medially, the examiner advances his left hand higher into the axilla. This technique is shown in Figure 13–9.

The technique of using small, circular motions of the fingers riding over the ribs is used for detecting adenopathy. Small, freely mobile, 3–5 mm nodes are common and are usually indicative of lymphadenitis secondary to minor trauma of the hand and arm. After one axilla is examined, the other is evaluated with the opposite hand.

Palpation

The woman is asked to lie down and is told that palpation of the breast is next. The examiner stands at the right side of the patient's bed. Although the examiner can usually palpate each breast from the patient's right side, it is often better in large-breasted women to examine the left breast from the left side.

The breast is best palpated by allowing it to lie evenly distributed over the chest wall. Small-breasted women may lie with their arms at their sides; larger-breasted women should be instructed to place their hands behind their head. A pillow placed beneath the shoulder on the side being examined will facilitate the examination.

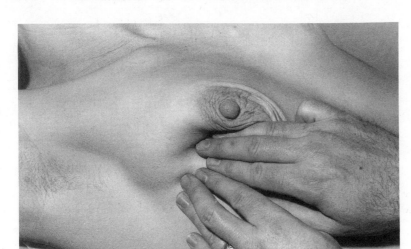

FIGURE 13–10. Technique for breast palpation.

Palpate the Breast

In palpation of the breast, the examiner should use both the flat of the hand and the fingertips, as shown in Figure 13–10. Palpation should be performed methodically by either the "spokes of a wheel" or the "concentric circles" approach. The "spokes of a wheel" method starts at the nipple. The examiner should start the palpation by moving outward from the nipple to the 12 o'clock position. The examiner then should return to the nipple and move along the 1 o'clock position, and continue the palpation around the breasts. The "concentric circles approach" also starts at the nipple, but the examiner moves from the nipple in a continuous circular manner around the breast. Any lesion found by either technique is described as being a certain distance from the nipple in clock time: for example, 3 cm from the nipple along the 1 o'clock line. These techniques are illustrated in Figure 13–11.

The examiner should be careful when evaluating the *inframammary fold*. This fold is commonly observed in older women and is the area where the mammary tissue is bound tightly to the chest wall. Often this ridge may be mistaken for breast pathology.

Describe the Findings

If a mass is palpated, the following characteristics should be described:

1. The *size* of the mass should be described in centimeters, and its position noted.
2. The *shape* of the mass is described.
3. The *delimitation* refers to the borders of the mass. Is it well delimited, as with a cyst? Are the edges diffuse, as with a carcinoma?
4. The *consistency* describes the "hardness" of the mass. A carcinoma is often stony hard. A cyst has some elastic qualities.
5. The *mobility* of the lesion is very important. Is the lesion movable in the tissue that surrounds it? Benign tumors and cysts are freely mobile. Carcinomas are generally fixed to the skin, underlying muscle, or chest wall.

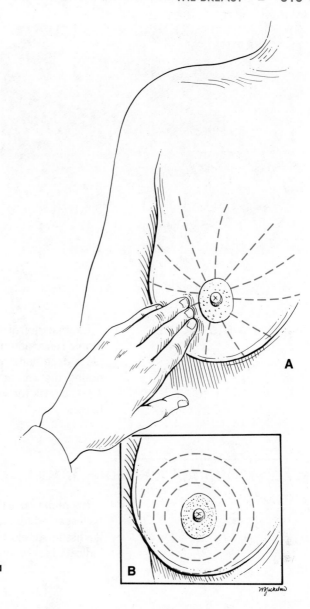

FIGURE 13–11. Methods of breast palpation. *A,* "Spokes of a wheel" approach. *B,* "Concentric circles" approach.

Evaluate for Retraction Phenomenon

If a mass is detected, *molding* of the skin may be useful to determine if the retraction phenomenon is present. The examiner should elevate the breast around the mass. Dimpling may occur if a carcinoma is present. Plate XI *C* shows the technique of molding and its result in a patient with carcinoma of the breast. Notice the marked dimpling of the breast. This patient also has metastatic lesions of breast carcinoma on her arm together with lymphedema. She presented to the clinic stating that she had discovered the swollen arm the day before.

Palpate the Subareolar Area

The subareolar area, or the area directly under the areola, should be palpated while the patient is lying supine. In the subareolar area, the breast tissue is less dense. An abscess of Montgomery's glands in the areola may cause a tender mass in this area.

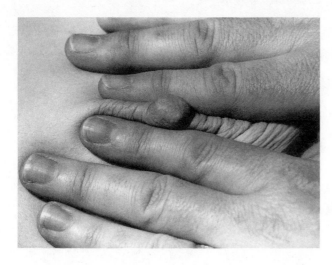

FIGURE 13-12. Technique for nipple examination.

Examine the Nipple

Examination of the nipple concludes the examination of the breast. Inspect for nipple retraction, fissures, and scaling. To examine for discharge, you should place each hand on either side of the nipple and gently compress the nipple, noting the character of any discharge. This technique is shown in Figure 13-12. Ask the woman if she would prefer to do this part of the examination herself.

Examination of the Male Breast

Examination of the breast should be performed on all men. The nipples should be inspected for swelling, discharge, or ulceration. The areola and the subareolar tissue should be palpated for any masses. The axillary examination is as indicated for women.

CLINICOPATHOLOGIC CORRELATIONS

Gynecomastia is the enlargement of one or both breasts in a man. It often occurs at puberty, occurs with aging, or is drug related. Plate XI *D* shows a 90 year old man who was treated with diethylstilbestrol for carcinoma of the prostate and developed gynecomastia.

TABLE 13-1. Limitations of Physical Examination and Mammography

Operating Characteristic	Physical Examination	Mammography
Sensitivity (%)	24	62
Specificity (%)	95	90

Data from Bond WH: *In* Jarrett AS (ed): Proceedings of a symposium on the treatment of carcinoma of the breast. Amsterdam, Excerpta Medica, 1968.

TABLE 13–2. Differentiation of Breast Masses

Characteristic	Cystic Disease	Benign Adenoma	Malignant Tumor
Patient age	25–60	10–55	25–85
Number	1 or more	1	1
Shape	Round	Round	Irregular
Consistency	Elastic, soft to hard	Firm	Stony hard
Delimitation	Well delimited	Well delimited	Poorly delimited
Mobility	Mobile	Mobile	Fixed
Tenderness	Present	Absent	Absent
Skin retraction	Absent	Absent	Present

TABLE 13–3. Characteristics of Breast Masses Suspicious for Cancer

Characteristic	Sensitivity (%)	Specificity* (%)
Fixed mass	40	90
Poorly delimited mass	60	90
Hard mass	62	90

* Based on the assumption that nonmalignant breast masses have benign characteristics.

Data from Venet L, et al: Cancer 28:1546, 1971.

The finding of a breast mass on palpation, even in the presence of a normal mammogram, requires a biopsy. However, breast palpation has a much lower true positive rate (sensitivity) than mammography. There are, unfortunately, many false negative findings in breast palpation. This is related to (1) the difficulty in palpating a small mass in large breasts, (2) the inherent properties of breast tissue, or (3) poor technique. The limitations of physical examination and mammography are shown in Table 13–1.

The physical examination is of great importance in determining the probability that a mass is cancerous. Any lump detected by either the patient or the examiner carries a 20% risk of cancer (Baker, 1982). As indicated in Table 13–2, benign lesions generally are freely mobile, have well-delimited borders, and feel soft or cystic. However, of all breast cancers, 60% are freely mobile, 40% have well-delimited borders, and 50% feel soft or cystic. A fixed lesion has a 50% chance of malignancy. If this lesion had irregular borders, the likelihood of malignancy rises to 60%. The sensitivity and specificity of certain physical findings in evaluating a breast mass for malignancy are shown in Table 13–3.

WRITING UP THE PHYSICAL EXAMINATION

Listed here are examples of the write-up for the examination of the breast.

The breasts are symmetrical with both nipples pointing outward. The overlying skin is normal. There is no dimpling present. There are no masses or discharge present. Axillary examination reveals no lymphadenopathy.

The left breast is slightly larger than the right. There is a serosanguineous discharge from the left nipple. When the patient presses her arms against her hips, a dimple is seen 4 cm from the nipple at the 2 o'clock position of the left breast. Palpation reveals a 2 × 3 cm stony mass under the area of dimpling. The mass appears fixed to the underlying muscle and overlying skin. Axillary examination of the left axilla reveals numerous hard, fixed lymph nodes.

The right breast is larger than the left. The skin is erythematous and warm to the touch, especially around the areola. The right nipple is inverted. There are no masses felt. Dimpling cannot be appreciated. No axillary adenopathy is present.

The breasts are pendulous and symmetrical. Both nipples are everted. There are multiple round, freely mobile masses in both breasts, more on the right. The masses are 2–3 cm in diameter, elastic in consistency, and somewhat tender. Skin retraction is absent. No discharge is present. No axillary adenopathy is present.

USEFUL VOCABULARY

Listed here are the specific roots that are important in order to understand the terminology related to breast disease.

ROOT	PERTAINING TO	EXAMPLE	DEFINITION
gyne(co)-	woman	*gyneco*mastia	Excessive development of the male breast
lact(o)-	milk	*lact*ation	The secretion of milk
mammo-	breast	*mammo*graphy	X-ray visualization of the breast
mast(o)-	breast	*mast*itis	Inflammation of the breast

BIBLIOGRAPHY

Baker LH: Breast Cancer Detection Demonstration Project: Five-year summary report. CA 32:194, 1982.

Bond WH: The treatment of carcinoma of the breast. *In* Jarrett AS (ed): Proceedings of a symposium on the treatment of carcinoma of the breast. Amsterdam, Excerpta Medica, 1968.

Feig SA, Schwartz GF, Nerlinger R, Edeiken J: Prognostic factors of breast neoplasms detected on screening by mammography and physical examination. Radiology 133:577, 1979.

Haagensen CD: Diseases of the Breast, 3rd ed. Philadelphia, WB Saunders Co, 1986.

Hicks MJ, Davis JR, Layton JM, Present AJ: Sensitivity of mammography and physical examination of the breast for detecting breast cancer. JAMA 242:2080, 1979.

Venet L, Strax P, Venet W, Shapiro S: Adequacies and inadequacies of breast examinations by physicians in mass screening. Cancer 28:1546, 1971.

THE ABDOMEN

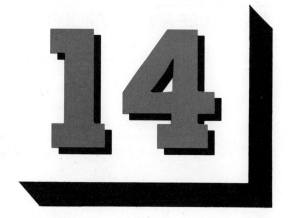

A good eater must be a good man; for a good eater must have good digestion, and good digestion depends upon a good conscience.

Benjamin Disraeli
1804–1881

GENERAL CONSIDERATIONS

Diseases of the abdomen are extremely common. In the United States, approximately 10% of the adult male population is affected by peptic ulcer disease. Five per cent of the population over the age of 40 years has diverticular disease. Cancer of the large bowel is the second most common malignant neoplasm affecting Americans (skin cancer is the first). Approximately 120,000 new cases are diagnosed yearly, and nearly 60,000 mortalities occur annually.

In the general American population, the probability of developing colorectal cancer from birth to age 70 years is approximately 4%. The risk for this type of cancer differs widely among individuals. Some patients, such as those with congenital polyposis or ulcerative colitis, have a predisposition to develop cancer of the colon, frequently at an early age. The lifetime risk of developing colonic cancer in patients with polyposis coli is 100% (Mulvihill, 1983). The incidence of polyposis in the population of the United States varies from 1 in 7000 to 1 in 10,000 live births. The risk of developing colonic cancer in patients with ulcerative colitis is 20% per decade.

Diet has been shown to have a relationship to the incidence of colonic cancer. Individuals on a low fiber and high fat diet are at higher risk.

Better physical diagnosis has been clearly shown to lower the mortality rates for colorectal cancer.

319

STRUCTURE AND PHYSIOLOGY

The abdominal cavity is generally divided into four quadrants for descriptive purposes. Two imaginary lines cross at the umbilicus to divide the abdomen into the right upper and lower quadrants and the left upper and lower quadrants. One line is drawn from the sternum to the pubic bone through the umbilicus. The second line is at right angles to the first at the level of the umbilicus. The four quadrants formed and the abdominal organs within each quadrant are shown in Figure 14–1.

Another method of description divides the abdomen into nine areas: *epigastric, umbilical, suprapubic,* right and left *hypochondriac,* right and left *lumbar,* right and left *inguinal.* Two imaginary lines are drawn by extending the midclavicular lines to the middle of the inguinal ligaments. These lines form the lateral extent of the rectus abdominus muscles. At right angles to these lines, two parallel lines are drawn: one at the costal margins and the other at the anterosuperior iliac spines. Only the names of the three middle areas are commonly used. The nine area system is shown in Figure 14–2.

It is important for the examiner to recognize the abdominal structures that are located in each area. Table 14–1 lists the organs present in each of the four quadrants.

Because the kidneys, duodenum, and pancreas are posterior organs, it is unlikely that abnormalities in these organs can be felt in the adult. In the child, in whom the abdominal muscles are less developed, renal masses can be felt.

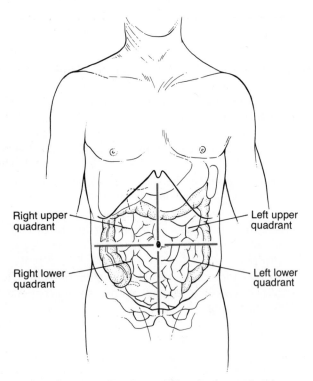

FIGURE 14–1. The four abdominal quadrants.

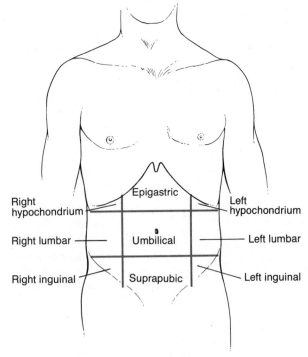

FIGURE 14–2. The nine abdominal areas.

TABLE 14–1. Abdominal Structures by Quadrants

Right	Left
Upper	
Liver	Liver: left lobe
Gallbladder	Spleen
Pylorus	Stomach
Duodenum	Pancreas: body
Pancreas: head	Left adrenal
Right adrenal	Left kidney: upper pole
Right kidney: upper pole	Splenic flexure
Hepatic flexure	Transverse colon: portion
Ascending colon: portion	Descending colon: portion
Transverse colon: portion	
Lower	
Right kidney: lower pole	Left kidney: lower pole
Cecum	Sigmoid colon
Appendix	Descending colon: portion
Ascending colon: portion	Left ovary
Right ovary	Left fallopian tube
Right fallopian tube	Left ureter
Right ureter	Left spermatic cord
Right spermatic cord	Uterus (if enlarged)
Uterus (if enlarged)	Bladder (if enlarged)
Bladder (if enlarged)	

A detailed description of the pathophysiology of the gastrointestinal system is beyond the scope of this text. A brief statement regarding the basic physiology will serve to integrate the signs and symptoms of abdominal disease.

As food passes into the esophagus, an obstructing lesion can produce *dysphagia,* or difficulty in swallowing. Gastroesophageal reflux can lead to heartburn. Upon entry of partially digested food into the stomach, relaxation of the stomach occurs. A failure of this relaxation may lead to early satiety, or pain. The stomach functions as a food reservoir secreting gastric juice and providing peristaltic activity with its muscular wall. Two to three liters of gastric juice are produced daily by the stomach lining and affect the digestion of proteins. The semifluid, creamy material produced by gastric digestion of food is called *chyme.* Secretion of gastric juice may produce pain if a gastric ulcer is present. Intermittent emptying of the stomach occurs when intragastric pressure overcomes the resistance of the pyloric sphincter. Emptying is normally complete within 6 hours after eating. Any obstruction to gastric emptying may produce vomiting.

The entry of chyme from the stomach into the duodenum stimulates the secretion of pancreatic enzymes and contraction of the gallbladder. The flow of pancreatic juice is maximal approximately 2 hours after a meal; the daily output is 1–2 liters. Its three enzymes, lipase, amylase, and trypsin, are responsible for the digestion of fats, starches, and proteins, respectively. In cases of pancreatic insufficiency, the stool is pale and bulky and has more of an offensive odor. The chyme and the neutralizing effect of these enzymes reduce the acidity of the duodenal contents and relieve the pain of peptic duodenal ulcer. The pain from an acutely inflamed gallbladder or from pancreatitis will worsen at this phase of the digestive cycle.

The digested food continues its course through the small intestine, where further digestion and absorption occur. Failure of bile production or its release from the gallbladder will result in decreased digestion and absorption of fats, leading to diarrhea. Gallstones may form as a result of diet or hereditary predisposition.

The liver functions to produce bile; to detoxify the byproducts of the digestion of food; and to metabolize proteins, lipids, and carbohydrates. The daily output of bile is about 1 liter. In the absence of normal liver function, jaundice, ascites, and coma may result.

The jejunum and ileum further digest and absorb the nutrients. Bile acids and vitamin B_{12} are absorbed in the ileum. The color of stool is due to the presence of stercobilin, a metabolite of bilirubin, which is secreted in the bile. If bile does not flow into the small intestine, the stools become clay-colored and are called *acholic,* or free from bile.

The colon functions to remove much of the remaining water and electrolytes from the chyme. Approximately 600 ml of fluid enters the colon daily, and only 200 ml of water is excreted in the stool daily. Abnormal colonic function leads to diarrhea or constipation. Aneurysmal pouches of colonic mucosa may cause bleeding; if infected, pain results. Colonic obstruction produces severe pain. Tumors may cause obstruction or bleeding.

REVIEW OF SPECIFIC SYMPTOMS

The most common symptoms of abdominal disease are as follows:

- Pain
- Nausea and/or vomiting
- Change in bowel movements
- Rectal bleeding
- Jaundice
- Abdominal distention
- Mass
- Pruritus (itching)

Pain

Pain is probably the most important symptom of abdominal disease. Although abdominal neoplasia may be painless, most abdominal disease manifests itself with some degree of pain. Pain can result from mucosal irritation, smooth muscle spasm, peritoneal irritation, capsular swelling, or direct nerve stimulation. Abdominal pain calls for speedy diagnosis and therapy. When a patient complains of abdominal pain, ask the following questions:

"Where is the pain?"
"Has the pain changed its location since it started?"
"Do you feel the pain in any other part of your body?"

"How long have you had the pain?"
"Have you had recurrent episodes of abdominal pain?"
"Did the pain start suddenly?"
"Can you describe the pain? Is it sharp? . . . burning? . . . cramping?"
"Is the pain continuous?"
*"Has there been any change in the severity or nature of the pain since it
     began?"*
"What makes it worse?"
"What makes it better?"
*"Is the pain associated with nausea? . . . vomiting . . . sweating? . . .
     . . . constipation? . . . diarrhea? . . . bloody stools? . . . abdomi-
     nal distention? . . . fever? . . . chills? . . . eating?"*
"Have you ever had gallstones? . . . kidney stones?"
If the patient is a woman, *"When was your last period?"*

It is important to note the exact *time* at which the pain started and what the patient was doing at that time. Sudden, severe pain awakening a patient from sleep may be associated with acute perforation, inflammation, or torsion of an abdominal organ. A stone in the biliary or renal tract will also cause intense pain. The *acuteness* of the pain is likewise important. Acute rupture of a fallopian tube by an ectopic pregnancy, perforation of a gastric ulcer, peritonitis, or acute pancreatitis causes such severe pain that fainting may result.

It is critical to determine the *location* of the pain at its onset, its *localization,* its *character,* and its *radiation.* Commonly when an abdominal organ ruptures, pain is felt "all over the belly," without localization to a specific area. Pain arising from the small intestine is commonly felt in the umbilical or epigastric regions: for example, pain from acute appendicitis begins at the umbilicus.

After a period of time, pain may become localized to other areas. Pain from acute appendicitis travels from the umbilicus to the right lower quadrant in about 1–3 hours after the initial event. Pain in the chest followed by abdominal pain should raise the suspicion of a dissecting aortic aneurysm.

The nature of the pain is important. Perforated gastric ulcer pain is often described as "burning"; dissecting aneurysm as "tearing"; intestinal obstruction as "gripping"; pyelonephritis as "dull, aching"; biliary or renal colic as "crampy, constricting."

Referred pain often provides insight as to the cause. Referred pain is a term used to describe pain originating in the internal organs but described by the patient as being located in the abdominal or chest wall, shoulder, jaw or other areas supplied by the somatic nerves. Pain appears to originate in areas supplied by the somatic nerves entering the spinal cord at the same segment as the sensory nerves from the organ responsible for the pain. For example, right shoulder pain may result from acute cholecystitis; testicular pain may result from renal colic or from appendicitis. The common sites for referred pain are shown in Figure 14–3. The location of pain in abdominal disease is summarized in Table 14–2.

The time of occurrence and factors that aggravate or alleviate the symptoms (e.g., meals or defecation) are particularly important. Periodic epigastric pain occurring 1/2 to 1 hour after eating is a classic symptom of gastric peptic ulcers. Patients with a duodenal peptic ulcer have pain 2–3 hours after eating or before the next meal. Food tends to lessen the pain, especially in duodenal ulcers.

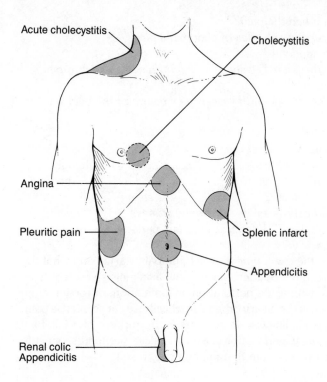

FIGURE 14–3. Common areas of referred pain. The dotted area is on the posterior chest.

Perforation of a duodenal ulcer to the pancreas may produce backache simulating an orthopedic problem. *Nocturnal pain* is a classic symptom of duodenal peptic ulcer disease. Pain after eating may also be associated with vascular disease of the abdominal viscera. These patients are older and have postprandial pain, anorexia, and weight loss. This triad is seen in *abdominal angina* resulting from obstructive vascular disease in the celiac axis or the superior mesenteric artery. Table 14–3 provides a summary of the important ameliorating factors in abdominal pain.

TABLE 14–2. Location of Pain in Abdominal Disease

Area of Pain	Affected Organ	Clinical Example
Substernal	Esophagus	Esophagitis
Shoulder	Diaphragm	Subphrenic abscess
Epigastric	Stomach	Peptic gastric ulcer
	Duodenum	Peptic duodenal ulcer
	Gallbladder	Cholecystitis
	Liver	Hepatitis
	Bile ducts	Cholangitis
	Pancreas	Pancreatitis
Right scapula	Biliary tract	Biliary colic
Midback	Aorta	Aortic dissection
	Pancreas	Pancreatitis
Periumbilical	Small intestine	Obstruction
Hypogastrium	Colon	Ulcerative colitis
		Diverticulitis
Sacrum	Rectum	Proctitis
		Perirectal abscess

TABLE 14–3. Ameliorating Factors in Abdominal Pain

Maneuver	Affected Organ	Clinical Example
Belching	Stomach	Gastric distention
Eating	Stomach, duodenum	Peptic ulcer
Vomiting	Stomach, duodenum	Pyloric obstruction
Leaning forward	Retroperitoneal structures	Pancreatic cancer Pancreatitis
Flexion of knees	Peritoneum	Peritonitis
Flexion of right thigh	Right psoas muscle	Appendicitis
Flexion of left thigh	Left psoas muscle	Diverticulitis

Nausea and Vomiting

Vomiting is usually caused by severe irritation of the peritoneum resulting from (1) the perforation of an abdominal organ; (2) obstruction of the bile duct, ureter, or intestine; or (3) toxins. Vomiting resulting from a *perforation* is rarely massive. *Obstruction* of the bile duct or other tube produces stretching of the muscular wall resulting in episodic vomiting occurring at the height of the pain. Intestinal obstruction prevents the intestinal contents from passing distally; consequently, vomiting may result in intestinal contents being vomited. *Toxins* generally cause persistent vomiting. It is important to recognize that not all abdominal emergencies cause vomiting. Intraperitoneal bleeding may occur in the absence of vomiting. Ask the following questions if a patient complains of nausea and/or vomiting:

> *"For how long have you had nausea or vomiting?"*
> *"What is the color of the vomitus?"*
> *"Is there an unusually foul odor to the vomitus?"*
> *"How often do you vomit?"*
> *"Is vomiting related to eating?"* If so, *"How soon after eating do you vomit? Do you vomit only after eating certain foods?"*
> *"Do you have nausea without vomiting?"*
> *"Is the nausea or vomiting associated with abdominal pain? . . . constipation . . . diarrhea? . . . a loss of appetite? . . . a change in the color of your stools? . . . a change in the color of your urine? . . . fever? . . . chest pain?"*
> *"Have you noticed a change in your hearing ability?"*
> *"Have you noticed ringing in your ears?"*
> If the patient is a woman, *"When was your last period?"*

The relationship of the pain to vomiting is important and may help in providing the diagnosis. In acute appendicitis, pain precedes the vomiting usually by a few hours. The character of the vomit may aid in determining its cause. Acute gastritis causes the patient to vomit stomach contents. Biliary colic produces bilious, or greenish-yellow, vomitus. Intestinal obstruction often causes the patient to vomit bilious vomitus followed by feculent smelling fluid. Remember that *feculent vomitus* is usually due to intestinal obstruction.

Nausea without vomiting is a common symptom in patients with hepatocellular disease, pregnancy, and metastatic disease. Nausea may be associated with a hearing loss and tinnitus in patients with Ménière's disease.

Change in Bowel Movements

A careful history of bowel habits is important. A change in bowel movements requires further elaboration. Ask these questions of the patient with *acute* onset of diarrhea:

> *"How long have you had the diarrhea?"*
> *"How many bowel movements do you have a day?"*
> *"Did the diarrhea start suddenly?"*
> *"Did the diarrhea begin after a meal?"* If so, *"What did you eat?"*
> *"Are the stools watery? . . . bloody? . . . malodorous?"*
> *"Is the diarrhea associated with abdominal pain? . . . loss of appetite? . . . nausea . . . vomiting?"*

The acute onset of diarrhea after a meal suggests an acute infection or toxin. Watery stools are often associated with inflammatory processes of the small bowel. Shigellosis is a self-limited disease of the small bowel producing bloody diarrhea. Amebiasis is also associated with bloody diarrhea.

The patient with *chronic* diarrhea should be asked the following:

> *"How long have you had diarrhea?"*
> *"Do you have periods of diarrhea alternating with constipation?"*
> *"Are the stools watery? . . . loose? . . . floating? . . . malodorous?"*
> *"Have you noticed blood in the stools? . . . mucus? . . . undigested food?"*
> *"What is the color of the stools?"*
> *"How many bowel movements do you have a day?"*
> *"Does the diarrhea occur after eating?"*
> *"What happens when you fast? Do you still have diarrhea?"*
> *"Is the diarrhea associated with abdominal pain? . . . abdominal distention? . . . nausea? . . . vomiting?"*
> *"Have you noticed that the diarrhea is worse at certain times of the day?"*
> *"How is your appetite?"*
> *"Has there been any change in your weight?"*

The alternation of diarrhea and constipation is frequently seen in patients with colon cancer or diverticulitis. Loose bowel movements are common in diseases of the left colon, whereas watery movements are seen in severe inflammatory bowel disease and protein losing enteropathies. Floating stools may result from malabsorption syndromes. Patients with ulcerative colitis commonly have stool mixed with blood and mucus. Any inflammatory process of the small bowel or colon can present with blood mixed with stool or undigested food. Irritable bowel syndrome classically produces more diarrhea in the morning.

Patients complaining of constipation should be asked these questions:

> *"For how long have you been constipated?"*
> *"How often do you have a bowel movement?"*
> *"What is the size of your stools?"*
> *"What is the color of your stools?"*
> *"Is the stool ever mixed with blood? . . . mucus?"*
> *"Have you noticed periods of constipation alternating with periods of diarrhea?"*

"Have you noticed a change in the caliber of the stool?"
"Do you have much gas?"
"How's your appetite?"
"Has there been any change in your weight?"

Change in the *caliber* of the stool is significant. "Pencil" diameter stools may result from an anal or distal rectal carcinoma. A change in the color of stools is important. As will be discussed later, clay-colored stools indicate an absence of bile. This can be due to an obstruction to bile flow from the gallbladder or to decreased production of bile. Weight changes are important with the symptom of constipation. An increase in weight may indicate a decreased metabolism seen in hypothyroidism; a decrease in weight may be associated with cancer of the colon.

Rectal Bleeding

Rectal bleeding may be manifested by bright red blood; blood mixed with stool; or black, tarry stools. Bright red blood per rectum, also known as *hematochezia,* can occur from colonic tumors, diverticular disease, or ulcerative colitis. It is often abbreviated as *BRBPR.* Blood mixed with stool can be the result of ulcerative colitis, diverticular disease, tumors, or hemorrhoids. Ask the patient who describes rectal bleeding the following questions:

"For how long have you noticed bright red blood in your stools?"
"Is the blood mixed with the stool?"
"Are there streaks of blood on the surface of the stool?"
"Have you noticed a change in your bowel habits?"
"Have you noticed a sensation in your rectum that you have to move your bowels but cannot?"

Tenesmus is the painful, continued, and ineffective straining at stool. It is caused by inflammation or tumor at the distal rectum or anus. Hemorrhoidal bleeding is a common cause of hematochezia and streaking of stool with blood.

Melena is a black, tarry stool that results from bleeding above the first section of the duodenum with partial digestion of the hemoglobin. Inquiring about the presence of melena is important. A useful way of questioning is to show the patient the black tubing on the stethoscope and ask, "Have your bowel movements *ever* been this color?" If asked directly whether he has ever had a black bowel movement, the patient may answer in the affirmative, equating dark (normal) stools with black stools. Ask the patient who describes melena these questions:

"Have you passed more than one black, tarry stool?" If so, *"When?"*
"How long have you been having black, tarry stools?"
"Have you noticed that you were lightheaded?"
"Have you had any nausea associated with these stools? . . . any vomiting? . . . diarrhea? . . . abdominal pain? . . . sweating?"

The answers to these questions can provide some information regarding the acuteness and the amount of the hemorrhage. Lightheadedness, nausea, and diaphoresis are seen with a rapid gastrointestinal bleed and hypotension.

The presence of *silver-colored stools* is rare but pathognomonic of acholic stools with melena, a condition resulting from cancer of the ampulla of Vater in the duodenum. The cancer produces biliary obstruction, and the cancerous fronds are sloughed, causing melena.

Jaundice

The presence of jaundice (icterus) must alert the examiner that there is either liver parenchymal disease or an obstruction to bile flow. The presence of icterus, or jaundice, results from a decreased excretion of conjugated bilirubin into the bile. This can result from intrahepatic biliary obstruction, known as "medical jaundice" or from extrahepatic biliary obstruction, known as "surgical jaundice." In any patient with icterus, the examiner should search for clues by asking the following questions:

"How long have you been jaundiced?"
"Did the jaundice develop rapidly?"
"Is the jaundice associated with abdominal pain? . . . loss of appetite? . . . nausea? . . . vomiting? . . . distaste for cigarettes?"
"In the past year have you had any transfusions? . . . tattooing? . . . inoculations?"
"Do you use any 'recreational drugs'?" If so, *"Any intravenously?"*
"Do you eat raw shellfish? . . . oysters?"
"Have you traveled abroad in the past year?" If so, *"To where?" "Did you drink any unclean water?"*
"Have you been jaundiced before?"
"Has your urine changed color since you noticed that you were jaundiced?"
"What is the color of your stools?"
"Is the jaundice associated with abdominal pain? . . . nausea? . . . vomiting? . . . chills? . . . fever? . . . itching? . . . weight loss?"
"Do you have any friends or relations who are also jaundiced?"
"What type of work do you do?" "What other types of work have you done?"
"What are your hobbies?"

Viral hepatitis is associated with a loss of appetite, an aversion to smoking, nausea, and vomiting. Hepatitis A has a fecal-oral route of transmission with an incubation period of 2–6 weeks. It can be associated with ingestion of raw shellfish. Hepatitis B is blood borne with an incubation period of 1–6 months. Health professionals are at increased risk for hepatitis. Any contact with an individual with viral hepatitis places one at a higher risk of contracting viral hepatitis. Slowly developing jaundice that is associated with clay-colored stools and "Coca-Cola" colored urine is obstructive jaundice, either intra- or extrahepatic. Jaundice associated with fever and chills is cholangitis until proved otherwise. Cholangitis may result from stasis of bile in the bile duct resulting from a gallstone or from cancer of the head of the pancreas. It is important to determine whether chemicals are used in a patient's occupation or in his hobbies, as they may be related to the cause of the jaundice. There are many industrial chemicals and drugs that have been associated with liver disease. These agents may be responsible for a viral hepatitis–like illness, cholestasis, granulomas, or hepatic tumors. Occupational exposure to carbon tetrachloride and vinyl chloride is well known to cause liver disease. Questions related to alcohol abuse are also important to ask. These are described in Chapter 1, The Interviewer's Questions.

Abdominal Distention

Abdominal distention may be related to increased gas in the gastrointestinal tract or to the presence of ascites. Increased gas can result from malabsorption, irritable colon, or air swallowing *(aerophagia)*. Ascites can be caused by a variety of etiologies, such as cirrhosis, congestive heart failure, portal hypertension, peritonitis, or neoplasia. To try to identify the cause of abdominal distention, ask these questions:

"How long have you noticed your abdomen to be distended?"
"Is the distention intermittent?"
"Is the distention related to eating?"
"Is the distention lessened by passing gas from above or below?"
"Is the distention associated with vomiting? . . . a loss of appetite? . . . weight loss? . . . a change in your bowel habits? . . . shortness of breath?"

Gaseous distention related to eating is intermittent and is relieved by the passage of flatus or belching. A patient with ascites has the insidious development of increased abdominal girth noted by a progressive increase in belt size. Loss of appetite is often associated with cirrhosis and malignancy, although end stage congestive heart failure may produce this symptom as well. Shortness of breath and ascites may be symptoms of congestive heart failure, but the shortness of breath may be the result of a decreased pulmonary capacity owing to ascites from another cause. Questions related to alcoholic abuse are most appropriate and are outlined in Chapter 1.

Mass

An abdominal mass may be a neoplasm or a hernia. An abdominal *hernia* refers to a protrusion from the peritoneal cavity into which peritoneal contents are extruded. The contents may be omentum, intestine, or bladder wall. An abdominal hernia may be inguinal, femoral, umbilical, or internal, depending upon its location. The most common complaint is swelling, which may or may not be painful. An inguinal hernia may present as a mass in the groin or scrotum. The major complications of a hernia are intestinal obstruction and intestinal strangulation from interference of blood supply. A hernia is termed "reducible" when it can be emptied of its contents by pressure or a change in posture.

A symptom of a pulsatile abdominal mass should alert the examiner to the possibility of an aortic aneurysm.

Pruritus

Pruritus, or itching, is a common symptom. Generalized itching may be a symptom of a diffuse skin disorder,* or a manifestation of chronic renal or hepatic disease. Intense pruritus may be associated with lymphoma or Hodgkin's disease, as well as with malignancies of the gastrointestinal tract. In the

---

* For example, dermatitis herpetiformis, a blistering disease predominantly on the buttocks, shoulders, elbows, and knees.

older individual, pruritus may also be caused by dry skin alone. *Pruritus ani* is localized itching of the anal skin. It has many causes, which include fistulae, fissures, psoriasis, parasites, poor hygiene, and diabetes.

IMPACT OF INFLAMMATORY BOWEL DISEASE ON THE PATIENT

Inflammatory bowel disease constitutes a group of diseases of unknown etiology. The symptoms produced depend upon the location, extent, and acuteness of the inflammatory lesion(s). The common presenting features are a febrile illness, anorexia, weight loss, abdominal discomfort, diarrhea, rectal urgency, and rectal bleeding. It is a chronic, potentially disabling illness, often resulting in multiple surgeries, fistula formation, and cancer.

Inflammatory bowel disease may lead to long periods of absence from school and work, disruption of family life, malabsorption, malnutrition, and multiple hospitalizations. As a consequence, patients with inflammatory bowel disease have many psychological problems. Imagine having 10–30 watery or bloody bowel movements each day! The psychological impact is enormous, particularly in the young adult. Sexual development may be delayed as a result of malnutrition. Social development is also retarded. The necessity of constantly having to remain near a bathroom inhibits the patient's ability from developing normal dating patterns. These patients frequently are socially immature, and social introversion is common. By necessity, they remain at home. Their lives revolve around their bowel habits.

In most cases, there is a positive correlation between the severity of the physical disease and the degree of emotional disturbance. *Dependency* is the most reported characteristic of patients with inflammatory bowel disease. Repressed rage, suppression of feelings, and anxieties are also common. It is described that many patients have a constant desire to rid themselves of events in their lives. This characteristic can be acted out through their diarrhea. Another important characteristic of these patients is to be *obsessive-compulsive*. The marked obsessive character becomes even more obvious when the patient is ill. It is typical for the patient to worry incessantly about what is happening within his bowels. The patients are intelligent, having often read much literature, including medical textbooks, about their disease.

Denial is generally not a prominent symptom. In contrast, these patients concentrate obsessively on the details of their bowel habits.

Sexual problems are common. Interest and participation in sexual activity tend to be at a low level. Many of these individuals prefer to be fondled like a child and largely reject any genital contact. Patients are prone to regard sexual activity in anal terms, such as "dirty," "unclean," or "soiling." They are squeamish about body contact, odors, and secretions. The loss of libido and decreased sexual drive may be related to their fear of bowel action during intercourse, perineal pain, or that sexual intercourse may have some effect in further damaging the bowel.

The frequent hospitalizations cause anxiety and depression, which exacerbate the disease. The fear of cancer may be the basis of depression, which is a common response to their disease. It is well established that emotional factors are important in maintaining and prolonging an existing attack. School work declines as the young adult is forced to miss more and more school, further increasing his anxiety.

An often unappreciated major complication of inflammatory bowel disease is substance abuse. As a result of chronic pain, as many as 5% of patients with inflammatory bowel disease are physically addicted to oral narcotics. Many more are psychologically dependent upon their pain medication.

Many patients with ulcerative colitis require an ileostomy. The fear of disfigurement, the loss of self-confidence, the potential lack of cleanliness, and the dread of unexpected spillage are common.

Time for listening and an interest in the patient's problem are important in gaining the patient's confidence. Listening may reveal and help unravel the emotional problem, which may be the source of the exacerbation of the bowel disease. Talking to the patient may be more efficacious than anti-inflammatory agents or tranquilizers. Careful and thoughtful discussion of the illness will strengthen the doctor-patient relationship as well as produce immeasurable therapeutic benefit.

PHYSICAL EXAMINATION

> The equipment necessary for the examination of the abdomen and rectum is the following: a stethoscope, gloves, lubricant, tissues, and occult blood testing card and reagent.

The patient should be lying flat in bed, and his abdomen should be fully exposed from the sternum to the knees. His arms should be at his sides, and his legs flat. Frequently patients will tend to place their arms behind their head, which will tighten the abdominal muscles and make the examination more difficult. Placing a pillow beneath the knees often aids in relaxation. The examiner should be standing on the patient's right side. A sheet or towel is placed over the genitalia, as illustrated in Figure 14–4.

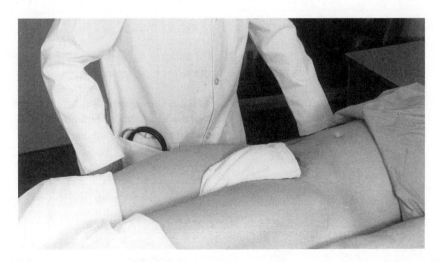

FIGURE 14–4. Technique for inspecting the abdomen.

If the patient has complained of abdominal pain, it is important that the area of pain be examined *last*. If the examiner touches the area of maximal pain, the abdominal muscles will tighten and the examination will be more difficult.

The physical examination of the abdomen includes the following:

- Inspection
- Auscultation
- Percussion
- Palpation
- Rectal examination
- Special techniques

Inspection

Evaluate General Appearance

The general appearance of the patient will often furnish valuable information as to the nature of his condition. Patients with renal or biliary *colic* are seen literally writhing in bed. They squirm constantly and can find no comfortable position. In contrast, patients with *peritonitis* who have intense pain on movement characteristically remain still in bed because any slight motion worsens the pain. They may be lying in bed with their knees drawn up to help relax the abdominal muscles and reduce intra-abdominal pressure. Patients who are pale and sweating may be suffering from the initial *shock* of pancreatitis or a perforated gastric ulcer.

Determine Respiratory Rate

The respiratory rate is increased in patients with generalized peritonitis, intra-abdominal hemorrhage, or intestinal obstruction.

Inspect the Skin

Inspect the skin and sclera for *jaundice* (icterus). Whenever possible, the patient should be evaluated for jaundice in natural light, as incandescent light frequently will mask the existence of icterus.

Inspect for *spider angiomas*. Spider angiomas have a high degree of sensitivity in patients with alcoholic cirrhosis but are non-specific because they are also seen in pregnancy and collagen vascular disorders.

Inspect the Hands

Is there muscle loss in the small muscles of the hands? This is associated with wasting.

The nails are examined for changes in the nail bed, especially an increase in the size of the lunula. The fingers of a patient with cirrhosis showing "half and half" nails are shown in Plate XI *E*.

Inspect the Facies

Are the eyes sunken? Is there temporal wasting present? These are signs of wasting and poor nutrition.

The skin around the mouth and oral mucosa may provide evidence of gastrointestinal disorders. Melanin deposition around and in the oral cavity, especially the buccal mucosa, suggests *Peutz-Jeghers* syndrome. Telangiectasias of the lips and tongue are suggestive of *Osler-Weber-Rendu* syndrome. In this syndrome, multiple telangiectasias are present throughout the gastrointestinal tract. These may bleed insidiously, causing anemia. The classic oral lesions of a patient with Osler-Weber-Rendu syndrome are shown in Plate XI *F*.

Inspect the Abdomen

The contour of the abdomen should be assessed. A *scaphoid,* or concave, abdomen may be associated with cachexia; a *protuberant* abdomen may result from gaseous distention of the intestines, ascites, organomegaly, or obesity. When a patient with ascites stands, the fluid sinks into the lower abdomen; when he lies supine, the fluid bulges in the flanks. If a patient with ascites lies on his side, the fluid flows to the lower side. A patient with a protuberant abdomen as a result of carcinomatous ascites is shown in Plate XII *A*.

The examiner should focus his attention on the abdomen to describe adequately the presence of any asymmetry, distention, masses, or visible peristaltic waves. The examiner should then observe the abdomen from above, looking for the same signs. Inspection of the abdomen for striae and scars may provide valuable data. Silver striae are stretch marks consistent with weight loss. Pinkish-purple striae are classic signs of adrenocortical excess. Plate XII *B* shows a patient with Cushing's disease showing the characteristic purplish striae.

Is the umbilicus everted? An everted umbilicus is often a sign of increased abdominal pressure, usually from ascites or a large mass. An umbilical hernia may also cause an everted umbilicus.

Are there ecchymoses on the abdomen or on the flanks? Massive ecchymoses may occur in these areas as a result of hemorrhagic pancreatitis or strangulated bowel. This finding bears the name *Grey Turner's sign.*

Cullen's sign is a bluish discoloration of the umbilicus resulting from hemoperitoneum of any cause.

Recognition of classic surgical scars may be very helpful. Figure 14–5 shows the locations of some common surgical scars.

Inspect for Hernias

With the patient is lying in bed, he should be asked to cough while the examiner inspects the inguinal, umbilical, and femoral areas. This maneuver, by increasing intra-abdominal pressure, may produce a sudden bulging in these areas, which may be related to a hernia. If the patient has had surgery, coughing may show a bulging along the abdominal scar related to an incisional hernia. In addition, coughing may elicit pain localized to a specific area. This technique will permit the examiner to identify the area of maximal tenderness and to perform most of the abdominal examination without too much discomfort to the patient. A patient with ascites secondary to metastatic breast carcinoma and an umbilical hernia is shown in Plate XII *C*.

Inspect the Superficial Veins

The venous pattern of the abdomen is usually barely perceptible. If visible in the normal individual, the drainage of the lower two thirds of the abdomen will be downward. In the presence of vena caval obstruction, superficial veins may dilate and the veins drain cephalad, or toward the head. In patients with portal

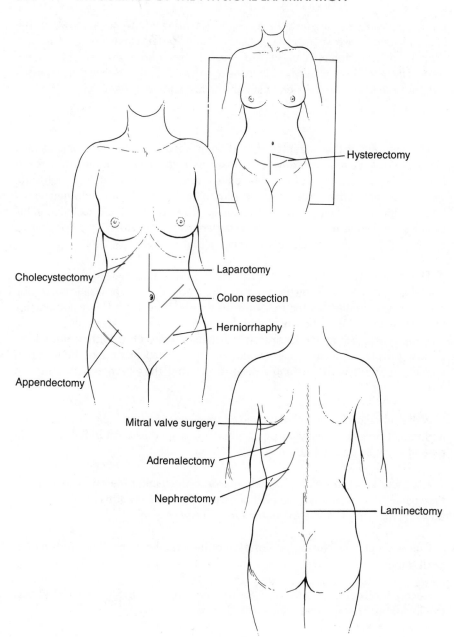

Hysterectomy

Cholecystectomy

Laparotomy

Colon resection

Herniorrhaphy

Appendectomy

Mitral valve surgery

Adrenalectomy

Nephrectomy

Laminectomy

FIGURE 14–5. Locations of common surgical scars.

hypertension, the dilated veins appear to radiate from the umbilicus. This is due to backflow through the collateral veins within the falciform ligament. This pattern is called *caput medusae.*

If the superficial veins are distended, evaluate the direction of drainage by the following technique: Place the tips of your index fingers on a vein that is oriented cephalad-caudad, not transverse, and compress it. Using continuous pressure, the index fingers should be slid apart for about 3–4 inches. Remove one finger and observe the time it takes to fill the vein. Repeat this procedure, but this time remove the other finger and observe the filling time. The direction of flow is in the direction of the faster filling.

Auscultation

Auscultation of bowel sounds can provide information about the motion of air and liquid in the gastrointestinal tract. Many examiners will perform auscultation of the abdomen before percussion or palpation, in contrast to the usual order. It is felt by these examiners that percussion or palpation may change the intestinal motility; therefore, they believe that auscultation should be performed first in order to produce a more accurate assessment of the existing bowel sounds.

Evaluate Bowel Sounds

The patient is placed in a supine position. Auscultation of the abdomen is performed by placing the diaphragm of the stethoscope over the midabdomen while the examiner listens for bowel sounds. This technique is shown in Figure 14–6.

Normal bowel sounds occur approximately every 5–10 seconds and have a high-pitched sound. If after 2 minutes no bowel sounds are heard, the statement "absent bowel sounds" may be made. The absence of bowel sounds suggests a paralytic ileus that is due to diffuse peritoneal irritation. There may be rushes of high-pitched "tinkles" termed *borborygmi*, which is associated with hyperperistalsis. This is frequently seen in early acute intestinal obstruction.

Rule Out Obstructed Viscus

A *succussion splash* may be detected in a distended abdomen as a result of the presence of gas and fluid in an obstructed organ. The examiner applies his stethoscope over the abdomen while shaking the patient from side to side. The presence of a sloshing sound generally indicates distention of the stomach or colon. This technique is illustrated in Figure 14–7.

Rule Out Abdominal Bruits

Auscultation is also useful for determining the presence of bruits. Each quadrant should be evaluated for their presence. Bruits may result from stenosis of the renal artery or the abdominal aorta.

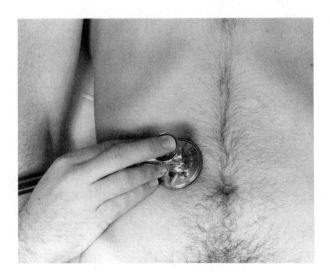

FIGURE 14–6. Technique for evaluating bowel sounds.

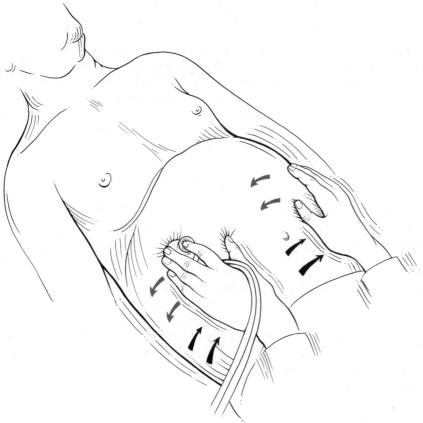

FIGURE 14-7. "Succussion splash" technique for assessing distention of abdominal viscera.

Rule Out Peritoneal Rubs

A peritoneal friction rub, like a pleural or pericardial rub, is a sound that indicates inflammation. During respiratory motion, a friction rub may be heard in the right or left upper quadrants in the presence of hepatic or splenic pathology.

Percussion

Percussion is used to demonstrate the presence of gaseous distention, fluid, or solid masses. In the normal examination, generally only the size and location of the liver and spleen can be determined. Some examiners prefer to palpate before percussion, especially if the patient complains of abdominal pain; either approach is correct. The technique of percussion is discussed in Chapter 10, The Chest.

Percuss the Abdomen

The patient lies supine. All four quadrants of the abdomen are evaluated by percussion. Tympany is the most common percussion note in the abdomen. This is due to the presence of gas within the stomach, small bowel, and colon. The suprapubic area may be percussed as dull if the urinary bladder is distended or, in a woman, if the uterus is enlarged.

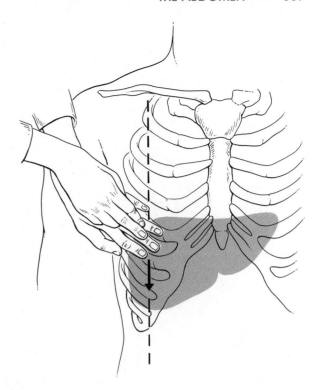

FIGURE 14-8. Technique for liver percussion.

Percuss the Liver

The upper border of the liver is percussed in the right midclavicular line, starting in the mid-chest. As one percusses from the chest downward, the resonant note of the chest becomes dull as the liver is reached. As one continues still further, this dull note becomes tympanic because the percussion is now over the colon. The upper and lower borders of the liver should be no more than 10 cm apart. Distention of the colon in the right upper quadrant may obscure the lower liver dullness. The examiner may, therefore, *under*estimate liver size. The technique is illustrated in Figure 14-8.

Percuss the Spleen

Although the area of the spleen is more difficult to percuss, determination of splenic size should be attempted. *Traube's space* is the area of the gastric air bubble in the left upper quadrant. Just lateral to Traube's space is an area of dullness related to the presence of the spleen. This area is approximately at the tenth rib, posterior to the midaxillary line.

Rule Out Ascites

On patients in whom ascites is thought to be present, a special percussion test for *shifting dullness* may be performed. While the patient is lying on his back, the examiner determines the borders of tympany and dullness. The level of tympany is present above the level of dullness. This is due to gas in the bowel that is floating on top of the ascites. The patient is then asked to turn on his side, and the examiner again determines the borders of the percussion notes. If ascites is present, dullness will "shift" to the more dependent position; the area around the umbilicus that was initially tympanic will now become dull. Shifting dullness

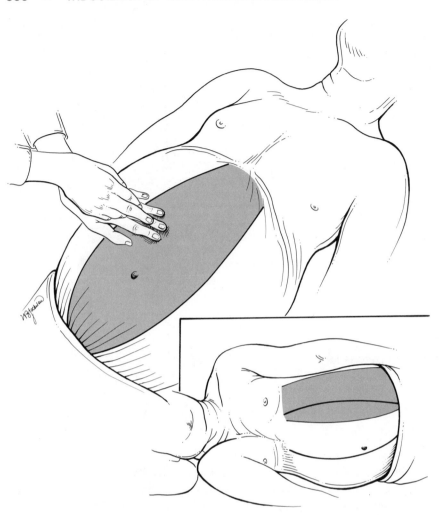

FIGURE 14–9. Technique for testing for shifting dullness. The colored areas represent the areas of tympany.

has a sensitivity of 83% and a specificity of 56%. The test for shifting dullness is illustrated in Figure 14–9.

An additional test for ascites is the presence of a *fluid wave*. Another examiner's hand or the patient's own hand is placed in the middle of his abdomen. Indenting the abdominal wall will stop transmission of an impulse by the subcutaneous adipose tissue. The examiner then taps one flank while palpating the other side. Detection of a fluid wave suggests ascites and is the most specific of

TABLE 14–4. Characteristics of Physical Signs for Detection of Ascites

Physical sign	Sensitivity (%)	Specificity (%)
Bulging flanks	78	44
Flank dullness	94	29
Shifting dullness	83	56
Fluid wave	50	82

Data from Cattau EL Jr, et al: JAMA *247*:1164, 1982.

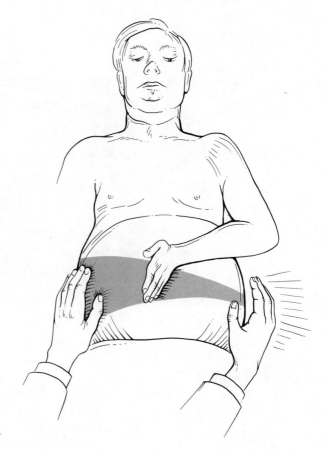

FIGURE 14–10. Technique for testing for a fluid wave.

all physical diagnostic tests for ascites. The presence of a fluid wave has a specificity of 82% (Cattau et al, 1982) but a sensitivity of only 50%. A false positive result may occur in obese patients, and a false negative may result when the ascites is small to moderate. This technique is illustrated in Figure 14–10.

The presence of flank dullness to percussion bilaterally is the most sensitive sign of ascites. The sensitivity is 94%, with a specificity of only 29%. If no flank dullness is detected, there is a 90% accuracy that ascites is absent. The sensitivities and specificities of the most important physical diagnostic tests are summarized in Table 14–4.

Palpation

Abdominal palpation is commonly divided into the following:

- Light palpation
- Deep palpation
- Liver palpation
- Spleen palpation
- Kidney palpation

The patient is supine during palpation. Always begin palpation in an area furthest away from the location of pain.

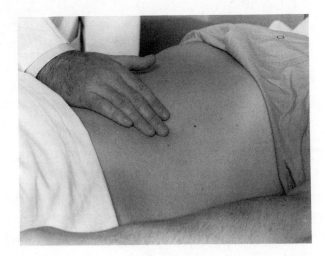

FIGURE 14–11. Technique for light palpation.

Light Palpation

Light palpation is used to detect tenderness and areas of muscular spasm or rigidity. The entire abdomen should be systematically palpated by using the flat part of the right hand or the pads of the fingers, *not* the fingertips. The fingers should be together, and sudden jabs are to be avoided. The hand should be lifted from area to area instead of sliding over the abdominal wall. Light palpation is demonstrated in Figure 14–11.

With patients who are ticklish, it may be useful to have them hold their hand over the examiner's hand, as shown in Figure 14–12.

During expiration, the rectus muscles usually relax and soften. If there is little change, *rigidity* is said to be present. Rigidity is involuntary spasm of the abdominal muscles and is indicative of peritoneal irritation. Rigidity may be

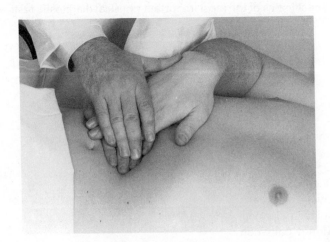

FIGURE 14–12. Technique to be used for ticklish patients. Notice that the patient's hand is sandwiched between the examiner's hands.

diffuse, as in diffuse peritonitis, or *localized,* as over an inflamed appendix or gallbladder. Patients with generalized peritonitis have an abdomen described as ''board-like.''

In patients who are complaining of abdominal pain, palpation should be performed gently. Lightly stroking the abdomen with a pin may detect an area of increased sensation that is due to inflamed visceral or parietal peritoneum. This is termed *hyperesthesia.* The patient is asked to determine whether the pin feels sharper on one side of the abdomen compared with the corresponding area on the other side. Although useful, the presence or absence of this finding must be considered in light of all other findings.

Deep Palpation

Deep palpation is used to determine organ size as well as the presence of abnormal abdominal masses. In deep palpation, the flat portion of the right hand is placed on the abdomen and the left hand is placed over it. The fingertips of the left hand exerts the pressure, while the right hand should appreciate any tactile stimulation. Pressure should be applied to the abdomen gently but steadily. The technique of deep palpation is shown in Figure 14–13.

During deep palpation, the patient should be instructed to breathe quietly through his mouth and to keep his arms at his sides. Asking the patient to open his mouth when breathing seems to aid in generalized muscular relaxation. The palpating hands should be warm, because cold hands may produce voluntary muscular spasm called *guarding.* Engaging the patient in conversation often aids in relaxing the patient's abdominal musculature. Patients with well-developed rectus muscles should be instructed to flex their knees in order to relax the abdominal muscles. Any tender areas must be identified.

Rule Out Rebound Tenderness

In a patient with abdominal pain, it should be determined whether rebound tenderness is present. Rebound tenderness is a sign of peritoneal irritation and can be elicited by palpating deeply and *slowly* in an abdominal area away from

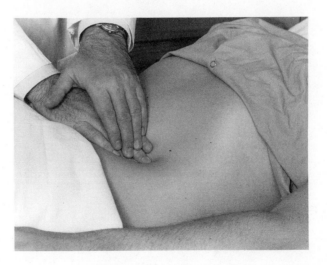

FIGURE 14–13. Technique for deep palpation.

the suspected area of local inflammation. The palpating hand is then quickly removed. The sensation of pain on the side of the inflammation that occurs on release of pressure is called rebound tenderness. If generalized peritonitis is present, pain will be felt in the area of palpation. The patient should be asked, "Which hurts more, *now* . . . (while pressing) or *now* . . . (during release)?" This is a very useful test, but because generalized pain will be elicited in the patient with peritonitis, the maneuver should be performed near the conclusion of the abdominal examination.

Palpate the Liver

Palpation of the liver is performed by placing the left hand posteriorly between the right twelfth rib and the iliac crest, lateral to the paraspinal muscles. The right hand is placed in the right upper quadrant parallel and lateral to the rectus muscles and below the area of liver dullness. The patient is instructed to take a deep breath as the examiner presses inward and upward with his right hand and pulls upward with his left hand. The liver edge may be felt to slip over the fingertips of the right hand as the patient breathes. It is important to start as low as the pelvic brim and gradually work upward. If the examination does not start low, a markedly enlarged liver edge will be missed. The technique of liver palpation is illustrated in Figure 14–14.

The normal liver edge has a firm, regular ridge, with a smooth surface. If the liver edge is not felt, repeat the maneuver after readjusting the right hand closer to the costal margin. Enlargement of the liver results from vascular congestion, hepatitis, neoplasm, or cirrhosis.

Another technique for liver palpation is known as the "hooking" method. The examiner stands near the patient's head and places both hands together below the right costal margin and the area of dullness. The examiner presses inward and upward and "hooks" around the liver edge as the patient is instructed to inhale deeply. The technique of hooking the liver is shown in Figure 14–15.

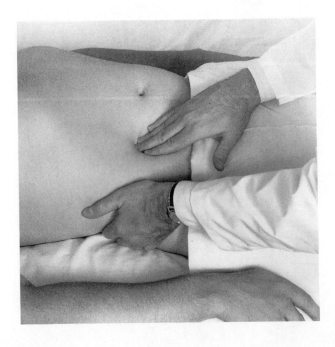

FIGURE 14–14. Technique for liver palpation.

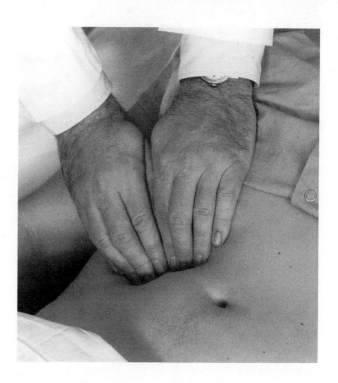

FIGURE 14–15. Technique for "hooking" the liver.

Occasionally, the liver appears to be enlarged but the actual border is difficult to determine. The *scratch test* may be helpful in ascertaining the liver's edge. The bell of the stethoscope is held with the left hand and is placed below the right costal margin over the liver. While the examiner listens through the stethoscope, the right index finger "scratches" the abdominal wall at points in a semicircle equidistant from the stethoscope. As the finger scratches over the liver's edge, there will be a marked increase in the intensity of the sound. The technique is illustrated in Figure 14–16.

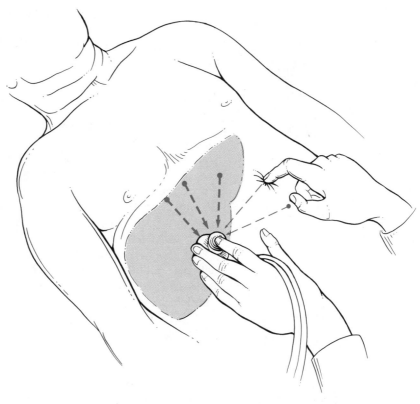

FIGURE 14–16. The scratch test for determining liver size.

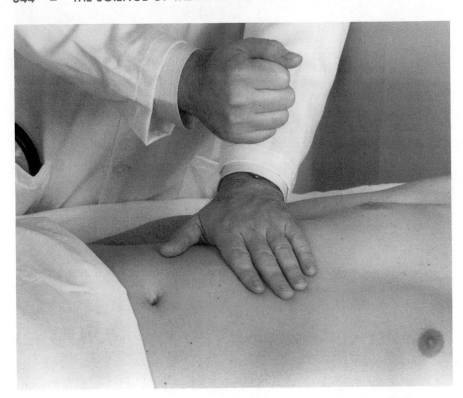

FIGURE 14–17. The liver tap for assessing liver tenderness.

Rule Out Hepatic Tenderness

Hepatic tenderness is elicited by placing the palm of the left hand over the right upper quadrant and *gently* striking it with the ulnar surface of the fist of the right hand. Inflammatory processes involving the liver or gallbladder will produce tenderness on fist palpation. Figure 14–17 illustrates this technique.

Occasionally during liver palpation, pain will be elicited during inspiration and the patient will suddenly stop his inspiratory effort. This is called *Murphy's sign* and is suggestive of acute cholecystitis. Upon inspiration, the inflamed gallbladder descends against the palpating hand; pain is produced, and there is inspiratory arrest.

Palpate the Spleen

Palpation of the spleen is more difficult than palpation of the liver. The patient lies on his back, with the examiner at the patient's right side. The examiner places his left hand over the patient's chest and elevates the patient's left rib cage. The right hand is placed flat below the left costal margin and presses inward and upward toward the anterior axillary line. The left hand exerts an anterior force to displace the spleen anteriorly. Figure 14–18 illustrates the positions of the hands for splenic palpation.

The patient is instructed to take a deep breath as the examiner presses inward with his right hand. The examiner should attempt to feel the tip of the spleen as it descends during inspiration. The tip of an enlarged spleen will lift the fingers of the right hand upward.

The examination of the spleen is repeated with the patient lying on his right side. This maneuver allows gravity to help bring the spleen anterior and downward into a more favorable position for palpation. The examiner places his left

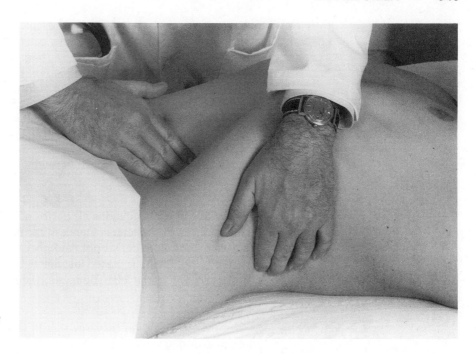

FIGURE 14-18. Technique for splenic palpation.

hand on the left costal margin while the right hand palpates in the left upper quadrant. The technique is shown in Figure 14-19.

Because the spleen enlarges diagonally in the abdomen from the left upper quadrant toward the umbilicus, it is important that the right hand always palpate near the umbilicus and gradually move toward the left upper quadrant.

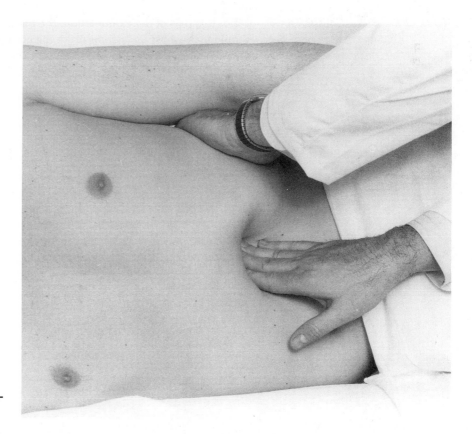

FIGURE 14-19. Another technique for splenic palpation.

This is particularly important if the spleen is massively enlarged, because starting the palpation too high may cause the examiner to miss the splenic border.

The spleen is not palpable under normal conditions, but both techniques should be utilized to attempt to palpate it. Splenic enlargement may be due to hyperplasia, congestion, infection, or infiltration by tumor or myeloid elements. Massive splenomegaly in a patient with chronic myelocytic leukemia is shown in Plate XII *D*.

Palpate the Kidneys

Palpation of the right kidney is performed by deep palpation below the right costal margin. The examiner stands at the patient's right side and places his left hand behind the patient's right flank, between the costal margin and the iliac crest. The right hand is placed just below the costal margin with the tips of the fingers pointing to the left. The method of kidney palpation is shown in Figure 14–20.

Very deep palpation may reveal the lower pole of the right kidney as it descends during inspiration. The lower pole may be felt as a smooth, rounded mass.

The same procedure is used for the left kidney except that the examiner is on the patient's left side. Because the left kidney is more superior than the right, the lower pole of a normal left kidney is rarely palpable. Occasionally, the spleen may be mistaken for an enlarged left kidney. The medial notch of the spleen is helpful in its differentiation from the kidney (see Plate XII *D*). More often than not, neither kidney can be palpated in the adult.

Rule Out Renal Tenderness

For this part of the examination, the patient should be seated. The examiner should make a fist and *gently* strike the area overlying the costovertebral angle on each side. Figure 14–21 illustrates the technique. Patients with pyelone-

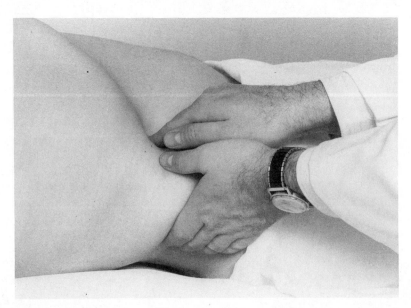

FIGURE 14–20. Technique for kidney palpation.

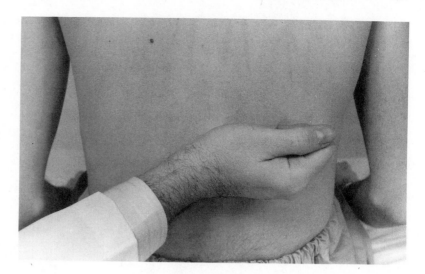

FIGURE 14–21. Assessing costovertebral angle tenderness.

phritis usually have extreme pain even on slight percussion in these areas. If pyelonephritis is suspected, only digital pressure should be used. As is described in Chapter 19, Putting the Examination Together, this portion of the abdominal examination is usually performed when the posterior chest is examined.

Rectal Examination

The routine abdominal examination concludes with the digital examination of the rectum. Because the anterior rectum has a peritoneal surface, the rectal examination may reveal tenderness if peritoneal inflammation is present.

Patient Positioning

The examination of the rectum may be performed with the patient lying on his back; lying on his left side; or standing, bent over the examination table. The modified lithotomy position (patient on his back with knees flexed) is used when the patient has difficulty standing or when a detailed examination of the anus is not required. The examiner passes his right hand under the patient's right thigh. The index finger in the rectum is used in conjunction with the examiner's left hand, which is placed on the abdomen. This bimanual approach is useful and causes minimal disturbance of the sick patient. The left lateral prone position, called the *Sims position,* is used commonly in women or when the patient is very weak and confined to bed. In this position, the right upper leg should be flexed while the left lower leg is semiextended. The modified lithotomy and left lateral prone positions are shown in Figure 14–22.

The standing position is the one most commonly used and allows for thorough inspection of the anus and palpation of the rectum. The patient is instructed to stand bent over with his shoulders and elbows supported on the bed or examination table. The examiner uses a gloved right hand to examine the anus and the tissue surrounding it while the left hand carefully spreads the buttocks. If infection is suspected, the examiner should wear gloves on both hands. The anal skin is inspected for signs of inflammation, excoriation, fissures, nodules, fistulae, scars, tumors, or hemorrhoids. Any abnormal areas should be palpated.

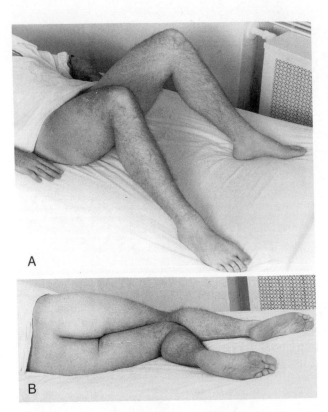

FIGURE 14–22. Positions for the rectal examination. *A,* Modified lithotomy position. *B,* Sims position.

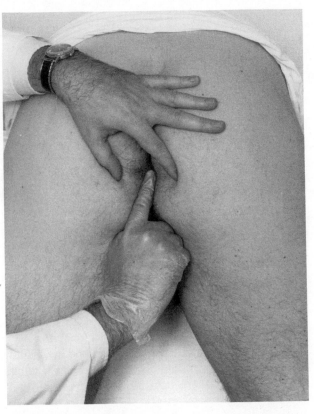

FIGURE 14–23. Technique of the rectal examination. Notice that the digit is inserted with the palm of the hand facing downward.

The patient is asked to strain while the examiner inspects the anus for hemorrhoids or fissures.

The Technique

The patient is told that a rectal examination will now be performed. The examiner should tell the patient that a cold feeling lubricant will be used, and this will be followed by the sensation that he will have to move his bowels; the patient should be assured that he will not do so.

The examiner lubricates his right gloved index finger and places his left hand on the patient's buttocks. As the left hand spreads the patient's buttocks, the right index finger is gently placed on the anal verge. The sphincter should be relaxed by gentle pressure with the palmar surface of the finger, as shown in Figure 14–23. Figure 14–24A also illustrates the procedure.

The patient is instructed to take a deep breath, at which time the right index finger is inserted into the anal canal as the anal sphincter relaxes. The sphincter should close completely around the examining digit. The sphincter tone should be assessed. The finger should be inserted as far as possible into the rectum, although 10 cm is the probable limit of digital exploration. The left hand can now be moved to the patient's left buttock, while the right index finger examines the rectum. The examination is illustrated in Figure 14–24B, and the position of the hands is shown in Figure 14–25.

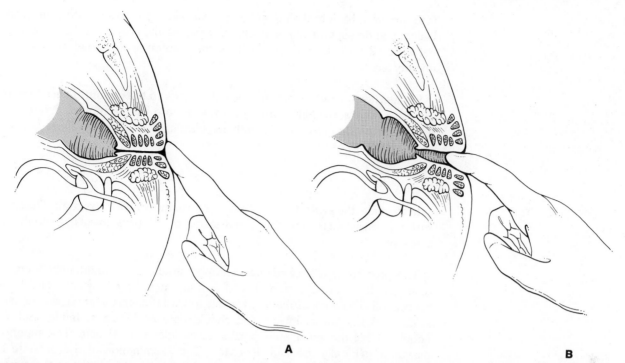

FIGURE 14–24. Illustration of the rectal examination. *A,* Sphincter is relaxed by gentle pressure with the palmar surface of the examiner's finger. *B,* With the left hand spreading the patient's buttocks, examination is carried out using the right index finger.

Palpate the Rectal Walls

The lateral, posterior, and anterior walls of the rectum are palpated. The lateral walls are felt by rotating the digit along the sides of the rectum. The ischial spines, coccyx, and lower sacrum can easily be felt. The walls are palpated for polyps, which may be sessile (attached by a base) or pedunculated (attached by a stalk). Any irregularities or undue tenderness should also be noted. The only way to examine the entire circumference of the rectal wall fully

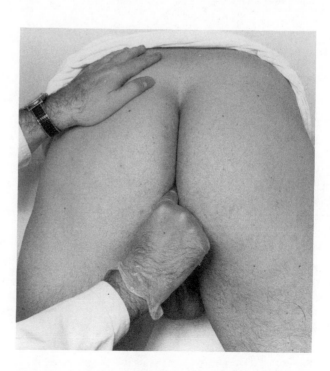

FIGURE 14–25. Technique for performing the rectal examination. Note position of the examiner's left hand.

is to turn your back to the patient, which will allow you to supinate your hand. Unless you do so, you will be unable to examine the portion of the rectal wall between 12 o'clock and 3 o'clock. A small lesion in this quadrant may go undetected.

Intraperitoneal metastases may be felt anterior to the rectum. These tumors are hard, and a shelf-like structure projects into the rectum as a result of infiltration of Douglas' pouch with neoplastic cells. This is referred to as *Blumer's shelf.*

Palpate the Prostate Gland

In the male, the prostate gland lies anterior to the wall of the rectum. The size, surface, consistency, sensitivity, and shape of the prostate gland should be assessed.

The prostate is a bilobed, heart-shaped structure approximately 4 cm in diameter. It is normally smooth and firm and has the consistency of a hard rubber ball. The apex of the heart points toward the anus. Identify the median sulcus and the lateral lobes. You should note any masses, tenderness, or nodules. Only the lower apex portion of the gland is palpable. The superior margin is generally too high to reach. The examination of the prostate is illustrated in Figure 14-26. The size of the prostate in relation to the examiner's finger is shown in Figure 14-27.

A hard, irregular nodule will produce asymmetry of the prostate gland and is suggestive of cancer. Carcinoma of the prostate frequently involves the posterior lobe, which can easily be identified during rectal examination. Benign prostatic hypertrophy (BPH) produces a symmetrically enlarged, soft gland that protrudes into the rectal lumen. This diffuse enlargement is very common over

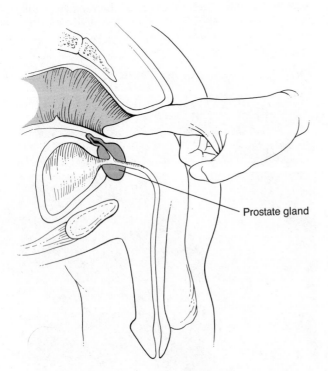

Prostate gland

FIGURE 14-26. Examination of the prostate.

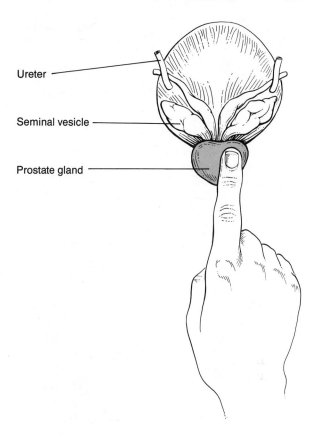

Ureter

Seminal vesicle

Prostate gland

FIGURE 14–27. Relationship of the size of the prostate gland to the examining finger.

the age of 60 years. A boggy, fluctuant, or tender prostate may indicate acute prostatitis. The seminal vesicles lie superior to the prostate gland and are rarely felt, unless they are enlarged.

In the female, the cervix lies anterior to the rectum. Generally, the examination of the rectum is performed *after* the pelvic examination. If a pelvic examination is not to be performed, the rectal examination may be done at this time.

The rectal examination is concluded by informing the patient that you are now going to withdraw your finger. Gently remove the examining finger and give the patient tissues to wipe himself.

TABLE 14–5. Clinical Comparison of Ulcerative Colitis and Crohn's Disease

	Ulcerative Colitis	Crohn's Disease
Diarrhea	Present	Present
Hematochezia	Common	Rare
Extraintestinal manifestations	Common	Common
Perirectal disease	Fissures	Fistulae Abscesses
Rectal disease	Present	Absent
Anal disease	Absent	Present

TABLE 14–6. Clinical Comparison of Cancer of the Stomach, Pancreas, and Colon

	Cancer of Stomach	Cancer of Pancreas	Cancer of Colon
Major Symptoms	Upper abdominal pain Occult bleeding Weight loss Vomiting Anorexia Dysphagia	Upper abdominal pain Back pain Weight loss Jaundice	Change in bowel habits Gastrointestinal bleeding Lower abdominal pain
Risk Factors	Adenomatous polyps Pernicious anemia Family history Immigrants from Japan	Smoking Alcoholism (?)	Adenomatous polyps Ulcerative colitis Familial polyposis Gardner's syndrome Villous adenomas

Test Stool for Occult Blood

The examining digit should be inspected. The color of the fecal material should be noted, and any fecal material should be examined with the occult blood testing card and reagent. A sample of stool should be placed on the testing card.

The guaiac or benzidine test detects occult blood. If blood is present, a chemical reaction will result in a blue coloration on the card. The reaction is graded by the intensity of the blue color, from light blue (trace blood) to dark blue (4+ positive).

Although the examination for inguinal hernias is part of the abdominal examination, it is discussed in Chapter 15, Male Genitalia and Hernias.

Special Techniques

Intra-abdominal inflammation may involve the psoas muscle. A special test performed when there is suspicion of intra-abdominal inflammation is the *iliopsoas test*. The patient is asked to lie on the unaffected side and extend his other leg at the hip against the resistance of the examiner's hand. A *positive psoas sign* is abdominal pain with this maneuver. Irritation of the right psoas muscle by an acutely inflamed appendix will produce a right psoas sign. This test is illustrated in Figure 14–28.

TABLE 14–7. Variation of Symptoms of Cancer of the Right Colon, Left Colon, and Rectum

Symptom	Cancer of Right Colon	Cancer of Left Colon	Cancer of Rectum
Pain	Ill defined	Colicky*	Steady, gnawing
Obstruction	Infrequent	Common	Infrequent
Bleeding	Brick red	Red mixed with stool	Bright red coating stool
Weakness†	Common	Infrequent	Infrequent

* Worse with ingestion of foods.
† Secondary to anemia.

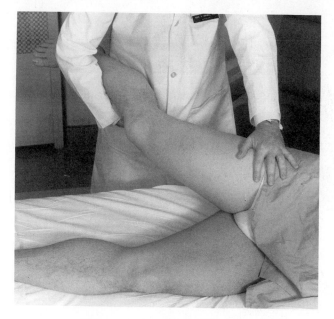

FIGURE 14-28. The iliopsoas test.

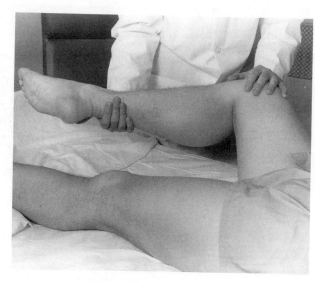

FIGURE 14-29. The obturator test.

Another useful test for inflammation is the *obturator test*. While the patient is lying on his back, the examiner flexes the patient's thigh at the hip, with knees bent, and rotates the leg internally and externally at the hip. If there is an inflammatory process adjacent to the obturator muscle, pain will be elicited. The obturator test is shown in Figure 14-29.

CLINICOPATHOLOGIC CORRELATIONS

Table 14-2 lists the classic locations of pain referred from abdominal structures. Table 14-3 summarizes the ameliorating factors in abdominal pain. Table 14-4 summarizes the sensitivities and specificities of the various maneuvers used to detect ascites. Table 14-5 is a comparison of the clinical manifestations of Crohn's disease and ulcerative colitis. Table 14-6 lists the clinical features of cancer of the stomach, pancreas, and colon. Table 14-7 lists the variation of symptoms in right-sided and left-sided colon cancer and in rectal cancer. The clinical manifestations of cirrhosis are numerous. Table 14-8 compares the symptoms and signs as they relate to hepatocellular failure and portal hypertension.

TABLE 14-8. Signs and Symptoms of Cirrhosis

Hepatocellular Failure	Portal Hypertension
Spider angiomata	Ascites
Gynecomastia	Varices: esophageal
Palmar erythema	Hemorrhoids
Ascites	Caput medusae
Jaundice	Splenomegaly
Testicular atrophy	
Impotence	
Bleeding problems	
Changes in mental function	

USEFUL VOCABULARY

Listed here are the specific roots that are important in order to understand the terminology related to abdominal disease.

ROOT	PERTAINING TO	EXAMPLE	DEFINITION
aer(o)-	air; gas	*aero*phagia	Air swallowing
celi(o)-	abdomen	*celi*ac	Pertaining to the abdomen
chol(e)-	bile	*chole*lith	Gallstone
cyst-	sac containing liquid	chole*cyst*itis	Inflammation of the gallbladder
enter(o)-	intestines	*enter*itis	Inflammation of the small intestines
gastr(o)-	stomach	*gastr*ectomy	Surgical removal of the stomach
lapar(o)-	loin; flank	*lapar*otomy	Surgical incision through the flank; generally, any abdominal incision
-phago-	eating	*phago*cyte	Any cell that ingests other cells or microorganisms

WRITING UP THE PHYSICAL EXAMINATION

Listed here are examples of the write-up for the examination of the abdomen.

The abdomen is scaphoid without scars. Bowel sounds are present. The liver is felt 2 finger breaths below the right costal margin for a total span of 10 cm. Neither the spleen nor any masses are felt. The kidneys are not palpable. Rectal examination reveals normal sphincter tone. The prostate is soft, without any masses. The walls of the rectum are smooth, without masses. Testing of the stool for blood is negative. No costovertebral angle tenderness* is present.

The abdomen has a scar in the right upper quadrant. Bowel sounds are absent. Marked tympany is present throughout the abdomen. Rigidity is present throughout. Marked tenderness is present in the abdomen, especially in the left lower quadrant. Examination of the rectum reveals tenderness in the same area. Stool guaiac is 4+ positive. The liver, spleen, and kidneys are not felt. No CVAT is present.

The abdomen is obese. Bowel sounds are present. Percussion notes are normal. There is an area of significant pain in the right lower quadrant, immediately above the right mid-position of the inguinal ligament. Rectal examination discloses severe pain in the same area. The obturator and straight leg raising signs are positive on the right. Stool guaiac is negative. Right CVAT is present. No organomegaly is felt.

The abdomen is protuberant, with a midline, well-healed scar. Bowel sounds are present. Shifting dullness and a fluid wave are present. A large mass 8 × 15 cm is felt in the right upper quadrant. Examination of the rectum is unremarkable except for a trace positive stool guaiac. There is no hepatosplenomegaly.

The abdomen is scaphoid and soft, without guarding, rigidity, or tenderness. Bowel sounds are present. The liver measures 12 cm in span in the midclavicular line. The spleen tip is felt below the left costal margin. No masses are present. Rectal examination reveals a 2 cm hard nodule in the posterior lobe of the prostate, which is nontender. Stool guaiac is negative.

* Often abbreviated as CVAT.

BIBLIOGRAPHY

Brooks FP: Gastrointestinal Pathophysiology. New York, Oxford University Press, 1978.

Cattau EL Jr, Benjamin SB, Knoff TE, Castell DO. The accuracy of the physical examination in the diagnosis of suspected ascites. JAMA 247:1164, 1982.

Helzer JE, Chammas S, Norland CC, Stillings WA, Alpers DH: A study of the association between Crohn's disease and psychiatric illness. Gastroenterology 86:324, 1984.

Koretz RL: Practical Gastroenterology. New York, John Wiley and Sons, 1982.

Latimer PR: Crohn's disease: A review of the psychological and social outcome. Psychol Med 8:649, 1978.

Lindner AE: Emotional Factors in Gastrointestinal Illness. New York, American Elsevier Company, 1973.

McKegney FP, Gordon RO, Levine SM: A psychosomatic comparison of patients with ulcerative colitis and Crohn's disease. Psychosom Med 32:153, 1970.

Mulvihill JJ: The frequency of hereditary large bowel cancer. In Ingall JRF, Mastromarino AJ (eds): Prevention of Hereditary Large Bowel Cancer. New York, Alan R Liss, 1983.

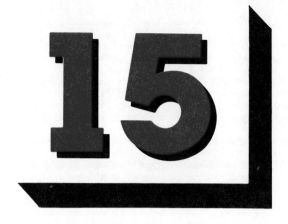

MALE GENITALIA AND HERNIAS

If a man's urine is like the urine of an ass, like beer yeast, like wine yeast or varnish, that man is sick . . . and through a bronze tube in the penis pour oil and beer and licorice.

From the Sushruta Samhita
ca. 3000 BC

GENERAL CONSIDERATIONS

Since the beginning of recorded history, the external genitalia and the urologic system have been of special interest to mankind. Kidney stones and urologic surgery were well described in antiquity. One of the earliest reported kidney stones was found in a young boy dating back to 7000 BC.

Although *circumcision* has been considered as a measure of hygiene, there is much evidence that it was a ritualistic act. Circumcision was often depicted on the walls of temples dating from 3000 BC. In the Egyptian Book of the Dead, it is written, "The blood falls from the phallus of the Sun God as he starts to incise himself." The Hindus regarded the penis and testicles as a symbol of the center of life and sacrificed the prepuce as a special offering to the gods.

The Bible has many urologic references. In Genesis 17:7, Abraham makes a covenant with God for the Jews. He is told in Genesis 17:14, "And the uncircumcised male who is not circumcised in the flesh of his foreskin, that soul shall be cut off from his people; he hath broken My covenant." In Leviticus 12:3, the Jews were told, "And in the eighth day the flesh of his foreskin shall be circumcised." Leviticus 15:2–17 deals with discharges that render a man unclean.

The Bible, Hindu literature, and Egyptian papyruses all described a disease we now presume was gonorrhea. The Mesopotamian tablets described a variety of cures, such as: "If a man's penis on occasions of his pleasure hurts him, boil beer and milk and anoint him from the pubis." Avicenna's Canon Medicae in 1000 AD was considered the authoritative text on medicine for centuries and described placing a louse in the penis to counteract a penile discharge.

Gonorrhea was probably first named by Galen in the second century AD. Gonorrhea is the Greek translation of "a flow of offspring." Galen apparently thought that the purulent discharge was a leakage of semen. Many terms have been used to describe gonorrhea over the years. Perhaps the most common is "the clap," a name used for the past 400 years. It is thought that the term "the clap" was derived from the red-light district in Paris, called "Le Clapier."

It is unclear when the scourge of *syphilis* actually began. There was much confusion between syphilis and gonorrhea. It was felt that gonorrhea was the first stage of syphilis. The etiology of these diseases was also unknown. Many believed that syphilis was due to floods, eating disguised human meat, or poisoning of the water. It was not until 1500, when syphilis was pandemic in Europe, that the venereal origins of both diseases were understood. It is now believed that syphilis was introduced on the European continent in 1492 by the returning sailors who had been traveling with Columbus. Following the invasion of Italy and the siege of Naples by France in 1495, syphilis became rampant throughout Europe. The "King's pox" and the "French pox" were the common terms used for syphilis.

Cancer of the genitourinary system is very common. In the United States, it is estimated that prostatic cancer accounts for 19% of all cancers in men, and urinary tract cancers account for an additional 9%. Prostatic cancer accounts for 10% of all cancer deaths, whereas other genitourinary malignancies account for 5%. There were over 90,000 new cases of prostatic cancer in 1986, making this diagnosis the second most common malignancy in men (lung cancer is the first). Approximately 95% of all prostatic cancers arise from the area of the gland that can be readily detected by rectal examination.

Although testicular cancer accounts for only 1% of all cancers in men, testicular carcinoma represents the most common cancer in men in the 15–35 year old age group. Approximately 90% of all testicular tumors present as an asymptomatic testicular mass. Once detected and treatment is begun, the cure rate can approach 90%. The most important prognostic factor has been shown to be early detection by routine physical examination.

STRUCTURE AND PHYSIOLOGY

Cross-sectional and frontal views of the male genitalia are shown in Figure 15–1.

The *penis* is composed of three elongated, distensible structures: two paired *corpora cavernosa* and a single *corpus spongiosum*. The urethra runs through the corpus spongiosum. The penis has two surfaces, dorsal and ventral (urethral), and consists of the root, the shaft, and the head. The shaft is composed of erectile tissue, which when engorged with blood produces a firm erection necessary for sexual intercourse. The corpora cavernosa also contain smooth muscle that contract rhythmically during ejaculation.

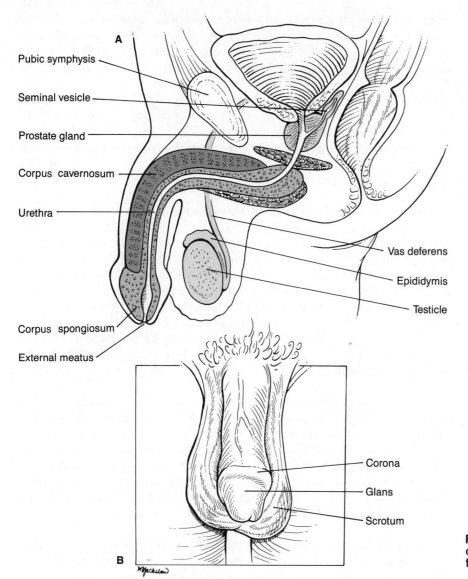

Pubic symphysis

Seminal vesicle

Prostate gland

Corpus cavernosum

Urethra

Vas deferens

Epididymis

Testicle

Corpus spongiosum

External meatus

Corona

Glans

Scrotum

FIGURE 15–1. Labeled diagrams of male genitalia. *A*, Cross-sectional view. *B*, Frontal view.

On the dorsal aspect in the midline of the penis runs the dorsal vein with an artery and nerve on either side. The distal end of the corpus spongiosum expands to form the head, or *glans penis.* The glans penis covers the end of the corpora cavernosa. The glans has a prominent margin on its dorsal aspect, called the *corona.* A slit-like opening on the tip of the glans is the *external meatus* of the urethra.

The skin of the penis is smooth, thin, and hairless. At the distal end of the penis, a free fold of skin called the *prepuce* (foreskin) covers the glans. Mucus secretion and sloughed epithelial cells called *smegma* collect between the prepuce and the glans, providing a lubricant during sexual intercourse. The prepuce can be retracted to expose the glans as far as the corona. During circumcision, the prepuce is removed.

The root of the penis lies deep to the scrotum, in the perineum. At the root, the corpora cavernosa diverge from each other. Each corpus cavernosum is

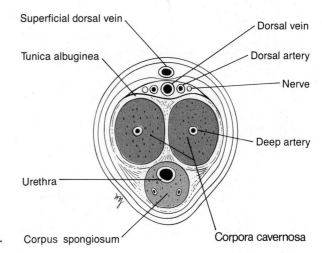

FIGURE 15–2. Cross-sectional view through the penis.

enveloped in a dense, fibroelastic covering called the *tunica albuginea,* and these tunicae fuse to form the median septum of the penis. A cross-section through the penis is shown in Figure 15–2.

The blood supply to the penis is from the internal pudendal artery, from which the dorsal and deep arteries of the corpora cavernosa are derived. The veins drain into the dorsal vein of the penis. In the flaccid state, the venous channels and arteriovenous anastomoses are widely patent, whereas the arteries are partially constricted. In the erect state, the arteriovenous channels are closed and the arteries are widely opened. Muscular pillars are present in the walls of the arteries, veins, and arteriovenous anastomoses, which aid in occluding the lumens. The physiology of erection is illustrated in Figure 15–3.

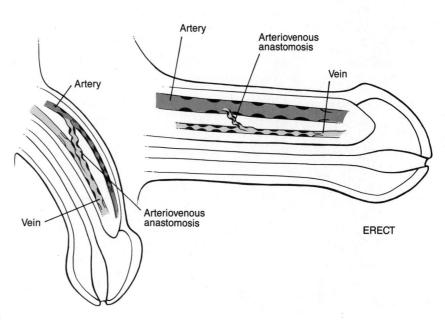

FIGURE 15–3. The physiology of erection.

The *urethra* extends from the internal urinary meatus of the bladder to the external meatus of the penis. The urethra can be divided into three portions: the prostatic (posterior) portion, the membranous portion, and the cavernous (anterior) portion. The short posterior portion passes through the prostate gland. The common ejaculatory duct as well as several prostatic ducts enters at the distal end of this portion. The external urethral sphincter surrounds the membranous urethra, and on either side lie Cowper's bulbourethral glands. The anterior urethra is the longest and passes through the corpus spongiosum. The ducts of Cowper's glands enter the anterior urethra near its proximal end.

The *scrotum* is the pouch containing the testes, which is suspended externally from the perineum. It is divided into halves by the interscrotal septum, one testis lying on each side. The wall of the scrotum contains involuntary smooth muscle and voluntary striated muscle. A major role of the scrotum is temperature regulation of the testes. The testes are maintained about 2° C lower than the peritoneal cavity, a condition necessary for spermatogenesis. The size of the scrotum is variable according to the individual and his response to ambient temperature. During exposure to cold temperatures, the scrotum is contracted and very rugated. In a warm environment, the scrotum becomes pendulous and smoother.

The *testes* are ovoid, smooth, and approximately 3.5–5 cm in length. The left testicle commonly lies lower than the right. The testes are covered with a tough fibrous coat called the *tunica albuginea testis*. Each testicle has a long axis directed slightly anteriorly and upward. Each contains long, microscopic, convoluted seminiferous tubules that produce sperm. The tubules end in the *epididymis*, which is comma shaped and located on the posterior border of the testis. It consists of a head that is swollen and overhangs the upper pole of the testicle. The inferior portion or tail of the epididymis continues into the *vas deferens*. The testicular artery enters the testicle in its posterior midportion. The veins draining the testicle form a dense network called the *pampiniform plexus*, which drains into the testicular vein. The right testicular vein drains directly into the inferior vena cava, whereas the left drains into the left renal vein. The lymphatic drainage of the testes is to the preaortic and precaval nodes, not to the inguinal

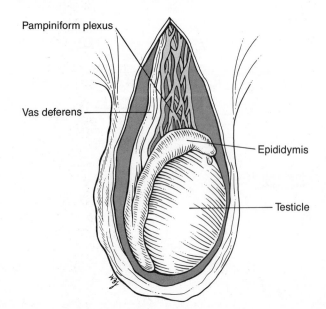

Pampiniform plexus

Vas deferens

Epididymis

Testicle

FIGURE 15–4. Anatomy of the testicle and epididymis.

nodes. This is important to recognize, because the testes are embryologically intra-abdominal organs, and neoplasms and inflammations of the testis produce adenopathy of these nodal chains. Generally, inguinal adenopathy is rare.

The relationship of the testicle and epididymis is shown in Figure 15–4.

The vas deferens is a cord-like structure, easily felt in the scrotum. The vas deferens, testicular arteries, and veins form the *spermatic cord,* which enters the inguinal canal. The vas deferens passes through the internal ring and after a convoluted course reaches the fundus of the bladder. It passes between the rectum and the bladder and approaches the vas deferens of the opposite side near the seminal vesicles. Near the base of the prostate, the vas deferens joins with the duct of the corresponding seminal vesicle to form the *ejaculatory duct,* which passes through the prostate gland to enter the posterior urethra.

The *prostate gland* is about the size of two almonds. It is approximately 3.5 cm long by 3 cm wide. Traversing through the gland in the midline is the posterior urethra. On either side is an ejaculatory duct. The prostate is commonly divided into five lobes. The posterior lobe is important, because carcinoma frequently affects this lobe. In the presence of cancer, the midline groove between the two lateral lobes may be obliterated. The middle and lateral lobes are above the ejaculatory ducts and are typically involved with benign hypertrophy. The anterior lobe is of little clinical importance.

The male genitalia showing the sources and direction of seminal fluid flow are illustrated in Figure 15–5.

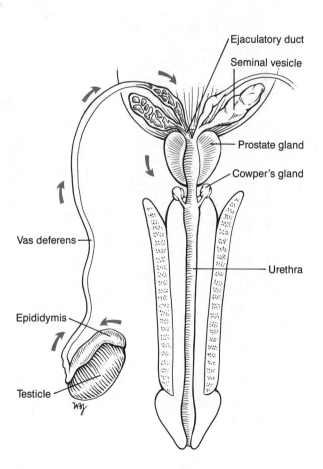

FIGURE 15–5. The sources and direction of seminal flow.

The descent of the testes is important to review at this time. In the normal full term male, both testes are in the scrotum at birth. The testes descend to this position just prior to birth. About the twelfth week of gestation, the *gubernaculum* develops in the inguinal fold and grows through the body wall to an area that will ultimately lie in the scrotum. This tract marks the location of the future inguinal canal. A dimple forms in the peritoneum called the *processus vaginalis,* which follows the course of the gubernaculum. By the seventh month of gestation, the processus vaginalis has reached the aponeurosis of the external oblique muscle. Each testis then begins its descent from the abdominal cavity through the internal ring to lie in the abdominal wall. During the eighth month, the testes descend along the inguinal canal; at birth, they are located in the scrotum. At birth, the gubernaculum is barely distinguishable and the processus vaginalis becomes obliterated within the spermatic cord. In about 5% of male infants, there is imperfect descent of the testis (cryptorchidism). The descent of the testes is illustrated in Figure 15–6.

The genital development stages for boys are illustrated and discussed in Figure 20–11 (Chapter 20, The Pediatric Patient).

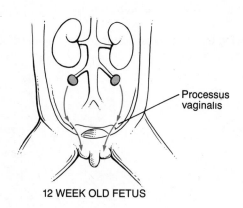

Processus
vaginalis

12 WEEK OLD FETUS

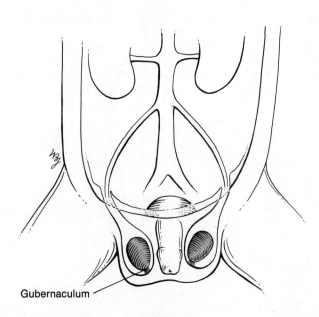

Gubernaculum

NEWBORN

FIGURE 15–6. The descent of the testes.

REVIEW OF SPECIFIC SYMPTOMS

The most common symptoms of male genitourinary disease are as follows:

- Pain
- Dysuria (burning on urination)
- Changes in urine flow
- Red urine
- Discharge
- Penile lesions
- Enlargement of scrotal contents
- Swelling or mass in the groin
- Impotence
- Infertility

Pain

Sudden distention of the ureter, renal pelvis, or bladder may cause flank pain Any patient with flank pain should be asked the following questions:

"When did the pain begin?"
"Where did the pain begin?" "Can you point to the area?"
"Do you feel the pain in any other area of your body?"
"Did the pain start suddenly?"
"Have you ever had this type of pain before?"
"Is the pain constant?"
"What seems to make the pain worse? . . . less?"
"Has the color of your urine changed?"
*"Is the pain associated with nausea? . . . vomiting? . . . abdominal disten-
    tion? . . . fever? . . . chills? . . . burning on urination?"*

Gradual enlargement of these structures is usually painless. An aching pain in the costovertebral angle may be related to sudden distention of the renal capsule, which results from acute pyelonephritis or obstructive hydronephrosis. The spasmodic, colicky pain from upper ureteral dilatation may cause referred pain to the testis on the same side. Lower ureteral dilatation may cause pain referred to the scrotum. The pain of ureteral distention is very severe, and the patient is restless and uncomfortable in any position. Bladder distention causes lower abdominal fullness and suprapubic pain with an intense desire to urinate. Pain is the groin may result from pathology of the spermatic cord, testicle, or prostate gland; lymphadenitis of any cause; hernia; herpes zoster, or may be neurologic in origin.

Testicular pain can result from nearly any disease of the testis or epididymis. This includes epididymitis, orchitis, hydrocele, spermatic cord torsion, or tumor. Referred pain from the ipsilateral ureter must always be considered. *Priapism* is a painful, persistent erection of the penis that is not a result of sexual excitation. The sustained erection results from thrombosis of the corpora cavernosa. This occurs in patients with sickle cell anemia or leukemia. The exact mechanism is unknown but appears to result from a blockage of venous drainage from the penis, while the arteries remain patent. Chronic priapism often results in organic impotence.

Dysuria

Pain on urination, called dysuria, is frequently described as "burning." Dysuria is evidence for inflammation of the lower urinary tract. The patient may describe discomfort in the penis or in the suprapubic area. Dysuria also implies difficulty in urination. This may result from external meatal stenosis or from a urethral stricture. Painful urination is usually associated with urinary frequency and urgency. When the patient describes pain or difficulty in urination, ask the following questions:

"How long have you noticed burning on urination?"
"How often do you urinate each day?"
"How does your urination feel different?"
"Is your urine clear?"
"Does the urine smell bad?"
"Do you have a discharge from your penis?"
"Does the urine seem to have gas bubbles in it?"
"Have you noticed any solid particles in your urine?"
"Have you noticed pus in your urine?"

Pneumaturia is the passage of air in the urine producing what the patient describes as "bubbles of gas in the urine." The air or gas is emitted usually at the end of urination. Normally, there is no gas in the urinary tract. The symptom of pneumaturia is important because it indicates the introduction of air by instrumentation; a fistula to the bowel; or a urinary tract infection by gas forming bacteria, such as *Escherichia coli* or clostridia.

Fecaluria is the presence of fecal material in the urine and is rare. The passage of feculent smelling material results from either an intestinovesicular fistula or a urethrorectal fistula. These fistulae occur as a consequence of ulceration from the bowel to the urinary tract. Diverticulitis, carcinoma, and Crohn's disease are frequent causes.

Pus in the urine, *pyuria,* is the body's response to inflammation of the urinary tract. Bacteria is the most common cause of inflammation resulting in pyruria, although pyuria is also seen in patients with neoplasms and kidney stones. Cystitis and prostatitis are common causes of pyuria.

Changes in Urine Flow

Changes in urine flow include frequency and incontinence. Urinary *frequency* is the most common symptom of the genitourologic system. Frequency is defined as passing urine more often than normal. *Nocturia* is urinary frequency at night. There are several causes of frequency: decreased bladder size, bladder wall irritation, and increased urine volume. If an obstructed bladder cannot be completely emptied at each voiding, its effective capacity is diminished. The following questions, in addition to the ones under dysuria, should be asked to help define the problem:

"Do you find that you must wake up at night to urinate?"
"Can you estimate the amount of urine passed each time you urinate?"
"Do you have sudden urges to urinate?"
"Have you found that despite an urge to urinate you cannot start the stream?"

"Has there been a change in the caliber of the stream?"
"Have you found that you must wait longer for the stream to start?"
"Do you have the sensation that after urination has stopped you still have the urge to urinate?"
"Do you have to strain at the end of urination?"
"Have you been drinking more fluids recently?"

Prostatic hypertrophy is the most common cause of reduced usable bladder capacity. Most bladder diseases, such as cystitis, cause frequency that is due to irritation of the bladder mucosa. *Polyuria,* or voiding large amounts of urine, is usually accompanied by excessive thirst, known as *polydipsia.* Diabetes mellitus and diabetes insipidus are common causes.

Urinary *incontinence* refers to the inability of the patient to retain his urine voluntarily. The urge to urinate may be so intense that incontinence may result. In addition to the questions regarding dysuria and frequency, ask the following:

"Do you lose involuntarily small amounts of urine?"
"Do you lose your urine constantly?"
"Do you lose your urine when lifting heavy objects? . . . laughing? . . . coughing? . . . bending over?"
"Do you have to press on your abdomen to urinate?"

In patients who have chronically distended bladders, as in patients with prostatic hypertrophy, there is always a large amount of residual urine. The pressure within the bladder is constantly elevated. A slight increase in intra-abdominal pressure raises the intravesicular pressure sufficiently to overcome bladder neck resistance, and urine escapes. Leakage may be steady or intermittent. This type of incontinence is termed *overflow* incontinence. *Stress* incontinence is leakage only when the patient strains. The primary defect is a loss of muscular support in the urethrovesicular region. Residual urine is insignificant. Any increase in intra-abdominal pressure causes leakage. This type of incontinence is more common in women and is further discussed in the next chapter.

Polyuria is the symptom of increased amounts of urination, frequently greater than 2 – 3 liters per day. The normal daily urine output varies from 1 to 2 liters. The most important diseases to differentiate are diabetes mellitus, diabetes insipidus, and psychological diabetes insipidus. Ask the following questions:

"For how long have you been passing large amounts of urine?"
"Was the onset sudden?"
"How often do you have to urinate at night?"
"Is there any variability to the urine flow from day to day?"
"Do you have an excessive thirst?"
"Do you prefer water or other fluids?"
"What happens if you don't drink? Will you still have to urinate?"
"How is your appetite?"
"Do you have any visual problems? . . . headaches?"
"Are you aware of any emotional problems?"

Patients with diabetes mellitus have a high osmotic load and have polyuria. The increased appetite is also very common. Diabetes insipidus is due to a vasopressin deficiency related to a lesion in the hypothalamus or pituitary. These patients cannot concentrate their urines despite a rise in plasma osmolality. Patients with psychogenic diabetes insipidus, which is more common, have polyuria related to compulsive drinking of water. It is seen in patients with psychological problems. The abrupt onset of polyuria is seen in psychogenic diabetes insipidus. These patients also have no preference for the type of fluid they drink. In contrast, patients with true diabetes insipidus prefer water. Because true diabetes insipidus is related to intracranial lesions, it is not surprising that these individuals suffer from headaches and visual disturbances, especially visual field abnormalities.

Red Urine

Red urine is an important symptom to evaluate because it often indicates *hematuria,* or blood in the urine. There are many causes of red urine, and it should not be automatically assumed that red urine indicates bleeding. Drugs, such as pyridium; vegetable dyes; and excessive ingestion of beets can cause red urine. When it is determined that the urine is red as a result of the presence of blood, the hematuria is termed *gross hematuria.* Hematuria may be the first symptom of serious disease of the urinary tract. Ask the following questions of any patient with the symptom of red urine:

> *"How long have you noticed red urine?"*
> *"Have you had red urine previously?"*
> *"Have you noticed that the urine starts red and then clears? . . . starts clear and then turns red? . . . is red throughout?"*
> *"Have you noticed clots of blood in the urine?"*
> *"Have you done any severely strenuous physical activity recently, such as prolonged hiking, running, or marching?"*
> *"Did you have an upper respiratory infection or a sore throat a few weeks ago?"*
> *"Is the red urine associated with flank pain? . . . abdominal pain? . . . burning on urination? . . . fever? . . . weight loss?"*
> *"Are you aware of any bleeding problems?"*
> *"Are you taking any medications?"*
> *"Do you eat beets often?"*

Individuals who participate in very strenuous activities may traumatize blood cells as these cells travel through the small vessels on the feet. A condition called *march hemoglobinuria* may result, causing intravascular hemolysis and hemoglobinuria. The temporal relationship of blood in the urine is an important factor. Blood only at the beginning, *initial* hematuria, usually has a source in the urethra. Blood only at the end of urination, *terminal* hematuria, indicates pathology at the bladder neck or at the posterior urethra. Blood evenly distributed throughout urination is called *total* hematuria and implies disease above the prostate gland or a massive hemorrhage at any level. Blood staining of undergarments without blood in the urine indicates pathology of the external urethral meatus. Weight loss and hematuria are seen in renal cell carcinoma. Red urine that has occurred 10–14 days after an upper respiratory infection may indicate acute glomerulonephritis.

Penile Discharge

Discharge from the penis is a continuous or intermittent flow of fluid from the urethra. It is important to ask the man if he has ever had a discharge, and if he has, whether it has been bloody or purulent. Bloody penile discharges are associated with ulcerations, neoplasms, or urethritis. Purulent discharges are thick, yellowish-green, and may be associated with gonococcal urethritis or chronic prostatitis. It is important to determine when the discharge was first noted.

Tactful direct questioning of any history of or exposure to sexually transmitted diseases is essential. The interviewer should determine the patient's sexual orientation and the type of sexual exposure — oral, vaginal, or anal — as this information will help to determine the types of bacteriologic cultures necessary. It is appropriate to ask whether the patient has more than one partner and if the partner(s) have any known illnesses. The sexual history questions suggested in Chapter 1 may be helpful.

Penile Lesions

A history of lesions on the penis should alert the examiner of the possibility of venereal disease. It is important to ask the man whether he has had gonorrhea, syphilis, herpes, trichomoniasis, or other venereal disease. Review the previous questions and those in Chapter 1.

Scrotal Enlargement

It is not uncommon for a man to complain of enlargement of his scrotum. It is often difficult for the man to determine which anatomic structures in the scrotum are enlarged. Ask these questions:

"When did you first notice the enlargement?"
"Is it painful?"
"Have you sustained any injury to your groin?"
"Does the enlargement change in size?"
"Have you ever had it before?"
"Have you ever had a hernia?"
"Have you had any problems with fertility?"

Swellings in the scrotum can be related to testicular or epididymal enlargement, a hernia, a varicocele, a spermatocele, or a hydrocele. Testicular enlargement can result from inflammation or tumor. Most of the time, enlargement is unilateral. Painful scrotal enlargements can result from acute inflammation of the epididymis or testis, torsion of the spermatic cord, or a strangulated hernia. Varicoceles are often a cause of decreased fertility.

Groin Mass or Swelling

If a patient describes a mass in the groin, ask the following questions:

"When did you first notice it?"
"Is the mass painful?"
"Does it change in size with different positions?"
"Have you had any venereal disease?"

The most common cause of swelling in the groin is a hernia. Hernias will be reduced in size after the patient has been lying down. Adenopathy from any infection of the external genitalia may produce inguinal swelling. Carcinoma of the testis will produce inguinal node enlargement only if the scrotal skin is involved.

Impotence

Erectile impotence is an important symptom because it frequently provides an insight into emotional problems of the patient. A delicate approach to the patient must be taken. It is necessary to use tact and appropriate language that will be understood by the patient. Explaining that impotence is a common problem often sets the tone. Deep-seated problems require careful questioning. Sometimes the interviewer will discover latent homosexuality. Guilt and taboos during early life may leave a lasting impression on sexual performance. Key and direct questions are important. It is appropriate to ask the following:

"Do you have early morning erections or nighttime emissions?"
"Do any women other than your wife (or girlfriend) arouse you?"
"Are you able to masturbate to an erection or climax?"

An affirmative answer to any of these questions will allow the interviewer to be reassured that the impotence is psychological in origin. Allowing the patient to discuss his problems may serve to vent some of his anxieties. The patient's confidence must be secured by guaranteeing confidentiality. The interviewer must resolve his own sexual anxieties in order to have a confident and straight-forward discussion. An open dialogue about the anxieties surrounding sexual intercourse may be fruitful. The interviewer must be careful not to impose his own moral standards on the patient. Improving communication between partners is helpful.

Infertility

Infertility refers to the inability to conceive or to cause pregnancy. Infertility is a common problem found in as many as 10% of all marriages. A couple is said to be infertile when after 1 year of normal intercourse pregnancy does not occur. It has been estimated that almost 30% of all infertility is due to a "male" factor. Any patient with the history of infertility should be questioned regarding a past history of mumps, testicular injury, venereal disease, exposure to x-rays, or any urologic surgical procedure. Frequency of sexual intercourse and difficulty in achieving or maintaining an erection are important factors to determine. A careful history of general work habits, alcoholic consumption, and sleeping habits is important.

IMPACT OF IMPOTENCE ON THE MAN

Impotence may be described as the inability of a man to achieve or maintain an erection sufficient to accomplish the coital act. Impotence may be either erectile or ejaculatory. This inability may also be partial or complete. Males may complain of difficulty in achieving or maintaining an erection, or of premature ejaculations. The incidence of some degree of impotence ranges from 20 to 30% of the married population. As the man ages, there is a natural loss of both libido and potency. Generally this does not occur before the age of 50 years. Some men remain sexually vigorous well into old age. If a patient suffering from impotence has occasional erections or can achieve orgasm during masturbation, he may have a primary emotional problem. In almost 90% of patients complaining of impotence, the inadequacy is found to be caused by emotional rather than anatomic factors.

Hearing about a friend's sexual activities, especially if they are exaggerated, will deflate a patient's ego and heighten his sense of inadequacy. The cultural environment of the patient must set the standard for adequacy. It is almost impossible to compare the cultural patterns of Occidentals with those of Orientals. In 1948, Kinsey and his group obtained factual data on Anglo-American sexual patterns. The frequency of sexual intercourse varied from once per week to four times per week. The period of maximum sexual activity existed between the ages of 20 and 30 years. It was shown that there were marked variations among individuals as well as among socioeconomic groups. The lower the socioeconomic group, the more frequent were the sexual encounters.

Boredom, anxiety, peer pressure, aging, deterioration of the stereotypical male role, and female "aggressiveness" are factors contributing to psychogenic impotence. Diabetes mellitus is one of the more common causes of organic impotence. Patients with multiple sclerosis, spinal cord tumors, degenerative diseases of the spinal cord, or local injury suffer from a gradual loss of potency. Certain medications can cause impotence: beta-blockers, carbonic anhydrase inhibitors, and antihypertensive agents, for example.

Guilt, anxiety, and hypochondriasis are common in the man with psychogenic impotence. The frigid woman may make the male feel further insecure in his own marital adjustment, worsening his impotence. The self-image of the man may be low. It is common for the man with marginal difficulties to worry incessantly about his next attempt. His fear of failure generates enormous anxiety, which reinforces his inadequacy, and a vicious cycle is begun. Each failure worsens the next attempt. If the act of coitus is not satisfactory to the patient or his partner, embarrassment and guilt develop.

Some men may be able to maintain an erection but have difficulty in ejaculation. These men may become physically exhausted and may have to stop intercourse before ejaculation. The ejaculatory ducts may become so inflamed or even ulcerated that if ejaculation does occur, blood is present in the semen. This produces further anxiety and emotional upset that aggravate the situation.

Regardless of the cause, impotence has vast implications. The man may feel emasculated with an inferiority complex. Anger and depression are common. If the patient's impotence is associated with an anatomic defect, there may be additional changes in his self-image related to the physical disease state. If sexual problems are not resolved, the patient may develop personality changes. His fear of losing his sexual partner interferes with his work. Sleep and rest are disturbed. If sexual maladjustment continues, neurotic complaints may ensue. Without proper guidance, the man may become completely impotent, and suicidal tendencies can develop.

Severe psychiatric disturbances must be treated by a trained psychiatrist or sexual therapist. Success depends to a great extent upon the ability of the physician and the patient's sexual partner to inspire confidence in the patient.

PHYSICAL EXAMINATION

> The only equipment necessary for the examination of the male genitalia is latex gloves.

Many students are concerned about the possibility of the patient having an erection during the examination. Although possible, it is rare for the man to become sexually excited, since he will usually be nervous under these circumstances. If the examination is performed in an objective manner, it should not be a source of stimulation to the patient.

Though the wearing of protective gloves may decrease the examiner's sensitivity, disposable latex gloves should be worn.

Examination of the male genitalia is performed with the patient first lying and then standing. This postural change is important, because hernias or scrotal masses may not be apparent in the lying position.

The examination of the male genitalia consists of the following:

- Inspection and palpation with the patient lying
- Inspection and palpation with the patient standing
- Hernia examination

Inspection and Palpation with the Patient Lying

Inspect the Skin and Hair

While the patient is lying, the skin in the groin should be inspected for the presence of a superficial fungal infection, excoriations, or other rashes. Excoriations may indicate a scabies infection.

Observe the distribution of hair. Inspect the pubic hair for the presence of crab lice or nits (egg cases) attached to the hair.

Inspect the Penis and Scrotum

In the examination of the penis and scrotum, note the following:

- Is the man circumcised?
- Observe the size of the penis and scrotum.
- Are there any lesions on the penis? Is there penile edema?

The scrotum is inspected for any sores or rashes. Pinpoint, dark red, slightly raised, telangiectatic lesions on the scrotum are common in individuals over the age of 50 years. They are called *angiokeratomas* and are benign. There is a disease called *Fabry's disease,* which is an inborn error of glycosphingolipid metabolism. This rare, sex-linked condition is characterized by pain, fevers, and diffuse angiokeratomas in a "bathing suit" distribution, especially around the umbilicus and scrotum. A patient with Fabry's disease and multiple angiokeratomas is shown in Plate XII *E.*

The scrotum is elevated by the examiner to inspect the perineum carefully for any inflammation, ulceration, warts, abscesses, or other lesions. Normally, none should be present.

Palpate the Inguinal Nodes

By rolling the fingers along the inguinal ligament, the examiner may assess the presence of inguinal adenopathy. Commonly, small (0.5 cm), freely mobile lymph nodes are present in this area. Because the lymphatics from the perineum, legs, and feet drain into this area, it is not surprising that small lymph nodes are frequently encountered.

Inspect for Groin Mass

Ask the patient to cough or strain while you inspect the groin. A sudden bulge may indicate an inguinal or femoral hernia.

Inspection and Palpation with the Patient Standing

The man is now asked to stand while the examiner assumes a seated position in front of him.

Inspect the Penis

If the man is not circumcised, the foreskin should be retracted. Some examiners prefer the patient to retract it himself, whereas others would rather determine the tightness of the foreskin. The cheesy, white material under the foreskin is smegma and is normal.

Phimosis is present when the foreskin cannot be retracted and prevents adequate examination of the glans. Because the glans also cannot be cleaned, smegma builds up, leading to possible inflammation of the glans and prepuce called *balanoposthitis*. Inflammation of the glans penis alone is called *balanitis*. This chronic irritation may be a causative factor in cancer of the penis.

The glans is inspected for any ulcers, warts, nodules, scars, or signs of inflammation.

Inspect the External Meatus

The examiner should note the position of the external urethral meatus. It should be central on the glans. The meatus is evaluated by the examiner placing his hands on either side of the glans penis and opening the meatus. The technique for examining the meatus is illustrated in Figure 15–7.

The meatus should be observed for any discharge, warts, or stenosis. Venereal warts, called *condylomata acuminata,* may be found near the meatus, on the glans, in the perineum, at the anus, or on the shaft of the penis. Typically, they have a verrucous surface resembling a cauliflower. A patient with meatal condylomata acuminata is shown in Plate XII *F.*

Occasionally, the urethral meatus will open on the ventral surface of the penis, a condition called *hypospadias.* A less common condition is *epispadias,* a condition in which the meatus is located on the dorsal surface of the penis.

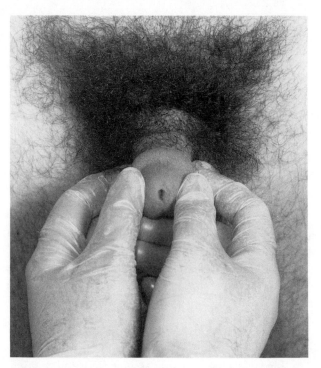

FIGURE 15–7. Technique for inspecting the external urethral meatus.

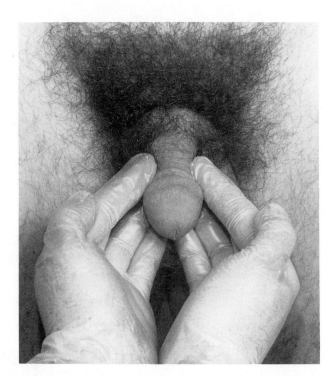

FIGURE 15–8. Technique for palpation of the penis.

Palpate the Penis

Palpate the shaft from the glans to the base of the penis. The presence of any scars, ulcers, nodules, induration, or signs of inflammation must be noted. Palpation of the corpora cavernosa is performed by holding the penis between the fingers of both hands and using the index fingers to note any induration. Figure 15–8 illustrates the method of palpation of the penis.

The presence of nontender induration or fibrotic areas under the skin of the shaft suggests *Peyronie's disease*. Patients with this condition may also complain of penile deviation on erection.

Palpate the Urethra

The urethra should be palpated from the external meatus through the corpus spongiosum to its base. In order to palpate the base of the urethra, the examiner elevates the penis with the left hand while the right index finger invaginates the scrotum in the midline and palpates deep to the base of the corpus spongiosum. The pad of the right index finger should palpate the entire corpus spongiosum from the meatus to its base. This technique is shown in Figure 15–9. If a discharge is present, "milking the urethra" may allow a drop to be placed on a glass slide for microscopic evaluation.

The foreskin, if retracted, should be replaced. *Paraphimosis* is a condition in which the foreskin can be retracted but cannot be replaced and becomes caught behind the corona.

Inspect the Scrotum

The scrotum is now re-evaluated in the standing position. Observe the contour and contents of the scrotum. Two testicles should be present. Normally the left testicle is lower than the right. The presence of any fullness not seen while the patient was lying should be noted.

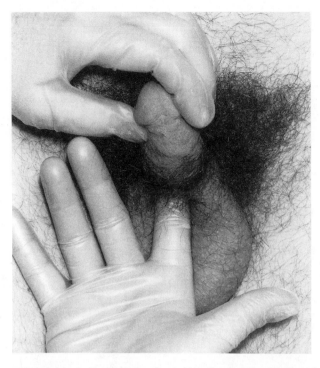

FIGURE 15-9. Technique for palpation of the base of the urethra.

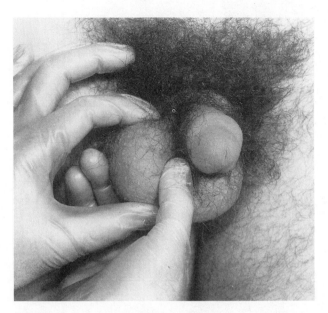

FIGURE 15-10. Technique for palpation of the testicle.

Palpate the Testes

Each testis is palpated separately. Use both hands to grasp the testicle gently. While the left hand holds the superior and inferior poles of the testicle, the right hand palpates the anterior and posterior surfaces. The technique for palpation of the testicle is shown in Figure 15-10.

Note the size, shape, and consistency of each testicle. There should be no tenderness or nodularity present. Normal testicles have a firm, rubbery consistency. The size and consistency of one testicle is compared with those of the other. Does one testicle feel heavier than the other? If a mass is present, can the examining finger get above the mass within the scrotum? Because inguinal hernias arise from the abdominal cavity, you will be unable to get above such a mass. In contrast, the examining finger can frequently get above a mass that is arising from within the scrotum.

Palpate the Epididymis and Vas Deferens

Next, locate and palpate the epididymis on the posterior aspect of the testicle. The head and tail should be carefully palpated for tenderness, nodularity, or masses.

The spermatic cord is palpated from the epididymis up to the external abdominal ring. The patient is asked to elevate his penis gently. If the penis is elevated too much, the scrotal skin will be reduced and the examination will be more difficult. The examiner should hold the scrotum in the midline by placing both thumbs in front of and both index fingers on the perineal side of the scrotum. Using both hands, the examiner should simultaneously palpate both spermatic cords between the thumbs and index fingers as the fingers are pulled laterally over the scrotal surface. The most prominent structure in the spermatic cord is the vas deferens. The vasa are felt as firm cords about 2-4 mm in diameter and feel like partially cooked spaghetti. The sizes are compared, and any tenderness or beading is noted. An absent vas deferens on one side is often

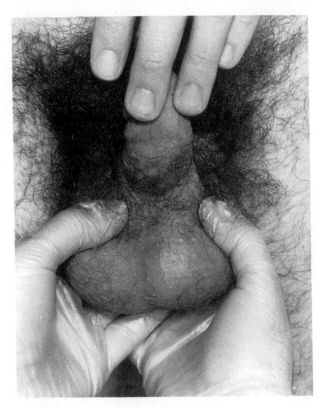

FIGURE 15-11. Technique for palpation of the spermatic cord.

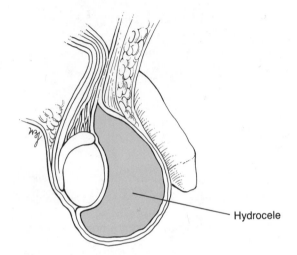

FIGURE 15-12. Cross-section through a hydrocele, showing its anatomy.

associated with an absent kidney on the same side. The technique of spermatic cord palpation is shown in Figure 15-11.

A common enlargement of the spermatic cord that is due to a dilatation of the pampiniform plexus is called a *varicocele*. These varicosities are usually on the left side, and the impression on palpation has been likened to that of feeling a "bag of worms." Because the varicocele is gravity dependent, it is usually visible only while the patient is standing or straining. The patient is asked to turn his head and cough while the spermatic cords are held between the fingers as indicated previously. A sudden pulsation, especially on the left side, confirms the diagnosis of a varicocele. Although the diagnosis is usually made by palpation, large varicoceles may be discovered by mere inspection, as can be seen in the patient shown in Plate XIII *A*.

Transilluminate Any Scrotal Masses

If a scrotal mass is detected, transillumination is necessary. In a darkened room, a light source is applied to the side of any scrotal enlargement. Vascular structures, tumors, blood, a hernia, and a normal testicle do not transilluminate. The transmission of the light as a red glow indicates a serous fluid – containing cavity, such as a *hydrocele* or a *spermatocele*. A hydrocele is a abnormal collection of clear fluid in the tunica vaginalis. The testicle is contained within this cystic mass, preventing actual palpation of the testis itself. By transillumination, it may even be possible to view the relationship of the normal-sized testicle within the hydrocele. A spermatocele is a pea-sized, nontender, mass containing spermatozoa usually attached to the upper pole of the epididymis. A patient with a hydrocele, seen only as massive scrotal enlargement, is shown in Plate XIII *B*. Transillumination of a hydrocele in another patient is depicted in Plate XIII *C*. An illustration of a hydrocele is shown in Figure 15–12.

Hernia Examination

Inspect Inguinal and Femoral Areas

Although hernias may be defined as any protrusion of a viscus, or part of it, through a normal or abnormal opening, 90% of all hernias are located in the inguinal area. Commonly, a hernial impulse is better seen than felt.

Instruct the patient to turn his head to the side and to cough or strain. You should inspect the inguinal and femoral areas for any sudden swelling during coughing, which may indicate a hernia. If a sudden bulge is seen, ask the patient to cough again and compare the impulse with that of the other side. If the patient complains of pain while coughing, determine the location of the pain and re-evaluate the area.

Palpate for Inguinal Hernias

Palpation for inguinal hernias is performed by having the examiner place his right index finger in the scrotum above the left testis and invaginate the scrotal skin. There should be sufficient scrotal skin to reach the external inguinal ring. The finger should be placed with the nail facing outward and the pad of the finger inward. This is shown in Figure 15–13. The examiner's left hand may be placed on the patient's right hip for better support.

The examiner's right index finger should follow the spermatic cord laterally into the inguinal canal parallel to the inguinal ligament and upward toward the

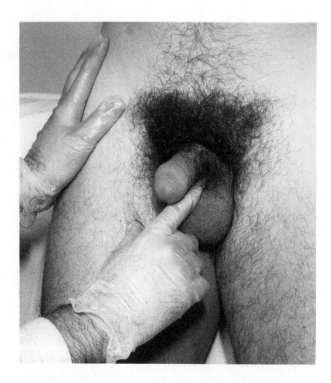

FIGURE 15–13. Technique for examination for inguinal hernias. Notice that the examiner's right index finger is directed inward and the examiner's left hand is placed on the patient's hip for support and better patient contact.

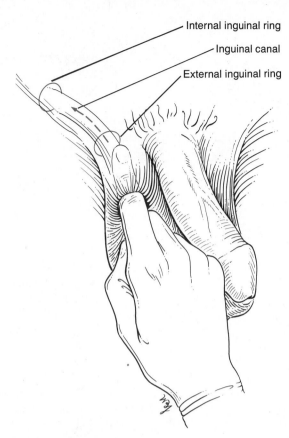

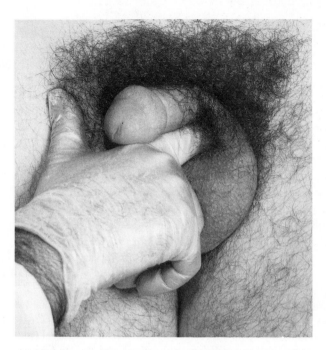

FIGURE 15–14. Technique for palpation of inguinal hernias.

FIGURE 15–15. Position of examining finger in the inguinal canal.

external inguinal ring, which is superior and lateral to the pubic tubercle. The external ring may be dilated and allow the finger to enter. The correct position of the right hand is shown in Figure 15–14 and is illustrated in Figure 15–15.

With the index finger placed either against the external ring or in the inguinal canal, ask the patient to turn his head to the side and to cough or strain down. Should a hernia be present, a sudden impulse against either the tip or the pad of the examining finger will be felt. If a hernia is present, have the patient lie down and observe if it can be reduced by gentle, sustained pressure on the mass. If the hernia examination is performed with adequate scrotal skin and is done *slowly,* it is painless. A discussion of the characteristics of hernias follows in the next section.

After the left side is evaluated, the procedure is repeated using the right index finger to examine the right side. Some examiners prefer to use the right index finger for examining the patient's right side, and the left index finger for the patient's left side. Try both techniques and see with which one you feel more comfortable.

If a large scrotal mass that does not transilluminate is present, an indirect inguinal hernia may be present in the scrotum. Auscultation of the mass may be used to determine whether bowel sounds are present in the scrotum, a sign useful in diagnosing an indirect inguinal hernia.

Examination of the prostate is discussed in the previous chapter. If the rectal examination has not yet been performed, this would be the appropriate time to examine the rectum and prostate.

TABLE 15 – 1. Causes of Hematuria by Age and Sex

Age (yr)	Male	Female
Under 20	Congenital urinary tract anomaly Acute glomerulonephritis Acute urinary tract infection	
20 – 40	Acute urinary tract infection Kidney stone Bladder tumor	
40 – 60	Bladder tumor Kidney stone Acute urinary tract infection	Acute urinary tract infection Kidney stone Bladder tumor
Over 60	Prostatic pathology Bladder tumor Acute urinary tract infection	Bladder tumor Acute urinary tract infection

CLINICOPATHOLOGIC CORRELATIONS

Gross hematuria that is usually painless is often the first indication of a urinary tract tumor, commonly located in the bladder. Table 15 – 1 lists the common causes of gross hematuria in different age groups and by sex.

Scrotal pathology is relatively common. Table 15 – 2 provides a differential diagnosis of common scrotal swellings.

Sexually transmitted diseases are extremely common. Out of every 100 outpatient visits to a venereal disease clinic, 25% of men have gonorrhea, another 25% have nongonococcal urethritis, 4% have venereal warts, 3.5% have herpes, 1.7% have syphilis, and 0.1% have chancroid. The incidence of both gonococcal and nongonococcal urethritis has increased dramatically over the past two decades. On college campuses, 85% of urethritis is nongonococcal in origin.

Genital lesions of venereal diseases may be ulcerative or nonulcerative. The incidence of genital lesions has changed greatly over the years. At one time, chancroid was common and herpes was rare; today, herpes is common and chancroid is rare. Anal ulcerative lesions are being seen more commonly, particularly in the male homosexual population. Table 15 – 3 lists a differential diagnosis of genital papular lesions.

TABLE 15 – 2. Differential Diagnosis of Common Scrotal Swellings

Diagnosis	Usual Age (yr)	Transillumination	Scrotal Erythema	Pain
Epididymitis	Any	No	Yes	Severe
Torsion of testis	<35	No	Yes	Severe
Testis tumor	<35	No	No	Minimal
Hydrocele (see Plate XIII B)	Any	Yes (see Plate XIII C)	No	None
Spermatocele	Any	Yes	No	None
Hernia (see Plates XIII F and XIV A)	Any	No	No	None to moderate*
Varicocele (see Plate XIII A)	>15	No	No	No

* Unless incarcerated, at which time pain may be severe.

TABLE 15 – 3. Differential Diagnosis of Genital Papules

Condition	Appearance	Pain	Lymphadenopathy
Herpes	Multiple, ulcers, vesicles	Present	Present
Condylomata lata (see Plate XIII E)	Multiple, moist, flat, round	Painful	Present
Condylomata acuminata (see Plate XII F)	Multiple, verrucous	Absent	Absent
Molluscum contagiosum	1 – 5 mm umbilicated papules, often in clusters; caseous material expressible from center	Painful	Rarely

The skin lesions of secondary syphilis are important to recognize. The classic papulosquamous rash on the palms and soles and the condylomata lata in the perineum are the hallmarks of secondary syphilis. Plate XIII D shows a patient with typical skin lesions on the feet. Plate XIII E shows condylomata lata in the same patient. The healing chancre of primary syphilis is also seen on the penis.

DIFFERENTIAL DIAGNOSIS OF HERNIAS

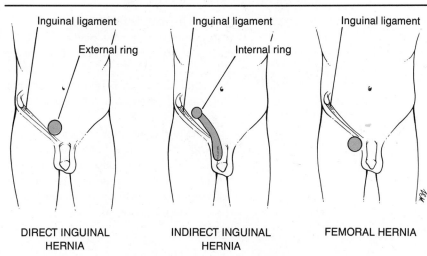

DIRECT INGUINAL HERNIA   INDIRECT INGUINAL HERNIA   FEMORAL HERNIA

Feature	Direct Inguinal*	Indirect Inguinal†	Femoral
Occurrence	Middle-aged and elderly men	All ages	Least common: more frequently found in women
Bilaterality	55%	30%	Rarely
Origin of swelling	Above inguinal ligament. Directly behind and through external ring.	Above inguinal ligament. Hernial sac enters inguinal canal at internal ring and exits at external ring.	Below inguinal ligament
Scrotal involvement	Rarely	Commonly	Never
Impulse location	At side of finger in inguinal canal	At tip of finger in inguinal canal	Not felt by finger in inguinal canal; mass below canal

* See Plate XIV A.
† See Plate XIII F.

FIGURE 15 – 16.

Hernias are extremely common. The major types of external hernias are the indirect and direct inguinal, and the femoral hernias. Plate XIII *F* shows a patient with a massive left indirect inguinal hernia. Plate XIV *A* shows a patient with a small right direct inguinal hernia. Figure 15–16 illustrates and lists the major differences in the differential diagnosis of hernias.

USEFUL VOCABULARY

Listed here are the specific roots that are important in order to understand the terminology related to urologic disease.

ROOT	PERTAINING TO	EXAMPLE	DEFINITION
andr-	man	*andr*ogen	Substance possessing masculinizing properties
litho-	stone	*litho*tomy	Incision of an organ for the removal of a stone
nephro-	kidney	*nephro*pathy	Disease of the kidneys
orchi(o)-	testes	*orchi*tis	Inflammation of the testis
pyel(o)-	pelvis of kidney	*pyelo*gram	X-ray of the kidney and ureter
ureter(o)-	ureter	*uretero*lith	A stone lodged or formed in the ureter
urethr(o)-	urethra	*urethro*plasty	Plastic surgery of the urethra
ur(o)-	urine	*ur*ology	Study of medicine concerning the urinary tract and the genital organs

WRITING UP THE PHYSICAL EXAMINATION

Listed here are examples of the write-up for the examination of the male genitalia.

The penis is circumcised. Both testes are in the scrotum and are within normal limits. There are no abnormal scrotal masses. No inguinal hernias are present. No inguinal adenopathy is present.

The penis is uncircumcised. The foreskin is easily retracted. The left hemiscrotum is markedly enlarged by a painless mass, which transilluminates. The left testicle cannot be palpated. The right testicle is within normal limits. No inguinal hernias are present. A small 2 × 2 soft, nonfixed, nontender lymph node is present in the right inguinal area.

The penis is circumcised. There is a 1–2 cm verrucous mass at the external meatus. A thick, yellow, purulent urethral discharge, which can be milked from the urethra, is seen at the meatus. The scrotal contents are within normal limits. No inguinal hernias are present.

The penis is uncircumcised. The foreskin is tight, although it can be retracted by the patient. A large amount of smegma is present behind the corona. There is a large mass of nontender, dilated veins present in the left hemiscrotum seen and felt when the patient stands. An impulse is felt in the left spermatic cord upon coughing. No inguinal hernias are present.

The penis is circumcised. The left testicle is soft and measures 2 × 3 cm. The right testicle appears normal. The scrotal contents are within normal limits. The hernia examination on the left side reveals a prominent impulse when the patient coughs. This impulse is felt at the tip of the examiner's finger.

The penis is circumcised. There is a 1 cm painless ulcer with a clean, nonpurulent base at the corona. The ulcer is indurated and has a smooth, regular, sharply defined border. Painless, firm, movable inguinal lymphadenopathy is present bilaterally. The testes are normal, as are the other scrotal contents. No inguinal hernias are present.

BIBLIOGRAPHY

Herman JR: Urology: A View Through The Retrospectroscope. Hagerstown, MD, Harper and Row, 1973.

Kinsey AC, Pomeroy WB, Martin CE: Sexual Behavior In The Human Male. Philadelphia, WB Saunders Co, 1948.

Marshall VF: Textbook of Urology. New York, Harper and Row, 1964.

McConnell EA, Zimmermann MF: Care of Patients with Urologic Problems. Philadelphia, JB Lippincott Co, 1983.

Murphy LJT: The History Of Urology. Springfield, IL, Charles C Thomas, 1972.

FEMALE GENITALIA

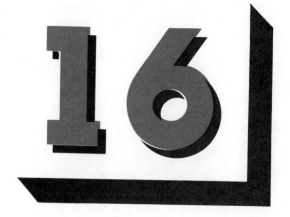

*In young girls, as I said, and in women past
childbearing, it (the uterus) is without blood, and
about the size of a bean. In a marriageable virgin it
has the magnitude and form of a pear. In women who
have borne children, and are still fruitful, it equals in
bulk a small gourd or a goose's egg; at the same time,
together with the breasts, it swells and softens,
becomes more fleshy, and its heat increased. . . .*

William Harvey
1578–1657

GENERAL CONSIDERATIONS

Gynecology and obstetrics had their beginnings with the origin of the human race. From a statistical analysis of worldwide populations in 1982, more than 4.7 million live births have occurred each year: over 12,000 each day, over 600 each hour, and over 10 every minute. Almost 98% of all live-born infants survive. At this rate, the population will double by the year 2010.

Records of obstetrics and gynecology date back to the time of Hippocrates in 400 BC. He was probably the first physician to describe midwifery, menstruation, sterility, symptoms of pregnancy, and puerperal (the period after labor) infections. Most of the early gynecologic history stems from Soranus in the second century AD. His works included chapters on anatomy, menstruation, fertility, signs of pregnancy, labor, care of the infant, dysmenorrhea (painful menstruation), uterine hemorrhage, and even the use of vaginal specula.

It should be remembered that William Harvey, the "father" of the theory of blood circulation, was also responsible for a monumental treatise on obstetrics. This work, which was published in 1651, included a detailed assessment of uterine changes throughout life.

The eighteenth century saw a further understanding of pregnancy, labor, and fertility. However, it was not until the nineteenth century that diseases of the female genitalia were better understood. As recently as 1872, Noeggerath published his investigations on gonorrhea, which ultimately changed the opinion of the medical world about the significance of this disorder. He was the first to suggest that "latent gonorrhea" was associated with sterility in women. Although the first cesarean section was described in 1596 by Mercurio, the development of the present day technique of Max Sänger was described as recently as 1882.

Over the past 30 years, deaths from cancer of the uterus and cervix in the United States have declined by 57%, predominantly as a result of better physical diagnosis. Cancer of the uterus and cervix now accounts for 13% of all cancers and 5% of all cancer deaths in women. The decline in mortality from cervical cancer is largely attributed to early detection by physical examination. Of the many risk factors that have been evaluated, the age of first sexual intercourse and sexual relations with multiple partners seem to be the most important ones associated with an increased risk of cervical cancer.

Although ovarian carcinoma accounts for only 4% of all cancers in women, over 5% of cancer deaths in women are due to ovarian cancer. Among the gynecologic malignancies, cancer of the ovary accounts for nearly 50% of all deaths that are due to cancer. The carefully performed pelvic examination has been shown to be the cornerstone of diagnosis of ovarian cancer.

STRUCTURE AND PHYSIOLOGY

The external female genitalia are shown in Figure 16–1. The *vulva* consists of the *mons veneris*, the *labia majora*, the *labia minora*, the *clitoris*, the *vestibule* and its glands, the *urethral meatus*, and the *vaginal introitus*. The mons veneris is a rounded prominence of fat tissue overlying the pubic symphysis. The labia majora are two wide skin folds that form the lateral boundaries of the vulva. They meet anteriorly at the mons veneris to form the anterior commissure. Both the labia majora and the mons have hair follicles and sebaceous glands. The labia majora correspond to the scrotum in the male. The labia minora are two narrow, pigmented skin folds lying between the labia majora and enclose the vestibule, which is the area lying between the labia minora. Anteriorly, the two labia minora form the prepuce of the clitoris. The clitoris, analogous to the penis, consists of erectile tissue and a rich supply of nerve endings. It has a glans and two corpora cavernosa. The external urethral meatus is located in the anterior portion of the vestibule below the clitoris. Paraurethral glands, or *Skene's glands,* are small glands that open lateral to the urethra. Secretion of sebaceous glands in this area protects the vulnerable tissues against urine.

The major vestibular glands are known as *Bartholin's glands,* or vulvovaginal glands. These glands correspond to the Cowper's glands in the male. Each pea-sized gland lies posterolaterally to the vaginal orifice. During sexual intercourse, a watery fluid is secreted that serves as a vaginal lubricant.

Inferiorly, the labia minora unite at the posterior commissure to form the *fourchette*. The *perineum* is the area between the fourchette and the anus.

The *hymen* is a circular fold of tissue that partially occludes the vaginal introitus. There are marked variations in its size as well as the number of openings in it.

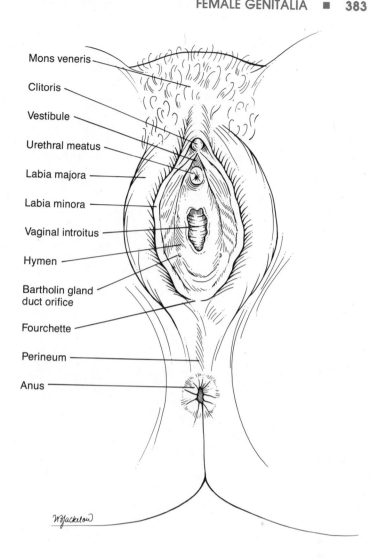

Mons veneris

Clitoris

Vestibule

Urethral meatus

Labia majora

Labia minora

Vaginal introitus

Hymen

Bartholin gland
duct orifice

Fourchette

Perineum

Anus

FIGURE 16–1. The external female genitalia.

The blood supply to the external genitalia and perineum is predominantly from the internal pudendal arteries. The lymphatic drainage is into the superficial and deep inguinal nodes.

The vaginal introitus is the border between the external and internal genitalia and is located in the lower portion of the vestibule.

The internal genitalia are shown in Figure 16–2. The *vagina* is a muscularly walled, hollow canal that passes upward and slightly backward, at a right angle to the uterus. The vagina lies between the urinary bladder anteriorly and the rectum posteriorly. The vaginal walls are thrown into transverse rugae, or folds. The lower portion of the cervix projects into the upper portion of the vagina and divides it into four fornices. The anterior fornix is shallow and is just posterior to the bladder. The posterior fornix is deep and is just anterior to the rectovaginal pouch, known as the *cul-de-sac (pouch) of Douglas*. The pelvic viscera lie immediately above this pouch. The lateral fornices contain the broad ligaments. The fallopian tubes and ovaries may be palpated in the lateral fornices. The superficial cells of the vagina contain glycogen, which is acted upon by the normal vaginal flora to produce lactic acid. This is in part responsible for the resistance of the vagina to infection.

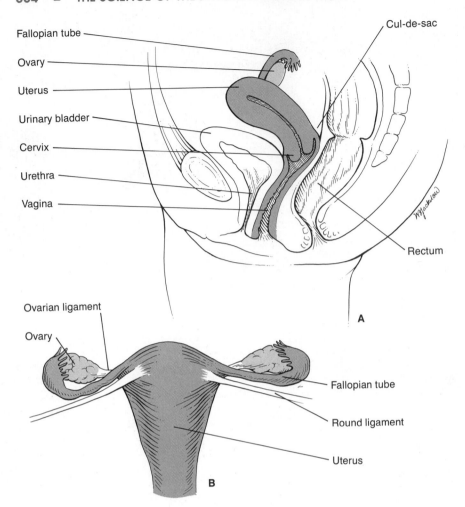

Fallopian tube

Ovary

Uterus

Urinary bladder

Cervix

Urethra

Vagina

Cul-de-sac

Rectum

A

Ovarian ligament

Ovary

Fallopian tube

Round ligament

Uterus

B

FIGURE 16–2. *A,* Cross-section of the internal female genitalia. *B,* Frontal view of uterus, fallopian tubes, and ovaries.

The arterial supply to the vagina is derived from the internal iliac, uterine, and middle hemorrhoidal arteries. The lymphatics of the lower third of the vagina drain into the inguinal nodes. The lymphatics of the upper two thirds enter the hypogastric and sacral nodes.

The *uterus* is a hollow muscular organ with a small central cavity. The lower end is the *cervix;* the upper portion is termed the *fundus.* The size of the uterus is different during various stages of life. At birth, the uterus is only 3–4 cm long. The adult uterus is 7–8 cm long and 3.5 cm wide, with an average wall thickness of 2–3 cm. The growth of the uterus and the relationship of the size of the fundus to the size of the cervix are shown in Figure 16–3.

The triangular uterine cavity is 6–7 cm in length and is bounded by the *internal cervical os* inferiorly and the entrances of the fallopain tubes superiorly. Normally, the long axis of the uterus is bent forward on the long axis of the vagina. This is termed *anteversion.* The fundus is also bent slightly forward on the cervix. This is termed *anteflexion.*

The uterus is freely mobile and is located centrally in the pelvic cavity. It is supported by the broad and uterosacral ligaments as well as by the pelvic floor. The peritoneum covers the fundus anteriorly down to the level of the internal cervical os. Posteriorly, the peritoneum covers the uterus down to the pouch of

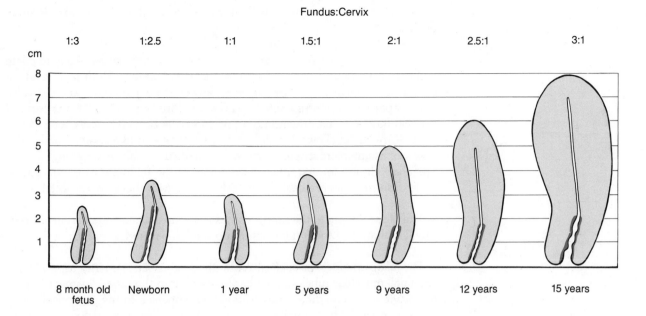

FIGURE 16–3. The growth of the uterus and changes in the fundus : cervix ratio with development. The darker red area represents the length of the cervix.

Douglas. The function of the uterus is childbearing. A detailed anatomy of the uterus is shown in Figure 16–4.

The cervix is the vaginal portion of the uterus. The greater portion of the cervix has no peritoneal covering. The cervical canal extends from the *external cervical os* to the *internal cervical os,* where it continues into the cavity of the fundus. The external cervical os in women who have not had children is small

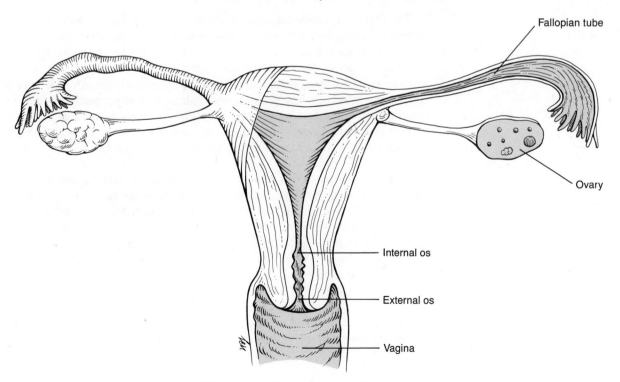

FIGURE 16–4. The anatomy of the uterus.

and circular. In women who have had children, the external cervical os is linear or oval.

With increasing levels of estrogens, the external cervical os begins to dilate and cervical mucus secretion becomes clear and watery. With high levels of estrogens, cervical mucus, when placed between two glass slides and the slides pulled apart, can be stretched 15–20 cm before breaking. This property of cervical mucus to be drawn into a fine thread is termed *spinnbarkeit*. When cervical mucus is allowed to dry on a glass slide and is examined under low power of a light microscope, a *fern pattern* made up of salt crystals may be seen. Spinnbarkeit and ferning reach a maximum at the midpoint of the menstrual cycle. Sperm can more easily penetrate mucus with these characteristics.

The blood supply to the uterus comes from the uterine and ovarian arteries. The lymphatics of the fundus enter into the lumbar nodes.

The *fallopian tubes,* or *oviducts,* enter the fundus at its superior aspect. They are small muscular tubes that extend outward into the broad ligament toward the pelvic wall. The other end of the oviduct opens into the peritoneal cavity near the ovary. These endings are surrounded by fringed-shaped projections called *fimbriae.* The primary function of the fallopian tube is to provide a conduit for and convey the egg from the corresponding ovary to the uterus, a trip that takes several days. Sperm traverse the oviduct in the opposite direction, and it is usually here that fertilization takes place.

The *ovaries* are almond-shaped structures about 3–4 cm long and are attached to the broad ligament. The primary functions of the ovary are oogenesis and hormone production.

The ovaries, fallopian tubes, and supporting ligaments are termed the *adnexa.*

The female reproductive system is under the influence of the hypothalamus, whose releasing factors control the secretion of the anterior pituitary gonadotropic hormones, *follicle stimulating hormone (FSH)* and *luteinizing hormone (LH).* In response to these hormones, the ovarian graafian follicle secretes estrogens and discharges its ovum. After ovulation, the ovarian follicle is termed the corpus luteum, which secretes both estrogens and progesterone. With the secretion of progesterone, the basal body temperature rises. This is a reliable sign of ovulation. Under the influence of the ovarian hormones, the uterus and breasts undergo the characteristic changes of the menstrual cycle.

If pregnancy does not occur, the corpus luteum regresses and the level of ovarian hormones begins to fall. At this time, many women have symptoms of weakness, depression, and irritability prior to menstruation. Breast tenderness is also common. These symptoms are termed *premenstrual syndrome (PMS).* About 5 days after the fall in the level of the hormones, the menstrual period begins. Menstruation over the entire 5 day period measures about 50–150 ml, only half of which is blood. The remainder is mucus. Because menstrual blood does not contain fibrin, it does not clot. When the menstrual flow is heavy, as it is on days 1–2, "clots" may be described. These "clots" are not fibrin clots but are combinations of red cells, glycoproteins, and mucoid substances that are believed to form in the vagina rather than in the uterine cavity.

Some of the cyclic hormone-dependent changes related to the menstrual cycle are shown in Figure 16–5.

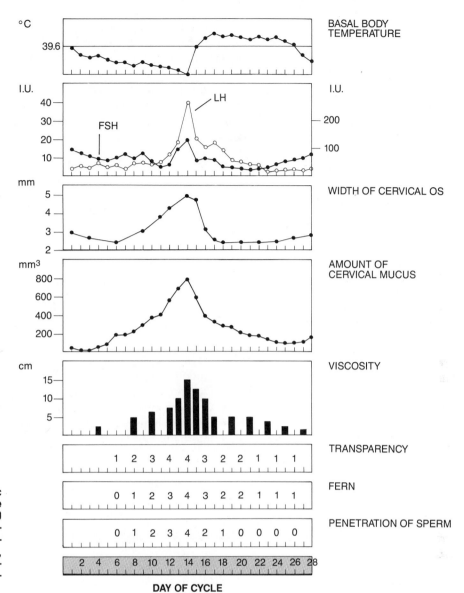

FIGURE 16-5. Physiologic changes associated with the menstrual cycle. The numbers 0 to 4 indicate an increasing characteristic of cervical mucus. Notice that ferning, transparency, and the ability for sperm penetration are maximal at midcycle.

About 1½ years prior to puberty, gonadotropins are measurable in the urine. The ovaries enter a period of rapid growth at age 8 – 9, which marks the onset of puberty. Estrogens begin to increase rapidly at about the age of 11 years. Concomitant with estrogen production, the sexual organs begin to mature. During puberty, the secondary sex characteristics begin to develop. The breasts enlarge, hair develops on the pubis, the vulva enlarges, the labia minora become pigmented, and the body contour changes. Puberty lasts for approximately 4 – 5 years. The first menstrual cycle, known as *menarche,* occurs at the end of puberty at about 12½ years of age. There is, however, a wide variation in the age of menarche. The cycles continue approximately every 28 days, with a flow lasting 3 – 5 days. The first day of the period is taken to be the first day of the cycle. It is rare for a woman to be absolutely regular, and cycles of 25 – 34 days may be considered normal.

At the time of menarche, the menstrual cycle is usually anovulatory* and irregular. After a period of 1–2 years, ovulation begins. After stabilization of the menses, ovulation occurs about mid-cycle in a woman with a regular cycle.

Menopause marks the ends of menstruation. Menopause is defined as the last uterine bleeding induced by ovarian function. It usually occurs between 45 and 55 years of age. Ovulation and corpus luteum formation no longer occur, and the ovaries decrease in size. The period after menopause is termed *postmenopausal*.

REVIEW OF SPECIFIC SYMPTOMS

The most common symptoms of female genitourinary disease are as follows:

- Abnormal vaginal bleeding
- Dysmenorrhea (painful menstruation)
- A mass or lesion
- Vaginal discharge
- Vaginal itching
- Abdominal pain
- Dyspareunia (pain occurring with sexual intercourse)
- Changes in hair distribution
- Changes in urinary pattern
- Infertility

Abnormal Vaginal Bleeding

Ask these questions of any woman with abnormal vaginal bleeding:

"How long have you noticed the vaginal bleeding?"
"What types of contraceptive do you use?"
"How often are your periods?"
"What is the duration of your menstrual flow?"
"How many tampons or napkins do you use on each day of your flow?"
"Are there any clots of blood?"
"When was your last period?"
"Have you noticed bleeding between your periods?"
"Do you have abdominal pain during your periods?"
"Do you have hot flashes? . . . cold sweats?"
"Do you have children?" If so, *"When was your last one born?"*
"Do you think you might be pregnant?"
"Are you under any unusual emotional stress?"
"Have you noticed an intolerance to cold? . . . heat?"
"Have you noticed a change in your vision?"
"Have you had any headaches? . . . nausea? . . . change in hair pattern? . . . milk discharge from your nipples?"
"What is your diet like?"

---

* Not accompanied by the release of an ovum from the ovary.

Abnormal bleeding, also known as dysfunctional uterine bleeding, includes amenorrhea, menorrhagia, metrorrhagia, and postmenopausal bleeding. *Amenorrhea* is the cessation or nonappearance of menstruation. Prior to puberty, amenorrhea is physiologic, as it is during pregnancy and after menopause. Primary amenorrhea is menstruation that has never occurred; secondary amenorrhea is menstruation that has occurred but has ceased, as in pregnancy. Long distance joggers, anorectics, or any woman with abnormally low body fat may have secondary amenorrhea. Diseases of the hypothalamus, pituitary, ovary, uterus, and thyroid gland are associated with amenorrhea. Galactorrhea, or milk discharge from the nipples, is commonly seen in many individuals, with pituitary tumors. Chronic disease is also frequently associated with secondary amenorrhea.

Menorrhagia is excessive bleeding at the time of the menstrual cycle. It may be increased flow of normal duration, normal flow of increased duration, or both. Asking a patient how many pads or tampons she uses each day of the cycle will help to quantify the flow. Menorrhagia in some cases may be associated with blood disorders such as leukemia, inherited clotting abnormalities, and decreased platelet states. Uterine fibroids are a leading cause of menorrhagia. This is related to the large surface area of the endometrium from which bleeding occurs.

Metrorrhagia is uterine bleeding of normal amount at irregular noncyclic intervals. Foreign bodies such as intrauterine devices (IUD) as well as ovarian and uterine tumors can cause metrorrhagia. Often there is increased bleeding between cycles as well as heavier periods. This is termed *menometrorrhagia*.

Postmenopausal bleeding (PMB) occurs after a 6–8 month period of amenorrhea after menopause. Any postmenopausal bleeding must be investigated. Uterine fibroids or tumors of the cervix, uterus, or ovary may be responsible.

Dysmenorrhea

Dysmenorrhea, or painful menstruation, is a common symptom. It is often difficult to define as abnormal, because many healthy women have some degree of menstrual discomfort. In most women, these mild, crampy pains subside soon after the commencement of the menstrual flow. There are two types of dysmenorrhea: primary and secondary. Primary dysmenorrhea is far more common. It begins shortly after menarche, is associated with colicky uterine contractions, and occurs with every period. Childbirth frequently marks the end-point of this state. Secondary dysmenorrhea is caused by acquired disorders within the uterine cavity (such as intrauterine devices, polyps, or fibroids), obstruction to flow (cervical stenosis, for example), or disorders of the pelvic peritoneum.* It usually occurs after several years of painless periods. Regardless of its cause, dysmenorrhea is described as intermittent, crampy pain accompanying the menstrual flow. The pain is felt in the lower abdomen and back, sometimes radiating down the legs. In severe cases, fainting, nausea, or vomiting may occur.

---

* Endometriosis or pelvic inflammatory disease, for example. Endometriosis is the presence of endometrial tissue outside the uterus and is a cause of chronic pelvic pain.

Masses or Lesions

Masses or lesions of the external genitalia are common. They may be related to venereal diseases, tumors, or infections. Ask these questions of any woman with a lesion on the genitalia:

"When did you first notice the mass (lesion)?"
"Is it painful?"
"Has it changed since you first noticed it?"
"Have you ever had it before?"
"Have you been exposed to anyone with venereal disease?"

Syphilis may result in a chancre on the labia. Often unnoticed, it is a small, painless nodule or ulcer with a sharply demarcated border. Small, acutely painful ulcers may be chancroid. A patient with a Bartholin's gland abscess may present with an extremely tender mass in the vulva. Benign tumors, such as venereal warts (condylomata acuminata), or malignant conditions present as a mass on the external genitalia.

The patient may sometimes complain of a fullness or mass in the pelvis as a result of *pelvic relaxation*. Pelvic relaxation applies to the descent or protrusion of the vaginal walls or uterus through the vaginal introitus. This is caused by a weakening of the pelvic supports. The anterior vaginal wall can descend, producing a *cystocele* triggering urinary symptoms such as frequency and stress incontinence. The posterior vaginal wall can descend, causing a *rectocele,* which will produce bowel symptoms such as constipation, tenesmus, or incontinence. The uterus can also descend, causing uterine prolapse. In its most severe state, the uterus may lie outside the vulva with complete vaginal inversion, a condition known as *procidentia.* The consequences of pelvic relaxation are further discussed in Clinicopathologic Correlations later in this chapter.

Vaginal Discharge

Vaginal discharges, also known as *leukorrhea,* are very common. Is there an associated foul odor? Although a whitish discharge is often normally present, a fetid discharge often indicates a pathologic problem. The most common pathologic odor is a foul, fishy odor related to the volatilization of amines that are produced by anaerobic metabolism. Is itching also present? Women with moniliasis (candidiasis) complain of a white, dry discharge appearing as "cottage cheese" with intense pruritus. Has the woman taken any medications, such as antibiotics, recently? Antibiotics change the normal vaginal flora, and an overgrowth of Candida may result. Table 16–1 (at the end of the chapter) summarizes the important characteristics of vaginal discharge.

Vaginal Itching

Vaginal itching is associated with monilial infections, glycosuria,* vulvar leukoplakia, or any condition that predisposes the woman to vulvar irritation. Pruritus may also be a symptom of psychosomatic disease.

---

* High levels of glucose in the urine, as in diabetes.

Abdominal Pain

Ask the following questions in addition to those indicated in Chapter 14, The Abdomen, of any patient with abdominal pain:

"When was your last period?"
"Have you ever had any type of venereal disease?"
"Is the pain related to your menstrual cycle?" If so, *"At what time in your cycle does it occur?"*
"Do you experience burning when you urinate?"

Abdominal pain may be acute or chronic. Is the patient pregnant? Acute abdominal pain may be a complication of pregnancy. Spontaneous abortion, uterine perforation, and ectopic tubal pregnancy are all life-threatening situations. Acute inflammation by gonococci of the fallopian tubes and ovary, known as *salpingo-oophoritis,* can produce intense lower abdominal pain. Acute lower abdominal pain localized to one side that occurs at the time of ovulation is termed *mittelschmerz.* This pain is related to a small amount of intraperitoneal bleeding at the time of ovum release. Urinary tract infection may also cause acute pain. Patients with urinary tract infections usually have associated urinary symptoms of burning or frequency.

Chronic abdominal pain may result from ectopic endometrial tissue; chronic pelvic inflammatory disease (PID) of the fallopian tubes and ovaries; or pelvic muscle relaxation with protrusion of the bladder, rectum, or uterus.

Dyspareunia

Dyspareunia is the occurrence of pain during or after sexual intercourse. Dyspareunia may be physiologic or psychogenic. Infections of the vulva, introitus, vagina, cervix, uterus, fallopian tubes, and ovaries have been associated with dyspareunia. Tumors of the rectovaginal septum, uterus, and ovaries have been described in patients with painful sexual intercourse. Dyspareunia is often present in the absence of pathology. A history of painful pelvic examinations and fears about pregnancy are common in these patients. Women may have "penetration anxiety" until they are assured that their vagina can be penetrated by a penis. In these individuals, dyspareunia may lead to *vaginismus,* a condition of severe pelvic pain and spasm when the labia are merely touched. In other women, dyspareunia may develop during times of stress or emotional conflicts. The examiner can obtain valuable information by asking, "What else is going on in your life now?" Dryness of the vagina and labia may cause irritation that can result in dyspareunia.

Changes in Hair Distribution

Hair loss or change in hair distribution may occur during certain states of hormonal imbalance. *Hirsutism* is defined as an excessive growth of hair on the upper lip, face, ear lobes, upper pubic triangle, trunk, and limbs. *Virilization* is extensive hirsutism associated with receding temporal hair, a deepening of the voice, and clitoral enlargement. Increased androgen production by the adrenal glands or ovaries may be responsible for these phenomena. Tumors of the ovary are usually associated with amenorrhea, rapidly developing hirsutism, and virilization. Polycystic ovarian disease is associated with menstrual irregularities, infertility, obesity, and hirsutism. It is important to determine whether the patient is taking any medications. A drug used to treat hypertension has been found to have the unexpected side-effect of causing diffuse hair growth on the face.

Hair loss is a distressing problem. *Alopecia* is the term used to describe hair loss. Many drugs may have a profound effect on hair growth. The interviewer must inquire whether the patient has taken any chemotheraputic agents or has been exposed to radiation. Different areas of the head seem to respond differently to androgens. The top and front of the scalp respond to increased androgen production by hair loss, whereas the face responds with increased hair growth. Has the patient been dieting? Because the hair has a high metabolic rate, crash diets and infectious diseases reduce the nutrients available for hair growth. Secondary alopecia may result.

Changes in Urinary Pattern

Changes in the patterns of urination are common. Chapter 15, Male Genitalia and Hernias, reviews many of the symptoms of changes in the urinary pattern. These symptoms may occur in the woman as well.

Stress incontinence is incontinence of urine on straining or coughing. Stress incontinence is more common in women than in men. The female urinary bladder and urethra are maintained in position by several muscular and fascial supports. It has been postulated that estrogens may, at least in part, be responsible for a weakening of the pelvic support. With aging, the support of the bladder neck, the length of the urethra, and the competence of the pelvic floor are weakened. Repeated vaginal deliveries, strenuous exercise, and chronic coughing increase the chance for stress incontinence. Ask these questions:

> *"Do you lose your urine on straining? . . . coughing? . . . lifting? . . . laughing?"*
> *"Do you lose your urine constantly?"*
> *"Do you lose small amounts of urine?"*
> *"Are you aware of a full bladder?"*
> *"Do you have to press on your abdomen to void?"*
> *"Are you aware of any weakness in your limbs?"*
> *"Have you ever had a loss of vision?"*
> *"Do you have diabetes?"*

Patients with pure stress incontinence describe urine loss without urgency that occurs during any activity that momentarily increases intra-abdominal pressure. Although stress incontinence is very common in women, it is important to rule out other types of incontinence, such as neurologic, overflow, or psychogenic. Neurologic incontinence may result from cerebral dysfunction, spinal cord disease, or peripheral nerve lesions. *Multiple sclerosis* is a chronic relapsing neurologic disorder causing urinary incontinence. Most individuals suffer from an episode of temporary visual loss as an early symptom. Overflow incontinence occurs when the pressure in the bladder exceeds the urethral pressure in the absence of bladder contraction. This may occur in patients with diabetes and an atonic bladder. Patients with psychoses often complain of incontinence. Psychotic individuals have been known to urinate in bed at night to "warm" themselves or in the daytime in group settings to bring attention to themselves.

Infertility

Infertility may result from failure to ovulate, known as *anovulation,* or from inadequate function of the corpus luteum. Both of these conditions can occur in women with cyclic menstrual bleeding. Therefore, the fact of having a period does not indicate fertility. The woman with the symptom of infertility should be asked these questions:

"Do you have regular menstrual periods?"
"Have you kept a chart of your basal body temperature?"
"Have you ever had venereal disease?"
"Have you been tested for thyroid disease?"
"Have you taken any medications to promote fertility?"

Charting basal body temperatures is a reliable method for detecting ovulation. Gonococcal disease in the woman may lead to salpingo-oophoritis with scarring of the fallopian tubes and infertility. Hypothyroidism is well known to be responsible for infertility.

General Suggestions

Even in the absence of specific symptoms, all women, regardless of age, should be asked several important questions. The answers to the following questions will provide a complete gynecologic and obstetric history. The first group of questions is related to the *gynecologic history* and menstrual cycle:

"At what age did you start to menstruate?"
"How often do your periods occur?"
"Are they regular?"
"For how many days do you have menstrual flow?"
"How many pads or tampons do you use each day of your flow?"
"Do you experience any breast tenderness or breast pain during your menstrual cycle? . . . bloating? . . . swelling? . . . headache? . . . edema?"
"When was your last menstrual period?"

The *catamenia* refers to the menstrual history and summarizes the age of menarche, the cycle length, and the duration of flow. If a woman reached menarche at age 12 and has had regular periods every 29 days lasting for 5 days, the catamenia can be summarized as *CAT 12 × 29 × 5.* The date of the *last menstrual period* can be abbreviated as *LMP: June 13, 1988.*

The history of any recurrent, mid-cyclic symptoms associated with the menstrual period, such as breast tenderness, bloating, and so forth, is termed *molimen.* The presence of molimen correlates with ovulation, although not all women experience molimen when ovulation occurs. Therefore, molimen is a specific but nonsensitive sign of ovulation.

The next group of questions is related to the *obstetric history:*

"Have you ever been pregnant?"
"How many full term pregnancies have you had?"
"Have you had any children born prematurely?"
"Have you ever had a miscarriage or an elective abortion?"

"Were any of your children stillborn?"
"How many living children do you have?"
"How were your children delivered (vaginally, cesarean)?"
"What were the birth weights of your children?"

The obstetric history includes the number of pregnancies, known as *gravidity*, and the number of deliveries, known as *parity*. If a woman has had three full term infants (37 weeks or more gestation), two premature infants (less than 37 weeks gestation), one miscarriage (or abortion), and four living children, her obstetric history can be summarized as *para 3 — 2 — 1 — 4.* An easy way to remember this four digit parity code is with the mnemonic *Florida Power And Light.* This abbreviation stands for: *full term, premature, abortions* (miscarriages), *living.* In this example, the woman is *gravida 6.*

When asking a woman about the date of her last menstrual period, *never* assume that menopause has occurred. Even a 62 year old woman should be asked when her last menstrual period occurred. Allow the patient to say that she hasn't had a period in 12 years.

A careful sexual history is important. Chapter 1 provides several ways of broaching the topic. The interviewer might start by asking, "Are you satisfied with your sex life?" It is important for the examiner to determine the marital status of the patient. Is the patient married? How many times? For how long? Are there other partners? If the patient is not married, is she currently having sexual relationship(s)? What type of birth control is being used?

It is important to determine whether the patient's mother was given DES* during her pregnancy.

It is important for the interviewer to speak using words that will be understood by the patient. It may be necessary to use such terms as "lips" to refer to the labia or "privates" to refer to the genitalia.

IMPACT OF INFERTILITY ON THE WOMAN

The problem of infertility is not new. From ancient times, cultures have practiced fertility rites to ensure the continuation of their people. Many societies considered a woman's worth in terms of her ability to have children. The "barren woman" was frequently banished.

The average time taken for a woman to conceive is 4–5 months. The American Fertility Society defines infertility as the inability to conceive "after one year of regular coitus without contraception." During this period, over 80% of women will conceive. After 3 years of regular sexual intercourse, 98% of women will become pregnant.

---

* Diethylstilbestrol (DES) was given to many pregnant women between 1940 and 1975 for a variety of reasons, such as a threatened abortion and premature labor. Vaginal involvement by adenosis often developed in the exposed daughter. Carcinoma of the vagina or cervix has also been occasionally reported in the offspring, as well as cervical incompetence.

It has been estimated that approximately one out of six couples in the United States has some problem with fertility. Infertility should be considered a problem of both men and women. It was previously thought that infertility was *functional* (no demonstrable organic pathology) in 30–50% of all cases, but it is now recognized that over 90% of infertile couples have a pathologic cause. However, only about 50% of these couples will achieve pregnancy. Fifty per cent of infertility is related to a female problem,* 30% to a male problem,† and 20% to a combined problem.

Infertility is one of the several important developmental crises of adult life. The impact of infertility on a woman can be monumental. The influence of the higher nervous system upon ovulation is well known but only partially understood. When the woman is told that she is infertile, she may be shocked, distressed, and upset about the loss of an important function of her body. This ''narcissistic'' injury lasts for a variable period of time. Often the woman feels defective or inadequate. This extends to her interactions with others, in addition to her desire for sexual intercourse. Her attitude toward her job may change; her productivity in her work may decline. There is a significant decrease in sexual desire. Depression, the loss of libido, and the concern of whether conception will ever occur all contribute to making sex a less pleasurable activity, and all decrease the possibility of normal ovulation. A period of mourning and frustration usually occurs.

Anxiety may be very high. Often the woman becomes preoccupied with her menstrual periods. When will the next one come? Is she pregnant? Did she have any symptoms of ovulation? When the next menstrual cycle occurs, the woman suffers further grief.

The infertile woman may fear that her partner will actually resent her, and she may feel ''cut off'' from him. She may experience jealousy and resentment toward friends or relations who have children. Her infertility lowers her self-esteem and may make her feel that she is unfit to be a parent.

Regardless of the cause of infertility, the treatment must work to lessen the psychological side-effects. Both partners must be encouraged to communicate. Education regarding the physical problem is important throughout the medical work-up. An open line of communication between the partners and the physician is paramount. The patient needs to be protected from her own insecurities while given empathy and compassion.

In some women, psychogenic factors may be the sole cause of infertility. Such factors may act at various phases in the reproductive process. These women may have an infantile personality and fear the responsibilities of motherhood. They use their infertility as a defense mechanism. In other cases, emotional conflicts may lead to somatic symptoms and signs. Vaginismus is the most common psychosomatic disorder causing infertility. In this condition, the introitus may become so constricted that it inhibits the penis from entering. Vaginismus protects the patient from conception. Many of these women view sexual intercourse as exploitative and degrading. Intercourse is feared because it is painful. These patients do well with psychotherapy that allows them to express their fears about intercourse, genitalia, and childbearing.

---

* Generally fallopian tubal patency or ovulation problems.

† Vas deferens obstruction, varicocele, chromosomal defects, testicular infection, autoimmune states, and decreased sperm count are the most important.

PHYSICAL EXAMINATION

> The equipment necessary for the examination of the female genitalia and rectum is the following: vaginal speculum, lubricant, cervical scrapers, cotton-tipped applicators, gloves, glass slides, occult blood testing card and reagent, culture media (as appropriate), fixative, tissues, and a light source.

General Considerations

Unlike most other parts of the physical examination, the pelvic examination is often viewed with apprehension by the patient. This is frequently related to a previous bad experience. An examination performed slowly and gently with adequate explanations will go a long way in developing a good doctor-patient relationship. It is important for the examiner to talk to the patient and tell her exactly what is going to be done. Eye contact is also necessary to decrease the patient's anxiety. A relaxed patient will provide a more accurate and less traumatic examination.

If the examiner is a male, he should examine the female genitalia in the presence of a female attendant. The woman attendant is important for assistance as well as for medicolegal considerations. Although not required by law, the presence of a female attendant is important, especially when the patient appears overly upset or seductive. At times, the woman may request that a family member be present. The examiner should generally grant such a request, if there is no other attendant available.

Throughout the world, there are preferred patient positions to facilitate the pelvic examination. These include having the woman lie on her back on an examining table, having the patient lie in bed on her left side, having the woman lie on her back in bed with her legs abducted, and having the woman sit upright in a chair with her legs abducted. In the United States, the examination is usually performed on an examination table with stirrups. This position is uncomfortable and demeaning. Male students should try lying in this position.

Preparation for the Examination

The patient should be instructed to empty her bladder and rectum prior to the examination. The patient is assisted onto an examination table with her buttocks placed near its edge. The stirrups of the table are extended, and the patient is instructed to place her heels in them. If possible, some cloth should be placed over the stirrups. They are cold. The head of the examination table should be elevated so that eye contact with the patient will occur. A sheet is usually draped over the lower abdomen and knees of the patient. Some patients prefer not to have the sheet used. The patient should be asked for her preference.

The knees are drawn up sufficiently to relax the abdominal muscles as the thighs are abducted. Ask the patient to let her legs fall to the sides. *Never* tell a patient to spread her legs!

Gloves should be worn for the examination of the female genitalia. The examiner should be seated on a stool between the legs of the patient. Good lighting, including a light source directed into the vagina, is essential.

The examination of the female genitalia consists of the following:

- Inspection and palpation of external genitalia
- Speculum examination
- Bimanual palpation
- Rectovaginal palpation

Inspection and Palpation of External Genitalia

Inspect the External Genitalia and Hair

To make the woman more comfortable during inspection of the external genitalia, it is often useful to touch the patient. Tell the patient that you are going to touch her leg. Use the *back* of your hand to touch the inside of the patient's thigh.

The external genitalia should be carefully inspected. The mons veneris is inspected for any lesions or swelling. The hair is inspected for its pattern and for the presence of any pubic lice or nits. The skin of the vulva is inspected for redness, excoriation, masses, leukoplakia, or pigmentation. Any lesions should be palpated for tenderness. *Kraurosis vulvae* is a condition in which the skin of the vulva shows a uniform reddened, smooth, shiny, almost transparent appearance. Although most common in the postmenopausal woman, it may be seen in patients of all ages. White patches of hyperkeratosis, known as *leukoplakia vulvae,* frequently appear on the labia and perineum. Its principal importance lies in the fact that this lesion commonly precedes carcinoma. Leukoplakia is less common than kraurosis vulvae. Plate XIV *B* shows a patient with an ulcerated lesion of squamous cell carcinoma of the vulva.

Inspect the Labia

Tell the patient that you are now going to spread the labia. With your right hand, the labia majora and minora are spread apart between the right thumb and index fingers, as shown in Figure 16–6. The vaginal introitus is inspected.

Any inflammatory lesion, ulceration, discharge, scarring, warts, trauma, swelling, atrophic changes, or masses are noted. Plate XIV *C* shows a woman with condylomata acuminata of the labia.

Inspect the Clitoris

The clitoris is inspected for size and for any lesions. The clitoris is normally 3–4 mm in size.

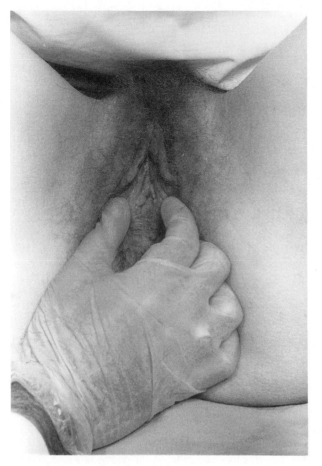

FIGURE 16–6. Technique for inspecting the labia.

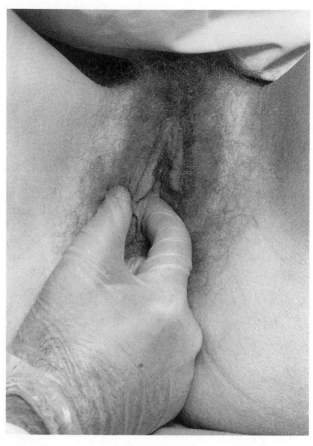

FIGURE 16–7. Technique for palpation of Bartholin's glands.

Inspect the Urethral Meatus

Is pus or inflammation present? If pus is present, determine its source. Dip a cotton-tipped applicator into the discharge and spread it on a microscope slide for later evaluation.

Inspect the Area of Bartholin's Glands

Tell the patient that you are going to palpate the glands of the labia. Palpate the area of the right gland (at 7 – 8 o'clock) by grasping the posterior portion of the right labia between the right index finger in the vagina and the right thumb on the outside, as shown in Figure 16 – 7. Is any tenderness, swelling, or pus present? Normally, Bartholin's glands can be neither seen nor felt. Use the left hand to examine the area of the left gland (at 4 – 5 o'clock).

Plate XIV *D* shows a patient with a left Bartholin's gland abscess.

Inspect the Perineum

The perineum and anus are inspected for any masses, scars, fissures, or fistulae. Is the perineal skin reddened? The anus should be inspected for hemorrhoids, irritation, or fissures.

Test for Pelvic Relaxation

With the labia spread widely, the patient is asked to bear down or cough. If vaginal relaxation is present, ballooning of the anterior or posterior walls may be seen. Bulging of the anterior wall is associated with a cystocele; bulging of the posterior wall indicates a rectocele. If stress incontinence is present, the coughing or bearing down may cause a spurt of urine from the urethra.

Speculum Examination

The Preparation

The speculum examination is performed in order to inspect the vagina and cervix. There are several types of specula. The metal Cusco, or bivalve, speculum is the most popular. This speculum consists of two blades that are introduced closed and are then opened by squeezing the handle mechanism. The vaginal walls are held apart by the blades, and adequate visualization of the vagina and cervix is achieved. There are basically two types of bivalve specula: the Graves and the Pedersen. The *Graves speculum* is the more common one and is used for most adult women. The blades are wider and are curved on the sides. The *Pedersen speculum* has narrower, flat blades and is used for a woman with a small introitus. The plastic, disposable bivalve speculum is becoming more commonly used. A disadvantage to its use is a loud click that is made as the lower blade is disengaged during removal from the vagina. If a plastic speculum is used, the patient should be informed that this sound will occur.

Before using the speculum in a patient, practice opening and closing it. If the patient has never had a speculum examination, show the speculum to her. You should warm the speculum with warm water and then touch it to the back of your hand to determine that the temperature is suitable. Jelly lubricant should not be used, because it may interfere with cervical cytologic determination and gonococcal cultures. Tell the patient that you are now going to perform the speculum part of the internal examination.

The Technique

While the examiner uses his left index and middle fingers to separate the labia and firmly depress the perineum, the closed speculum, held by the examiner's right hand, is introduced at an oblique angle *slowly* into the introitus over the left fingers. This procedure is shown in Figures 16–8 and 16–9 and is illustrated in

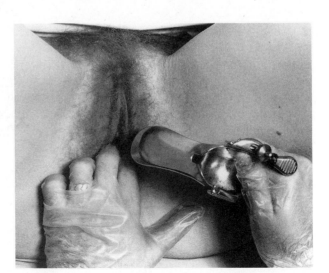

FIGURE 16–8. Technique for insertion of the vaginal speculum. Note the examiner's fingers pressing downward on the perineum.

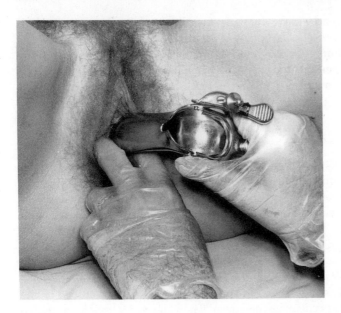

FIGURE 16-9. Technique for insertion of the vaginal speculum. Notice that the speculum rides over the examiner's fingers, avoiding contact with the external urethral meatus and clitoris.

Figure 16–10. It is important not to introduce the speculum vertically, because injury to the urethra or meatus may occur.

Inspect the Cervix

The speculum is introduced as far into the vagina as possible. When it is completely inserted, the speculum is rotated to the transverse position, with the handle now pointing downward, and is opened *slowly*. With the blades open, the vaginal walls and cervix can be visualized. The cervix should rest within the blades of the speculum. This is shown in Figure 16–11 and illustrated in Figure 16–12. In order to keep the speculum open, the set screw can be tightened. If

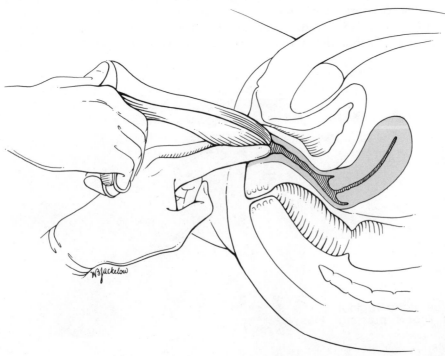

FIGURE 16-10. Cross-section of the speculum examination.

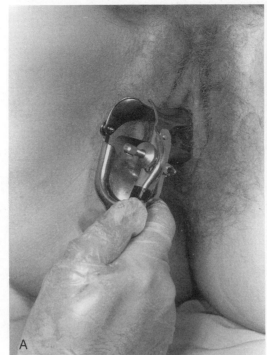

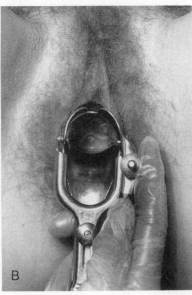

A

B

FIGURE 16–11. Technique for inspecting the cervix. *A* shows the opening of the speculum blades after it has been fully inserted and rotated to the transverse position. *B* shows the internal view of the cervix when the speculum is correctly inserted.

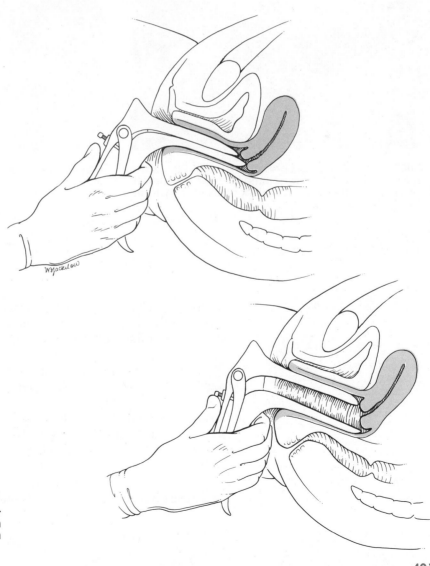

FIGURE 16–12. Cross-section illustrating the position of the speculum during inspection of the cervix with the speculum.

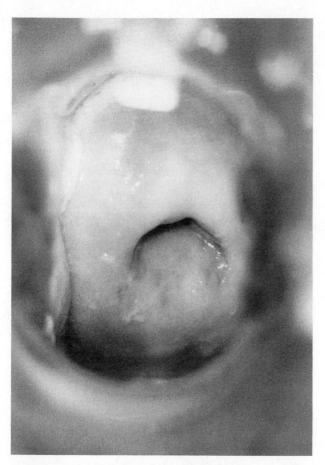

FIGURE 16–13. A normal cervix. Note the linear external cervical os, which is commonly seen in women with children. The external cervical os in a woman without children is perfectly round.

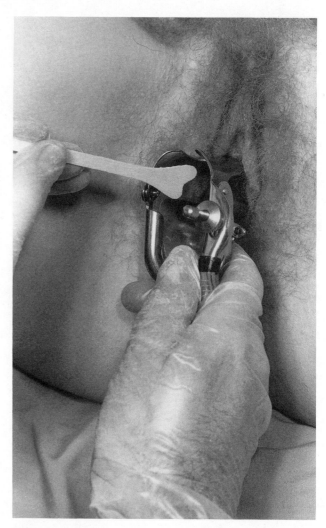

FIGURE 16–14. Technique for obtaining a smear for the Pap test.

the cervix is not immediately seen, gently turn the blades in various directions to expose the cervix. The most common reason for not visualizing the cervix is failure to insert the speculum far enough before opening it.

If there is a discharge obscuring any part of the vaginal walls or cervix, it should be removed with a cotton-tipped applicator and spread onto a glass slide.

Inspect the cervix for any discharge, erythema, erosion, ulceration, leukoplakia, or mass. What is the shape of the external cervical os? What is the color of the cervix? A bluish discoloration may be an indication of pregnancy or a large tumor.

A normal cervix is seen in Figure 16–13. Notice that the external cervical os is linear, which is characteristic of a cervix of a woman who has had a vaginal delivery.

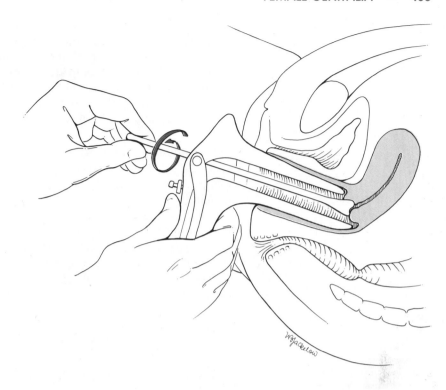

FIGURE 16–15. Obtaining smear for the Pap test. Notice that the longer end of the wooden spatula is placed in the cervical os.

The Pap Smear

A Pap* smear is obtained using a wooden spatula inserted through the speculum, as shown in Figure 16–14. The longer end of the spatula is inserted into the external cervical os (Fig. 16–15). The spatula is then rotated 360° while scraping off cells from the external cervical os. Other specimens are taken by using a cotton-tipped applicator from the posterior and lateral vaginal fornices and from the endocervix. The specimens are smeared separately onto glass slides and are fixed either by dropping them in a solution of equal parts of 95% methyl alcohol and ether or by spraying them with a rapidly drying fixative.

Inspect the Vaginal Walls

The patient is told that the speculum will now be removed. The set screw is released with the right index finger, and the speculum is rotated back to the original oblique position. As the speculum is slowly withdrawn and closed, the vaginal walls are inspected for masses, lacerations, leukoplakia, or ulcerations. The walls should be smooth and nontender. A moderate amount of colorless or white mucus will usually be present.

Bimanual Palpation

The bimanual examination is used for palpation of the uterus and adnexa. In this examination, the hands are placed in the vagina and on the abdomen and the pelvic structures are palpated between the hands. The choice of which hand to use vaginally is a matter of preference. Generally, the right hand is inserted into the vagina and the left hand palpates the abdomen.

---

* Pap is the abbreviated name for Dr. Papanicolaou, who developed this screening technique. The properly performed test can accurately lead to the diagnosis of cervical carcinoma in 98% of cases and can detect 80% of cases of endometrial carcinoma.

The Technique

The physician should be positioned between the patient's legs. If the right hand is to be used vaginally, the examiner places his right foot on a small footrest or stool. A suitable jelly lubricant is held in the left hand, and a small amount is dropped from the tube onto the examiner's gloved right index and middle fingers. The examiner should not touch the tube of lubricant to the gloves, because contamination of the lubricant will occur. The patient is told that the "internal examination" will now begin.

As the bimanual examination is being performed, observe the patient's face. Her expression will quickly reveal if the examination is painful. Tell the woman that you are again going to touch her leg as you begin the examination. The back of your left hand should touch the inside of the patient's right thigh. The labia are spread, and the lubricated right index and middle fingers are introduced vertically into the vagina. A downward pressure toward the perineum is applied. The right fourth and fifth fingers are flexed into the palm of the hand. The right thumb is extended. The area around the clitoris should not be touched. You may now rest your right elbow on your right knee so that undue pressure is not placed on the patient.

The correct position of the physician, assistant, and patient is shown in Figure 16–16.

The vaginal walls are palpated for nodules, scarring, or induration.

Once inserted into the vagina, the right hand is rotated 90° clockwise so that the palm is facing upward. Some physicians prefer not to rotate the vaginal hand, because this may decrease the depth of penetration. The left hand is now placed on the abdomen approximately one third the way to the umbilicus from the pubic symphysis. The wrist of the abdominal hand should not be flexed or supinated. The right (vaginal) hand brings the pelvic organs up out of the pelvis and stabilizes them while they are palpated by the left (abdominal) hand. It is the abdominal, not the vaginal, hand that performs the palpation. The technique for the bimanual examination is shown in Figure 16–17 and is illustrated in Figure 16–18.

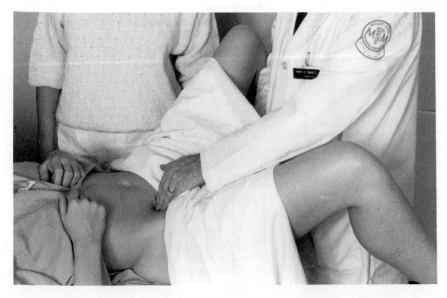

FIGURE 16–16. The positions of the examiner, assistant, and patient for the pelvic examination.

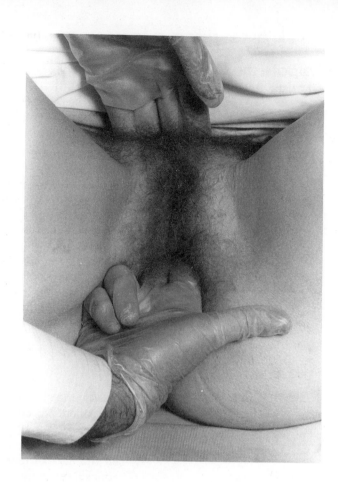

FIGURE 16–17. Technique for the bimanual examination.

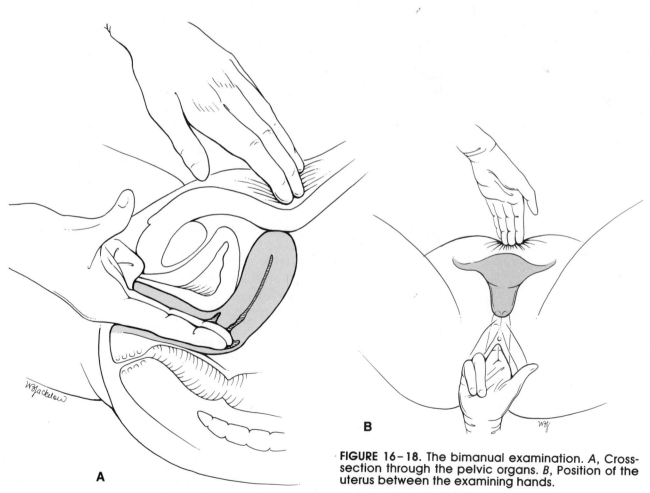

FIGURE 16–18. The bimanual examination. *A*, Cross-section through the pelvic organs. *B*, Position of the uterus between the examining hands.

Palpate the Cervix and Uterine Body

The cervix is palpated. What is its consistency (soft, firm, nodular, friable)?

Tell the patient that she will now feel you move her cervix and uterus, but this should not be painful. The cervix can usually be moved 2–4 cm in any direction. The cervix is pushed backward and upward toward the abdominal hand as the abdominal hand pushes downward. Any restriction of motion or the development of pain on movement should be noted. Pushing the cervix up and back tends to tip an anteverted, anteflexed uterus forward into a position that is more easily palpated. The uterus should then be felt between the two hands. Carefully describe its *position, size, shape, consistency, mobility,* and *tenderness.* Determine whether the uterus is anteverted or retroverted, enlarged, firm, and mobile. Are any irregularities felt? Is there any tenderness when the uterus is moved?

Palpation by the bimanual technique is possible only if the uterus is anteverted and anteflexed, which is the most common uterine position. A retroverted uterus is directed toward the spine and is not easily felt by bimanual palpation.

Palpate the Adnexa

After the uterus has been evaluated, the right and left adnexa are palpated. If the patient has complained of pain on one side, start the examination on the other side. The right hand should move to the left lateral fornix while the left (abdominal) hand moves to the patient's left lower quadrant. The vaginal fingers lift the adnexa toward the abdominal hand, which attempts to palpate the adnexal structures. This is illustrated in Figure 16–19.

The adnexa should be explored for any masses. Describe the *size, shape, consistency,* and *mobility,* as well as any *tenderness* of the structures in the adnexa. The normal ovary is sensitive to pressure when squeezed. After the left side is examined, the right adnexa are palpated by moving the right (vaginal) hand to the right lateral fornix and the left (abdominal) hand to the right lower quadrant of the patient.

In many individuals, the adnexal structures cannot be palpated. In thin women, the ovaries are frequently palpable. Adnexal tenderness or enlargement is relatively specific for a pathologic state.

After completion of the examination of the adnexa, the examining vaginal fingers move to the posterior fornix to palpate the uterosacral ligaments and the pouch of Douglas. Marked tenderness and nodularity suggest the presence of endometriosis.

If the patient has had children, the examiner should have no difficulty in using both the right index and middle fingers in the vagina for bimanual palpation. If the introitus is small, the examiner should introduce the right middle finger first and gently push downward toward the anus. By stretching the introitus, the right index finger can then be introduced with little discomfort. If the patient is a virgin, only the right middle finger should be used.

Rectovaginal Palpation

Palpate the Rectovaginal Septum

Tell the patient that you will now examine the vagina and rectum. The rectovaginal examination allows for better evaluation of the posterior portion of the pelvis and the cul-de-sac than the bimanual examination alone. You can

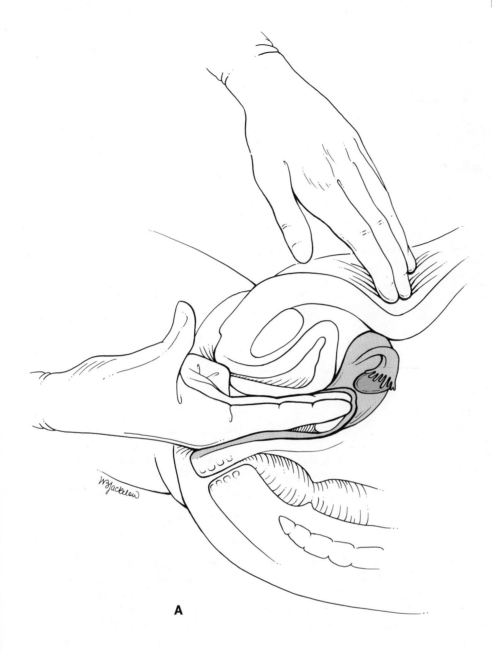

A

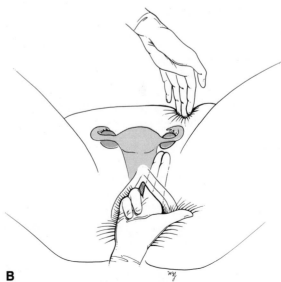

B

FIGURE 16–19. Technique for palpating the left ad-nexa. *A,* Cross-section through the pelvic organs. *B,* Position of the ovary and fallopian tube between the examining hands.

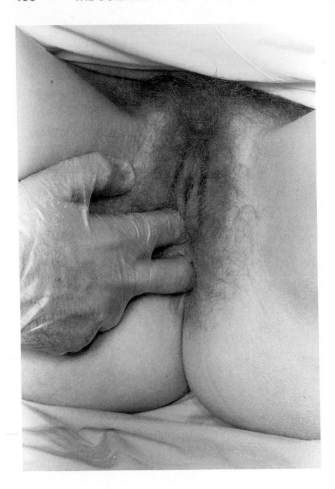

FIGURE 16-20. Technique for performing the recto-vaginal examination.

often get 1-2 cm higher into the pelvis by the rectovaginal examination. The right hand, still in the vagina, is slightly withdrawn so that the right middle finger can be removed from the vagina. The patient is asked to bear down, at which time the right middle finger is slowly inserted into the rectum. The examining right index finger is positioned as far up the posterior surface of the vagina as possible. This technique is shown in Figure 16-20 and is illustrated in Figure 16-21.

The rectovaginal septum is palpated. Is it thickened or tender? Are nodules or masses present? The right middle finger should feel for tenderness, masses, or irregularities in the rectum.

The patient is told that the "internal examination" is completed and that you are about to remove your hand. When you withdraw your fingers, inspect them for discharge or blood. Offer the woman a tissue to wipe off any excess lubricant.

Test Stool for Occult Blood

Any fecal material on the middle (rectal) finger should be tested with the occult blood testing card and reagent. If the patient is menstruating, it is important to change gloves prior to the rectovaginal examination so that vaginal blood will not be confused with rectal blood.

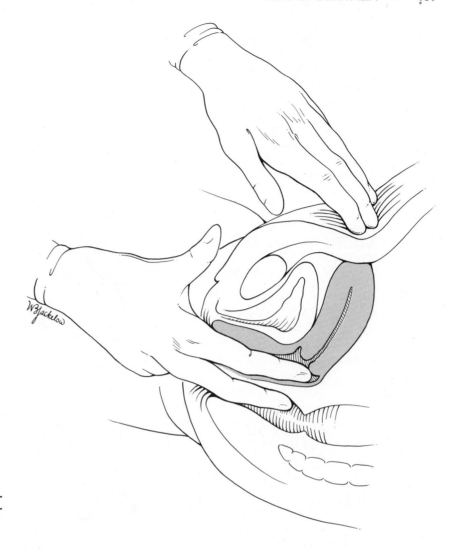

FIGURE 16-21. Cross-section illustrating the rectovaginal examination.

Ask the woman to move back on the examination table, remove her legs from the stirrups, and then sit up slowly. You should now remove your gloves and wash your hands. This concludes the examination of the female genitalia.

CLINICOPATHOLOGIC CORRELATIONS

Figure 16-22 shows several of the common uterine positions.

As had been indicated, pelvic relaxation is a common problem. The consequences include cystocele, rectocele, and uterine prolapse. Figure 16-23 illustrates these sequelae of relaxation of the pelvic floor.

A summary of dysfunctional uterine bleeding is illustrated in Figure 16-24.

Table 16-1 lists the characteristics of common vaginal discharges. Table 16-2 summarizes the clinical features of genital ulcerations.

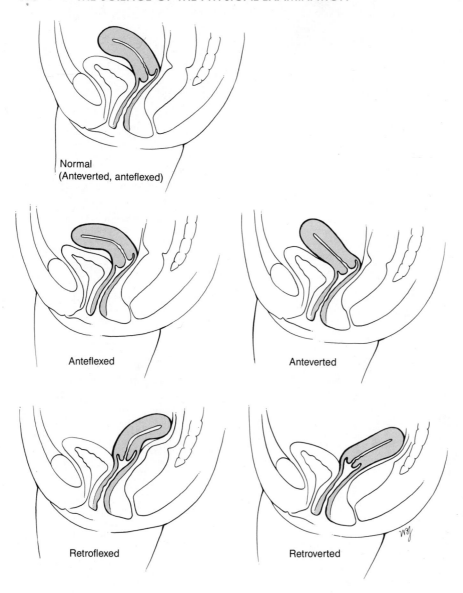

Normal
(Anteverted, anteflexed)

Anteflexed

Anteverted

Retroflexed

Retroverted

FIGURE 16–22. Common uterine positions.

TABLE 16–1. Characteristics of Common Vaginal Discharges

Feature	Physiologic Discharge	Nonspecific Vaginitis (NSV)	Trichomonas	Candida	Gonococcal
Color	White	Gray	Grayish yellow	White	Greenish yellow
Fishy odor	Absent	Present	Present	Absent	Absent
Consistency	Nonhomogeneous	Homogeneous	Purulent, often with bubbles	"Cottage cheese"	Mucopurulent
Presence	Dependent	Adherent to walls	Often pooled in fornix	Adherent to walls	Adherent to walls
Discharge at introitus	Rare	Common	Common	Common	Common
Vulva	Normal	Normal	Edematous	Erythematous	Erythematous
Vaginal mucosa	Normal	Normal	Usually normal	Erythematous	Normal
Cervix	Normal	Normal	May show red spots	Patches of discharge	Pus in os

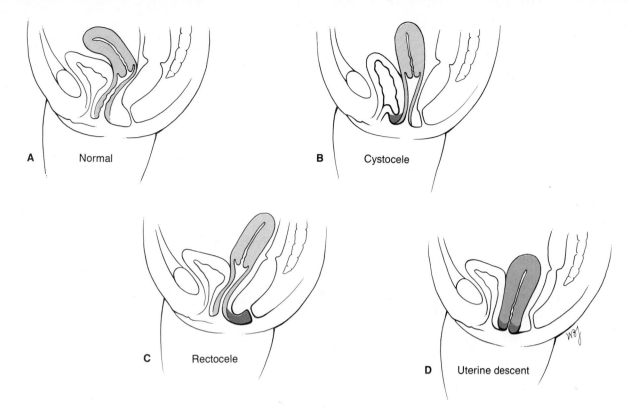

FIGURE 16–23. Sequelae of pelvic floor relaxation. *A*, Normal anatomy. *B*, A cystocele, which is a protrusion of the wall of the urinary bladder through the vagina. *C*, A rectocele, which is a protrusion of the rectal wall through the vagina. *D*, Uterine descent, which is a protrusion of the uterus through the vagina.

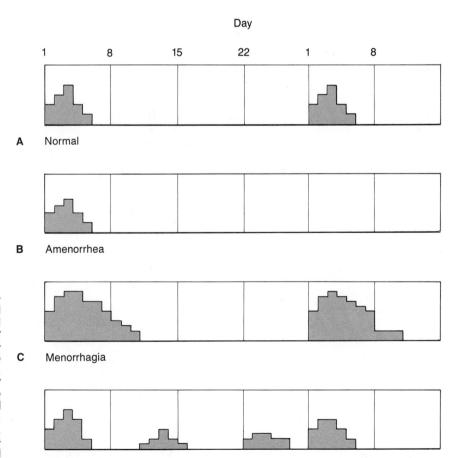

FIGURE 16–24. Types of dysfunctional uterine bleeding. *A*, Normal 28 day cycle. Note that menstrual flow occurs on day 1 and lasts for approximately 5 days. *B*, Amenorrhea. After a menstrual flow of 5 days, the period does not recur. *C*, Menorrhagia. Note that the flow occurs at 28 day intervals but the amount of the flow is heavier and its duration is longer than normal. *D*, Metrorrhagia. In this condition, flow is regular but there is bleeding between the normal menstrual flow cycles.

411

TABLE 16–2. Clinical Features of Genital Ulcerations

Feature	Genital Herpes	Primary Syphilis	Chancroid
Incubation period	3–5 days	9–90 days	1–5 days
Number of ulcers	Multiple	Single	Multiple
Appearance at onset	Vesicle	Papule	Papule/pustule
Later appearance	Small, grouped	Round, indurated	Irregular, ragged
Ulcer pain	Present	Absent	Present
Inguinal adenopathy	Present, tender	Present, painless	Present, painful
Healing	Within 2 weeks	Slowly over weeks	Slowly over weeks
Recurrence (even if not infected)	Common	Rare	Common

USEFUL VOCABULARY

Listed here are the specific roots that are important in order to understand the terminology related to diseases of the female genitalia.

ROOT	PERTAINING TO	EXAMPLE	DEFINITION
gyn(e)-	woman	*gyne*cology	Branch of medicine that deals with treating diseases of the genital tract in women
hyster(o)-	uterus	*hyster*ectomy	Surgical removal of the uterus
metro-	uterus	*metro*rrhagia	Uterine bleeding
oophor(o)-	ovary	*oophoro*tomy	Incision of an ovary
ov-	egg	*ov*ulation	The discharge of an egg from the ovary
salping(o)-	fallopian tube	*salping*itis	Inflammation of the fallopian tube

WRITING UP THE PHYSICAL EXAMINATION

Listed here are examples of the write-up for the examination of the female genitalia.

Examination of the vulva is within normal limits. There are no lesions present. The cervix appears pink, smooth, and nulliparous. There is no discharge from the external cervical os. The vaginal walls appear normal. Bimanual palpation reveals an anteverted, anteflexed uterus without masses or tenderness. The adnexa are unremarkable. Rectovaginal examination reveals a thin rectovaginal membrane without tenderness. Stool guaiac is negative.

Examination of the vulva reveals groups of tense vesicles and scattered erosions that are covered with exudate. The cervix is pink and multiparous. No cervical lesions are present. No discharge is present. The vagina is within normal limits. The uterus is anteverted and anteflexed. A 6 × 6 cm mass is felt with the uterus. The ovaries and tubes are unremarkable. Rectovaginal examination is within normal limits.

The vulva appears within normal limits without masses or lesions. The cervix has an erosion with a thick, white, cottage cheese discharge in the vagina. The discharge is adherent to the vaginal walls. The uterus is retroverted and cannot be adequately examined. There is a walnut-sized mass felt in the left adnexa. It appears rubbery and is freely mobile. The rectovaginal examination is normal. Stool guaiac is negative.

The vulva is normal. Upon straining, a rectocele becomes apparent. The vagina is normal. The cervix is smooth, pink, and multiparous. The uterus is anteverted and anteflexed and is not enlarged. The adnexa are difficult to assess because of obesity of the patient. No tenderness is present.

BIBLIOGRAPHY

Magee J: The pelvic examination: A view from the other end of the table. Ann Intern Med *83*:563, 1975.

Mazor MD, Simons HF (eds): Infertility: Medical, Emotional and Social Considerations. New York, Human Sciences Press, 1984.

Peckham BM, Shapiro SS: Signs and Symptoms in Gynecology. Philadelphia, JB Lippincott, 1983.

Priest RG: Psychological Disorders in Obstetrics and Gynaecology. London, Butterworths, 1985.

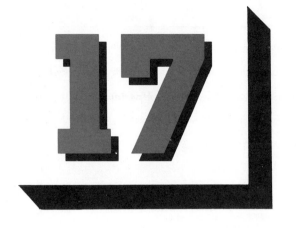

THE MUSCULOSKELETAL SYSTEM

The hand of the Lord was upon me . . . and set me down in the midst of the valley which was full of bones. . . . behold, there were very many in the open valley; and, lo, they were very dry. . . . Thus saith the Lord God unto these bones: Behold, I will cause breath to enter into you, and ye shall live. And I will lay sinews upon you, and will bring up flesh upon you, and cover with skin, and put breath in you, and ye shall live. . . . there was a noise, and behold a commotion, and the bones came together, bone to bone. . . . and skin covered them . . . and the breath came into them, and they lived, and stood up upon their feet. . . .

Ezekiel XXXVII: 1–10

GENERAL CONSIDERATIONS

Diseases of the musculoskeletal system rank first among disease conditions that alter the quality of life. This is related to limitation of activity, disability, and impairment. In the United States, one out of *every seven persons* suffers from some sort of musculoskeletal disorder, the cost of which *exceeds 60 billion dollars annually*. This includes lost earnings and medical expenses.

Diseases of the musculoskeletal system fall into two categories: systemic diseases and local diseases. Patients with systemic disease, such as rheumatoid arthritis, systemic lupus erythematosis, and polymyositis, may appear chronically ill with generalized weakness, pain, and episodic stiffness of their joints. Patients with local disease are basically healthy individuals who suffer restriction of motion and pain from a single area. Included in this group of patients are those suffering from back pain, tennis elbow, arthritis, or bursitis. Despite the fact that these patients may have only local symptoms, their disability can greatly limit their work capacity and the disease can have monumental impact.

Diseases of the musculoskeletal system rank first in cost to workers' compensation insurance carriers. Nearly 100,000 workers receive disability payments annually, with a total cost to the carriers of over 200 billion dollars annually.

It has been estimated that musculoskeletal-related problems rank second (after cardiovascular disorders) in the number of visits to internists and rank third in the number of surgical procedures in hospitals.*

Although not primarily fatal disorders, musculoskeletal conditions affect the quality of life. Studies have indicated that backache is experienced by greater than 80% of all Americans at some time in life. Patients with backache for longer than 6 months constitute a large portion of permanently disabled individuals. Over 50% of these patients never return to work. Over 25 million Americans suffer from arthritis that requires medical attention. Arthritis ranks second to cardiac disease as a cause of limitation of activity.

In the United States, at least 10% of the population experience a bone fracture, dislocation, or sprain annually. Each year, there are over 1.2 million fractures sustained by women over the age of 50 years. There are over 200,000 hip fractures annually, and these are associated with prolonged disability. Osteoporosis† is the most common musculoskeletal disorder in the world and is second only to arthritis as a leading cause of morbidity in the geriatric population. Postmenopausal osteoporosis and age-related osteoporosis increase the risk of fractures in the older population. There are over 40 million women in the United States over the age of 50 years, more than 50% of whom have evidence of spinal osteoporosis. Almost 90% of women over the age of 75 years have significant radiographic evidence of osteoporosis.

The high prevalence of musculoskeletal disease in the elderly requiring nursing care assistance has a significant impact on the American economy. It is expected that by 1990 the cost for nursing home care will be almost 75 billion dollars (Freeland et al, 1980). Over 10 million individuals in the United States have some form of inflammatory arthritis, the most prevalent being rheumatoid arthritis. It is estimated that greater than 7 million of these patients have this form of arthritis.

Although trauma to the spinal cord producing paraplegia or quadriplegia is rare, the average total lifetime cost per patient exceeds $150,000.

Musculoskeletal problems have their most significant financial effect on the aged population. Over one billion dollars are spent annually by Medicare for hospitalizations of patients with these conditions. This represents 20% of all Medicare payments.

STRUCTURE AND PHYSIOLOGY

The principal functions of the musculoskeletal system are to provide support and protection of the body and to bring about movement of the extremities for locomotion and for the performance of tasks.

The parts of the musculoskeletal system are composed of variable forms of dense connective tissue, which include the following:

---

* Gynecologic surgery is first, followed by abdominal surgery.
† Osteoporosis refers to a state of decreased density of normal mineralized bone.

- Bone
- Skeletal muscle
- Ligaments and tendons
- Cartilage

Bone is composed of an organic matrix that consists of collagen fibers embedded in a cementing gel made up of calcium and phosphate. Bone is an actively changing tissue constantly undergoing *remodeling* while reappropriating its mineral stores and matrix according to mechanical stresses. Normal bone is composed of collagen fibers aligned parallel to the tension stresses to which the bone is exposed. The long bones in the adult are composed of tubes of *cortical,* or compact, bone surrounding a medullary cavity of *cancellous,* or spongy, bone. Cortical bone exists in areas where support is necessary, whereas cancellous bone is found in areas where hematopoesis or bone formation occurs. In cortical bone, the bone cells, or *osteocytes,* are enclosed in lacunae, which are spaces in the sheets of bone tissue called *lamellae.* Several lamellae are arranged concentrically around a vascular channel and are termed an *haversian canal.* In cancellous bone, the lamellae are not arranged in haversian systems, but are organized into a spongy network called *trabeculae.* These trabeculae align along lines of stress.

The ends of the long bones, known as *epiphyses,* are expanded near the articular surfaces and are composed of spongy bone. The shaft of the long bone, known as the *diaphysis,* is covered with a layer of *periosteum.* The inner cavity of the long bone is lined with *endosteum* and is filled with marrow.

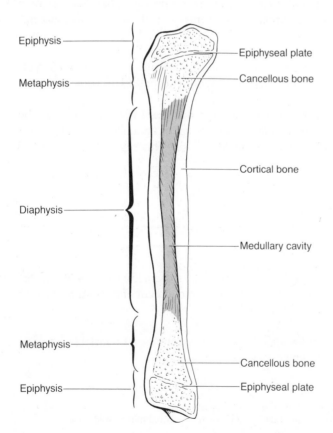

FIGURE 17–1. Anatomy of a long bone.

For a period of time, a layer of cartilage exists between the diaphysis and the epiphysis. This cartilage is known as the *growth plate* or *epiphyseal plate*. The purpose of the growth plate is to determine the longitudinal growth of the bone. The parts of a long bone are illustrated in Figure 17–1.

Cells in the periosteum can develop into *osteoblasts*, which lay down new bone, or into *osteoclasts*, which resorb bone. Trauma, infection, or tumors stimulate the development of osteoblasts. Osteoblasts secrete the matrix that is refashioned into lamellae and is arranged to meet the mechanical stresses to which the bone is subjected.

A pathologic process that interferes with the normal architecture of bone will tend to weaken it. Paget's disease is a disease of bone in which there is a disruption of the normal architecture. Patients with this condition are extremely susceptible to pathologic fractures.

Skeletal muscle is an organ, the contraction of which produces movement.

Ligaments attach bone to bone, whereas *tendons* attach muscle to bone. Both are dense connective tissues that offer great resistance to a pulling force.

Cartilage is a type of connective tissue with great resilience. It plays an important role in joint function and in determining bone length.

The basic functional unit of the musculoskeletal system is the *joint*. A joint is a union of two or more bones. There are several types of joints in the body. They include joints that are

- Immovable
- Slightly movable
- Movable

Immovable joints are joints fixed as a result of fibrous tissue banding. Examples of this type of joint are the sutures of the skull. *Slightly movable joints* are termed *symphyses*. In this type of joint, there is fibrocartilage joining the articulating bones. The pubic symphysis is an example of a slightly movable joint. The most common type of joint is the *movable joint*. The body has many different types of movable joints, also known as *synovial joints*. In synovial joints, the bone structures come in contact with each other and are covered with hyaline articular cartilage. A capsule surrounds the joint by attaching to the bones on either side of the joint. Within the capsule is a small amount of synovial fluid, which plays a role in joint lubrication and nourishment of the articular cartilage. Synovial joints are classified according to the type of movement their structure permits. The classifications include the following:

- Hinge joint
- Pivot joint
- Condyloid joint
- Saddle joint
- Ball-and-socket joint
- Plane joint

A *hinge joint* permits movement in only one axis, namely flexion or extension. The axis is transverse. An example of a hinge joint is the elbow. A *pivot joint* permits rotation in one axis. The axis is longitudinal along the shaft of the bone.

One bone moves around a central axis without any displacement from that axis. An example of a pivot joint is the proximal radioulnar joint. A *condyloid joint* permits movement in two axes. In this type of joint, the articular surfaces are oval and have been described as an "egg-in-spoon joint." One axis is the long diameter of the oval, whereas the other axis is the short diameter of the oval. The wrist joint is an example of a condyloid joint. A *saddle joint* is also a biaxial joint. In this type of joint, the articular surfaces are saddle shaped with the movements similar to those of the condyloid joint. The carpometacarpal joint of the thumb is an example of the saddle joint. The *ball-and-socket joint* is an example of a polyaxial joint; motion is possible in many axes. In a ball-and-socket joint, the articular surfaces are reciprocal segments of a sphere. The hip and shoulder joints are examples of ball-and-socket joints. A *plane joint* is also a

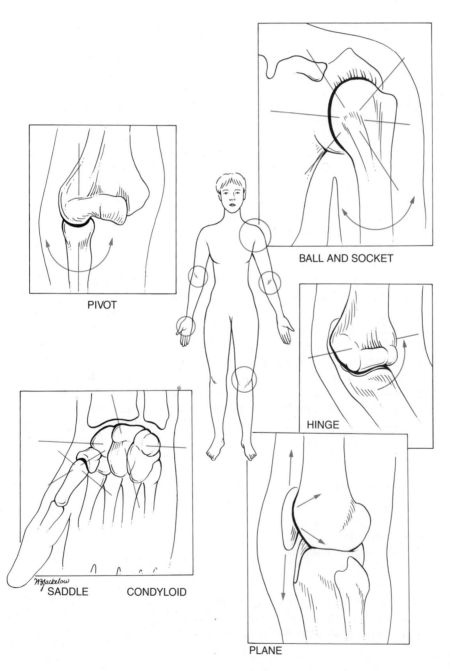

PIVOT

BALL AND SOCKET

HINGE

SADDLE   CONDYLOID

PLANE

FIGURE 17–2. Types of movable joints.

polyaxial joint. In the plane joint, the articular surfaces are flat and one bone merely rides over the other in many directions. The patellofemoral joint is an example of a plane joint. These different types of movable joints are shown in Figure 17–2 according to the movement permitted.

The stability of a joint is dependent upon the following:

- The shape of the articular surfaces
- The ligaments
- The associated muscles

There are certain anatomic terms that refer to positions with which the reader must be familiar (Table 17–1). The *median plane* bisects the body into a right and left half. A plane parallel to the median plane is a *sagittal plane*. *Medial* and *lateral* are used in reference to the sagittal plane. A position closer to the median plane is medial; further from the median plane is lateral. In the upper limb, *ulnar* is often subsituted for medial and *radial* is used to denote lateral. In the lower limb, *tibial* is used to denote medial and *peroneal* or *fibular* is substituted for lateral.

The anatomic terms are illustrated in Figure 17–3.

The front of the body is the *anterior,* or *ventral,* surface, whereas the part of the body nearest the back is the *posterior,* or *dorsal,* side. The *palmar* or *volar* aspect of the hand is the anterior surface. The dorsal aspect of the foot faces upward, whereas the *plantar* aspect is the sole of the foot. *Proximal* refers to the part of an extremity that is closest to its root; *distal* refers to the part farthest from the root.

The most important terms relating to deformities of the bone structure are *valgus* and *varus.* In a valgus deformity, the distal portion of the bone is displaced away from the midline and angulation is toward the midline. In a varus deformity, the distal portion of the extremity is displaced toward the midline and angulation is away from the midline. The name of the deformity is determined by the joint involved. An example of a valgus deformity of the knees is called knock-knee, also known as *genu valgum.* An example of a varus deformity of the knee is known as bowleg, technically termed *genu varum.*

In the evaluation of a joint, the *range of motion* is critical to assess. Each joint has a characteristic range of motion that can be measured passively and actively. *Passive* range of motion is the motion elicited by the examiner as a result of the examiner moving the patient's body. *Active* range of motion is the motion that the patient performs as a result of moving his musculature. The passive range of motion usually equals the active range of motion except in paralysis of muscles or in ruptured tendons. The range of motion of individual joints is

TABLE 17–1. Anatomic Terms for the Upper and Lower Limb

Limb	Medial	Lateral
Upper	Ulnar	Radial
Lower	Tibial	Peroneal Fibular

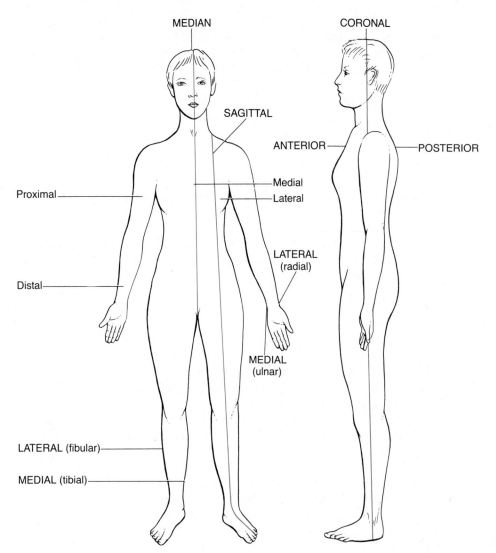

FIGURE 17–3. Anatomic terms.

discussed later in this chapter. Joint motion is measured in degrees of a circle with the joint at the center. If a limb is extended with the bones in a straight line, the joint is said to be at *zero position*. The zero position is the neutral position of the joint. As the joint is flexed, the angle increases. The concept of range of motion is illustrated in Figure 17–4.

There are six basic types of joint motion. They are as follows:

- Flexion and extension
- Dorsiflexion and plantar flexion
- Adduction and abduction
- Inversion and eversion
- Internal and external rotation
- Pronation and supination

The definitions of these motions and the joints at which the motions are seen are summarized in Table 17–2.

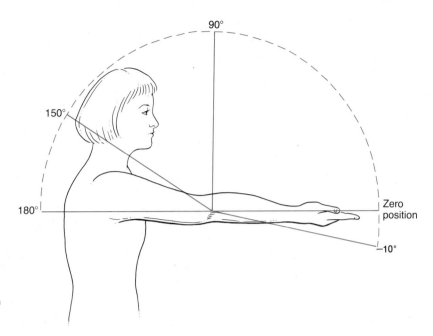

FIGURE 17–4. The concept of range of motion.

TABLE 17–2. Joint Motion

Motion	Definition	Example
Flexion	Motion away from the zero position	Most joints
Extension	Return motion to the zero position*	Most joints
Dorsiflexion	Movement in the direction of the dorsal surface	Ankle, toes, wrist, fingers
Plantar (or palmar) flexion	Movement in the direction of the plantar (or palmar) surface	Ankle, toes (wrist, fingers)
Adduction	Movement toward the midline†	Shoulder, hip, metacarpophalangeal, metatarsophalangeal joints
Abduction	Movement away from the midline	Shoulder, hip, metacarpophalangeal, metatarsophalangeal joints
Inversion	Turning of the plantar surface of the foot inward	Subtalar and midtarsal joints of the foot
Eversion	Turning of the plantar surface of the foot outward	Subtalar and midtarsal joints of the foot
Internal rotation	Turning of the anterior surface of a limb inward	Shoulder, hip
External rotation	Turning of the anterior surface of a limb outward	Shoulder, hip
Pronation	Rotation so that the palmar surface of the hand is directed downward	Elbow, wrist
Supination	Rotation so that the palmar surface of the hand is directed upward	Elbow, wrist

* If motion goes beyond the zero position, *hyperextension* is said to be present.
† In the hand or foot, the midline is a line drawn through the middle finger or middle toe, respectively.

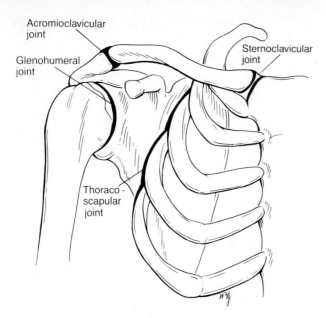

FIGURE 17-5. Anatomy of the shoulder joint.

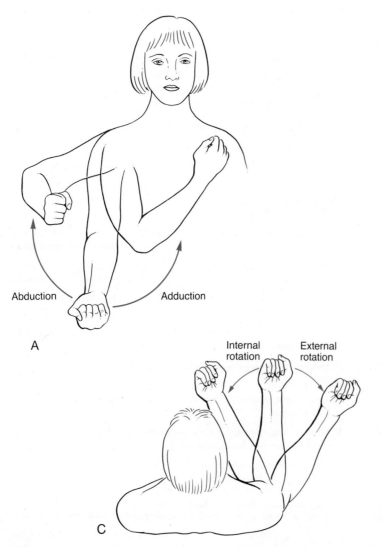

FIGURE 17-6. Range of motion at the shoulder. *A*, Abduction and adduction. *B*, Flexion and extension. *C*, Internal and external rotation.

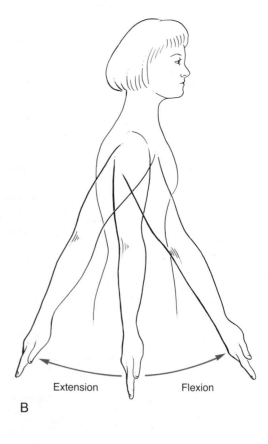

422

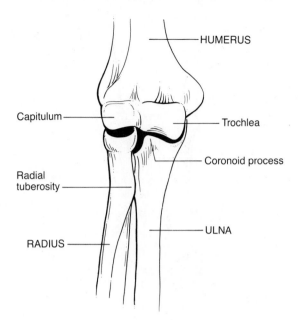

FIGURE 17-7. Anatomy of the elbow joint.

The anatomy of the *shoulder joint* is illustrated in Figure 17-5. The joint movements at the shoulder are abduction and adduction, flexion and extension, and internal and external rotation. These motions are illustrated in Figure 17-6.

The anatomy of the *elbow joint* is shown in Figure 17-7. The joint movements at the elbow are flexion and extension, and supination and pronation. These motions are illustrated in Figure 17-8.

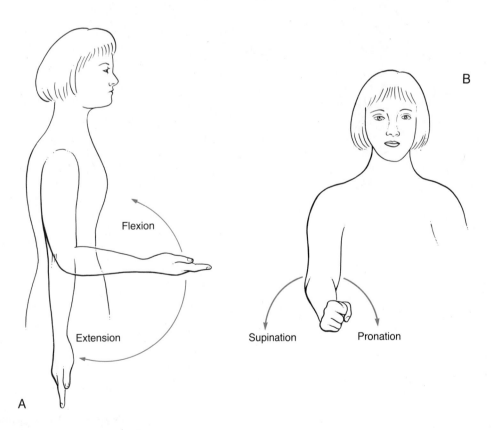

FIGURE 17-8. Range of motion at the elbow joint. *A*, Flexion and extension. *B*, Supination and pronation.

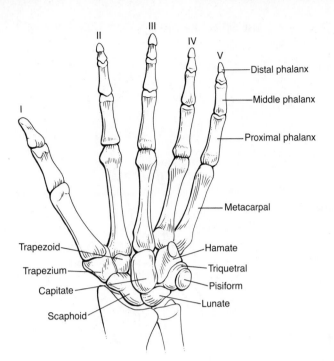

FIGURE 17-9. Anatomy of the wrist and fingers.

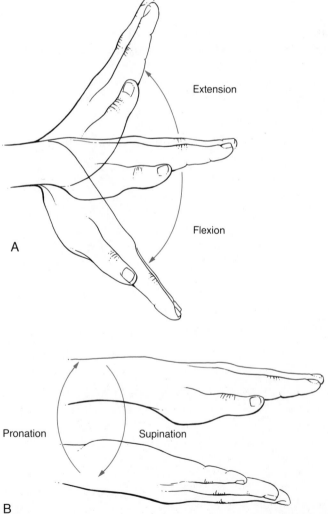

FIGURE 17-10. Range of motion at the wrist joint. *A*, Dorsiflexion (extension) and palmar flexion. *B*, Supination and pronation.

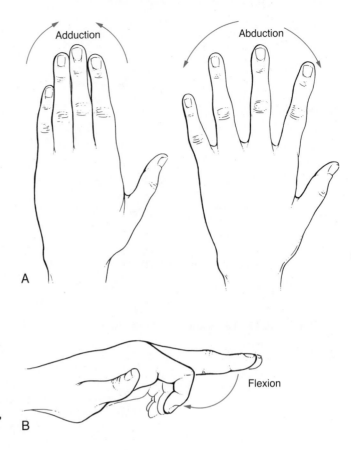

FIGURE 17-11. Range of motion at the finger joints. *A,* Abduction and adduction. *B,* Flexion.

The anatomy of the *wrist and fingers* is illustrated in Figure 17-9. The joint movements at the wrist are dorsiflexion (or extension) and palmar flexion, and supination and pronation. These motions are illustrated in Figure 17-10. The joint movements at the fingers are abduction and adduction, and flexion. These motions are illustrated in Figure 17-11.

The joint movements of the *thumb* are flexion and extension, and opposition. These motions are illustrated in Figure 17-12.

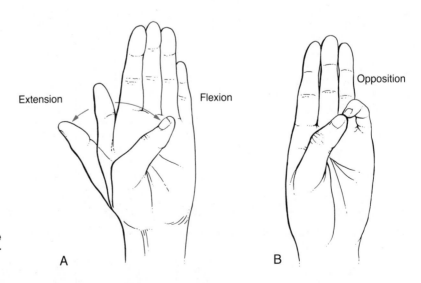

FIGURE 17-12. Range of motion of the thumb. *A,* Flexion and extension. *B,* Opposition.

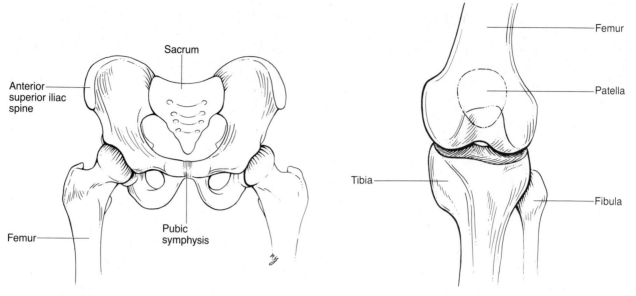

FIGURE 17–13. Anatomy of the hip joint.

FIGURE 17–15. Anatomy of the knee joint.

The anatomy of the *hip* is illustrated in Figure 17–13. The joint movements at the hip are flexion and extension; abduction and adduction; and internal and external rotation. These motions are illustrated in Figure 17–14.

The anatomy of the *knee* is shown in Figure 17–15. The joint movements at the knee are flexion and hyperextension. These motions are illustrated in Figure 17–16.

The anatomy of the *ankle and foot* is illustrated in Figure 17–17. The joint movements at the ankle are dorsiflexion and plantar flexion, and eversion and inversion. These motions are illustrated in Figure 17–18.

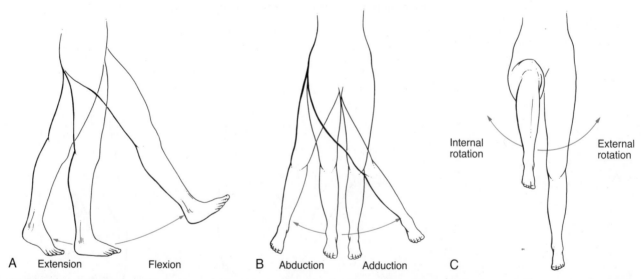

FIGURE 17–14. Range of motion at the hip joint. *A,* Flexion and extension. *B,* Abduction and adduction. *C,* Internal and external rotation.

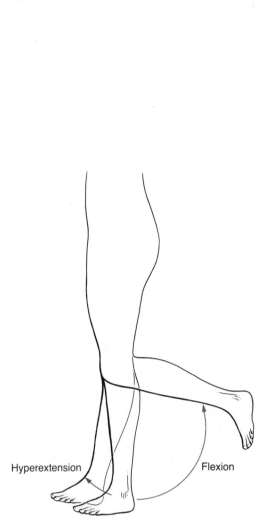

FIGURE 17-16. Range of motion at the knee joint: flexion and hyperextension.

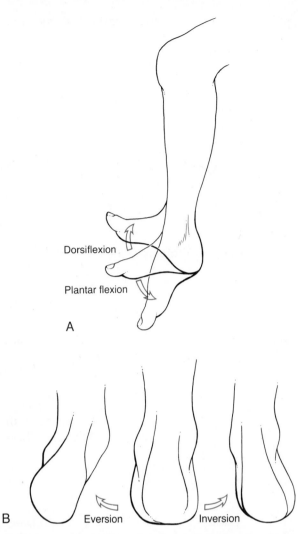

A

B   Eversion   Inversion

FIGURE 17-18. Range of motion at the ankle and foot joints. *A*, Dorsiflexion and plantar flexion. *B*, Eversion and inversion.

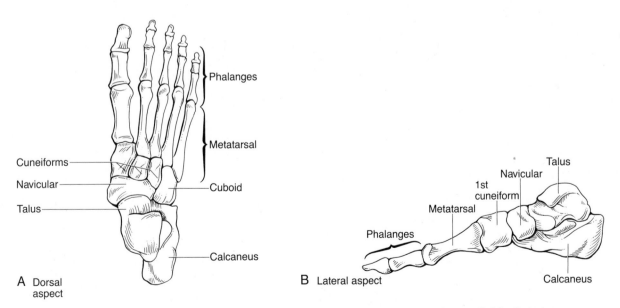

A Dorsal aspect

B Lateral aspect

FIGURE 17-17. Anatomy of the ankle and foot joints. *A*, View from above. *B*, Medial view.

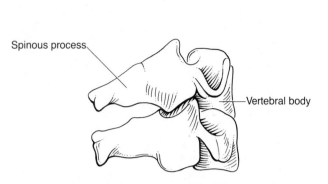

Spinous process

Vertebral body

FIGURE 17–19. Anatomy of the cervical spine.

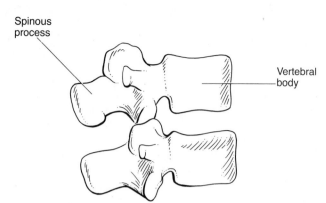

Spinous process

Vertebral body

FIGURE 17–21. Anatomy of the lumbar spine.

The anatomy of the *cervical spine* is shown in Figure 17–19. The joint movements of the neck are flexion and extension; rotation; and lateral flexion. These motions are illustrated in Figure 17–20.

The anatomy of the *lumbar spine* is illustrated in Figure 17–21. The joint movements of the lumbar spine are flexion and extension; rotation; and lateral extension. These motions are illustrated in Figure 17–22.

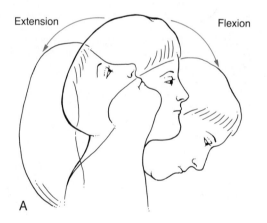

Extension

Flexion

A

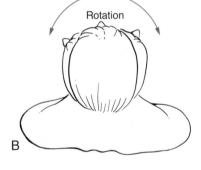

Rotation

B

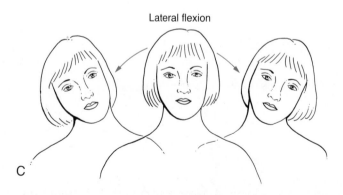

Lateral flexion

C

FIGURE 17–20. Range of motion at the cervical spine. *A,* Flexion and extension. *B,* Rotation. *C,* Lateral flexion.

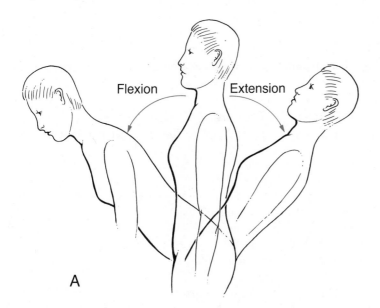

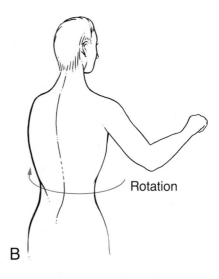

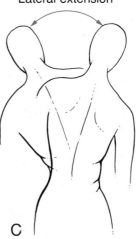

FIGURE 17–22. Range of motion at the lumbar spine. *A*, Flexion and extension. *B*, Rotation. *C*, Lateral extension.

REVIEW OF SPECIFIC SYMPTOMS

The most common symptoms of musculoskeletal disease are as follows:

- Pain
- Weakness
- Deformity
- Limitation of movement
- Stiffness
- Joint clicking

The location, character, and onset of each of these symptoms must be ascertained. It is important for the interviewer to determine the time course of any of these symptoms carefully.

Pain

Pain can result from pathology of the bone, muscle, or joint. Ask the following questions:

> *"When did you first become aware of the pain?"*
> *"Where do you feel the pain? Point to the most painful spot with one finger."*
> *"Did the pain occur suddenly?"*
> *"Does the pain occur daily?"*
> *"During which part of the 24 hour day is your pain worse? . . . morning?. . . afternoon?. . . evening?"*
> *"Did a recent illness precede the pain?"*
> *"What makes the pain worse?"*
> *"What do you do to relieve the pain?"*
> *"Is the pain relieved by rest?"*
> *"What kind of medications have you taken to relieve the pain?"*
> *"Have you noticed that the pain changes according to the weather?"*
> *"Do you have any difficulty in putting on your shoes or coat?"*
> *"Does the pain ever awaken you from sleep?"*
> *"Does the pain shoot to another part of your body?"*
> *"Have you noticed that the pain moves from one joint to another?"*
> *"Has there been any injury, overuse, or strain?"*
> *"Have you noticed any swelling?"*
> *"Are other bones, muscles, or joints involved?"*
> *"Have you had a recent sore throat?"*

Bone pain may occur with or without trauma. It is typically described as "deep," "dull," "boring," or "intense." The pain may be so intense that the patient is unable to sleep. Typically, bone pain is not related to movement unless a fracture is present. Pain from a fractured bone is often described as "sharp." Muscle pain is frequently described as "crampy." It may last only for a brief period or may last longer. Muscle pain in the lower extremity on walking, described in Chapter 12, suggests ischemia of the calf or hip muscles. Muscle pain associated with weakness is suspicious for a primary muscular disorder. Joint pain is felt around or in the joint. In some conditions, the joint may be exquisitely tender. Movement usually worsens the pain, except with rheumatoid arthritis, in which movement often reduces the pain. Pain experienced over several years' duration rules out an acute septic process and usually malignancy. Chronic infection that is due to tuberculosis or fungal infections may smoulder for years before pain is present. The severity of the pain may often be assessed by the interval between the onset of the pain and the time the patient sought medical attention.

The time of the day when the pain is worse may be helpful in diagnosing the disorder. The pain of many rheumatic disorders tends to be accentuated in the morning, particularly upon arising. Tendinitis worsens during the early morning hours and eases off by midday. Osteoarthritis worsens as the day progresses.

Sudden onset of pain in a metatarsophalangeal joint is suspicious for gout. Entrapment syndromes are apt to radiate pain distally. Severe pain may awaken any patient from sleep. Rheumatoid arthritis and tendinitis often cause early awakening because of pain, particularly when the patient is lying on the affected limb.

Acute rheumatic fever, leukemia, gonococcal arthritis, sarcoidosis, and juvenile rheumatoid arthritis are commonly associated with *migratory polyarthritis,* in which one joint is affected, the disease subsides, and then another joint becomes involved.

Viral illnesses are commonly associated with muscle aches and pains. A recent history of a sore throat with joint pains occurring 10–14 days later is suspicious for rheumatic fever. If rest does not relieve the pain, serious musculoskeletal disease may be present. The interviewer should keep in mind the possibility of *referred pain.* Pain from hip pathology is frequently referred to the knee, especially in the child.

Weakness

Muscular weakness should always be differentiated from fatigue. It is important to ascertain which functions the patient is unable to perform as a result of "weakness." Is the weakness related to proximal or distal muscle groups? *Proximal* weakness is usually a myopathy; *distal* weakness is usually a neuropathy. The patient with the symptom of muscular weakness should be asked these questions:

"Do you have difficulty in combing your hair?"
"Do you have difficulty in lifting objects?"
"Have you noticed any problem with holding a pen or pencil?"
"Do you have difficulty in turning doorknobs?"
"Do you have trouble standing up after sitting in a chair?"
"Do you find that, as the day goes on, there is a change in the weakness?" If so, *"Does the weakness worsen or improve?"*
"Have you noticed any decrease in your muscle size?"
"Are the weak muscles stiff?"
"Do you have trouble with double vision? . . . swallowing? . . . chewing?"

The patient with proximal weakness of the lower extremity has difficulty in walking and crossing his knees. A proximal weakness of the upper extremity is manifested by difficulty in brushing hair or lifting objects. A distal weakness of the upper extremity is manifested by difficulty in turning doorknobs or buttoning a shirt or blouse. Patients with myasthenia gravis have generalized weakness and have difficulty with diplopia and in swallowing and chewing.

Deformity

Deformity may be the result of a congenital malformation or an acquired condition. In any patient with a deformity, it is important to determine the following:

"When was the deformity first noticed?"
"Did the deformity occur suddenly?"
"Did the deformity occur as a result of trauma?"
"Has there been any change in the deformity with time?"

Limitation of Motion

Limitation of motion may result from changes in the articular cartilage, scarring of the joint capsule, or muscle contractures. It is important to determine the types of motion that the patient can no longer easily perform, such as combing the hair, putting on shoes, or buttoning a shirt.

Stiffness

Stiffness is a very common symptom of musculoskeletal disease. For example, a patient with arthritis of the hip may have difficulty in crossing his legs to tie his shoes. It is important to ask the patient whether the stiffness is worse at any particular time of the day. Patients with rheumatoid arthritis tend to have stiffness after periods of joint rest. Typically these patients describe morning stiffness, which may take several hours to improve.

Joint Clicking

Joint clicking is commonly associated with specific movements in the presence of dislocations of the humerus, displacement of the biceps tendon from its groove, degenerative joint disease, damaged knee meniscus, and temporomandibular joint (TMJ) problems.

IMPACT OF MUSCULOSKELETAL DISEASE ON THE PATIENT

Musculoskeletal diseases have an enormous impact on the life of the patient and his family. The perturbation of the patient's personal life and his restriction of activities as a result of his diability are frequently more catastrophic than the muscle or joint pain itself.

Diseases of the musculoskeletal system range from minor aches and pains to severe crippling disorders, often associated with premature death. Rheumatoid arthritis is a crippling disorder striking many patients in the prime of life. In addition to having the joint pain and reduction of activity, the patient with rheumatoid arthritis fears the possibility of being crippled for the rest of his life. Greater dependence on others occurs as the disease progresses. The disability alters the patient's self-image and self-esteem. The altered body image may be devastating; the patient often becomes withdrawn.

The physical limitations of musculoskeletal disease, especially when accompanied by joint or muscle pain, threaten the integrity of the patient in his social world. Marital and familial ties may suffer as the patient becomes further debilitated and withdrawn. Because of the patient's disability, he may have to change occupations, which causes him further anxiety and depression. The loss of status and financial adjustments may further jeopardize his marital situation. The fear of loss of independence is extremely common. The patient is forced to make more demands but recognizes that this may only worsen his relationship with others.

Rehabilitation is important for the physical and psychological improvement of the patient. The patient is the key contributor to this rehabilitative process. Motivation may first be provided by those caring for the patient, but it is the patient's own attitude that will ultimately determine whether the rehabilitation process will be successful. The motivation of the patient to tackle his disability depends on many factors, which include his self-image as well as his own psychological, social, and financial resources. It is incumbent on the physician to gain the patient's confidence to help him overcome his disability.

PHYSICAL EXAMINATION

> There is no special equipment necessary for the examination of the musculoskeletal system.

The purpose of the internist's musculoskeletal examination is as a screening examination to indicate or exclude functional impairment of the musculoskeletal system. The examination should take only a few minutes and should be part of the routine examination of all patients. If an abnormality is noted or if the patient has specific symptoms referable to a particular joint, a more detailed examination of that area is indicated. The detailed description of the examination of specific joints follows the discussion of the screening examination.

The Screening Examination

The screening examination should pay specific attention to the following:

- Inspection
- Palpation
- Passive and active range of motion
- Muscle strength
- Integrated function

General Principles

During inspection, any asymmetry should be assessed. Nodules, wasting, masses, or deformities may be responsible for the absence of symmetry. Are there any signs of inflammation? *Swelling, warmth, redness,* or *tenderness* suggests inflammation. To determine a difference in temperature, use the back of your hand to compare one side with the other.

Palpation may reveal areas of tenderness or discontinuity of a bone. Is *crepitus* present? Crepitus is a palpable crunching sensation often felt in the presence of roughened articular cartilages.

The *assessment of range of motion* of specific joints is next. It is very important for you to *recognize* that inflamed or arthritic joints may be painful. Move these joints *slowly!*

Muscle function and *integrated function* are usually evaluated during the neurologic examination, and these topics are discussed in the next chapter.

Evaluate Gait

The first part of the screening examination consists of inspection of gait and posture. Ask the patient to disrobe to his underwear and walk barefoot to determine any eccentricity of gait. Have the patient walk away from you, then back to you on tiptoes, away from you on his heels, and finally back to you in tandem gait. If there is difficulty in gait, modification of these maneuvers must be performed.

Observe the rate, rhythm, and arm motion employed in walking. Does the patient have a staggering gait? Are the feet lifted high and slapped downward firmly? Does the patient walk with an extended leg that is swung laterally during walking? Are the steps short and shuffling? A complete discussion of gait abnormalities follows in Chapter 18, The Nervous System. Figure 18–57 illustrates the more common types of gait abnormalities.

Evaluate the Spine

Attention should then be focused on the spine to detect any abnormal spinal curvatures. Have the patient stand erect. You should now stand at the patient's side to inspect the profile of the patient's spine. Are the cervical, thoracic, and lumbar curves normal?

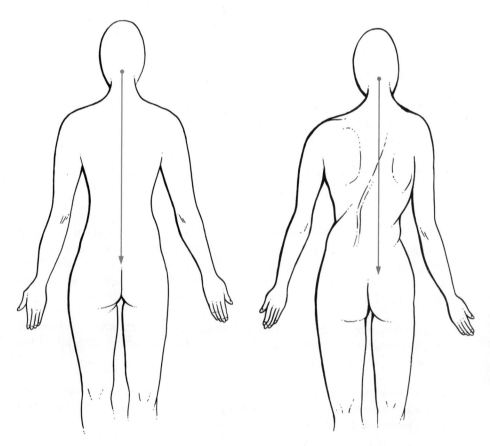

FIGURE 17–23. Technique of evaluating patient for "straightness" of the spine. The lateral deviation of the spine may be related to a herniated disc or to spasm of the paravertebral muscles. This functional deviation is often termed a **list.** True scoliosis may be due to an actual deformity of the spine. In many cases, the spine may actually twist in the opposite direction, so that a plumb line may actually be in the center.

You should move to inspect the patient's back. What is the level of the iliac crests? A difference may result from a leg length inequality, scoliosis, or flexion deformity of the hip. An imaginary line drawn from the posterior occipital tuberosity should fall over the intergluteal cleft. Any lateral curvature is abnormal. Figure 17–23 illustrates this point.

Ask the patient to bend forward, flexing at the trunk as far as possible with his knees extended. Note the smoothness of this action. This position is best for determining whether a scoliosis is present. As the patient bends forward, the lumbar concavity should flatten. A persistence of the concavity may indicate an arthritic condition of the spine called ankylosing spondylitis.

Ask the patient to bend to each side from the waist. Have the patient then bend backward from the waist to test *extension of the spine*, as shown in Figure 17–24A.

To test *rotation of the lumbar spine*, sit on a stool behind the patient and stabilize the patient's hips by placing your hands on them. Ask the patient to rotate his shoulders one way and then reverse, as shown in Figure 17–24B.

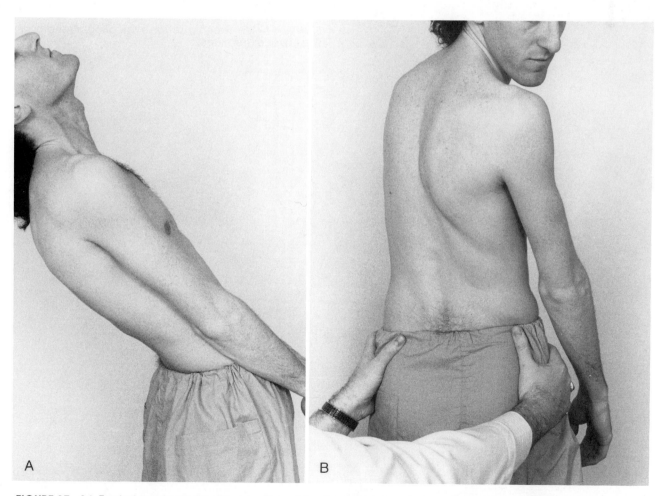

A

B

FIGURE 17–24. Technique for evaluating motion of the lumbar spine. *A,* Test for extension of the spine. *B,* Test for rotation of the spine.

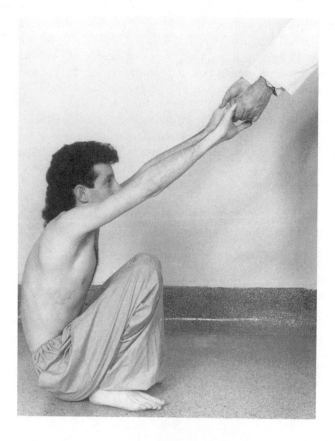

FIGURE 17–25. Technique for evaluating strength of the lower extremities.

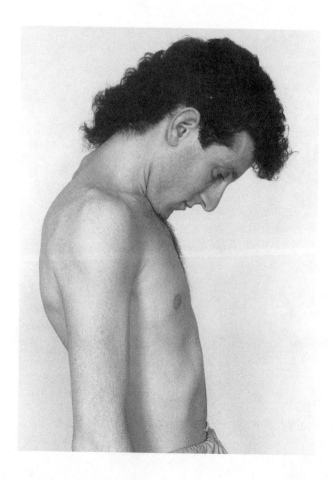

FIGURE 17–26. Technique for testing flexion of the neck.

Evaluate Strength of the Lower Extremities

To assess the function of all major joints of the lower extremities, stand in front of the patient and have him squat with his knees and hips fully flexed. Assist the patient by holding his hand to secure balance. This is shown in Figure 17–25. Ask the patient to then stand. Observing the manner in which the patient squats and then stands provides an excellent impression of the muscle strength and joint action of the lower extremities.

Evaluate Neck Flexion

The patient is instructed to sit, and the range of motion of the neck is assessed. The patient is asked to put his chin on his chest with his mouth closed, as shown in Figure 17–26. This tests full flexion of the neck.

Evaluate Neck Extension

To test full extension of the neck, place your hand between the occiput and the spinous process of C7. Instruct the patient to trap your hand by extending his neck. This is shown in Figure 17–27.

Evaluate Neck Rotation

Rotation of the neck is determined by asking the patient to rotate his neck to one side and have him touch his chin to his shoulder. This is shown in Figure 17–28. The examination is then repeated on the other side.

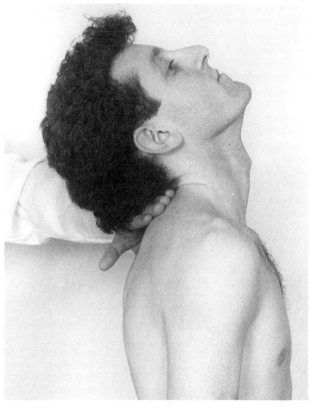

FIGURE 17–27. Technique for testing extension of the neck.

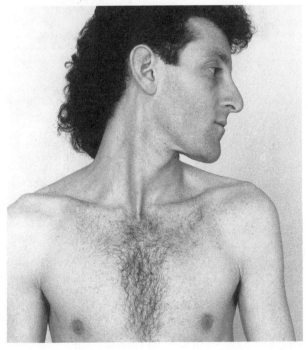

FIGURE 17–28. Technique for testing rotation of the neck.

Evaluate Intrinsics of the Hand

The patient is instructed to stretch out his arms in front of him with the fingers spread. The examiner then attempts to compress the fingers together against resistance, as shown in Figure 17–29. This tests the intrinsic muscles of the hands.

Evaluate External Rotation of the Arm

In order to test the functional range of external rotation of the humerus as well as the *shoulder, acromioclavicular,* and *sternoclavicular joints,* instruct the patient to abduct his arms fully and place his palms together above his head. The arms should touch the patient's ears with the head and cervical spine in the vertical position. This is shown in Figure 17–30.

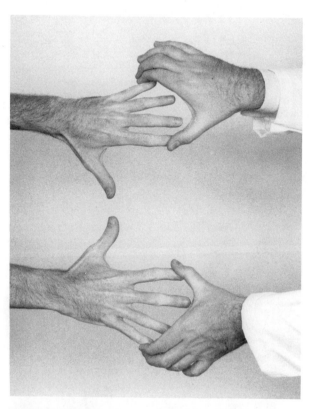

FIGURE 17–29. Technique for testing the intrinsic muscles of the hand.

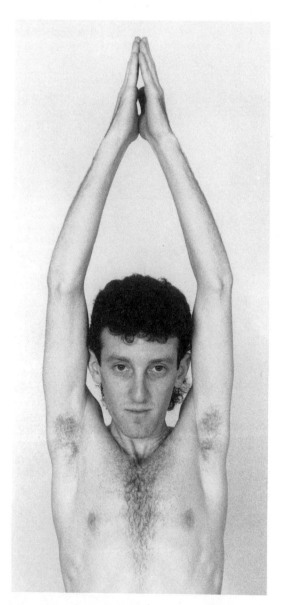

FIGURE 17–30. Technique for testing external rotation of the arm.

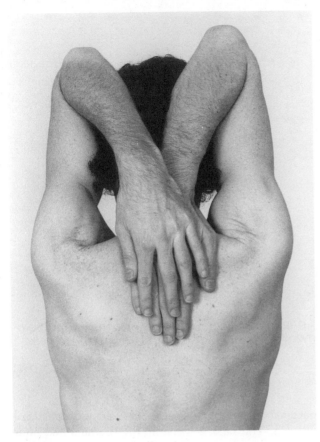

FIGURE 17–31. Technique for testing internal rotation of the arm.

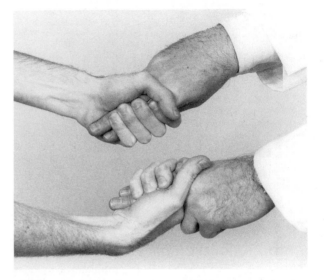

FIGURE 17–32. Technique for assessing strength in the upper extremities.

Evaluate Internal Rotation of the Arm

The patient is then asked to place his hands on his back between his scapulae. The hands should normally reach the level of the inferior angle of the scapulae. This is shown in Figure 17–31. This maneuver tests internal rotation of the humerus and the range of motion at the elbow.

Evaluate Strength of the Upper Extremities

The final test of the screening examination assesses the power of the major groups of muscles in the upper extremity. The patient is asked to grasp the index and middle fingers of the examiner in each hand. The patient is instructed to resist upward, downward, lateral, and medial movement by the examiner. This position is shown in Figure 17–32.

This completes the basic musculoskeletal screening examination. The remainder of this chapter describes the symptoms and examination of specific joints.

Examinations of Specific Joints

Any area must be inspected for evidence of swelling, atrophy, redness, or deformity, as well as palpated for swelling, muscle spasm, or local painful areas. The range of motion is assessed both actively and passively.

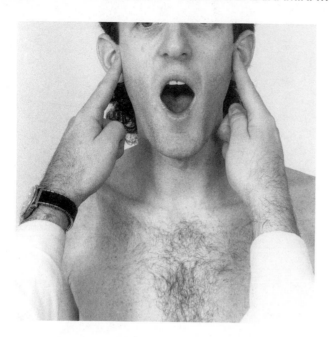

FIGURE 17–33. Technique for evaluating the temporo-mandibular joint.

Temporomandibular Joint
Symptoms

The patient with temporomandibular joint (TMJ) problems may complain of unilateral or bilateral jaw pain. The pain is worse in the morning and after chewing or eating. The patient may also complain of "clicking" of his jaw.

Examination

To examine the temporomandibular joint, the examiner should place his index fingers in front of the tragus and instruct the patient to open and close his jaw slowly. The examiner should observe the smoothness of the range of motion and note any tenderness. This is illustrated in Figure 17–33.

The Shoulder
Symptoms

Although shoulder pain may be related to a primary shoulder disorder, *always* consider the possibility of shoulder pain as being referred from either the chest or the abdomen. Coronary artery disease, pulmonary tumors, and gallbladder disease commonly are associated with referred pain to the shoulder.

Pain is the main symptom of shoulder disorders. Inflammation of the *supraspinatus muscle* causes pain that is usually worse at night or when the patient lies on the affected shoulder. The pain often radiates down the arm as far as the elbow. The pain is commonly referred to the lower part of the deltoid area and is characteristically aggravated by combing the hair, putting on a coat, or reaching into the back pocket. A diffusely tender shoulder associated with pain on moving the humerus posteriorly is associated with pathology of teres minor, infraspinatus, and subscapularis muscles. In this case, the pain usually does not radiate into the arm and is generally absent when the arm is dependent.

The movements of the shoulder occur at the glenohumeral, thoracoscapular, acromioclavicular, and sternoclavicular joints. The glenohumeral joint is a ball-and-socket joint. In contrast to the hip joint, which is also a ball-and-socket joint, in the glenohumeral joints the humerus sits into the very shallow glenoid socket. Therefore, the function of the joint depends upon the muscles surrounding the socket for stability. These muscles and their tendons form the *rotator cuff* of the shoulder. For this reason, many shoulder problems are muscular, and not actually bone or joint, in etiology.

Examination

Inspect the shoulder for any deformity, wasting, or asymmetry. The shoulder should be palpated for any local areas of tenderness. The range of motions for abduction, adduction, external and internal rotation, and flexion is evaluated and compared with that of the other side. Any pain is noted.

Special tests are required to determine specific diagnoses. The impingement syndrome, tears of the rotator cuff, and bicipital tendinitis are very common. The examinations for these conditions are described in this section.

The *impingement syndrome,* also known as *rotator cuff tendinitis,* is usually secondary to sports trauma. Irritation of the avascular portion of the supraspinatus tendon progresses to an inflammatory response known as *tendinitis.* This inflammatory response later involves the biceps tendon, subacromial bursa, and the acromioclavicular joint. With continued trauma, rotator cuff tears and calcification may occur. The most reliable test for the impingement syndrome is the reproduction of pain while the examiner forcibly flexes the patient's arm with the elbow extended against resistance.

Sudden onset of shoulder pain in the deltoid area within 6–10 hours after trauma suggests a *rotator cuff tear or rupture.* Extreme tenderness over the greater tuberosity of the humerus as well as pain and restricted motion at the glenohumeral joint is usually present. Active abduction of the glenohumeral joint is markedly reduced. When the examiner attempts to abduct the arm, pain and a characteristic *shoulder shrug* result.

Generalized tenderness anteriorly over the long head of the biceps associated with pain especially at night is suspicious for *bicipital tendinitis.* In this condition, there is normal abduction and forward flexion. The hallmark of bicipital tendinitis is the reproduction of anterior shoulder pain during resistance to forearm supination. The patient is asked to place his arm at his side with the elbow flexed 90°. The patient is then instructed to supinate his arm against the resistance by the examiner. If there is pain in the triceps area with resisted extension of the elbow, *tricipital tendinitis* may be present.

The Elbow

Symptoms

The most common symptom of elbow disorders is well-localized elbow pain.

Although a simple hinge joint, the elbow is the most complicated joint of the upper extremity. The distal end of the humerus articulates with the proximal ulna and radius. Flexion and extension of the elbow are effected through the humeroulnar portion of the joint. The radius plays little role in this action: its role is primarily in pronation and supination of the forearm. The ulnar nerve lies in a vulnerable position as it passes around the medial epicondyle of the humerus.

Examination

Palpate the elbow for any swelling, masses, tenderness, or nodules.

Test flexion and extension.

To test for pronation and supination, the elbows should be flexed at 90° and placed firmly on a table. The patient is asked to rotate his forearm and wrist

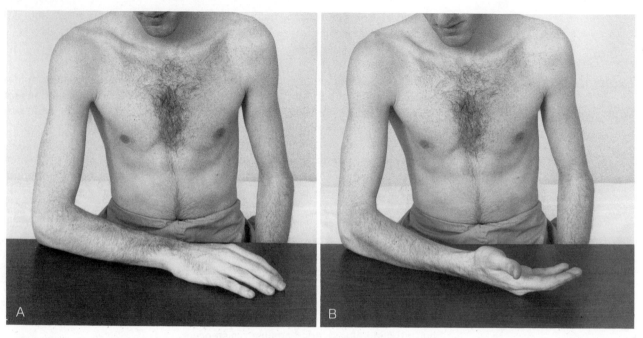

FIGURE 17–34. Technique for evaluating pronation and supination at the elbow. *A,* Pronation. *B,* Supination.

down (pronation), as shown in Figure 17–34*A*, and up (supination), as shown in Figure 17–34*B*. Any limitation of motion or pain is noted.

Tennis elbow, also known as *lateral epicondylitis,* is a common condition characterized by pain in the region of the lateral epicondyle of the humerus. The pain radiates down the extensor surface of the forearm. Patients with tennis elbow often experience pain when attempting to open a door or when lifting a glass. To test for tennis elbow, the examiner should flex the elbow and fully pronate the hand. Pain over the lateral epicondyle while extending the elbow is diagnostic of tennis elbow. Another test involves having the patient clench his fist, dorsiflex the wrist, and extend the elbow. In a patient with tennis elbow, pain will be elicited by trying to force the dorsiflexed hand into palmar flexion.

The Wrist

Symptoms

The symptoms of wrist disorders include pain in the wrist or hand, numbness or tingling in the wrist or fingers, loss of movement and stiffness, and deformities. It should be remembered that pain in the hand may be referred from the neck or elbow.

The wrist is composed of the articulation of the distal end of the radius with the proximal row of the carpal bones. The stability of the wrist is due to strong ligaments banding these bones together. The distal ulna does not articulate with any of the carpal bones. On the volar aspect of the wrist, the carpal bones are connected by the carpal ligament. The passage under this ligament is the *carpal tunnel,* through which the median nerve and all the flexors of the wrist pass. Entrapment of the nerve, known as *carpal tunnel syndrome,* produces symptoms of numbness and tingling.

Examination

Palpate the wrist joint between your thumb and index fingers, noting any tenderness, swelling, or redness (Fig. 17–35).

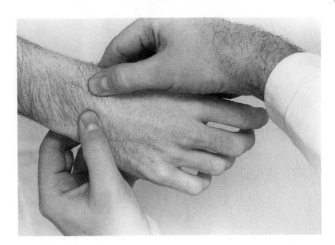

FIGURE 17–35. Technique for palpation of the wrist joint.

The range of motion of dorsiflexion and palmar flexion is noted. With the forearms fixed, the degree of supination and pronation is evaluated. Is there ulnar or radial deviation present?

When the diagnosis of carpal tunnel syndrome is suspected, a sharp tap or pressure directly over the median nerve may reproduce the paresthesias of the carpal tunnel syndrome. This has been termed *Tinel's sign*. Another useful test is for the examiner to stretch the median nerve by extending the patient's elbow and dorsiflexing the wrist. The development of pain or paresthesias suggests the diagnosis. A third test is to ask the patient to hold both wrists in a fully palmar-flexed position for 2 minutes. The development or exacerbation of paresthesias is suggestive of the carpal tunnel syndrome.

The Hand

Symptoms

Pain and swelling of joints are the most important symptoms of disorders of the hand.

Examination

Palpate the metacarpophalangeal joints and note any swelling, redness, or tenderness, as shown in Figure 17–36. Palpate the medial and lateral aspects

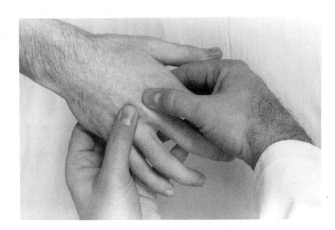

FIGURE 17–36. Technique for palpation of the metacarpophalangeal joints.

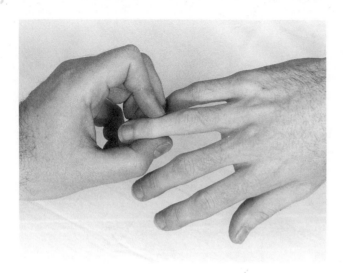

FIGURE 17–37. Technique for palpation of the inter-phalangeal joints.

of the proximal and distal interphalangeal joints between your thumb and index fingers, as shown in Figure 17–37. Note any swelling, redness, or tenderness.

The range of motion of the fingers includes the movements at the distal interphalangeal joint, the proximal interphalangeal joint, and the metacarpo-phalangeal joints of the fingers and the thumb.

Ask the patient to make a fist with the thumb across the knuckles and then extend and spread the fingers. The normal fingers should flex to the distal palmar crease. The thumb should oppose to the distal metacarpal head. Each finger should extend to the zero position in relation to its metacarpal.

de Quervain's disease is tenosynovitis of the thumb abductors and extensors. The patient complains of weakness of grip and of pain at the base of the thumb that is aggravated by certain movements of the wrist. To confirm the diagnosis, ask the patient to flex the thumb and close his fingers over it. You should now attempt to move the hand into ulnar deviation. Excruciating pain will accompany this maneuver if de Quervain's tenosynovitis is present.

The Spine

Symptoms

The most common symptom of pathology of the spine is pain. Pain from the thoracic spine often radiates around the trunk along the lines of the intercostal nerves. Pain from the upper lumbar spine may be felt in the front of the thighs and knees. Pain originating in the lower lumbar spine can be felt in the coccyx, hip, and buttocks as well as shooting down the back of the legs to the heel and foot. The pain is often intensified by movement. Patients with a herniated vertebral disc may complain of pain that is exacerbated by sneezing or coughing. It is important to determine whether there is associated numbness or tingling in the lower extremity, which is related to nerve root lesions.

Examination

The cervical spine may be examined with the patient seated. You should inspect the cervical spine from the front, back, and sides for any deformity or unusual posture. Test range of motion of the cervical spine. Palpate the para-vertebral muscles for tenderness or spasm.

The thoracolumbar spine is examined with the patient standing in front of the examiner. Inspect the spine for deformity or swelling. Inspect the spine from the

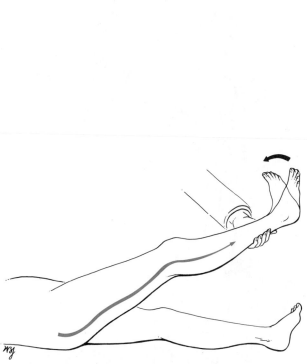

FIGURE 17-38. The straight leg raising test.

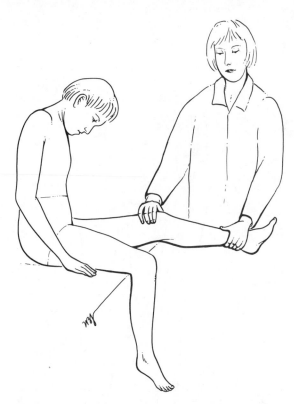

FIGURE 17-39. The sitting knee extension test.

side for abnormal curvature. Test range of motions. Palpate the paravertebral muscles for tenderness. Percuss each spinous process for tenderness.

The range of motions tested for the spine is composed of forward flexion, extension, lateral flexion, and rotation.

The presence of a *cervical rib* may cause coldness, discoloration, and trophic changes as a result of ischemia to an upper extremity. To test for a cervical rib, palpate the radial pulse. Move the arm through its range of motions. Obliteration of the pulse by this maneuver is suggestive of a cervical rib. Ask the patient to turn his head toward the affected side and take a deep breath while you are palpating the radial pulse on the same side. Obliteration of the pulse by this maneuver is also suggestive of a cervical rib. Often auscultation over the subclavian artery will reveal a bruit suggestive of mechanical obstruction by a cervical rib. With any of these tests, repeat them on the opposite side. Cervical ribs are rarely bilateral.

Pain from the sciatic nerve is called *sciatica*. Patients with sciatica describe pain, burning, or aching in the buttocks radiating down the posterior thigh to the posterolateral aspect of the calf. Pain is worsened by sneezing, laughing, or straining at stool. One of the tests for sciatica is the straight leg raising test. The patient is asked to lie supine while the examiner flexes the extended leg to the trunk at the hip. The patient is then asked to plantar flex and dorsiflex his foot. This test puts the sciatic nerve on stretch. If sciatica is present, this test will reproduce pain in the leg. The test is illustrated in Figure 17-38.

Another test for sciatica is the sitting knee extension test. In this test, the patient sits off the side of the bed and flexes his neck, placing his chin on his chest. The examiner fixes the thigh on the bed with one hand while the other hand extends the leg. If sciatica is present, pain will be reproduced as the leg is extended. This test is demonstrated in Figure 17-39.

445

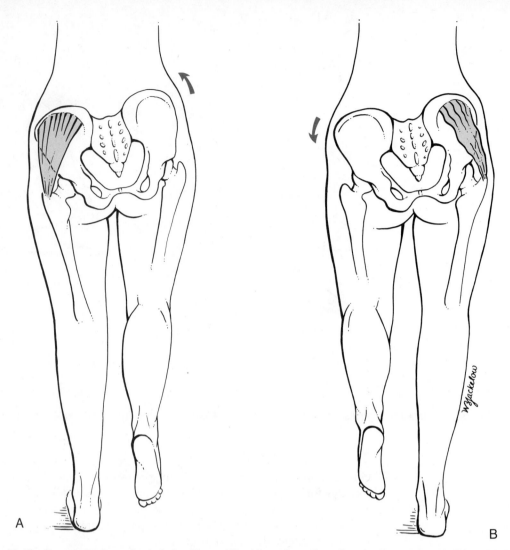

A   B

FIGURE 17–40. The Trendelenburg test. *A*, Position of the hips when standing on the normal left leg. Notice that the right hip elevates as a result of contraction of the left hip musculature. *B*, Position of the hips when standing on the abnormal right leg. Notice that the left hip falls as a result of lack of adequate contraction of the right hip muscles.

The Hip

Symptoms

The main symptoms of hip disease are pain, stiffness, deformity, and a limp. Hip pain may be localized to the groin or may radiate down the medial aspect of the thigh. Stiffness may be related to periods of immobility. An early symptom of hip disease is difficulty in putting on a shoe. This requires external rotation of the hip, which is the first motion to be lost with degenerative disease of the hip. This is followed by loss of abduction and adduction; finally, hip flexion is the last movement to be lost.

Examination

The examination of the hip is performed with the patient both standing and lying on his back.

Inspection of the hips and gait have already been described. The *Trendelenburg test* indicates pathology between the pelvis and the femur. The patient is asked to stand on his "good" leg, as illustrated in Figure 17–40A. The examiner should note that the pelvis on the opposite side elevates, demonstrating that the gluteal medius is working efficiently. When the patient is asked to stand on the "bad" leg, as shown in Figure 17–40B, the pelvis on the opposite side will fall. This is termed a positive Trendelenburg test.

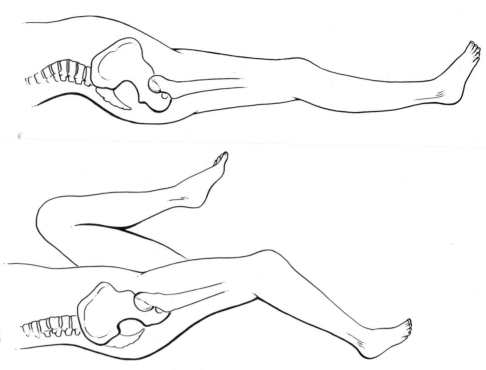

FIGURE 17–41. Evaluation for a flexion deformity of the hip.

Ask the patient to now lie on his back. The hip is acutely flexed on the abdomen to flatten the lumbar spine. A flexion of the opposite thigh suggests a flexion deformity of that hip. Figure 17–41 illustrates the technique.

Leg length measurements are useful in evaluating hip disorders. The distance between the anterior superior iliac spine to the tip of the medial malleolus is measured on each side and compared. A difference in leg length may be caused by hip joint disorders.

As indicated, loss of rotation of the hip is an early finding in hip disease. To test this movement, ask the patient to lie on his back. You should flex the hip and knee to 90° and rotate the ankle inward for external rotation, as illustrated in Figure 17–42A, and outward for internal rotation, as shown in Figure 17–42B. Restriction of this motion is a sensitive sign of degenerative hip disease.

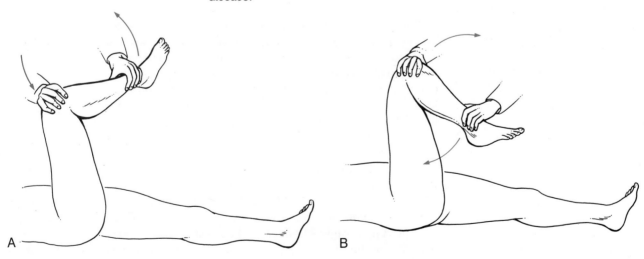

A   B

FIGURE 17–42. Testing the range of motion at the hip. The examiner flexes the hip and knee to 90° and rotates the ankle inward for external rotation (A), and outward for internal rotation (B).

The Knee
Symptoms

Although the knee is the largest joint in the body, it is not the strongest. The knee is a hinge joint between the femur and the tibia and permits flexion and extension. When flexed, a small degree of lateral motion is also normal. As with the shoulder, the knee depends on the strong muscles and ligaments around the joint for its stability.

Pain, swelling, joint instability, and limited movement are the main symptoms of knee pathology. Knee pain is exacerbated by movement and may be referred to the calf or thigh. Swelling of the knee indicates a synovial effusion or bleeding into the joint, also known as *hemarthrosis*. Knee trauma may result in hemarthrosis and limitation of joint motion. *Locking* of the knee results from small pieces of broken cartilage lodged between the femur and the tibia blocking full extension of the joint.

Examination

The examination of the knee is performed with the patient both standing and lying on his back.

While the patient is standing, any varus or valgus deformity should be noted. Is there wasting of the quadriceps muscle? Is there swelling of the knee? An early sign of knee joint swelling is the loss of the slight depressions on the lateral sides of the patella. You should inspect for any swelling in the popliteal fossa. A *Baker's cyst* in the popliteal fossa may be responsible for a swelling in the popliteal fossa causing calf pain.

The patient is then asked to lie on his back. The contours of the knee are evaluated. The patella is palpated in extension for tenderness. By stressing the patella against the femoral condyles, pain may be elicited. This occurs in osteoarthritis.

Testing for *knee joint effusion* is performed by pressing the fluid out of the suprapatellar pouch down behind the patella. Start about 15 cm above the superior margin of the patella and slide your index finger and thumb firmly downward along the sides of the femur, milking the fluid into the space between the patella and the femur. By maintaining pressure on the lateral margins of the patella, tap on the patella with the other hand. This technique is termed *ballottement*. In the presence of an effusion, a palpable tap will be felt and the transmitted impulse will be felt by the fingers on either side of the patella. This technique is shown in Figure 17–43.

There are several tests for the *collateral ligaments*. The knee is now flexed to 90° in order to palpate the tibiofemoral joint better. Allow the patient's foot to rest on the bed. You should grasp the patient's leg and press your thumbs lateral to the patellar tendon beneath the femoral epicondyles. The collateral ligaments may now be palpated. When an opening is detected on the medial aspect of the knee, damage of the medial collateral ligament is present; if the opening is on the lateral aspect, the lateral collateral ligament is ruptured. A medial collateral ligament rupture is illustrated in Figure 17–44.

Another test for *collateral ligament rupture* is performed by having the examiner place his left hand on the lateral aspect of the knee at the level of the joint. The knee is flexed about 25° and the lower leg is pushed outward by the examiner's right hand, using his left hand as a fulcrum. This maneuver attempts to "open up" the medial side of the knee joint. The finding should be compared with that of the other side. Abnormal lateral motion is seen in rupture of the medial collateral ligament, as illustrated in Figure 17–45. The maneuver may

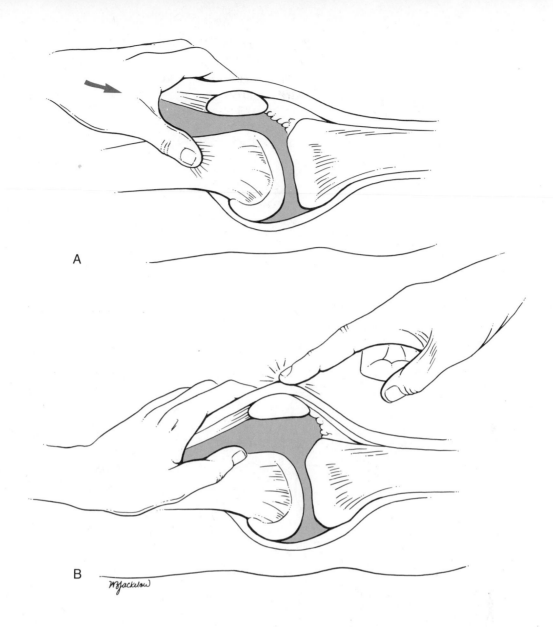

A

B

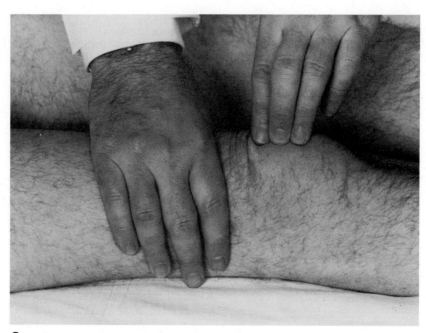

FIGURE 17–43. Technique for testing for a knee joint effusion. *A*, Position of the hand for pushing fluid out of the bursae. *B* and *C*, Position for tapping the patella.

C

449

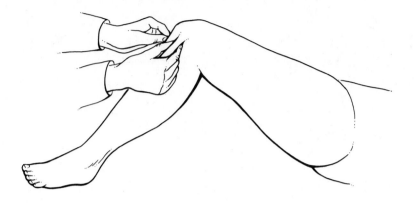

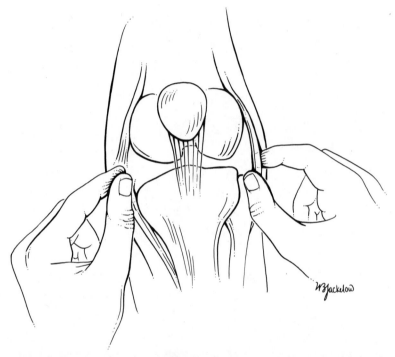

FIGURE 17–44. Technique for testing the collateral ligaments. Note the ruptured medial collateral ligament in the lower illustration.

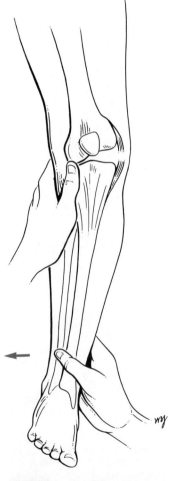

FIGURE 17–45. Another technique for testing the collateral ligaments.

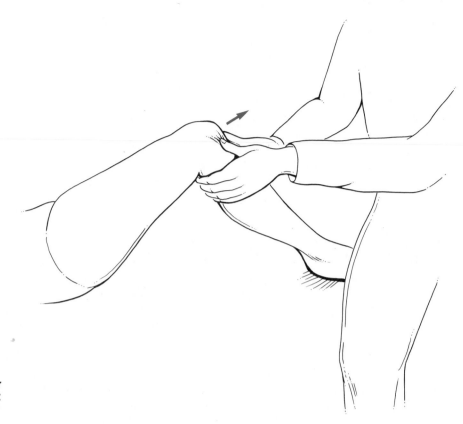

FIGURE 17-46. Technique for testing the cruciate ligaments: the drawer test.

be used to test for rupture of the lateral collateral ligament by reversing the positions.

The drawer test is used to test for rupture of the *cruciate ligaments*. The patient is instructed to flex his knee to 90°. The examiner should sit close to the foot to steady it. The examiner then grasps the leg just below the knee with both hands and jerks the tibia forward, as illustrated in Figure 17–46. Abnormal forward mobility of 2 cm or more suggests rupture of the anterior cruciate ligament. This maneuver may be used to test the posterior cruciate ligament by flexing the knee to 90°, steadying the foot, and attempting to jerk the leg backward. Abnormal backward motion of 2 cm or more indicates rupture of the posterior cruciate ligament.

The Ankle and Foot
Symptoms

Symptoms in the ankle and foot usually have a local etiology. These symptoms include pain, swelling, and deformities.

The patient's only complaint may be shoe wear. In normal sole wear, the sole is fairly evenly worn. The lateral sides may show maximum wear. Patients with flat feet wear down their soles on the medial side extending to the tip of the shoe. The outer portion of the heel is also worn out early. Scuff marks are usually present on the medial sides of the shoes. Patients with unusually high arches have excessive wear under the metatarsal head area. There is also excessive wear of the back of the heels.

The ankle is a hinge joint between the lower end of the tibia and the talus.

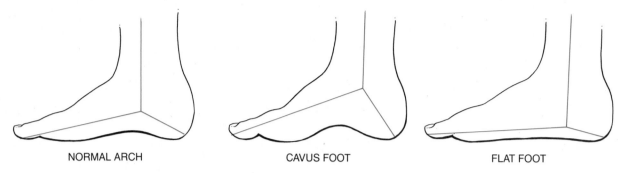

FIGURE 17–47. Common foot abnormalities.

Examination

The examination of the ankle and foot is performed with the patient standing and then sitting.

Ask the patient to stand. The ankles and feet are inspected for swellings and deformities. Abnormalities of the longitudinal arch are described. A *cavus foot* has an abnormallty high arch. A *flat foot* has the longitudinal arch flatter than normal. Common foot abnormalities are illustrated in Figure 17–47.

Ask the patient to sit with his feet dangling off the side of the bed. Palpate the medial and lateral malleoli. Palpate the Achilles tendon. Are there any nodules present? Is tenderness present?

Test the range of movements at the ankle, which includes dorsiflexion and plantar flexion.

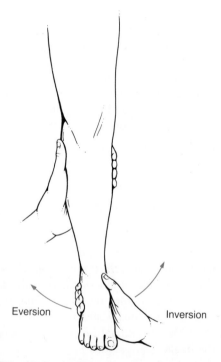

Eversion   Inversion

FIGURE 17–48. Evaluating the range of motions at the subtalar joint.

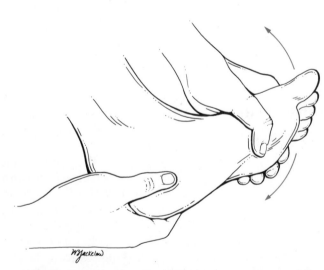

FIGURE 17–49. Evaluating the range of motion at the midtarsal joint.

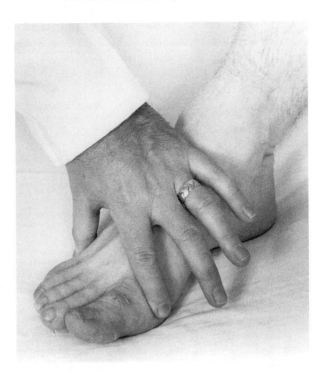

FIGURE 17–50. Technique for evaluating the metatarsophalangeal joints.

Test the range of movements at the subtalar joint, which includes eversion and inversion. You should hold the patient's leg in one hand and rotate the heel and foot with the other into eversion and inversion. This technique is shown in Figure 17–48.

Test the range of movements at the midtarsal joint, which includes eversion and inversion. Stabilize the heel with one hand and rotate the forefoot into eversion and inversion. This is demonstrated in Figure 17–49.

The movements of the metatarsophalangeal joints are tested individually. Palpate the head of each joint as well as the groove between them. Is tenderness present?

You should grasp the metatarsophalangeal joints between your thumb and index fingers and attempt to compress the forefoot. Pain elicted by this maneuver is often an early sign of *rheumatoid arthritis.* This test is demonstrated in Figure 17–50. Pain in the first metatarsophalangeal joint, a condition termed *podagra,* associated with redness and swelling suggests gout.

CLINICOPATHOLOGIC CORRELATIONS

Rheumatoid arthritis is a common musculoskeletal disorder and is the most destructive and disabling of the principal joint diseases. It is a condition of chronic inflammation not only of joints but also of many other organs. However, the joints display the most marked destructive changes. The most characteristic changes are found in the hands. In the early stages of the disease, there is swelling of the proximal interphalangeal, the metacarpophalangeal, and the wrist joints. As the disease progresses, there is bone erosion, which produces

TABLE 17–3. Clinical Features Differentiating Rheumatoid Arthritis from Osteoarthritis

Clinical Feature	Rheumatoid Arthritis*	Osteoarthritis†
Patient's age (yr)	3–80	Over 45
Morning stiffness	More than 1 hr	Less than 1 hr
Disability	Often great	Usually minimal
Joint distribution		
Distal interphalangeal joint	Rare	Very common
Proximal interphalangeal joint	Very common	Common
Metacarpophalangeal joint	Very common	Absent
Wrist	Very common	Absent
Soft tissue swelling	Very common	Rare
Interosseous muscle wasting	Very common	Rare
Swan-necking	Common	Rare
Ulnar deviation	Common	Absent

* See Plate XIV *E* and *F*.
† See Plate XV *A*.

the classic signs of the disease. The most characteristic deformity of the fingers is ulnar deviation at the metacarpophalangeal joints. The two main deformities of the interphalangeal joints are

- The swan-neck deformity
- The boutonnière deformity

The *swan-neck* deformity, which results from shortening of the interosseous muscles, produces flexion of the metacarpophalangeal joints, hyperextension of the proximal interphalangeal joints, and flexion of the distal interphalangeal joints. The *boutonnière* deformity is a flexion deformity of the proximal interphalangeal joints with hyperextension of the distal interphalangeal joints. Plate XIV *E* shows the hands of a woman with rheumatoid arthritis. Note the marked ulnar deviation of the metacarpophalangeal joints. Plate XIV *F* shows another patient with a characteristic swan-neck deformity.

TABLE 17–4. Clinical Features Differentiating Diseases Affecting the Hands and Wrists

Clinical Feature	Rheumatoid Arthritis	Psoriatic Arthritis*	Acute Gout	Osteoarthritis	Carpal Tunnel Syndrome
Age (yr)	3–80	10–60	30–80	50–80	40–80
Sex	F	M	M	F	M = F
Pain onset	Gradual	Gradual	Abrupt	Gradual	Gradual
Stiffness	Very common	Common	Absent	Common	Absent
Swelling	Common	Common	Common	Common	Common
Redness	Absent	Uncommon	Common	Uncommon	Absent
Deformity	Flexion of PIP and MCP; swan-neck;† boutonnière; ulnar deviation	Frequent DIP, PIP, and MCP involvement; "sausage" shaped digits	None in acute stage; resembles RA if deposits occur in tendon sheaths in chronic gout	Flexion and lateral deviation of DIP and PIP	Thenar muscle atrophy

* Needlepoint pitting of the nails is often associated with psoriatic arthritis. See Plate I *E* and Figure 5–7.
† See Plate XIV *F*.
Abbreviations: PIP = proximal interphalangeal joint; MCP = metacarpophalangeal joint; DIP = distal interphalangeal joint; RA = rheumatoid arthritis.

TABLE 17–5. Clinical Features Differentiating Diseases Affecting the Elbow

Clinical Feature	Rheumatoid Arthritis	Psoriatic Arthritis	Acute Gout*	Osteoarthritis	Tennis Elbow
Age (yr)	3–80	10–60	30–80	50–80	20–60
Sex	F	M	M	F	M = F
Pain onset	Gradual	Gradual	Abrupt	Gradual	Gradual
Stiffness	Very common	Common	Absent	Common	Occasional
Swelling	Common	Common	Common	Common	Absent
Redness	Absent	Uncommon	Common	Absent	Absent
Deformity	Flexion contractures, usually bilaterally	Flexion contractures, usually bilaterally	Flexion contractures only in chronic state	Flexion contractures	None

* See Plate XV *B*. This patient has chronic tophaceous gout with painless tophi on her elbows.

Osteoarthritis, or degenerative joint disease, is also very common. In most cases, the inflammatory response is minimal as compared with rheumatoid arthritis. The picture of osteoarthritis depends on the joints involved. One of the more frequently involved joints is the distal interphalangeal joint. Progressive enlargement of these joints has been termed *Heberden's nodes.* As the disease progresses, the proximal interphalangeal joints may become involved. The name often given to involvement of these joints is *Bouchard's nodes.* Plate XV *A* shows the hands of a woman with osteoarthritis.

Gout is a metabolic disease characterized by high levels of uric acid, recurrent attacks of acute arthritis, and deposition of urate crystals in and around the joints. The initial presentation is frequently acute pain in the first metatarsophalangeal joint (podagra), often awakening the patient from sleep. Even at rest, the pain is severe, but the slightest movement of the joint is agonizing. Within a few hours, the joint becomes swollen, shiny, and red. The higher the level of uric acid, the more likely the patient is to develop *tophi,* which are subcutaneous and periarticular deposits of urate crystals. The commonly involved sites are over the first metatarsophalangeal joint, the finger, the ear, the elbow, and the Achilles tendon. Plate XV *B* shows a patient with chronic tophaceous gout having large tophi on her elbows as well as smaller tophi on her hands.

Table 17–3 summarizes the important clinical features of rheumatoid arthritis and osteoarthritis. Table 17–4 summarizes some of the important features of diseases affecting the hands and wrists. Table 17–5 outlines the clinical features of important musculoskeletal disorders affecting the elbow. Table 17–6 lists the features of important diseases affecting the knee.

TABLE 17–6. Clinical Features Differentiating Diseases Affecting the Knee

Clinical Feature	Rheumatoid Arthritis	Psoriatic Arthritis	Acute Gout	Osteoarthritis	Torn Meniscus
Age (yr)	3–80	10–60	30–80	50–80	20–60
Sex	F	M	M	F	M
Pain onset	Gradual	Gradual	Abrupt	Gradual	Abrupt
Stiffness	Very common	Common	Absent	Common	Occasional
Swelling	Common	Common	Common	Common	Common
Redness	Absent	Uncommon	Common	Absent	Absent
Deformity	Flexion contractures	Flexion contractures	Flexion contractures only in chronic state	Flexion contractures	None

USEFUL VOCABULARY

Listed here are the specific roots that are important in order to understand the terminology related to musculoskeletal diseases.

ROOT	PERTAINING TO	EXAMPLE	DEFINITION
arthr(o)-	joint	*arthro*gram	An x-ray of a joint
myo-	muscle	*myo*pathy	Disease of muscle
oste(o)-	bone	*osteo*malacia	A condition marked by softening of the bones
scolio-	twisted	*scolio*sis	Lateral deviation of the spine
teno-	tendon	*teno*tomy	Surgical cutting of a tendon

WRITING UP THE PHYSICAL EXAMINATION

Listed here are examples of the write-up for the examination of the musculoskeletal system.

All of the joints have a full range of motion. No deformities, tenderness, or abnormalities are detected.

There is marked ulnar deviation of both hands associated with a flexion deformity of all the proximal interphalangeal joints and hyperextension of all the distal interphalangeal joints. Marked tenderness of both wrists is present.

There is abnormal forward mobility of the knee. There is 3–4 cm of motion detected.

The left first metatarsophalangeal joint is markedly erythematous and painful. The joint is shiny and edematous. There is also a large, 2 cm, hard, whitish mass on the pinna of the patient's right ear.

No joint deformities are noted. There is marked reduction of hip internal and external rotation. No pain is produced by these movements. There is pain produced by abduction of the right shoulder against resistance. The range of right shoulder abduction is reduced. The range of motion of the hands, wrists, spine, knees, and ankles is normal.

BIBLIOGRAPHY

Birnbaum JS: The Musculoskeletal Manual. Orlando, FL, Grune and Stratton, 1986.

Cooper BS, Rice DP: The economic cost of illness revisited. Sco Sec Bull *39*:21, 1976.

D'Ambrosia RD: Musculoskeletal Disorders: Regional Examination and Differential Diagnosis. Philadelphia, JB Lippincott, 1986.

Dieppe PA, Bacon PA, Bamji AN, Watt I: Atlas of Clinical Rheumatology. Philadelphia, Lea and Febiger, 1986.

Freeland M, Calat C, Schendler CE: Projections of national health expenditures, 1980, 1985, and 1990. Health Care Fin Rev *1*(3):1, 1980.

Gartland JJ: Fundamentals of Orthopaedics, 4th ed. Philadelphia, WB Saunders Co, 1987.

Kelsey JL, Pastides H, Bisbee GE Jr: Musculo-Skeletal Disorders: Their Frequency of Occurrence and Their Impact on the Population of the United States. New York, Prodist, 1978.

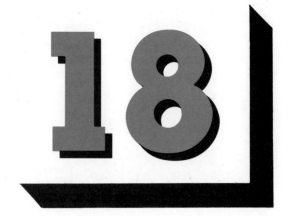

THE NERVOUS SYSTEM

As the debility increases and the influence of the will over the muscles fades, the tremulous agitation becomes more vehement. It now seldom leaves him for a moment; but even when exhausted nature seizes a small portion of sleep, the motion becomes so violent as not only to shake the bed-hangings, but even the floor and sashes of the room. The chin is now almost immovably bent down upon the sternum. The slops with which he is attempted to be fed, with the saliva, are continually trickling from the mouth. The power of articulation is lost. The urine and faeces are passed involuntarily; and at the last, constant sleepiness, with slight delirium, and other marks of extreme exhaustion, announce the wished-for release.

James Parkinson
1755 – 1824

GENERAL CONSIDERATIONS

By the second century AD, Galen had already described the cerebral ventricles, seven of the twelve cranial nerves, and the cerebral convolutions. There was, however, little further interest in the anatomy and physiology of the neurologic system until the sixteenth century. In 1543, Vesalius illustrated the basal ganglia, and in 1552, Eustachius described the cerebellar peduncles and the pons.

The seventeenth century saw the descriptions and illustrations by Willis of the cerebral circulation, the "striate body," and the internal capsule. Bartholin and others felt that the function of the cerebral cortex was to protect the blood vessels, whereas other investigators felt that the cerebrum possessed higher functions. Pourfour du Petit stressed that the cortex was responsible for motor activity. This concept, however, lay dormant until the end of the nineteenth century.

Careful anatomic descriptions of the tracts, nuclei, and gyri were described in the writings of the scientists of the eighteenth and early nineteenth centuries. Reil and Burdach provided names for the many gross anatomic structures that had been illustrated by others in the previous centuries. Reil has been credited with the naming of the insula, the capsule, the uncinate and cingular fasculi, and the tapetum. The uncus, lenticular nucleus, pulvinar, cingulate, and gyrus cinguli were named by Burdach. During this same period, Soemmering, Vicq d'Azyr, Gall, Gratiolet, and Rolando made many detailed illustrations of the cerebral convolutional patterns.

The early eighteenth century saw the beginnings of the descriptions of several disease states. In 1817, James Parkinson wrote an essay describing the "shaking palsy" that now bears his name. In 1829, Charles Bell wrote:

> . . . The next instance was in a man wounded by the horn of an ox. The point entered under the angle of the jaw and came out before the ear . . . He remains now a singular proof of the effects of the loss of function in the muscles of the face by this nerve being divided. The forehead of the corresponding side is without motion, the eyelids remain open, the nostril has no motion in breathing, and the mouth is drawn to the opposite side.

This is the classic description of facial nerve (seventh cranial nerve) palsy, also known as Bell's palsy.

In the mid-nineteenth century, an interest in microscopic neuroanatomy sprang up. Purkinje, Schwann, and Helmholtz were but a few of the many neuroanatomists who contributed valuable information about the intricacies of the nervous system. However, it was not until the late nineteenth century that specific staining techniques were developed by Golgi, Marchi, and Nissl, which lead the way to our current understanding of neuronal disease. The nerve cell had finally been discovered.

The twentieth century saw further progress in the description of the cerebral cortex, anterior commissure, thalamus, and hypothalamus. A major advance came from the work of Cajal in 1904. His careful histologic exploration clarified the complexities of the neuron. It was not until 1925 that the hypophyseo-hypothalamic connections were described, and even to this day, the function of the hypothalmus is not fully understood.

It has been suggested that over 40% of patients who present to the internist have symptoms referrable to neurologic disease. The internist must have the ability to identify the early signs and symptoms of neurologic disease in order to initiate the appropriate therapy. All too often, subtle signs and symptoms may be ignored and a diagnosis is not made until advanced disability is apparent.

The internist holds an important position because the patient with a neurologic problem will usually seek help from him first. A thorough knowledge of the basic neuroanatomy and physiology is the cornerstone of neurologic diagnosis.

STRUCTURE AND PHYSIOLOGY

The brain, which is enclosed in the cranium and surrounded by the meninges, is the center of the nervous system. The brain can be divided into the cerebral cortex, basal ganglia, thalamus and hypothalamus, midbrain, brain stem, and cerebellum.

The two *cerebral hemispheres* make up the largest portion of the brain. Each hemisphere may be subdivided into four major lobes named for the cranial bones that overlie them: frontal, parietal, occipital, and temporal. The fissures and sulci divide the cerebral surface. A deep midline, longitudinal fissure sepa-

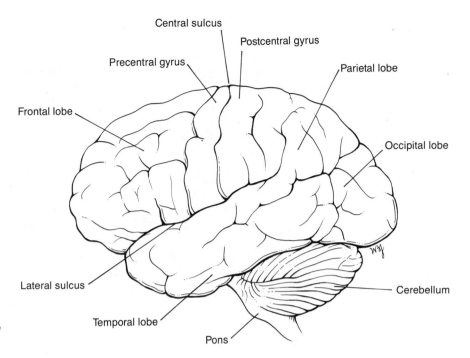

FIGURE 18-1. Lateral view of the left cerebral hemisphere.

rates the two hemispheres. The convolutions, or gyri, lie between the fissures. A lateral view of the left cerebral hemisphere is shown in Figure 18-1. Figure 18-2 shows a medial view of the right cerebral hemisphere. A basal view of the cerebral hemispheres is shown in Figure 18-3.

The cerebrum is responsible for motor, sensory, associative, and higher mental functions. The primary *motor cortex* is located in the precentral gyrus. Neurons in this area control voluntary movements of the skeletal muscle on the

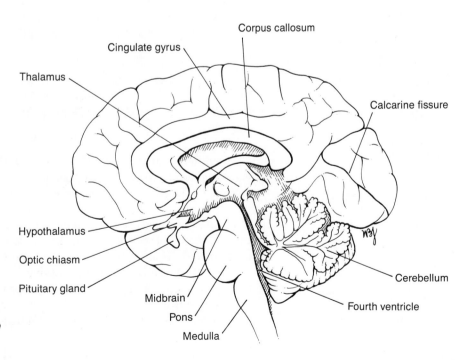

FIGURE 18-2. Medial view of the right cerebral hemisphere.

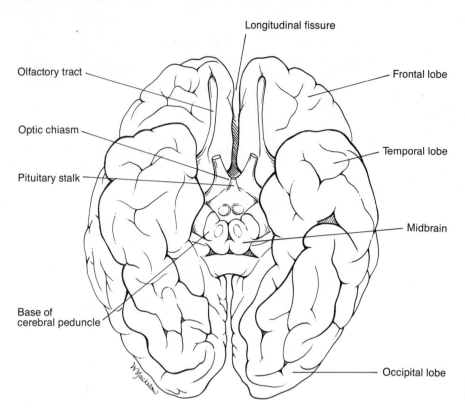

FIGURE 18–3. Basal view of the cerebral hemispheres.

opposite side of the body. An irritative lesion in this area may cause seizures or changes in consciousness. Destructive lesions in this area can produce contralateral flaccid paresis or paralysis.

The primary *sensory cortex* is located in the postcentral gyrus. Irritative lesions in this area may produce paresthesias (''numbness'' or ''pins and needles'' sensations) on the opposite side. Destructive lesions produce an impairment in cutaneous sensation on the opposite side.

The primary *visual cortex* is located in the occipital lobe along the calcarine fissure, which divides the cuneus from the lingual gyri. Irritative lesions in this area produce visual symptoms such as flashes of light or rainbows. Destructive lesions cause an homonymous hemianopsia on the contralateral side. Central macular vision is spared.

The primary *auditory cortex* is located in the temporal lobe along the transverse temporal gyrus. Irritative lesions in this area produce a buzzing or ringing in the ears. Destructive lesions rarely produce deafness.

The *basal ganglia* are situated deep to the cerebral hemispheres. The structures of the basal ganglia include the caudate and lenticular nuclei, the internal capsule, and the amygdala. These are important structures in the extrapyramidal system, which is concerned with modulating voluntary body movements, postural changes, and autonomic integration. The basal ganglia are especially involved with fine movements of the extremities. Disturbances of the basal ganglia can result in tremors and rigid movements.

The *thalamus* is a large mass located in the center of the brain, with the third ventricles lateral to it. The thalamus serves as a relay station for sensory and motor impulses traveling to the brain. All sensory impulses pass through the thalamus on the way to the cerebrum. The thalamus is also involved with the control of primitive responses such as fear and self-preservation. It appears that the thalamus may be the critical structure for the perception of pain and temperature, and that the cortex may only modify the thalamic impression.

The *hypothalamus* is located below the thalamus. It includes the optic chiasm and the neurohypophysis. The hypothalamus is responsible for many regulatory mechanisms, such as temperature regulation; neuroendocrine control of catecholamines, thyroid stimulating hormone, adrenocorticotropic hormone, follicle stimulating and luteinizing hormones, prolactin, and growth hormones; thirst; appetite; water balance; and sexual behavior.

The *midbrain* contains the superior and inferior colliculi; the cerebral peduncles; and the nuclei of the trochlear, oculomotor, and trigeminal nerves. The superior colliculi are associated with the visual system, whereas the inferior colliculi are associated with the auditory system. The cerebral peduncles converge from the inferior aspect of the cerebral hemispheres and enter the pons. A destructive lesion of the superior colliculi causes paralysis of upward gaze. Destructive lesions of the cranial nerve nuclei produce the classic paralysis of the affected nerve. A destructive lesion of the cerebral peduncle gives rise to spastic paralysis on the other side of the body. Destruction of still other tracts in the midbrain results in rigidity and involuntary movements. Figure 18–4 shows the external anatomy of the midbrain.

The *brainstem* consists of the *pons* and *medulla.* The brainstem is responsible for relaying all messages between the upper and lower levels of the central nervous system. Cranial nerves III through XII also arise from the brainstem. The brainstem, thalamus, and hypothalamus constitute the *reticular formation,* a network that provides for constant muscle stimulation to counteract the force of gravity. In addition to its anti-gravity effects, this area of the brain is essential

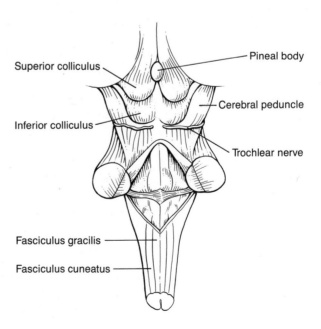

FIGURE 18–4. Anatomy of the midbrain.

for the control of consciousness. The neurons in the reticular activating system are capable of waking and arousing the entire brain.

The pons lies ventral to the cerebellum and rostral to the medulla. The abducens, facial, and acoustic (and vestibular) nuclei are found within the pons, and their nerves exit through a groove that divides the pons from the medulla. The motor and sensory nuclei of the trigeminal nerve are also located in the pons. At this level, the corticospinal tracts (also known as the pyramidal tracts) have not yet crossed, and a lesion at this level will produce loss of voluntary movement on the opposite side. Destructive lesions of the pons may produce a wide variety of clinical syndromes, such as the following:

- Contralateral hemiplegia with ipsilateral trigeminal hemiplegia (paralysis of the jaw muscles and loss of sensation over the same side of the face)
- Contraleral hemiplegia with ipsilateral facial palsy (Bell's palsy)
- Contralateral hemiplegia with ipsilateral facial palsy and ipsilateral abducens palsy (paralysis of the lateral rectus muscle on the same side of the face)
- Contralateral hemiplegia with ipsilateral abducens palsy
- Quadriplegia and nystagmus

The medulla is the portion of the brainstem between the pons and the spinal cord. The nuclei of the hypoglossal, vagus, glossopharyngeal, and spinal accessory nerves are located within the medulla. It should be remembered that it is within the medulla that the majority of the corticospinal tracts cross to the opposite side. Destructive lesions in the medulla produce symptoms that are referable to the tracts interrupted by the lesion. Some important clinical syndromes are as follows:

- Contralateral hemiplegia with ipsilateral hypoglossal palsy*
- Ipsilateral vagal palsy† with contralateral loss of pain and temperature sense
- Ipsilateral vagal palsy with ipsilateral spinal accessory palsy‡
- Ipsilateral vagal palsy with ipsilateral hypoglossal palsy
- Ipsilateral vagal palsy, ipsilateral spinal accessory palsy, and ipsilateral hypoglossal palsy

There are many more clinical syndromes, which are beyond the scope of this text. The reader is advised to review the neuroanatomy further in order to understand the complexities of these neurologic syndromes.

The *cerebellum* is located in the posterior fossa of the skull and is composed of a small midline lobe and two large lateral hemispheres. The cerebellum acts to keep the individual oriented in space and to halt or check motions. The cerebellum is also responsible for the fine movements of the hands. Essentially, the cerebellum coordinates and refines the action of muscle groups to produce steady and precise movements. Destructive lesions of the cerebellum will cause swaying, staggering, intention tremors,§ and the inability to change movements rapidly.

---

* Paralysis of the tongue muscles on the same side of the lesion. The tongue deviates to the side of the lesion when the patient is asked to stick out his tongue.

† Paralysis of the soft palate and difficulty in speaking, known as *dysarthria*.

‡ Paralysis of the sternocleidomastoid and/or trapezius muscles. This results in the inability to turn the head to the side opposite the lesion and to shrug the shoulder.

§ Tremors that result when the individual moves his hands to do something but may not be present at rest.

The blood supply to the brain is 80% through the internal carotid arteries and 20% through the vertebral basilar arteries. Each internal carotid artery terminates as the anterior cerebral and middle cerebral arteries. The posterior cerebral artery arises from the basilar artery, which joins with the posterior communicating artery, a branch of the internal carotid artery. The two anterior cerebral arteries are joined by the anterior communicating artery. This vascular network forms the circle of Willis, located at the base of the brain. This is illustrated in Figure 18–5.

Continuous with the medulla is the *spinal cord,* a cylindrical mass of neuronal tissue measuring 40–45 cm in length in the adult. Its distal end attaches to the first segment of the coccyx. The spinal cord is divided into two symmetrical halves by the anterior median fissure and the posterior median sulcus. Each half can be further subdivided into white and gray matter. This is illustrated in Figure 18–6.

In the center of the spinal cord is the *gray matter.* The anterior gray matter, the *anterior horn,* is the motor portion of the spinal cord and is composed of the cells of origin of the *anterior roots* of the peripheral nerves. The posterior gray matter, the *posterior horn,* is the receptor portion of the spinal cord.

The *white matter* of the spinal cords consists of tracts that serve to link segments of the spinal cord and to connect it to the brain. There are three main

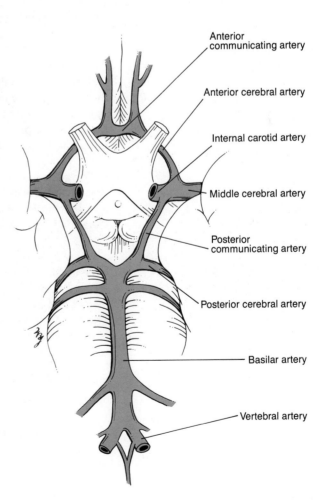

FIGURE 18–5. The circle of Willis.

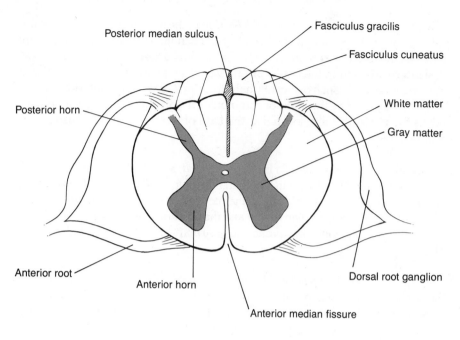

FIGURE 18-6. Cross-section through the spinal cord.

columns. Between the anterior median fissure and the anterolateral sulcus is the *anterior white column,* which contains the descending fibers of the *ventral corticospinal* tract and the ascending fibers of the *ventral spinothalamic* tract. The ventral corticospinal tract is involved with voluntary motion, whereas the ventral spinothalamic tract carries light touch.

The *lateral white column* is located between the anterolateral and posterolateral sulci and contains the descending fibers of the *lateral corticospinal* tract and the ascending *spinocerebellar* and *lateral spinothalamic* tracts. The lateral corticospinal tract is responsible for voluntary movement; the spinocerebellar tract carries reflex proprioception; the lateral spinothalamic tract carries pain and temperature sensation.

The *posterior white column* is located between the posterolateral and posterior median sulcus. The most important fibers in this column are the ascending fibers of the *fasciculus gracilis* and the *fasciculus cuneatus.* These tracts carry vibration sense, passive motion, joint position, and two-point discrimination.

There are 31 pairs of spinal roots, each having an anterior and posterior root. Each nerve consists of a sensory and a motor root. The anterior root consists of *efferent* nerve fibers, which have originated in the anterior and lateral gray matter and travel to the peripheral nerve and muscle. This is the motor root. The posterior root consists of *afferent* nerve fibers, which have their cell bodies in the *dorsal root ganglion.* This is the sensory root.

The *spinal nerves* are grouped into 8 cervical (C1–C8), 12 thoracic (T1–T12), 5 lumbar (L1–L5), 5 sacral (S1–S5), and 1 coccygeal nerve. These nerves are shown in Figure 18–7.

A *spinal reflex* involves an afferent neuron and an efferent neuron at the same level in the spinal cord. The basis for this reflex arc is an intact sensory limb, functional synapses in the spinal cord, an intact motor limb, and a muscle

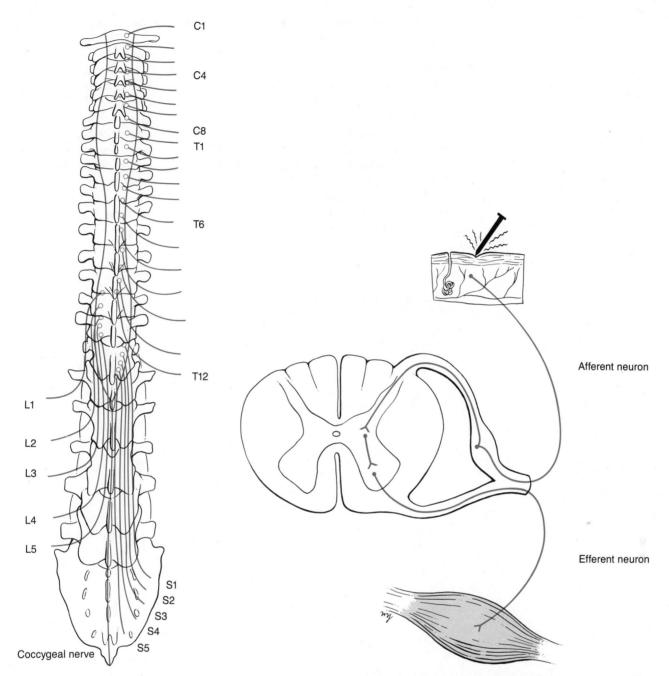

FIGURE 18–7. The spinal nerves.

FIGURE 18–8. The reflex spinal arc.

capable of responding. The afferent and the efferent limbs travel together in the same spinal nerve. When a stretched muscle is suddenly stretched further, the afferent sensory limb sends impulses through its spinal nerve that travel to the posterior root of that nerve. After synapsing in the gray matter of the spinal cord, the impulse is transmitted to the anterior nerve root. These impulses are then conducted through the anterior root to the neuromuscular junction, where a brisk contraction of the muscle completes the reflex arc. Figure 18–8 illustrates a reflex spinal arc.

The afferent sensory limb is not only important in the reflex arc but is also important in the conscious appreciation of sensation. Nerve fibers carrying pain and temperature sensation enter the spinal cord and cross to the other side within one or two spinal segments. They ascend in the contralateral *lateral spinothalamic tract*, travel through the brainstem and the thalamus, and end in the postcentral gyrus of the parietal lobe, as illustrated in Figure 18–9A. Fibers carrying *proprioceptive* sensation from muscles, joints, and tendons enter the posterior root and participate in the reflex arc. Other fibers carrying proprioceptive sensation pass directly into the *posterior columns* and ascend in the fasciculi gracilis and cuneatus to their ipsilateral nuclei, cross in the medial lemniscus, synapse in the thalamus, and end in the postcentral gyrus of the parietal lobe. Still other proprioceptive fibers ascend crossed and uncrossed in the spinocerebellar tracts to the cerebellum. These additional pathways are illustrated in Figure 18–9B.

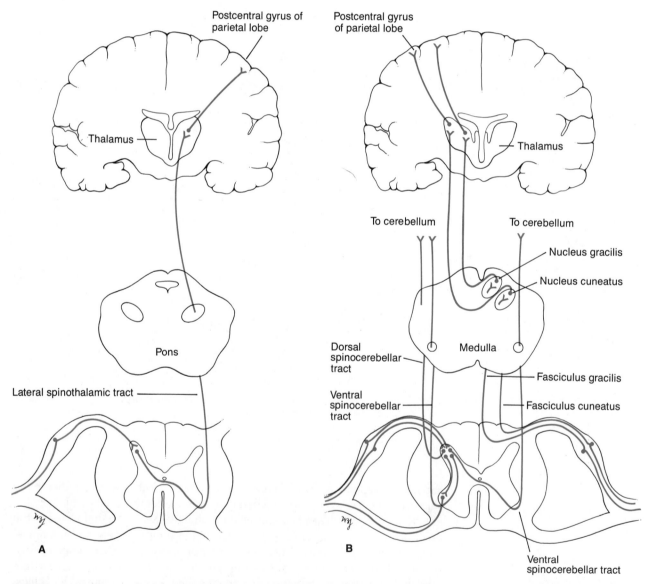

FIGURE 18–9. The conscious appreciation of sensation. *A*, Nerve pathways for pain and temperature sensation through the lateral spinothalamic tracts. *B*, Pathways of the fibers carrying proprioceptive sensation through the posterior columns and in the spinocerebellar tracts.

REVIEW OF SPECIFIC SYMPTOMS

The most common symptoms of neurologic disease are as follows:

- Headache
- Loss of consciousness
- "Dizziness"
- Ataxia (unsteadiness on the feet)
- Changes in consciousness
- Visual disturbances
- Dysphasia (speech abnormalities)
- Brain failure (failing memory, etc.)
- Cerebral vascular accidents (strokes)
- Gait disorders
- Tremor
- "Numbness"
- "Weakness"
- Pain

Headache

Headache is the most common neurologic symptom. It has been estimated that more than 35 million individuals in the United States suffer from recurrent headaches. Most of these patients have headaches that are related to migraine and muscle contraction or to tension. A headache pattern that is *unchanged* and has been present for several years is unlikely to be related to the present illness of the patient. Several points must be clarified in any patient complaining of a recent change in the frequency or severity of the headaches. Ask the following questions:

"For how long have you been having headaches?"
"When did you notice a change in the pattern or severity of your head-aches?"
"How has the pattern of your headaches changed?"
"How often does your headache occur?"
"How long does each headache last?"
"Which part of your head aches?"
"Describe what the headache feels like?"
"How quickly does the headache reach its maximum?"
"When you get the headache, do you have any other symptoms?"
"Are you aware of anything that produces the headache?"
"Are there any warning signs?"
"Does anything make the headache worse?"
"What makes the headache better?"

Patients complaining of a *sudden* onset of headache generally have more serious illnesses than patients with headaches of chronic duration. A continuous headache can be related to muscle spasm, whereas a *recurrent* headache may be migraine or cluster. A *throbbing* headache often has a vascular etiology. Certain headaches are associated with visual phenomena, nausea, or vomiting. In patients with increased intracranial pressure, any maneuver that increases the pressure, such as coughing or bending, may worsen the headache.

Migraine is a biphasic type of headache associated with a prodromal phase, called the *aura*, followed by the headache phase. During the aura, one or more physiologic events may occur. These include transient autonomic, visual, motor, or sensory phenomena. Common visual symptoms are photophobia, blurred vision, and scotomata. As the aura fades, the headache begins. It is usually unilateral, often described as pulsating, and lasts for hours to days. Migraine headaches are often triggered by stress, anxiety, the use of birth control pills, and hormonal changes. Patients frequently experience migraine headaches after a period of excitement. Other important triggers are hunger and the ingestion of certain foods such as chocolate, cheese, cured meats, and highly spiced foods. There is often a family history of migraine.

Cluster headaches are associated with oculosympathetic disturbances. The patient is frequently a middle-aged man complaining of recurrent episodes of pain centered around the eye lasting for up to 1 hour. Classically, cluster headaches awaken the patient from sleep on successive nights over a 2–4 week period. There is ipsilateral miosis, ptosis, conjunctival edema, tearing, and nasal stuffiness during the headache. It is thought that alcohol may precipitate such attacks.

It is important to remember that headache may be the result of referred pain from sinus infections, ocular disease, and dental disease. Systemic conditions such as viral infections, chronic obstructive pulmonary disease, and poisoning may produce headaches. It is vital to determine whether the patient is taking any medications that may be producing the head pain. (See Table 18–2, under Clinicopathologic Correlations, which provides an approach to the patient with the symptom of headache.)

Loss of Consciousness

Loss of consciousness—that is, syncope—may result from cardiovascular or neurologic causes. The cardiovascular causes are discussed in Chapters 11 and 12. The term "blackout" is very commonly used but may mean different conditions to the patient and interviewer. Any patient who uses this term should be asked to clarify its meaning. The term "to blackout" or "to fall out" is often used by the patient to indicate an actual loss of consciousness, dimming of vision, or a decreased awareness of the environment without an actual loss of consciousness.

A useful way to clarify the symptom of loss of consciousness is to ask the patient, "Have you ever lost consciousness, fainted, or felt that you were not aware of your surroundings?" If the patient answers in the affirmative, it is important to identify the cause of the loss of consciousness. Ask the following questions:

> *"Can you describe the attack to me? I want you to describe every event as it occurred until you lost consciousness."*
> *"Did anyone witness the attack?"**
> *"Were there any symptoms that preceded the attack?"*

---

* It is very important to obtain a history from an observer if possible.

"Were you told that there were body movements?"
"I would like you to describe everything you remember after the attack until you felt completely normal."
"Was there a period of sleepiness that followed?" If so, *"For how long did this period last?"*
"How did you feel after the attack? Where you confused?"
"Did you notice afterward that you had urinated or had a bowel movement during the attack?"

Epileptic seizures, or fits, may produce a loss of consciousness and are produced by the sudden excessive disorderly discharge of neurons. The first step in approaching the symptom of "seizure" is to identify its type. If the discharge is *focal,* the clinical seizure will reflect the effect of the excessive discharge in that area of the body. For example, if the discharge is located in the inferior precentral gyrus, involved with hand and arm motion, the seizure will result in involuntary motion of the hand and arm. A *generalized* seizure results from a discharge in the subcortical structures, such as the thalamocortical radiations. These have widespread bilateral cortical connections. There are three main types of generalized seizures:

- Petit mal
- Grand mal
- Myoclonic

A *petit mal* seizure is characterized by a sudden attack of unconsciousness lasting only about 10 seconds, usually without any warning. During the petit mal seizure, the patient appears to be staring or daydreaming. There is no associated falling or involuntary limb motion. The patient rapidly returns to normal activity without being aware of the attack. These seizures are most common in children between the ages of 5 and 15 years. Occasionally they may perist into adulthood.

A *grand mal* seizure is a generalized major motor convulsion. The patient loses consciousness and often falls rigidly to the floor. In 50% of patients with grand mal seizures, there is an aura of giddiness, involuntary twitching, change in mood, confusion, or epigastric discomfort as the seizure begins. Some patients may cry out initially. During this *tonic* phase, there is an increase in muscle tone resulting in first a rigid, flexed posture and then a rigid, extended posture. The patient may become apneic and cyanotic. The eyes may open and stare or may be deviated to one side. The *clonic* phases follows with involuntary movements of the body. These are often associated with salivation, eye rolling, and incontinence. Biting the tongue is common. Following the clonic phase, the individual passes into a phase resembling sleep from which he cannot be easily awakened. *Postictally,* or after the seizure, the patient may be confused and often falls into a deep sleep for hours. Accompanying muscle pain and headache are common.

The *myoclonic* seizure is a minor motor seizure characterized by sudden muscle contractions of the face and upper extremities. The eyelids and forearms are commonly affected. There is no detectable loss of consciousness.

Febrile convulsions are common in children between the ages of 6 months and 6 years and are similar to grand mal seizures. When a child has a high fever, a seizure lasting less than 10 minutes may occur. The younger the child at the time of the first febrile seizure, the greater the likelihood that a seizure will recur.

"Dizziness"

"Dizziness" is a term used frequently by the patient and should be avoided by the interviewer. "Dizziness" may be the patient's description of vertigo, ataxia, or lightheadedness. Any time the patient uses the term "dizziness," it must be clarified by additional questioning, because different pathophysiologic mechanisms may be responsible. It is important for the interviewer to differentiate vertigo from ataxia. If the patient complains of "dizziness," it is important to ask these questions:

> "Would you describe the 'dizziness' as a funny spinning sensation in your head?"
> "Did the room spin, or did it feel like you were spinning?"
> "Were you unsteady while walking?"

Vertigo is partially discussed in Chapter 8, The Ear and Nose. Vertigo is the hallucination of movement. Acute vertigo may be associated with nausea, vomiting, perspiration, and a sense of anxiety. It is important to ask a patient whether he has had the sensation that objects are moving around him or that he is spinning or moving. In addition to the questions in Chapter 8, ask the patient the following questions:

> "During the attack did you experience any nausea or vomiting?"
> "Have you noticed any problem with hearing or ringing in your ears?"
> "Have you ever been given an antibiotic called gentamicin?"

Ménière's disease can result in protracted attacks of severe vertigo associated with vomiting. Patients with Ménière's disease often have the associated symptoms of tinnitus and a hearing loss. During the attacks, the patient is very unsteady with horizontal nystagmus directed away from the affected ear. Certain drugs (such as gentamicin) are associated with changes in the labyrinth of the ear and cause vertigo and deafness.

Ataxia

Disruption of the vestibulo-ocular-cerebellar control mechanism produces ataxia. Ataxia is persistent unsteadiness on the feet. Any patient complaining of "dizziness" must be evaluated for abnormal function of the vestibular, visual, proprioceptive, and cerebellar systems. Equilibrium requires the integration of sensory input and motor output acting primarily at a reflex level for the maintenance of balance. The ears, eyes, their central connections in the brainstem, and the cerebellum are intimately involved in balance. Any patient with ataxia should be asked:

> "Are you unsteady when you walk, or are you clumsy with your hands?"
> "Have you noticed that the 'dizziness' is worse when your eyes are open or closed?"
> "What does your diet consist of? What did you eat yesterday?"
> "Have you ever had syphilis?"

Abnormal proprioceptive input from the lower extremities can cause ataxia. Severe posterior column damage from syphilis, vitamin B_{12} deficiency, or multiple sclerosis may produce a "sensory" ataxia resulting in a wide-based, high-stepping gait. The gait is worsened by having the patient close his eyes and is improved by having the patient observe his feet. Vitamin B_{12} deficiency may result from pernicious anemia or from inadequate intake, although poor nutrition is a rare cause. "Motor" ataxia results from an abnormality in the cerebellum and central vestibular pathways. It is characterized by wide-based, irregular placement of the feet and poor placement of the center of gravity with a lurching to either side.

Changes in Consciousness

Changes in consciousness may be related to changes in attention span, perception, arousal, or a combination. In *confusional states,* the patient has the ability to receive information normally but the processing is disturbed. In *delirium,* the individual perceives the information abnormally. Any patient, or member of the patient's family, who indicates that a change in consciousness has occurred should be asked the following:

> *"Has the change occurred suddenly?"*
> *"Have there been other symptoms associated with the change of consciousness?"*
> *"Do you use any medications? . . . depressants? . . . insulin? . . . alcohol? . . . street drugs?"*
> *"Is there a history of psychiatric illness?"*
> *"Is there a history of kidney disease? . . . liver disease? . . . thyroid disease?"*
> *"Have you ever had an injury to your head?"*

There are many factors that may produce changes in consciousness. The acuteness of the change in consciousness is often helpful in making a diagnosis. Hemiparesis, paresthesia, hemianopsia, garbled speech, and arm and leg weakness are common associated symptoms of supratentorial lesions. Brainstem lesions are often associated with changes in consciousness and with nystagmus, vomiting, double vision, nausea, and yawning. Drugs of any type are associated with acute changes in consciousness. A prior history of psychiatric illness is important. Toxic or metabolic changes are frequently associated with changes in consciousness. Liver or kidney failure, myxedema, and diabetic ketoacidosis are common causes of metabolic abnormalities. A history of head trauma may result in a subdural hematoma and produce a gradual change in consciousness.

Visual Disturbances

Visual disturbances are common neurologic presenting symptoms. The most important symptoms are acute visual loss, chronic visual loss, and double vision. It is important to ask any patient complaining of visual disturbances the following key questions:

> *"For how long have you noticed these visual changes?"*
> *"Is the visual loss associated with pain?"*
> *"Did it occur suddenly?"*
> *"Do you have a history of glaucoma?"*
> *"Have you ever been told that you have had a thyroid problem?"*
> *"Do you have diabetes?"*

Acute painless visual loss is caused by either a vascular accident or a retinal detachment. Acute narrow angle glaucoma may also be responsible for transient loss of vision associated with intense ocular pain. Painless loss of vision over a longer period is seen with compression of the optic nerve, tract, or radiation. Glaucoma is often the cause for chronic, insidious, painless loss of vision. Episodes of migraine may produce transient episodes of visual loss prior to the development of the headache. *Amaurosis fugax* is the transient visual loss lasting up to 3 minutes and is a feature of internal carotid artery disease.

Diplopia is discussed in Chapter 7, The Eye. Ocular motor palsies, thyroid abnormalities, myasthenia gravis, and brainstem lesions are well known causes of diplopia. Ocular motor palsies are seen in trauma, multiple sclerosis, myasthenia gravis, aneurysms of the circle of Willis, diabetes, and tumors. Ask the following questions of any patient complaining of diplopia:

> *"Are you diabetic?"*
> *"In which field of gaze do you have double vision?"*
> *"Did the double vision come on suddenly?"*
> *"Was there any pain associated with the double vision?"*
> *"Has there been any injury to the head or eye?"*
> *"Have you ever been told that your blood pressure has been elevated?"*
> *"Does the double vision get worse when you are tired?"*
> *"Have you been exposed to anyone with AIDS?"*

When a cranial nerve is affected resulting in an extraocular muscle palsy, a patient may complain of diplopia in one field of gaze when the affected eye is unable to move conjugately with the other. Ocular palsies involve the third, fourth, and sixth cranial nerves. A complete third nerve palsy causes ptosis, mydriasis, and the loss of all extraocular movements except abduction. Trauma, multiple sclerosis, tumors, and aneurysms are the most frequent causes. Aneurysms of the posterior communicating artery can involve the third nerve as this nerve passes near the artery on its way to the cavernous sinus. Cavernous sinus thrombosis, not infrequently seen today in patients suffering from AIDS, may also produce a complete third nerve palsy. Pupil sparing third nerve, trochlear nerve, and abducens nerve palsies are seen in diabetics and in patients with long standing hypertension. Patients with myasthenia gravis often have diplopia in the later part of the day as the muscles tire and weaken.

Dysphasia

Speech abnormalities, or dysphasia, may be either nonfluent (expressive) or fluent (receptive). In expressive aphasia, the speech pattern is hesitant and labored with poor articulation. The patient has no problem with comprehension. When asked to say, "No ifs, ands, or buts," the patient has great difficulty. In receptive aphasia, the speech is rapid and appears fluent but is full of syntax errors with the omission of many words. Handwriting changes are nonspecific but indicate an impairment of neuromuscular control. It is important to ask the following questions:

> *"Have you noticed any recent change in your speech pattern, such as slurring of your words?"*
> *"Do you have trouble understanding things that are said to you?"*
> *"Have you had any difficulty in finding the right word in conversation?"*
> *"Has you handwriting changed recently?"*

Brain Failure

An important symptom of neurologic disease is failing memory. The term "brain failure" has been introduced to replace "dementia." Brain failure can be defined as the progressive impairment of orientation, memory, judgment, and other aspects of intellectual function. Brain failure is a symptom rather than a specific disease entity. The most important cause of brain failure today is *Alzheimer's disease*. Other causes include Parkinson's disease, vascular disorders, metabolic disorders, drugs, tumors, vitamin B_{12} deficiency, and normal pressure hydrocephalus. It is not uncommon for patients with early brain failure to recognize an increasing failure to comprehend written material. It is important to ask the patient and his friends and family the following:

"Have you noticed any change in your memory lately?"
"What was the patient's personality like a few years ago?"
"When was the last time the patient seemed normal?"
"What does the patient's diet consist of?" "Does he eat well?"
"Can the patient live alone?"
"Do you have difficulty in reading or understanding what you have read?"

Cerebral Vascular Accidents

Strokes, or cerebral vascular accidents (CVA), are very common. Most are thromboembolic (80%), whereas others are hemorrhagic (20%). Thirty per cent of patients with a stroke die within the first month. Most patients with strokes have paresis of at least one limb. *Transient ischemic attacks* (TIA) are short episodes of focal neurologic dysfunction. They generally last only a few minutes, after which complete recovery occurs. The importance of transient ischemic attacks is that 30% of patients with TIA develop a stroke within 4–5 years.

Gait Disturbances

Gait disturbances may occur for a variety of reasons. Gait may be changed by local pain in the foot, pain in a joint, claudication of the hip or leg, bone disease, vestibular problems, or extrapyramidal disorders. Interruption of the corticospinal tracts in the cerebrum following a stroke produces a spastic weakness in the contralateral leg. The foot is dragged, and the whole leg appears stiff and extended. Lesions in the spinal cord may produce a spastic paralysis affecting both legs. The gait is slow and stiff with small steps. Patients suffering from Parkinson's disease walk stooped over with short, quick, shuffling steps. Any patient with a gait disturbance should be asked the following:

"Do you have pain in your leg or hip when you walk?"
"Do you have a history of diabetes?"
"Have you ever had syphilis?"
"What do you eat?" "Tell me everything you ate yesterday."

Patients with vascular occlusive disease of the hip or leg may experience pain while walking and may alter their gait. Diabetes, syphilis, and pernicious anemia may produce a sensory loss, and each condition may result in gait abnormalities.

Tremor

A tremor is a rhythmic motion of the distal parts of the limbs or head. A physiologic tremor has an oscillation of 10–12 cycles per second and is more obvious after exercise. A pathologic tremor is slower. *Parkinson's disease* is the most frequently encountered extrapyramidal movement disorder. In this condition, the tremor is present at rest and is decreased with action. It has a frequency of 3–6 cycles per second and is worsened by anxiety. An intention, or *ataxic*, tremor is very slow (at 2–4 cycles per second) and worsens on attempted movement. Multiple sclerosis is one of the many causes of an intention tremor. Metabolic problems from liver or kidney failure are frequently responsible. Withdrawal from alcohol or caffeine are often precipitating factors. Any patient with the symptom of a tremor should be asked these questions:

"Does the tremor worsen when you try to do something?"
"Is there a history of thyroid disease?"
"Have you been told of any problems with your liver or kidneys?"
"What is your daily consumption of alcoholic beverages?"
"How much coffee or tea do you drink?"
"How much chocolate do you eat?"

Chorea is involuntary jerky motions of the face and limbs. An important cause is *Huntington's chorea,* which causes chorea and brain failure. These patients frequently present with personality changes and symptoms of brain failure.

"Numbness"

"Numbness" is another term used by patients to indicate a variety of problems. "Numbness" can be used by patients to describe "pins and needles" sensations, coolness, pain, or clumsiness. The interviewer should be careful to clarify the meaning. The examiner must be careful during the physical examination to palpate the distal pulses in any patient complaining of "numbness," because arterial insufficiency is a possible cause.

"Weakness"

"Weakness" may be a symptom of the motor system. A patient with a *proximal arm* motor weakness complains of difficulty in brushing his hair, shaving, or reaching on shelves. A patient with *distal arm* weakness complains of difficulty in putting a button through a buttonhole, using keys, or writing with a pen or pencil. *Proximal leg* weakness is characterized by difficulty in climbing stairs or getting into bed or the bathtub. Foot drop is a classic sign of *distal leg* motor weakness. Chapter 17, The Musculoskeletal System, reviews some of the important questions relating to "weakness."

Pain

Pain is an infrequent symptom of neurologic disease, but it does deserve mention. *Trigeminal neuralgia,* also known as *tic douloureux,* is the occurrence of severe, jabbing pain lasting only seconds in the distribution of the maxillary or mandibular divisions of the trigeminal nerve. It is frequently provoked by motion, touch, eating, or exposure to cold temperatures. Another cause of facial pain is the cluster headache, already discussed. *Herpes zoster* infection of a nerve root, also known as *shingles,* presents with intense pain along a nerve root. Three to four days later, the classic linear, vesicular skin eruption develops along the distribution of the nerve. Look at the patient in Plate III *D,* showing the classic dermatologic manifestations of herpes zoster infection of spinal nerve T3.

Sciatica is intense pain shooting down the leg in the distribution of the sciatic nerve. In this condition, there is an impingement of portions of the sciatic nerve by the vertebrae. Arthritis of the lumbosacral spine is frequently the cause.

IMPACT OF CHRONIC NEUROLOGIC DISEASE ON THE PATIENT

The ramifications of chronic neurologic disease on the patient and his family are enormous. All family members experience emotional pain while observing the progressive clinical changes. The family bears an immense personal burden in assisting the patient to cope with his disability.

One example of a progressive neurologic condition is Alzheimer's disease. A devastating chronic disorder of unknown etiology, Alzheimer's disease is the most common diffuse brain degeneration causing brain failure.* This condition is characterized by progressive and widespread brain degeneration with a hopeless prognosis, at least at the present time.

Memory problems and impairment of intellectual function are the main symptoms of Alzheimer's disease. Depression is common. The patient may have significant cognitive impairment, preventing his ability to negotiate in his environment. He may forget where he lives. He might forget to turn off a gas burner on the stove or to put out a cigarette. He may wander aimlessly through the streets.

Patients with Alzheimer's disease represent a clinical spectrum from awareness of the disability to a vegetative state. Many patients with Alzheimer's disease have lost touch with reality. During an interview with such a patient, it may become clear that he has even lost his ability to describe his own medical history.

Early in the course of the disease, a patient may use a number of circumlocutions, substituting words when he cannot find the more appropriate ones. Another early change is the disorientation to time and place. Visual hallucinations are very common. Sexual disinterest is almost universal. Motor behavior diminishes progressively as impairment of consciousness increases. An important characteristic is the development of bizarre thoughts and fantasies that come to dominate consciousness. Delusions are common, especially delusions of persecution.

In the early stages of the disease, when the patient is still aware of his environment but has experienced the symptoms of memory loss, mild depression, anxiety, and irritability are common. As the disease progresses, apathy is

---

* Brain failure is the term now recommended to indicate dementia.

the dominant feature. The patient may actually appear indifferent and emotionally withdrawn. In other patients, in whom there is increased motor activity, anxiety and fear are common. In these individuals, terror and panic attacks are not uncommon. Hostility and paranoia develop rapidly. Regression and sudden displays of highly charged emotion are the responses to their frequent hallucinations.

In the milder cases, depression, hypochondriasis, and phobic features abound. Hysterical conversion reactions, such as hysterical blindness, may occur. Social interaction is lost, and the patient may suddenly explode with anger, anxiety, or tears. As the disease progresses, suicidal attempts are common. Emotional lability is often extreme, with periods of laughter followed by crying. With progressive disease, dullness of affect and a lack of an emotional response occur as gross neurologic disability develops. In their terminal stages, patients with Alzheimer's disease may show severe body wasting with profound dementia.

PHYSICAL EXAMINATION

> The equipment necessary for the neurologic examination is the following: safety pins, cotton-tipped applicators, 128 Hz tuning fork, gauze pads, familiar objects (coins, keys), and a reflex hammer.

The neurologic examination consists of assessment of the following:

- Mental status
- Cranial nerves
- Motor function
- Reflexes
- Sensory function
- Cerebellar function

Mental Status

The mental status examination consists of evaluation of the following:

- Level of consciousness
- Speech
- Orientation
- Knowledge of current events
- Judgment
- Abstraction
- Vocabulary
- Emotional responses
- Memory
- Calculation
- Object recognition
- Praxis (integration of motor activity)

Assess Level of Consciousness

The level of consciousness can be assessed as soon as you introduce yourself to the patient. Is the patient awake? Is he alert? Is the patient's sensorium clouded by exogenous or endogenous insults? Does the patient appear confused? If the patient does not respond to your introduction, hold the patient's hand and softly say, "Hello Mr. _____, can you hear me? If you hear me, squeeze my hand." If there is no response, try gently shaking the patient. If there is still no response and the patient appears obtunded, squeezing the nipple or applying pressure with your thumb to the bony ridge under the eyebrow is a painful maneuver that may rouse the patient. If these maneuvers fail to awaken the patient, the patient is in *coma*. Patients who are in coma are completely unconscious and cannot be roused even by painful stimuli. If either painful stimulus is used, be careful not to pinch the skin or bruise the patient. If there are friends or relatives present, make sure to indicate to them what you are doing.

Evaluate Speech

If the patient is awake and alert, you will have already observed his speech. The patient should now be asked to recite short phrases such as "no if, ands, or buts." Is dysarthria, dysphonia, dysphasia, or aphasia present? *Dysarthria* is difficulty in articulation. Generally, lesions of the tongue and palate are responsible for dysarthria. *Dysphonia* is difficulty in phonation. The result is an alteration in the volume and tone of the voice. Lesions of the palate and vocal cords are often responsible. *Dysphasia* is difficulty with comprehension or with speech as a result of cerebral dysfunction. Patients with a total loss of speech have *aphasia*. Different areas of the brain are responsible for the different types of aphasia. A motor, expressive, nonfluent aphasia is present when the patient knows what he wants to say but has motor impairment and cannot articulate properly. He understands written and verbal commands but cannot repeat them. A frontal lobe lesion is often the cause. A sensory, receptive, fluent aphasia is present when the patient articulates spontaneously but uses words inappropriately. The patient has difficulty in understanding written and verbal commands and cannot repeat them. A temporoparietal lesion is frequently the cause.

Introduction to Formal Mental Status Examination

During the interview, the examiner has already gained much insight into the mental status of the patient. The interviewer may have already been able to assess the patient's remote memory, affect, and judgment. The formal mental status portion of the neurologic examination is introduced by the examiner saying to the patient, "I would like to ask you a few routine questions. Some of them you will find very easy. Others will be more difficult. Do the best you can."

Evaluate Orientation

The patient's orientation to person, place, and time must be established. Orientation refers to the person's awareness of himself in relation to other persons, places, and time. Disorientation occurs in association with impairment of memory and attention span. The patient should be asked these questions:

> *"What is today's date?"*
> *"What is the day of the week?"*
> *"What is the name of this hospital (or building)?"*

Evaluate Knowledge of Current Events

A knowledge of current events can be assessed by asking the patient to name the last four Presidents of the United States. Asking the patient the name of the mayor or governor is also useful. If the patient is not American or unfamiliar with

American affairs, asking the patient about more general current events may be more useful. The ability to name current events requires an intact orientation, intact recent memory, and the ability to think abstractly.

Assess Judgment

Evaluation of judgment is performed by asking the patient to interpret a simple problem. Ask the patient the following:

> *"What would you do if you noticed an addressed envelope with an uncanceled stamp on it on the street near a mailbox?"*
> *"What would you do if you were in a crowded movie theatre and a fire started?"*

A correct response to the first question would be to pick up the letter and mail it. An example of an incorrect response might be, "I'd open the letter, read it, and keep the stamp." Judgment requires higher cerebral function.

Assess Abstraction

Abstraction is a higher cerebral function that requires comprehension and judgment. Proverbs are used commonly to test abstract reasoning. The patient should be asked to interpret the following:

> *"People who live in glass houses shouldn't throw stones."*
> *"A rolling stone gathers no moss."*

A patient with an abnormality in abstract reasoning might interpret the first quote by using a *concrete* interpretation such as, *"The glass will break if you throw a stone through it."* A concrete interpretation of the second proverb might be, *"Moss only grows under rocks that don't move and not under a rolling stone."* Concrete responses are common in patients with mental retardation or with brain failure. Schizophrenic patients often answer with concrete interpretations, but bizarre assessments are also common.

Another method of testing abstract reasoning is to ask the patient how a pair of items are similar or dissimilar. You might ask, *"What is similar about a dog and a cat?"* *"What is similar about a church and a synagogue?"* or *"What is dissimilar about an apple and a chicken?"*

Assess Vocabulary

Vocabulary is often very difficult to assess. It is based on many factors, which include the patient's education, background, work, environment, and cerebral function. It is, however, an important parameter in assessing intellectual capacity. Patients who are mentally retarded have a limited vocabulary, whereas those patients with mild brain failure have a well-preserved vocabulary. Patients should be asked to define words or use them in sentences. Any words can be used, but they should be asked with increasing levels of difficulty. The examiner may wish to consider these words in the following order:

> *"Car"*
> *"Ability"*
> *"Dominant"*
> *"Voluntary"*
> *"Telescope"*
> *"Reticent"*
> *"Enigma"*

Assess Emotional Responses

Although emotional response has probably already been informally observed, it is important to inquire specifically whether the patient has noticed any sudden mood changes. It is appropriate for the examiner to ask, "How are your spirits?" During the interview, the interviewer has already noticed the patient's *affect*. Affect is defined as the emotional response to an event. The response may be *appropriate, abnormal,* or *flat.* An appropriate response to a loved one's death may be to cry. An inappropriate response is to laugh. A flat response shows little emotional response. Patients with bilateral cerebral damage lose control of their emotions.

Assess Memory

In order to test memory, it is necessary to have the patient recall the recent and the remote past. *Recent* memory is easily tested by presenting three words to the patient and asking him to recall them 5 minutes later. For example, tell the patient, "Repeat these words after me and remember them. I will ask for them later: necklace, thirty-two, barn." Continue with the mental status examination. Five minutes later, ask the patient, "What were those words I asked you to remember?"

A simpler test of memory is to have the patient recall as many elements in a category as he can. Ask the patient,

> "Name as many flowers as you can."
> "Name as many occupations as you can."
> "Name as many tools as you can."

An abnormality in recent memory may be related to a lesion in the temporal lobe.

In order to test the *remote* past memory, ask the patient about well-known events in the past. Don't ask about events or things that you cannot verify.

Assess Calculation Ability

The ability to calculate depends on the integrity of the dominant cerebral hemisphere as well as on the patient's intelligence. Ask the patient to perform simple arithmetic problems, such as subtracting 7 from 100, then 7 from the result, then 7 from the result, and so forth. This is termed the *serial sevens* test. If the patient has difficulty with serial sevens, ask him to add or subtract several numbers such as *"How much is 5 plus 7? How much is 12 plus 9? How much is 27 minus 9?"*

Assess Object Recognition

Object recognition is termed *gnosia. Agnosia* is the failure to recognize a sensory stimulus despite normal primary sensation. Show the patient a series of well-known objects such as coins, pens, eyeglasses, or pieces of clothing and ask him to name them. If the patient has normal vision and fails to recognize the object, *visual agnosia* is said to be present. *Tactile agnosia* is the inability of a patient to recognize an object by palpation in the absence of a sensory deficit. This occurs with a lesion in the nondominant parietal lobe. *Autotopagnosia* is the term used to describe the inability to recognize a patient's own body part, such as his hand or leg.

Assess Integration of Motor Activity

Praxis refers to the ability to perform a motor activity. *Apraxia* is the inability of a patient to perform a voluntary movement in the absence of deficits in motor strength, sensation, or coordination. *Dyspraxia* is the decreased ability to perform the activity. The patient hears and understands the command, but he cannot integrate the motor activities that will complete the action. Ask a patient to pour water from his pitcher into a glass and drink the water. A patient with dyspraxia may either drink the water from the pitcher or may drink from the empty glass. A deep frontal lobe lesion is frequently responsible for this disorder.

Another type of apraxia is termed *constructional apraxia.* In this condition, the patient has an inability to construct or draw simple designs. The examiner draws a shape and asks the patient to copy it. Alternately, the patient can be asked to draw the face of a clock. Patients with constructional apraxia often have a lesion in the posterior portion of the parietal lobe.

Cranial Nerves

The examination of the cranial nerves should be carried out in an orderly fashion. Several of the cranial nerves have already been evaluated. Table 18–1 lists the cranial nerves, their functions, and the clinical findings when a lesion exists.

Cranial Nerve I: Olfactory

The olfactory nerve supplies nerve endings to the superior nasal concha and upper one third of the nasal septum. The olfactory nerve is not routinely tested. However, any patient in whom frontal lobe pathology is suspected should be evaluated.

TABLE 18–1. Cranial Nerves

Cranial Nerve	Function	Clinical Findings with Lesion
I: Olfactory	Smell	Anosmia
II: Optic	Vision	Amaurosis
III: Oculomotor	Eye movements; pupillary constriction; accommodation	Diplopia; ptosis; mydriasis; loss of accommodation
IV: Trochlear	Eye movements	Diplopia
V: Trigeminal	General sensation of face, scalp, and teeth; chewing movements	"Numbness" of face; weakness of jaw muscles
VI: Abducens	Eye movements	Diplopia
VII: Facial	Taste; general sensation of palate and external ear; lacrimal gland, and submandibular and sublingual gland secretion; facial expression	Loss of taste on anterior two thirds of tongue; dry mouth; loss of lacrimation; paralysis of facial muscles
VIII: Vestibulocochlear	Hearing; equilibrium	Deafness; tinnitus; vertigo; nystagmus
IX: Glossopharyngeal	Taste; general sensation of pharynx and ear; elevates palate; parotid gland secretion	Loss of taste on posterior one third of tongue; anesthesia of pharynx; partially dry mouth
X: Vagus	Taste; general sensation of pharynx, larynx, and ear; swallowing; phonation; parasympathetic to heart and abdominal viscera	Dysphagia; hoarseness; palatal paralysis
XI: Spinal accessory	Phonation; head, neck, and shoulder movements	Hoarseness; weakness of head, neck and shoulder muscles
XII: Hypoglossal	Tongue movements	Weakness and wasting of tongue

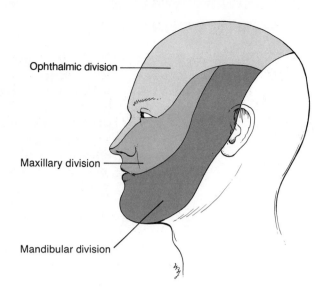

FIGURE 18-10. The divisions of the trigeminal nerve.

Test Olfaction

The patient is asked to close his eyes and one nostril as the examiner brings a test substance close to the patient's other nostril. The patient is instructed to sniff the test substance. The substance must be volatile and nonirritating, such as cloves, vanilla bean, freshly ground coffee, or lavender. The use of an irritating agent such as alcohol will involve cranial nerve V as well as cranial nerve I, and the test will be inaccurately performed.

Each nostril is tested separately. The examiner asks the patient to identify the test material. A unilateral loss of smell, known as unilateral *anosmia,* is more important than the bilateral loss, because it indicates a lesion affecting the olfactory tract on that side.

Cranial Nerve II: Optic

The optic nerve ends in the retina. The examinations for visual acuity as well as the ophthalmoscopic examination are discussed in Chapter 7, The Eye.

Cranial Nerve III: Oculomotor

The oculomotor nerve supplies the medial, superior, and inferior rectus muscles, and the inferior oblique muscles, which control most eye movements. The third nerve also innervates the intrinsic muscles, controlling pupillary constriction and accommodation.

Extraocular muscle movements are discussed in Chapter 7. A patient with an oculomotor palsy is shown in Figure 7-24. The pupillary light reflex depends on the function of cranial nerves II and III. This reflex is discussed in Chapter 7. Visual fields are part of both the eye examination and the neurologic examination. The technique for visual field testing is discussed in Chapter 7.

Cranial Nerve IV: Trochlear

The trochlear nerve is responsible for the movement of the superior oblique muscle. Extraocular muscle movements are discussed in Chapter 7.

Cranial Nerve V: Trigeminal

The trigeminal nerve is responsible for supplying sensation to the face, the nasal and buccal mucosa, and the teeth. The motor division supplies the muscles of mastication. There are three major subdivisions of the trigeminal nerve: the ophthalmic, the maxillary, and the mandibular nerves. These divisions are shown in Figure 18-10.

The *ophthalmic division* supplies sensation to the frontal sinuses, the conjunctiva, the cornea, the upper lid, the bridge of the nose, the forehead, and the scalp as far as the vertex of the skull. The *maxillary division* supplies sensation to the cheek, the maxillary sinus, the lateral aspects of the nose, the upper teeth, the nasal pharynx, the hard palate, and the uvula. The *mandibular division* supplies sensation to the chin, the lower jaw, the anterior two thirds of the tongue, the lower teeth, the gums and floor of the mouth, and the buccal mucosa of the cheek. The motor division supplies the muscles of mastication and the tensor tympani.

The examination of the trigeminal nerve consists of the following:

- The corneal reflex
- Testing the sensory division
- Testing the motor division

Test Corneal Reflex

The corneal reflex depends on the function of cranial nerves V and VII. In order to evaluate the corneal reflex, the examiner uses a cotton-tipped applicator, the tip of which has been pulled into a thin strand about 1/2 inch in length. The examiner then stabilizes the patient's head by placing his hand on the patient's eyebrow and head. The patient is asked to look to the right side as the cotton tip is brought in from the left side to touch the left cornea gently. This is shown in Figure 18–11. A prompt bilateral reflex closure of the lids is the normal response. The examination is repeated on the other side by reversing the directions.

The responses on the two sides are compared. The sensory limb of the corneal reflex is the ophthalmic division of the trigeminal nerve; the motor limb is conducted through the facial nerve.

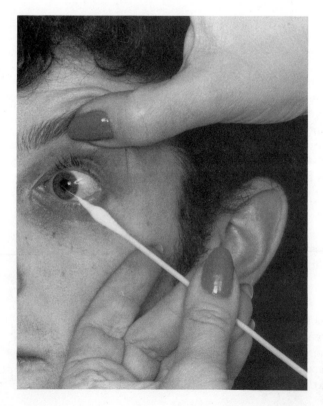

FIGURE 18–11. Technique for evaluating the corneal reflex.

In performing the corneal reflex, it is important to touch the cornea and not the eyelashes or conjuctiva, which will give an inaccurate result.

Test Sensory Division

The sensory division of the trigeminal nerve is tested by asking the patient to close his eyes and to respond when he feels that he is being touched. A piece of gauze is applied to one side of the forehead and then to the corresponding position on the other side. This test is then performed on the cheeks, and then on the jaw, testing all three subdivisions of the nerve. The patient is also asked if one side feels the same or different than the other side. The examination is shown in Figure 18–12.

The procedure is then repeated using a sharp pin, alternating between the sides.

Test Motor Division

The motor division of the trigeminal nerve is tested by having the patient bite down or clench his teeth while the masseter and temporalis muscles are palpated bilaterally. This is shown in Figure 18–13. Unilateral weakness will cause the jaw to deviate toward the side of the lesion.

Cranial Nerve VI: Abducens

The abducens nerve is responsible for movement of the lateral rectus muscle. Extraocular muscle movements are discussed in Chapter 7.

Cranial Nerve VII: Facial

The facial nerve innervates the facial muscles and supplies taste to the anterior two thirds of the tongue. A very small component also supplies general sensation to the external ear. The facial nerve also carries parasympathetic motor fibers to the salivary glands and chorda tympani. Testing for abnormalities of taste are generally not performed by the internist.

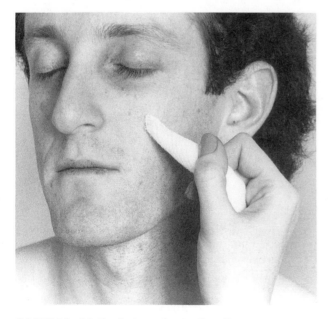

FIGURE 18–12. Technique for testing the sensory division of the trigeminal nerve.

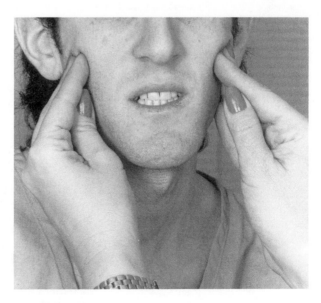

FIGURE 18–13. Technique for testing the motor division of the trigeminal nerve.

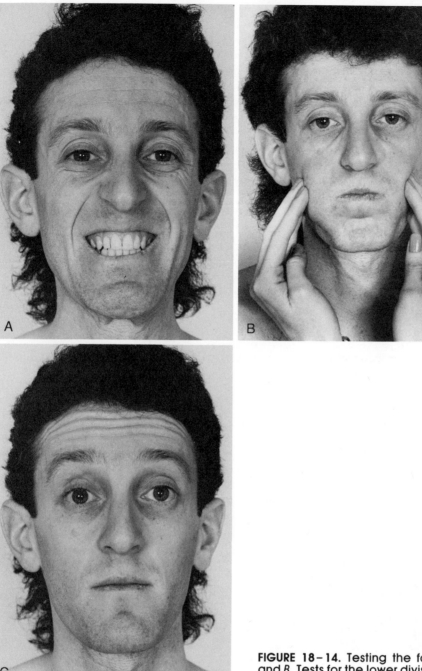

FIGURE 18–14. Testing the facial nerve. *A* and *B*, Tests for the lower division. *C*, Test for the upper division.

Test Function

The patient is asked to bare his teeth while the examiner observes for asymmetry. The patient is asked to puff out his cheeks against resistance and then to wrinkle his forehead. It is helpful if the examiner actually demonstrates these maneuvers for the patient. These maneuvers are shown in Figure 18–14.

The patient is then asked to close his eyes tightly while the examiner tries to open them. The patient is told to close his eyes as tight as he can. The examiner

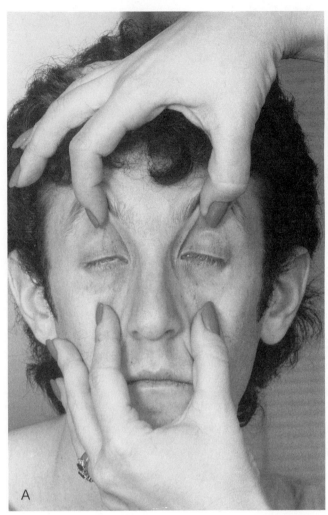

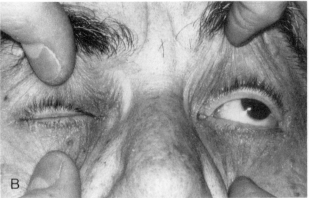

FIGURE 18-15. Testing the strength of eyelid closure. *A,* Normal response. Notice that the eyelids cannot be opened by the examiner. *B,* Test in a patient with a stroke that involved the facial nerve nucleus. Note the loss in strength of the muscle around the left eye.

can say, "Don't let me open them." This procedure is demonstrated in Figure 18-15*A.* Each eye is examined separately, and the strengths are compared. Normally the examiner should not be able to open the eyes. Look at the patient shown in Figure 18-15*B.* Notice the marked weakness of the left orbicularis oculi muscle as a result of a stroke involving the facial nucleus.

Facial Weakness

The innervations of the facial nerve are shown in Figure 18-16. There are two types of facial weakness. Upper motor neuron lesions such as a stroke involving the corticobulbar pathways will produce contralateral weakness of the lower face with normal function of the upper face. The patient will still be able to wrinkle his forehead. This is related to the bilateral innervation of the upper face by the corticobulbar fibers. The lower face has only unilateral innervation from contralateral cortical centers. This type of upper motor neuron lesion is illustrated by lesion "A" in Figure 18-16. The second type of facial weakness will produce total involvement of the ipsilateral facial muscles with no area being spared. This may result from lesions of the nerve as it exits from the skull or from involvement of the facial nucleus in the pons, as shown by lesion "B" in Figure 18-16.

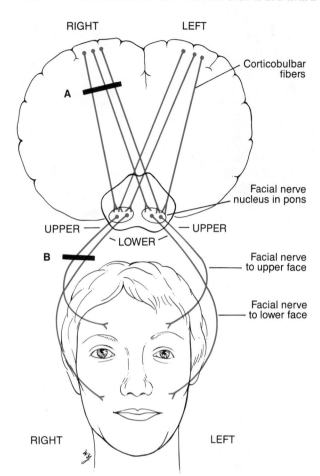

FIGURE 18–16. Types of facial weakness. Lesion "A" produces an upper motor nerve palsy that produces contralateral weakness of the lower face but spares the contralateral forehead. Lesion "B" produces a lower motor nerve palsy that produces total paralysis of the ipsilateral face.

Look at the patient shown in Plate XV *C*. When he was asked to smile, the right side of his face was drawn to the left. This patient has a right facial palsy, also known as a right Bell's palsy. Further maneuvers revealed that the entire right side of his face was involved as a result of a lesion affecting the right facial nucleus.

Cranial Nerve VIII: Vestibulocochlear

The vestibulocochlear nerve is responsible for hearing, balance, and an awareness of position. Auditory testing is discussed in Chapter 8, The Ear and Nose. Tests for the vestibular function of cranial nerve VIII are not generally performed.

Cranial Nerve IX: Glossopharyngeal

The glossopharyngeal nerve supplies sensation to the pharynx, posterior one third of the tongue, tympanic membrane, and secretory fibers to the parotid gland.

Test Function

Examination of the glossopharyngeal nerve involves the gag reflex. The examiner may use either a tongue blade or an applicator stick. By touching the posterior third of the tongue, the soft palate, or the posterior pharyngeal wall, the examiner should elicit a gag reflex. The sensory portion of the loop is through the glossopharyngeal nerve; the motor is mediated through the vagus nerve.

Another way of testing the nerve is to ask the patient to open his mouth widely and to say, "Ah . . . Ah . . . ." Symmetrical elevation of the soft palate demonstrates normal function of cranial nerves IX and X. The uvula should remain in the midline.

Taste sensation of the posterior third of the tongue is not routinely tested.

Cranial Nerve X: Vagus

The vagus nerve supplies parasympathetic fibers to the viscera of the chest and abdomen, motor fibers to the pharynx and larynx, and sensation to the external ear canal.

Examination of the vagus nerve has been performed with evaluation of the glossopharyngeal nerve.

Dysphonia or dysarthria may result from paralysis of the vagus nerve.

Cranial Nerve XI: Spinal Accessory

The spinal accessory nerve is a motor nerve supplying the sternocleidomastoid and trapezius muscles.

Test Function

The right spinal accessory nerve is examined by asking the patient to turn his head to the left against the resistance of the examiner's hand. This is shown in Figure 18–17. The left spinal accessory nerve is examined by reversing the directions.

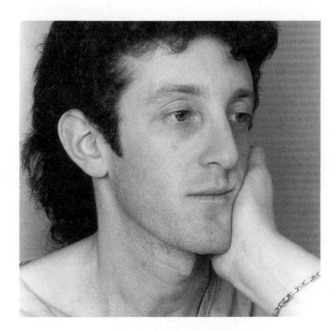

FIGURE 18–17. Technique for evaluating the spinal accessory nerve.

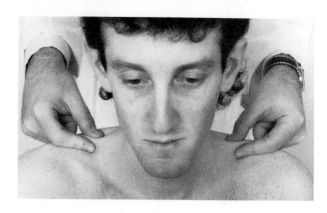

FIGURE 18–18. Alternate technique for evaluating the spinal accessory nerve.

An alternate test is to evaluate the trapezius muscles. The examiner places both hands on the trapezius muscles of the patient. Both muscles are palpated between the thumb and index fingers. The patient is then asked to shrug his shoulders against the resistance of the examiner's hands. Both sides should be equal. This technique is shown in Figure 18–18.

Cranial Nerve XII: Hypoglossal

The hypoglossal nerve supplies motor fibers to the muscles of the tongue. The examination of the hypoglossal nerve is performed by asking the patient to open his mouth with the tongue resting quietly at the floor of the mouth. Inspection for *fasciculations** is performed. Fasciculations are indicative of a hypoglossal lower motor neuron lesion.

Test Function

Ask the patient to open his mouth and stick out his tongue. Normally, the tongue is protruded and lies in the midline. This is shown in Figure 18–19. Deviation of the tongue to either side is abnormal. Because the tongue muscles

---

* Spontaneous contractions of groups of muscles visible on inspection.

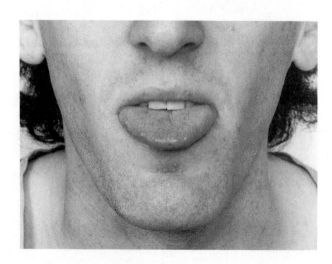

FIGURE 18–19. Technique for evaluation of the hypoglossal nerve.

push rather than pull, weakness of one side will result in the tongue being pushed by the normal side to the side of the lesion.

Look at the tongue of the patient shown in Plate XV *D*. Notice the marked scalloping of the tongue's surface. This is a patient with a chronic neurologic disease known as *amyotrophic lateral sclerosis*,* characterized by progressive degeneration of motor neurons. This patient had the typical features of a lower motor neuron bulbar palsy affecting the hypoglossal nucleus: wasting of the tongue with fasciculations.

Motor Function

Principles of Testing Motor Function

The motor system is evaluated for the following:

- Muscle bulk
- Muscle strength
- Muscle tone

The motor examination begins with inspection of each area being examined. Compare the contours of symmetrical *muscle masses*. Inspection is used to determine muscle atrophy and the presence of fasciculations.

Test *muscle strength* by having the patient move actively against your resistance. Compare one side against the other. The following is an arbitrary scale that is commonly used for the grading of muscle strength:

0: Absent   No contraction detected

1: Trace   Slight contraction detected

2: Weak   Movement with gravity eliminated

3: Fair   Movement against gravity

4: Good   Movement against gravity with some resistance

5: Normal   Movement against gravity with full resistance

If a muscle weakness is found, a comparison of the proximal and distal strengths is important. In general, proximal weakness is related to muscle disease; distal weakness is related to neurologic disease.

Tone can be defined as the slight residual tension in a voluntarily relaxed muscle. Tone is assessed by resistance to passive movement. Ask the patient to relax. Perform passive motion of the muscle. Compare one side with the other. It should be remembered that upper motor neuron lesions produce spasticity,† hyperreflexia, clonus,‡ and a Babinski§ sign. Lower motor neuron lesions produce atrophy, fasciculations, decreased tone, and hyporeflexia. Both types of lesions will result in weakness. Fasciculations may become more apparent by gently tapping the muscle with a reflex hammer.

---

* This disease is also called *Lou Gehrig's disease*, after the famous baseball star who was one of its victims.

† Spasticity is defined as an increase in muscle tone that results in continuous resistance to stretching. Spasticity is generally worse at extremes of range.

‡ Clonus is spasm in which there is alternating rigidity and relaxation in rapid succession.

§ Dorsiflexion of the big toe upon stimulating the sole of the foot.

It is impractical to test all muscles during the internist's neurologic examination. By testing key muscle groups, the examiner can determine if a gross deficit exists. Further testing of specific muscles and nerve roots may then be necessary. The student is referred to the many fine textbooks on neurology for these detailed examinations.

In the assessment of motor function, the upper extremities are examined first.

Inspect the Upper Extremities for Symmetry

Ask the patient to sit off the side of the bed facing you. Inspect both arms and hands for size differences, paying special attention to the size of the thumbs and the small muscles of the hands. Is muscle wasting present?

Test Flexion and Extension of the Arm

You should now test flexion and extension strength of the upper extremity by having the patient pull and push against your resistance. You might say, "Push down . . . relax." "Push up . . . relax." "Push back . . . relax." "Push forward . . . relax." It is important to say "Relax" after each direction so that the patient will not continue to push or pull after you have removed your hands. After one side is tested, the other is tested and the two sides are compared.

Test Arm Abduction

Ask the patient to hold out his arms in front of him with his palms facing down. Place your hands at the lateral aspect of the patient's arms. Instruct the patient to abduct his arms against resistance. This tests abduction of the arm by the *axillary nerve* from roots C5 – C6. This test is shown in Figure 18 – 20.

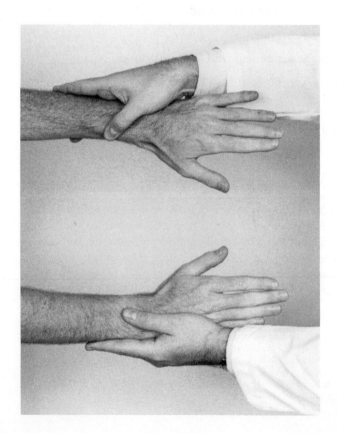

FIGURE 18 – 20. Technique for testing abduction of the arm.

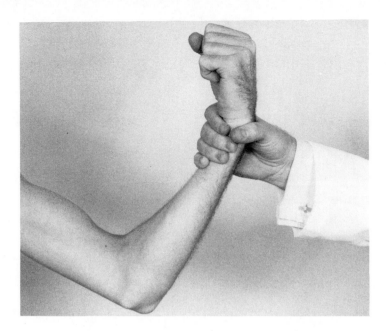

FIGURE 18-21. Technique for testing flexion of the forearm.

Test Forearm Flexion

Have the patient make a fist and flex his forearm. You should hold the patient's fist or wrist. Ask the patient to pull his arm toward himself against your resistance. This tests flexion of the forearm by the *musculocutaneous nerve* from roots C5–C6. This test is shown in Figure 18–21.

Test Forearm Extension

Ask the patient to abduct his arm and hold it midway between flexion and extension. Support the patient's arm by holding the wrist. Instruct the patient to extend his arm against your resistance. This tests extension of the forearm by the *radial nerve* from roots C6–C8. This is illustrated in Figure 18–22.

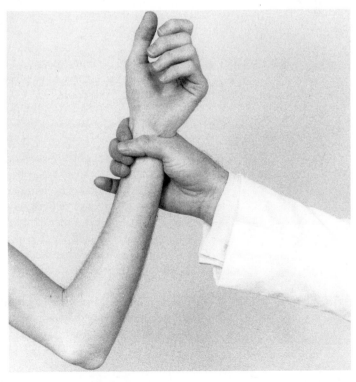

FIGURE 18-22. Technique for testing extension of the forearm.

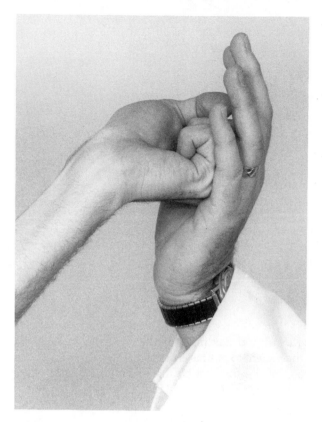

FIGURE 18-23. Technique for testing extension of the wrist.

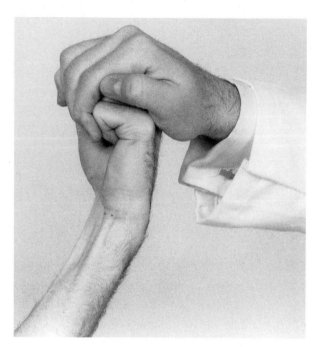

FIGURE 18-24. Technique for testing flexion of the wrist.

Test Wrist Extension

Instruct the patient to make a fist with his hand and extend his wrist while you attempt to push it up. This tests extension of the wrist by the *radial* nerve from roots C6–C8. This procedure is illustrated in Figure 18–23.

Test Wrist Flexion

The patient is asked to make a fist with his hand and flex his wrist while the examiner attempts to pull it down. This tests flexion of the wrist by the *median* nerve from roots C6–C7. This is shown in Figure 18–24.

Test Finger Adduction

The patient is asked to grasp the examiner's extended index and middle fingers and to squeeze them as hard as he can. The examiner should compare the strengths of both hands. It is important for the examiner to remove any rings on his fingers, which may produce discomfort. This tests adduction of the fingers by the *median* nerve from roots C7–T1. This procedure is shown in Figure 18–25.

Test Finger Abduction

Ask the patient to extend his hand with his palm down and to spread his fingers as widely as he can. Tell the patient to resist your attempt to bring the fingers together. This tests abduction of the fingers by the *ulnar* nerve from roots C8–T1. This is illustrated in Figure 18–26.

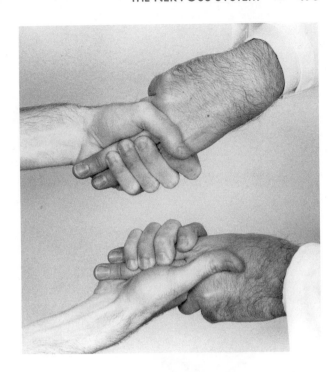

FIGURE 18-25. Technique for testing finger adduction.

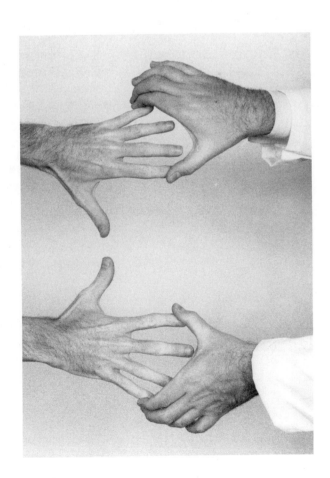

FIGURE 18-26. Technique for testing finger abduction.

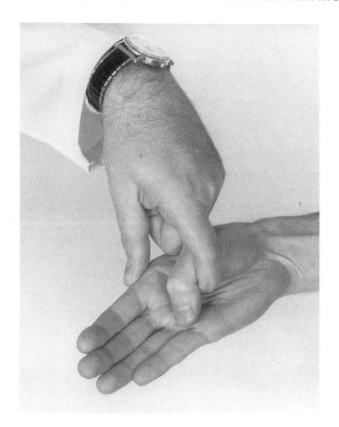

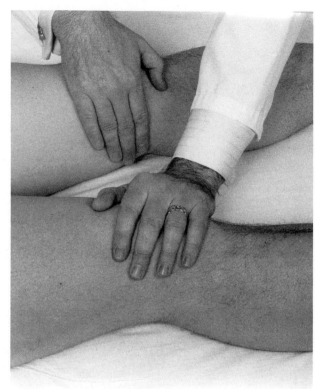

FIGURE 18–27. Technique for testing thumb adduction.

FIGURE 18–28. Technique for testing hip adduction.

Test Thumb Adduction

The patient is instructed to touch the base of the little finger with the tip of the thumb against resistance while the thumbnail remains parallel to the palm. This tests adduction of the thumb by the *median* nerve from roots C8–T1. This test is shown in Figure 18–27.

Assess Upper Extremity Tone

Tone is assessed in the upper limbs by passive flexing and extending the limbs to determine the amount of resistance to the examiner's movements. Increased resistance, as in muscle rigidity or spasticity, means increased muscle tone. Decreased resistance, as in limpness or flaccidity, means decreased muscle tone. Normal tone has a smooth sensation. In extrapyramidal disease, palpation of a proximal muscle during passive movement will detect the presence of *cogwheeling*, which is a ratchety jerkiness to the motion.

Inspect the Lower Extremities for Symmetry

The lower extremities are now examined for muscle bulk and muscle wasting. This examination is performed with the patient lying on his back in bed. As with the upper extremities, proximal and distal muscle strengths are compared as well as symmetry of one leg with the other.

Test Hip Adduction

Ask the patient to open his legs. Place your hands on the medial aspect of the patient's knees. Instruct the patient to close his legs against your resistance.

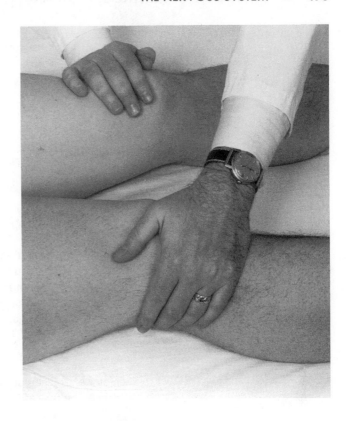

FIGURE 18–29. Technique for testing hip abduction.

This tests adduction of the hips by the *obturator* nerve from roots L2–L4. This procedure is shown in Figure 18–28.

Test Hip Abduction

Place your hands on the lateral margins of the patient's knees. Ask the patient to open his legs against your resistance. This tests abduction of the hips by the *superior gluteal* nerve from roots L4–S1. This is shown in Figure 18–29.

Test Knee Flexion

Ask the patient to elevate his knee with the foot resting on the bed. Instruct the patient to hold his foot down as you try to extend the leg. This tests flexion of the knee by the *sciatic* nerve from roots L4–S1. This is shown in Figure 18–30.

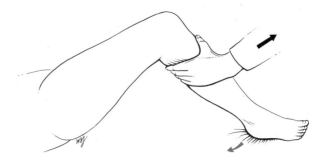

FIGURE 18–30. Technique for testing knee flexion.

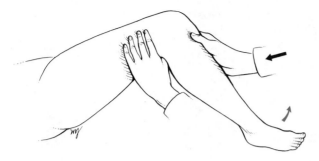

FIGURE 18-31. Technique for testing knee extension.

Test Knee Extension

Instruct the patient again to elevate his knee with the foot resting on the bed. Place your left hand under the knee. Ask the patient to straighten the leg against the resistance of your right hand, which is placed on the patient's shin. This procedure tests extension of the knee by the *femoral* nerve from roots L4–S1. This is shown in Figure 18–31.

Test Ankle Dorsiflexion

You next place your hands on the dorsum of the foot and ask the patient to dorsiflex the foot at the ankle against your resistance. This tests dorsiflexion of the ankle by the *deep peroneal* nerve from roots L4–L5. This maneuver is illustrated in Figure 18–32.

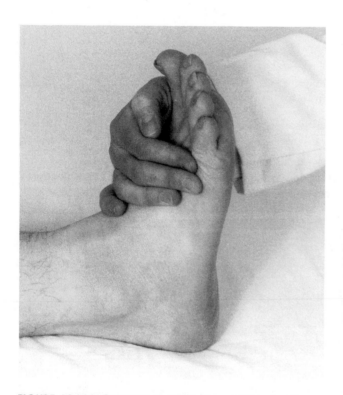

FIGURE 18-32. Technique for testing ankle dorsiflexion.

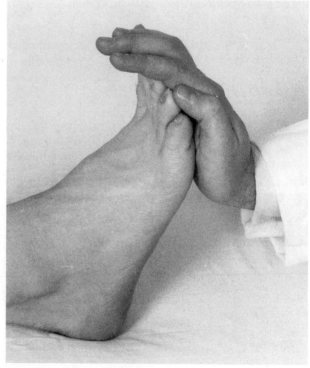

FIGURE 18-33. Technique for testing plantar flexion.

Test Ankle Plantar Flexion

Now place your hand on the sole of the foot and ask the patient to plantar flex the foot at the ankle against your resistance. This tests plantar flexion of the ankle by the *tibial* nerve from roots L5–S2. The test is shown in Figure 18–33.

Test Great Toe Dorsiflexion

Place your hand on the dorsal aspect of the big toe. Ask the patient to dorsiflex his big toe against your resistance. This tests dorsiflexion of the big toe by the *deep peroneal* nerve from roots L4–S1. This is demonstrated in Figure 18–34.

Test Great Toe Plantar Flexion

Now place your hand on the plantar surface of the big toe. The patient is asked to plantar flex his great toe against your resistance. This tests plantar flexion of the great toe by the *posterior tibial* nerve from roots L5–S2. This is shown in Figure 18–35.

Assess Lower Extremity Tone

Tone in the lower extremities is assessed as in the upper extremities.

The examiner should grasp the foot and passively dorsiflex and plantar flex it several times and end with dorsiflexion of the foot. If a sudden rhythmic involuntary dorsiflexion and plantar flexion occur, *ankle clonus* is said to be present. This frequently occurs in conditions of increased tone.

If there is any abnormality noted in the motor strength of the upper or lower extremity, a more detailed examination should be performed. Table 18–7, at the end of this chapter, lists the muscle innervations and their actions.

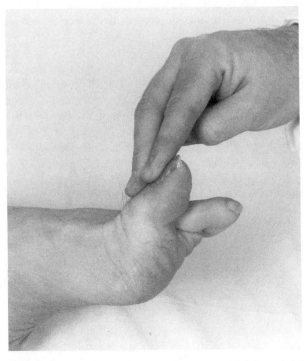

FIGURE 18–34. Technique for testing great toe dorsiflexion.

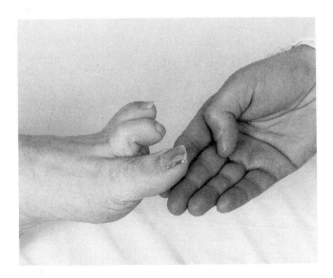

FIGURE 18–35. Technique for testing great toe plantar flexion.

Reflexes

Basic Principles

There are two main types of reflexes tested. They are the *stretch*, or deep tendon, reflexes and the *superficial* reflexes.

In order to elicit a stretch reflex, you should support the joint being tested so that the muscle is relaxed. The reflex hammer is held between the thumb and the index finger and is swung by motion at the wrist, not the elbow. In general, the pointed end of a triangular reflex hammer is used. A gentle tap over the tendon being tested should produce muscle contraction. It is often necessary to palpate as well as observe the muscle in order to assess its contraction. Test each reflex and compare it with the other side. Reflexes should be symmetrically equal.

There is a wide variation in the reflex response. Only with experience will the examiner be able to make an adequate assessment of normal reflexes. Reflexes are commonly graded on a 0–4+ scale as follows:

0 No response

1+ Diminished

2+ Normal

3+ Increased

4+ Hyperactive

Hyperactive reflexes are characteristic of pyramidal tract disease. Electrolyte abnormalities, hyperthyroidism, and other metabolic abnormalities may also be the cause of hyperactive reflexes. *Diminished* reflexes are characteristic of anterior horn cell pathology and myopathies. The examiner should always consider the strength of the reflex to the bulk of the muscle mass. A patient may have diminished reflexes as a result of a decrease in his muscle bulk. Patients with hypothyroidism have decreased relaxation after a deep tendon reflex, which is termed a *hung reflex*.

In a patient with a diminished reflex, the technique of *reinforcement* may be useful. By asking the patient to perform isometric contraction of other muscles, the generalized reflex activity may be increased. In testing reflexes on the upper extremities, have the patient clench his teeth or push down on the bed with his thighs. In testing reflexes on the lower extremities, have the patient lock his fingers and try to pull them apart at the time of testing. This procedure is sometimes called the *Jendrassik maneuver*. This is illustrated in Figure 18–36.

The deep tendon reflexes that are routinely tested are as follows:

- Biceps
- Brachioradialis
- Triceps
- Patellar
- Achilles

Test Biceps Tendon Reflex

The biceps tendon reflex is assessed by having the patient relax his arm and pronate the forearm midway between flexion and extension. The examiner should place his thumb firmly on the biceps tendon. The hammer is then struck

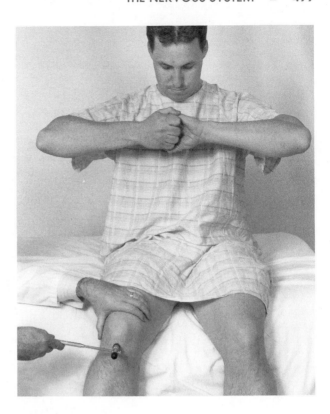

FIGURE 18-36. The Jendrassik maneuver.

on the examiner's thumb. This is illustrated in Figure 18-37. The examiner should observe for contraction of the biceps followed by flexion at the elbow. The examiner may also palpate the contraction of the muscle. This reflex tests the nerves at roots C5-C6.

Test Brachioradialis Tendon Reflex

The brachioradialis tendon reflex is performed by having the patient's forearm in semiflexion and semipronation. The arm should be rested on the patient's knee. If a triangular reflex hammer is used, the wide end should strike the

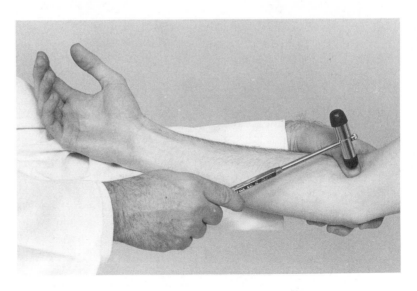

FIGURE 18-37. The biceps tendon reflex.

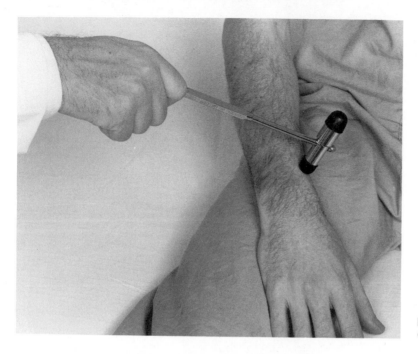

FIGURE 18–38. The brachioradialis tendon reflex.

styloid process of the radius about 1–2 inches above the wrist. The examiner should observe for flexion at the elbow and simultaneous supination of the forearm. The position is shown in Figure 18–38. This reflex tests the nerves at roots C5–C6.

Test Triceps Tendon Reflex

The triceps tendon reflex is tested by flexing the patient's forearm at the elbow and pulling the arm toward the chest. The elbow should be midway between flexion and extension. Tap the triceps tendon above the insertion of the

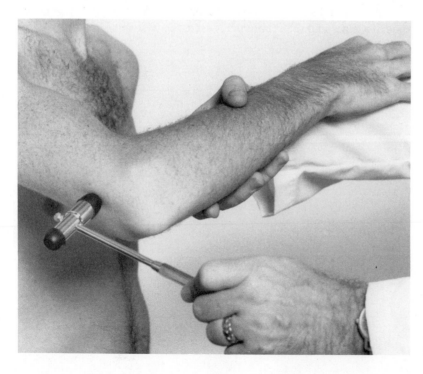

FIGURE 18–39. The triceps tendon reflex.

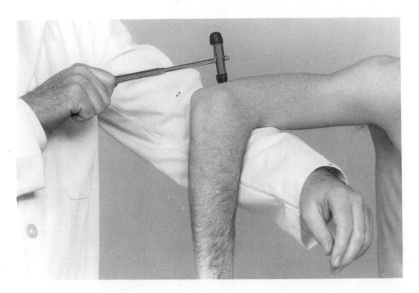

FIGURE 18–40. Another test for the triceps tendon reflex.

ulna's olecranon process about 1 – 2 inches above the elbow. There should be a prompt contraction of the triceps with extension at the elbow. This technique is shown in Figure 18 – 39. This reflex tests the nerves at roots C6 – C8.

If the triceps reflex cannot be elicited by this maneuver, try to hang the patient's arm over your arm, as shown in Figure 18 – 40. Tapping the triceps tendon in this position will often elicit the reflex.

Test Patellar Tendon Reflex

In order to perform the patellar reflex, also known as the knee jerk, have the patient sit with his legs dangling off the side of the bed. Place your hand on the patient's quadriceps muscle. Strike the patellar tendon firmly with the base of the reflex hammer. A contraction of the quadriceps should be felt and extension at the knee should be observed. This technique is shown in Figure 18 – 41. This reflex tests the nerves at roots L2 – L4.

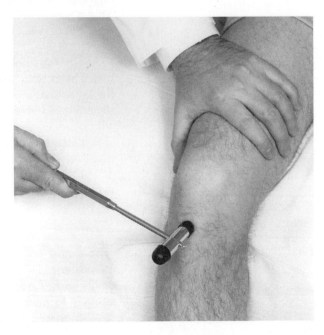

FIGURE 18–41. The patellar tendon reflex.

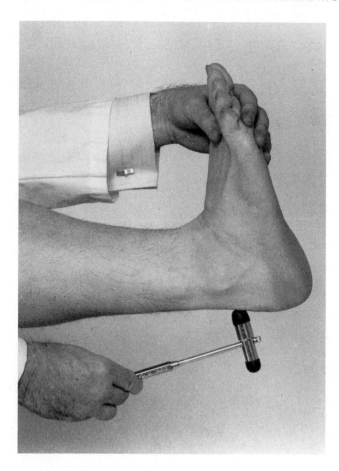

FIGURE 18–42. The Achilles tendon reflex.

Test Achilles Tendon Reflex

The Achilles reflex, also known as the ankle jerk, is elicited by having the patient with his feet dangling sit off the side of the bed. The leg should be flexed at the hip and the knee. The examiner should place his hand under the patient's foot to dorsiflex the ankle. The Achilles tendon is struck just above its insertion on the posterior aspect of the calcaneus with the wide end of the reflex hammer. This is shown in Figure 18–42. The result is plantar flexion at the ankle. This tests the nerves at roots S1–S2.

Another method of testing for the Achilles reflex is to have the patient lie in bed. The examiner should flex one leg at the hip and knee and externally rotate the leg so that it lies on the opposite shin. The examiner should again dorsiflex the ankle as the tendon is struck. This test is demonstrated in Figure 18–43*A*.

A patient with a depressed Achilles reflex should be asked to kneel, if possible, on the bed with his feet hanging off the side, as shown in Figure 18–43*B*. The examiner should tap the Achilles tendon and observe the reflex response in this position.

Test Superficial Reflexes

The most commonly tested superficial reflexes are the abdominal and the cremasteric. The *abdominal* superficial reflex is elicited by having the patient lie on his back. An applicator stick or tongue blade is quickly stroked horizontally laterally to medially toward the umbilicus. The result is a contraction of the

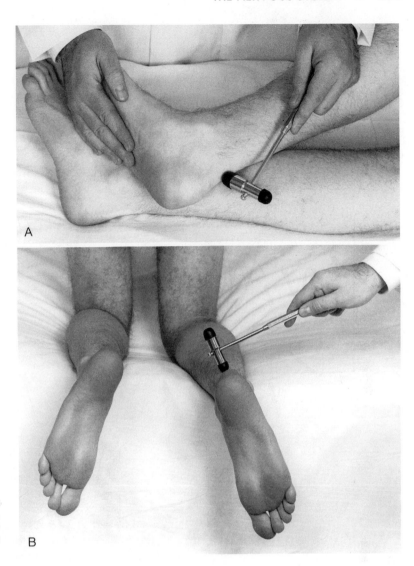

FIGURE 18–43. *A,* Alternate technique for evaluating the Achilles tendon reflex. *B,* Technique for assessing the Achilles tendon reflex when the reflex appears to be depressed.

abdominal muscles with the umbilicus deviating toward the stimulus. The abdominal reflex is frequently not seen in obese individuals. The *cremasteric* superficial reflex in males is elicited by lightly stroking the inner aspect of the thigh with an applicator stick or tongue depressor. The result is a rapid elevation of the testicle on the same side. Although the superficial reflexes are absent on the side of a corticospinal tract lesion, there is little clinical significance to their presence or absence. They are indicated here for completeness only.

Test for Abnormal Reflexes

Babinski's sign or reflex is a pathologic reflex. Normally when the lateral aspect of the sole is stroked from the heel to the ball of the foot and curved medially across the heads of the metatarsal bones, there is plantar flexion of the big toe. This tests the nerve roots at L5 – S2. The foot should be stroked with a noxious stimulus such as a key. A pin should *never* be used! In the presence of pyramidal tract disease, when the described movement is performed, there is a *dorsiflexion* of the big toe with fanning of the other toes. This is the Babinski reflex. Because the Babinski sign is an abnormal reflex, one should only comment that a Babinski sign is present; it is *never* absent. It is correct to describe

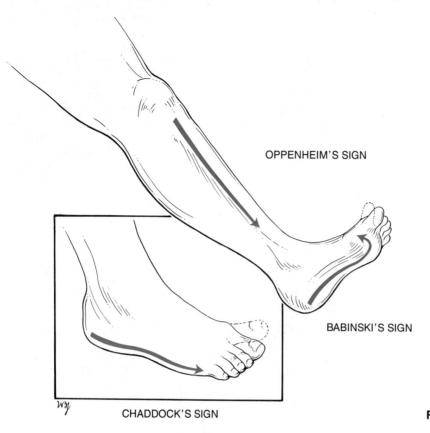

OPPENHEIM'S SIGN

BABINSKI'S SIGN

CHADDOCK'S SIGN

FIGURE 18–44. The plantar reflex.

the plantar reflex as either plantar flexion (normal) or dorsiflexion (abnormal, Babinski). The technique for evaluating the plantar reflex is shown in Figure 18–44.

Pyramidal tract disease is also suggested when the big toe dorsiflexes upon stroking the lateral aspect of the foot. This is *Chaddock's sign*. In the presence of pyramidal tract disease, downward pressure along the shin will also cause the big toe to dorsiflex. This is known as *Oppenheim's sign*. Both of these signs are less sensitive than stroking the plantar surface.

Another abnormal reflex associated with pyramidal tract disease is *Hoffmann's sign*. To elicit this sign, the patient's hand is pronated and the examiner grasps the terminal phalanx of the middle finger between the index finger and thumb. With a sharp jerk, the phalanx is passively flexed and suddenly released. A positive response consists of adduction and flexion of the thumb as well as flexion of the other fingers.

Sensory Function

Basic Principles

The sensory examination consists of testing for the following:

- Light touch
- Pain sensation
- Vibration sense
- Proprioception (position sense)
- Tactile localization
- Discriminative sensations (include two-point discrimination, stereognosis, graphesthesia, and point localization)

In a patient without any symptoms or signs of neurologic disease, the examination for sensory function can be performed by quickly assessing the presence of normal sensation on the distal fingers and toes. The examiner can choose to test for light touch, pain, and vibration sense. If these are normal, the details of the rest of the sensory examination are not required. If there are symptoms or signs referable to a neurologic disorder, complete testing is indicated.

As with the motor examination, the examiner compares side to side and proximal to distal. Neurologic disorders usually result in a sensory loss that is first seen more distally than proximally.

The hand is supplied by the median, ulnar, and radial nerves. The median nerve is the chief nerve of sensation because it supplies the palmar surfaces of the digits, the parts of the hand most commonly employed for feeling. The ulnar nerve supplies sensation only to the ulnar one and a half fingers. The radial nerve has its sensory distribution to the dorsum of the hand. There is considerable overlap in innervation. The clinically most reliable cutaneous areas for testing these nerves are illustrated in Figure 18–45. In these areas, there is the least likelihood of overlapping innervation.

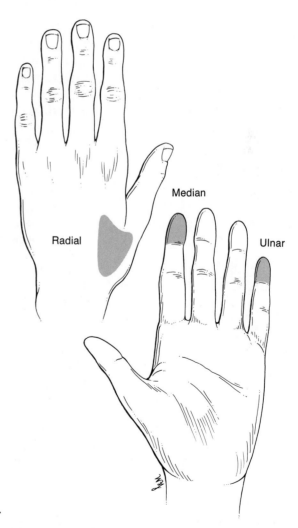

FIGURE 18–45. Hand sensation.

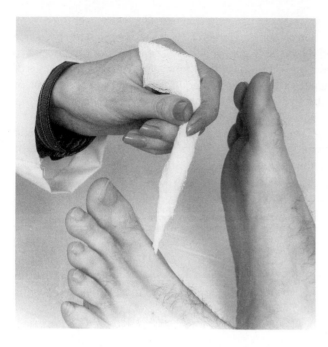

FIGURE 18-46. Technique for testing light touch.

Test Light Touch

Light touch is evaluated by lightly touching the patient with a small piece of gauze. Ask the patient to close his eyes and to tell you when he feels you touching him. Try touching the patient on the toes and fingers. This is illustrated in Figure 18-46. If sensation is normal, continue with the next test. If sensation is abnormal, work proximally until a *sensory level* can be determined. A sensory level is a spinal cord level below which there is a marked decrease in sensation. Figure 18-47 shows the segmental distribution of the spinal nerves that transmit sensation to the spinal cord.

Test Pain Sensation

Pain sensation is tested by using a safety pin and asking the patient if he feels it. Ask the patient to close his eyes. Open the safety pin and touch the patient with its tip. Tell the patient, "This is sharp." Now touch the patient with the blunt end of the pin and say, "This is dull." This is shown in Figure 18-48. Start testing pain sensation on the toes and fingers and say, "What is this, sharp or dull?" If the patient has no loss of sensation, proceed with the next examination. If there is a sensory loss to pain, continue proximally to determine the sensory level. A new pin should be used for each patient.

Test Vibration Sense

Vibration sense is tested using a 128 Hz tuning fork. Tap the tuning fork on the heel of your hand and place it on the patient on a bone prominence distally. Instruct the patient to inform you when he can no longer feel the vibration. Ask the patient to close his eyes. Place the vibrating tuning fork over the distal phalanx of the patient's finger and your own finger under the patient's finger, as shown in Figure 18-49A. In this fashion, you will be able to feel the vibration through the patient's finger to determine the accuracy of the patient's response. After the fingers are tested, test the big toes as shown in Figure 18-49B. If there is no loss of vibration sense, proceed with the next examination. If a loss is present, determine the level.

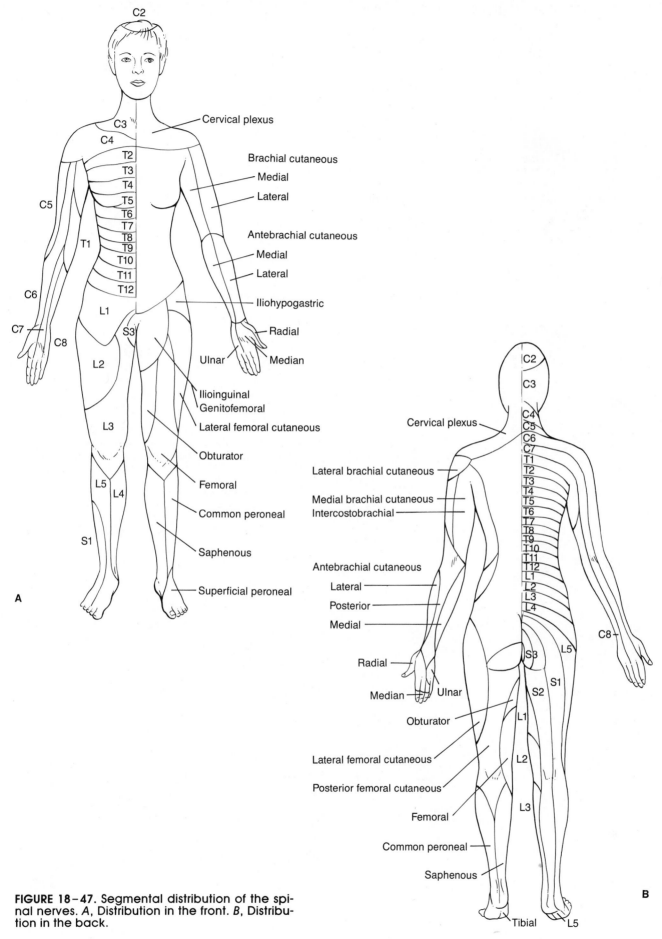

FIGURE 18–47. Segmental distribution of the spinal nerves. *A,* Distribution in the front. *B,* Distribution in the back.

507

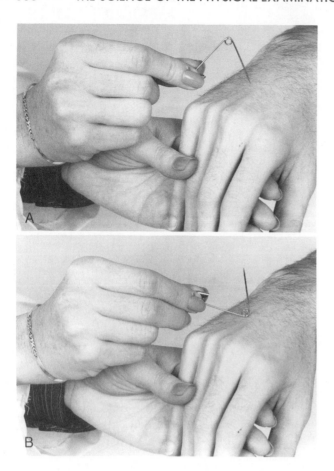

FIGURE 18–48. Technique for testing pain sensation. The examiner should hold the pin as shown in *A* and say, *"This is sharp." "This is dull"* is illustrated in *B*.

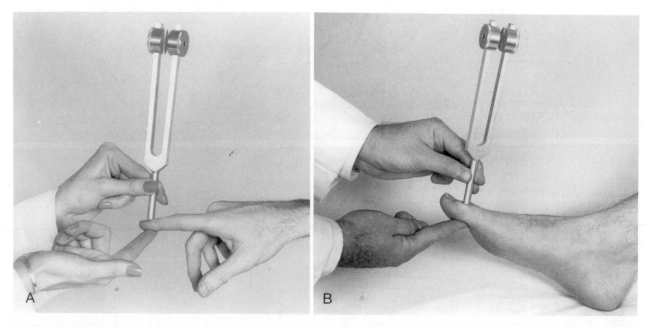

FIGURE 18–49. Technique for testing vibration sensation. *A,* Correct position for evaluating the vibration sensation in the finger. *B,* The technique for a toe.

Test Proprioception

Position sense, or proprioception, is tested by moving the distal phalanx. The examiner holds the distal phalanx at its *lateral* aspects and moves the digit up while telling the patient, "This is up." The examiner now moves the distal phalanx down and tells the patient, "This is down." With the patient's eyes closed, the examiner moves the distal phalanx up and down and finally stops and asks, "What is this, up or down?" This is shown in Figure 18–50A. It is important that the examiner grasp only the *sides* of the digit so that the patient will not have a clue by the pressure exerted on the digit. It is routine to test the terminal phalanx of a finger on each hand and the terminal phalanx of the toes (Fig. 18–50B). If no loss of position sense is detected, the examiner should continue with the rest of the examination. A loss requires further evaluation to determine the level of loss of proprioception.

Test Tactile Localization

Tactile localization, also known as double simultaneous stimulation, is assessed by having the patient close his eyes while asking him to identify where he was touched. The examiner can touch the patient on the right cheek and the left arm. The patient is then asked, "Where did I touch you?" This is demonstrated in Figure 18–51. Normally, patients will have no problem in identifying both

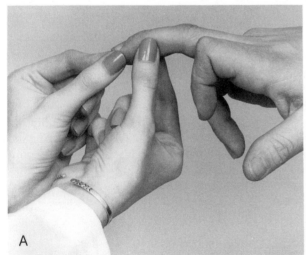

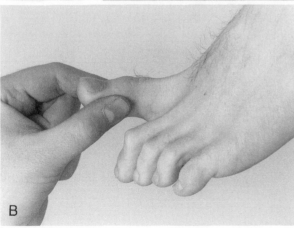

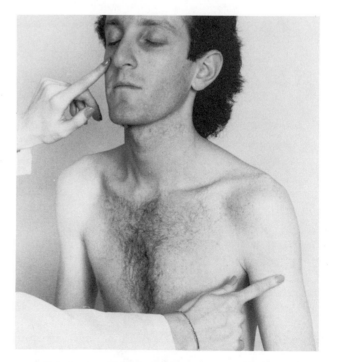

FIGURE 18–50. Technique for testing proprioception. *A,* Correct manner of holding the digit. *B,* Technique for the toe.

FIGURE 18–51. Technique for testing tactile localization.

areas. A patient with a lesion in the parietal lobe may feel the individual touches but may "extinguish" the sensation on the side contralateral to the side of the lesion. This is the phenomenon termed *extinction*.

Test Two-Point Discrimination

Two-point discrimination tests the ability of a patient to differentiate one stimulus from two. Gently hold two pins 2–3 mm apart and touch the patient's fingertip. Ask the patient to state the number of pins he feels. This is demonstrated in Figure 18–52. Compare this finding with the corresponding area on a fingertip on the other hand. Because different areas of the body have different sensitivities, it is important for the examiner to know these differences. At the fingertips, two-point discrimination is 2 mm apart. The tongue can discriminate 1 mm; the toes 3–8 mm; the palms 8–12 mm; the back 40–60 mm. The fingertips of the two hands are compared. A lesion in the parietal lobe will impair two-point discrimination.

Test Stereognosis

Stereognosis is the integrative function of the parietal and occipital lobes in which the patient attempts to identify an object placed in his hands. Have the patient close his eyes. Place a key, pencil, paper clip, or coin in the palm of the patient's hand and ask him to identify it. Test the other hand and compare the findings.

Test Graphesthesia

Graphesthesia is the ability to identify a number written in the palm one's hand. Ask the patient to close his eyes and extend his hand. Use the blunt end of a pencil to "write" numbers from 0 to 9 in the palm. The numbers should be oriented *facing* the patient. Normally, the patient will be able to identify the numbers. Compare one hand with the other. The inability to identify the numbers is a sensitive sign of parietal lobe disease. This is shown in Figure 18–53.

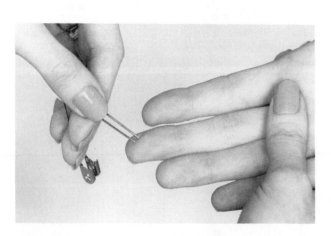

FIGURE 18–52. Technique for testing two-point discrimination.

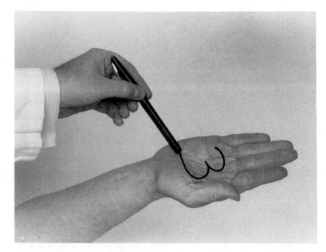

FIGURE 18–53. Technique for testing graphesthesia.

Test Point Localization

Point localization is the ability of a person to point to an area where he was touched. Have the patient close his eyes. Touch the patient. Ask the patient to open his eyes and "point" to the area where he was touched. Abnormalities of the sensory cortex will impair the ability to localize the area touched.

Cerebellar Function

Cerebellar function is tested by

- The finger-to-nose test
- The heel-to-knee test
- Rapid alternating movements
- The Romberg test
- Gait

Perform the Finger-to-Nose Test

The finger-to-nose test is performed by asking the patient to touch his nose and the examiner's finger alternately as quickly, accurately, and smoothly as possible. The examiner holds his finger at arm's length from the patient. The patient is instructed to touch the finger and then his nose. This is repeated several times, after which the patient is asked to perform the test with his eyes closed. This is demonstrated in Figure 18–54. Patients with cerebellar disease persistently overshoot the target, a condition known as *past pointing*. They may often have in addition a tremor as the finger approaches the target.

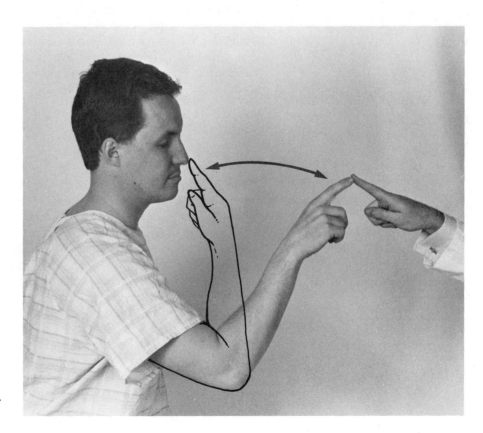

FIGURE 18–54. The finger-to-nose test.

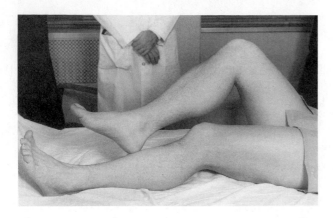

FIGURE 18–55. The heel-to-knee test.

Perform the Heel-to-Knee Test

The heel-to-knee test is performed by having the patient lie on his back. The patient is instructed to slide the heel of one lower extremity down the shin of the other, starting at the knee. A smooth movement should be seen, with the heel staying on the shin. This is shown in Figure 18–55. In patients with cerebellar disease, the heel wobbles from side to side.

Assess Rapid Alternating Movements

The ability to perform rapid alternating movements is known as diadochokinesia. These motions may be tested in the upper extremity or in the lower extremity. The patient may be asked to pronate and supinate one hand on the other hand rapidly. Another technique involves having the patient touch his thumb to each finger as quickly as possible. The patient may also be asked to slap his thigh, raise the hand, turn it over, and slap his thigh again rapidly. This pattern is repeated over and over as quickly as possible. These techniques are illustrated in Figure 18–56. An abnormality in performing rapid alternating movements is called adiadochokinesia.

Perform the Romberg Test

The Romberg test is performed by having the patient stand in front of the examiner with his feet together so that the heels and toes are touching. The examiner instructs the patient to extend his arms with his palms facing upward and to close his eyes. If the patient can maintain this posture without moving, the test is said to be "negative." A Romberg test is "positive" if the patient begins to sway and has to move his feet for balance. Another common finding is for one of the arms to drift downward with flexion of the fingers. This is called *pronator drift* and is seen in patients with a mild hemiparesis. The Romberg test examines the posterior columns rather than actual cerebellar function. It is important that the examiner be at the patient's side during this test, because occasionally a patient will suddenly sway and fall if assistance is not provided.

Assess Gait

Foremost in the examination of cerebellar function is the observation of gait. The patient is asked to walk straight ahead while the examiner observes his gait. He is then instructed to return on his tiptoes; walk away again on his heels; and

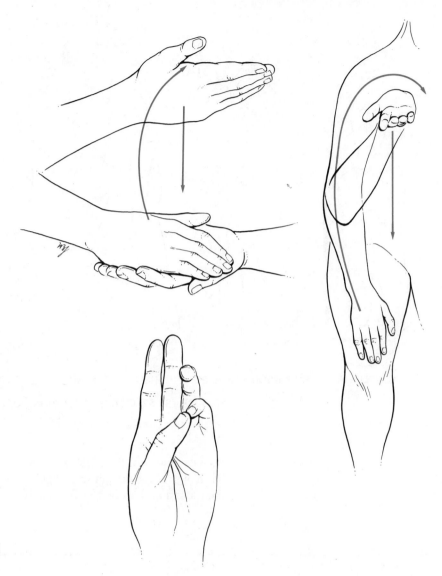

FIGURE 18–56. Techniques for testing rapid alternating movements.

finally return to the examiner by walking in tandem gait with one foot placed in front of the other; the heel of one foot touches the toes of each step. The examiner may wish to demonstrate this gait for the patient. The patient should have normal posture, and there should be normal associated movements of the arms. The examiner should pay special attention to the way in which the patient turns around. These maneuvers will often accentuate cerebellar ataxia as well as to indicate weakness in the lower extremities.

Many neurologic disorders produce striking and characteristic gaits. The patient with *hemiplegia* tends to drag or to circumduct his weak and spastic leg. The arm is frequently flexed at the elbow across the abdomen as the patient walks. The patient with *Parkinson's disease* shuffles with short, hurried steps. His head is bowed, with his back bent over. The patient with *cerebellar ataxia* walks with a wide-based gait. His feet are very far apart as he staggers from side to side. The patient with *foot drop* has a characteristic slapping gait resulting

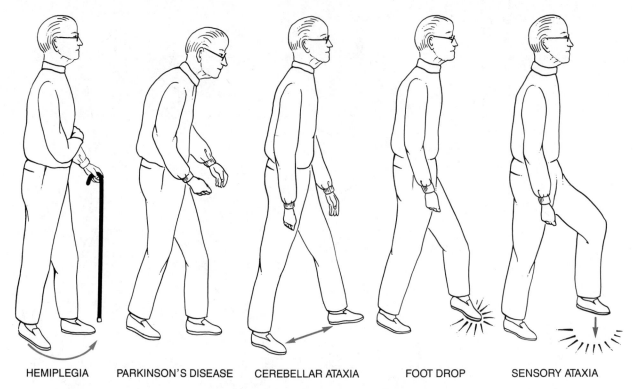

HEMIPLEGIA   PARKINSON'S DISEASE   CEREBELLAR ATAXIA   FOOT DROP   SENSORY ATAXIA

FIGURE 18–57. Common types of gaits.

from weakness of the dorsiflexors of the ankle. The patient with *sensory ataxia* has a high stepping gait. He slaps his feet down firmly as if he were not sure of their location. Figure 18–57 illustrates these gaits.

CLINICOPATHOLOGIC CORRELATIONS

The Comatose Patient

Coma is the state in which the patient is unable to respond to any stimuli. The causes of coma include the following:

- Meningeal infection
- Increased intracranial pressure of any cause
- Subarachnoid hemorrhage
- Focal cerebral lesion
- Brainstem lesion affecting the reticular system
- Metabolic encephalopathy*
- Status post-seizure activity

If the patient's friends or family is available, speak with them. They can help in the evaluation of the patient by giving valuable information. Is there a history of hypertension, diabetes, epilepsy, substance abuse, or recent head trauma?

---

* Common causes include electrolyte abnormalities, endocrine disorders, liver or kidney failure, vitamin deficiencies, poisoning, intoxications, and marked changes in body temperature.

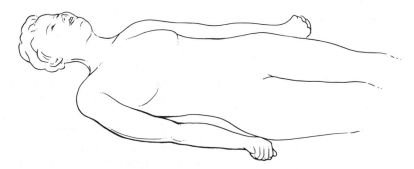

DECEREBRATE POSTURE

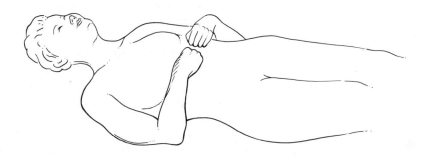

FIGURE 18–58. Postures of the comatose patient.

DECORTICATE POSTURE

If there is any evidence of head trauma, x-rays of the cervical spine must be taken before the examiner moves the patient's neck.

The physical examination of the comatose patient should start with inspection. The clothing, age, or evidence of chronic illness provides valuable clues as to the etiology of the coma. Does the patient have gingival enlargement consistent with anti-epileptic medical therapy?* Is there a characteristic odor to the breath? The sweet smell of ketones may be present in diabetic ketoacidosis. An odor of alcohol may be present. Are there stigmata of chronic liver disease?

What is the *posture* of the patient? Patients with cerebral hemispheric dysfunction or a destructive lesion of the pyramidal tracts maintain a *decorticate* posture, whereas those patients with a midbrain or pons lesion maintain a *decerebrate* posture. In decorticate rigidity, the arms are adducted and the elbows, wrists, and fingers are flexed. The legs are internally rotated. In decerebrate rigidity, the arms are also adducted but they are rigidly extended at the elbows and the forearms pronated. The wrists and fingers are flexed. In both postures, the feet are plantar flexed. These positions are shown in Figure 18–58.

The head should be evaluated for any areas of depression, as in a depressed skull fracture. Does the nose appear broken? Are there any broken teeth? Is there any clear, watery discharge from the nose or ear, suggestive of a leak of cerebrospinal fluid?

* Commonly related to phenytoin (Dilantin) therapy.

The *respiratory pattern* should be evaluated. Central neurogenic hyperventilation is seen in lesions of the midbrain or pons. This type of respiration consists of rapid, deep, regular breathing. *Cheyne-Stokes* breathing is characterized by rhythmic changes in the breathing pattern. Periods of rapid breathing are separated by periods of apnea. Cheyne-Stokes breathing is associated with brainstem compression or bilateral cerebral dysfunction.

The neurologic examination of the comatose patient is largely based on the pupillary size and the light reflexes. Small, reactive pupils are seen in bilateral cerebral dysfunction. Dilated pupils are seen following an overdose of hallucinogenic agents or central nervous system stimulants. A unilateral fixed and dilated pupil is suggestive of pressure on the ipsilateral oculomotor nerve. Pupillary dilation precedes paralysis of the extraocular muscles. This is due to the fact that the pupillary nerve fibers are located superficial to the fibers innervating the extraocular muscles and are more vulnerable to extrinsic stresses. This is an important sign of uncal herniation. In the presence of normally reactive pupils with absent corneal reflexes and absent extraocular movement, consider a metabolic abnormality as the cause of the coma.

The fundus of the eye may provide a clue as to the cause of the coma.

If there is no evidence of a fracture of the cervical spine, *oculocephalic reflexes* should be tested. If a comatose patient's head is rapidly turned to one side while the eyelids are held open, the eyes should move conjugately to the other side. This reflex has been termed *doll's eyes*. In a patient with a lesion in the brainstem, the doll's eyes reflex will be absent. The doll's eyes reflex can only be elicited in a comatose patient, because alert individuals will fixate on an object and override this reflex.

Caloric stimulation is used to enhance the doll's eyes reflex or to test movements in an individual with a broken cervical spine. The patient should be placed with his head flexed at 30°. This orients the semicircular canal in a horizontal position. A large bore syringe is filled with 20 – 30 ml of ice water, and the water is squeezed into one of the external auditory canals. The normal response is the development of nystagmus. Slowly the eyes will move conjugately to the ipsilateral side, followed by the rapid movement of the eyes back to the midline. Because nystagmus is named for the rapid component, the use of cold water causes nystagmus to the opposite side. If warm water is used, the eyes will show the rapid component toward the side being irrigated. This can easily be remembered by using the mnemonic *COWS*, which stands for *c*old *o*pposite, *w*arm *s*ame.

An absence of the caloric response is seen in patients with a disruption of the connections between the vestibular nuclei and the sixth nerve nucleus at the level of the brainstem.

Descriptions of Tables

As was indicated earlier in the chapter, headache is an important symptom of neurologic disease. Table 18 – 2 provides a differential diagnosis of headaches.

The correct assessment of a patient's motor activity can help to localize the site of a lesion. The term "extrapyramidal" refers to those parts of the motor

TABLE 18–2. Differential Diagnosis of Headache

Type	Epidemiology	Location	Signs and Symptoms
Migraine	Family history Young adults Females	Bifrontal	Nausea Vomiting Possible neurologic deficits
Cluster	Adolescent males	Orbitofrontal Unilateral	Unilateral nasal congestion Lacrimation
Tension	Females	Bilateral Generalized or occipital	
Hypertensive	Family history	Variable	Hypertensive retinopathy Possible papilledema
Increased intracranial pressure		Variable	Nausea Vomiting Papilledema
Meningitis		Bilateral Often occipital	Nuchal rigidity Fever
Temporal arteritis	Adults	Unilateral Over temporal artery	Tender temporal artery Loss of vision in ipsilateral eye

system that are not directly involved with the pyramidal tracts. The extrapyramidal system is composed of the basal ganglia, nuclei of the midbrain and reticular formation, and cerebellum. Table 18–3 lists the major areas and the specific motor problems associated with lesions of the lower motor neuron, the pyramidal tract, and the extrapyramidal tract. Table 18–4 summarizes the important signs and symptoms in five common chronic neurologic disorders.

A comparison of the *effects* of upper and lower motor neuron lesions is shown in Table 18–5.

Paraplegia and *quadriplegia* are upper motor neuron defects. They can involve lower motor neurons in addition. Injury of the spinal cord can produce partial or complete paralysis. In patients with cervical or thoracic lesions, spasticity will be present below the level of the lesion and flaccidity will be present in all muscles supplied from reflex arcs at the level of the lesion. In the presence of sacral lesions, a flaccid paralysis results. Table 18–6 summarizes motor involvement in spinal cord lesions.

TABLE 18–3. Effects of Various Lesions

	Lower Motor Neuron	Pyramidal Tract	Extrapyramidal Tract
Major effect	Flaccid paralysis	Spastic paralysis Hyperactive reflexes	No paralysis
Muscle appearance	Atrophy Fasciculations	Mild atrophy from disuse	Rest tremor
Muscle tone	Decreased	Increased	Increased
Muscle strength	Decreased or absent	Decreased or absent	Normal
Coordination	Absent or poor	Absent or poor	Slowed

TABLE 18–4. Common Neurologic Conditions and Their Signs and Symptoms

Condition	Age of Onset (yr)	Sex	Signs and Symptoms
Multiple sclerosis	30–35	Females	Nystagmus Diplopia Slurring of speech Muscular weakness Paresthesias Poor coordination Bowel and bladder dysfunction
Amyotrophic lateral sclerosis	50–80	Males	Irregular twitching of involved muscles Muscular weakness Muscle atrophy Absence of sensory or mental deficits
Parkinson's disease	60–80	Males	Rigidity Slowing of movements Involuntary tremor Difficulty in swallowing Tremor in upper extremities Jerky, "cogwheel" motions Slow, shuffling gait with loss of arm swing Mask-like facial expression Body in moderate flexion Excessive salivation
Myasthenia gravis	20–50	Females	Generalized muscular fatigue Bilateral ptosis* Diplopia Difficulty in swallowing Voice weakness
Huntington's chorea	35–50	Both	Choreiform movements Brain failure Rapid movements Facial grimacing Dysarthria Personality change

* See Plate V F.

Often a patient may complain of a decreased ability to perform a task. Physical examination may often reveal a decreased motor strength. Table 18–7 summarizes the major actions of the more common muscles and their corresponding cord segments.

Patients with *inflammation of the meninges* often complain of pain in the neck and a resistance to flexion of the neck. If meningitis is suspected, have the

TABLE 18–5. Comparison of Effects of Upper and Lower Motor Neuron Lesions

Effect	Upper Motor Neuron Lesion	Lower Motor Neuron Lesion
Voluntary control	Lost	Lost
Muscle tone	Spastic, increased	Flaccid, decreased
Reflex arcs	Present	Absent
Pathologic reflexes	Present	Not present
Muscle atrophy	Little or none	Significant

TABLE 18–6. Motor Involvement in Spinal Cord Lesions

Affected Cord Segment	Motor Involvement
C1–4	Paralysis of neck, diaphragm, intercostals, and all four extremities.
C5	Spastic paralysis of trunk, arms, and legs. Partial shoulder control.
C6–7	Spastic paralysis of trunk and legs. Upper arm control. Partial lower arm control.
C8	Spastic paralysis of trunk and legs. Hand weakness only.
T1–10	Spastic paralysis of trunk and legs.
T11–12	Spastic paralysis of legs.
L1–S1	Flaccid paralysis of legs.
S2–5	Flaccid paralysis of lower legs. Bowel, bladder, and sexual function affected.

patient lie on his back. Place your hand behind the patient's neck and flex it until the chin touches the sternum. In patients with meningitis, there is neck pain and resistance to motion. There may also be flexion of the patient's hips and knees. This has been called *Brudzinski's sign*. Another sign of meningeal irritation can be elicited while the patient lies on his back, and you flex one of the patient's legs at the hip and knee. If pain or resistance is elicited as the knee is straightened, a positive *Kernig's sign* is said to be present.

TABLE 18–7. Motor Function According to Cord Segments

Area of Body	Action Tested	Cord Segment
Shoulder	Flexion, extension, or rotation of neck	C1–C4
Arm	Adduction of arm	C5–C8, T1
	Abduction of arm	C4–C6
	Flexion of forearm	C5–C6
	Extension of forearm	C6–C8
	Supination of forearm	C5–C7
	Pronation of forearm	C6–C7
Hand	Extension of hand	C6–C8
	Flexion of hand	C7–C8, T1
Finger	Abduction of thumb	C7–C8, T1
	Adduction of thumb	C8, T1
	Abduction of little finger	C8, T1
	Opposition of thumb	C8, T1
Hip	Flexion of hip	L1–L3
	Extension of leg	L2–L4
	Flexion of leg	L4–L5, S1–S2
	Adduction of thigh	L2–L4
	Abduction of thigh	L4–L5, S1–S2
	Medial rotation of thigh	L4–L5, S1
	Lateral rotation of thigh	L4–L5, S1–S2
	Flexion of thigh	L4–L5
Foot	Dorsiflexion of foot	L4–L5, S1
	Plantar flexion of foot	L5, S1–S2
Toe	Extension of great toe	L4–L5, S1
	Flexion of great toe	L5, S1–S2
	Spreading of toes	S1–S2

USEFUL VOCABULARY

Listed here are the specific roots that are important in order to understand the terminology related to neurologic diseases.

ROOT	PERTAINING TO	EXAMPLE	DEFINITION
asthe-	feeling	an*esthe*sia	Loss of feeling
-gnosia	recognition	a*gnosia*	Loss of the power to recognize sensory stimuli
myelo-	spinal cord	*myelo*gram	An roentgenogram of the spinal cord
-paresis	weakness	hemi*paresis*	Muscular weakness affecting half of the body
-plegia	paralysis	ophthalmo*plegia*	Paralysis of the eye muscles
radicul(o)-	spinal nerve root	*radiculo*pathy	Disease of a spinal nerve root

WRITING UP THE PHYSICAL EXAMINATION

Listed here are examples of the write-up for the examination of the neurologic system.

The patient is oriented to person, time, and place. Cranial nerves II – XII are intact. Motor examination reveals normal gait, normal heel-to-toe movement, and normal strength bilaterally. Reflexes are equal bilaterally and are within normal limits. The sensory examination is normal, with pain, light touch, and stereognosis intact. Cerebellar function is normal.

The mental status examination is within normal limits. There is a marked weakness of the lower half of the right side of the face. The right nasolabial fold is flat, and the mouth droops downward on the right. There is no other cranial nerve abnormality. The motor and sensory examinations are within normal limits. Reflexes are normal. Romberg is negative.

The patient has an expressive aphasia and a right hemiplegia with ipsilateral trigeminal hemiplegia. Reflexes in the right lower extremity are hyperactive compared with the left. Sensory examination is difficult to assess. A Babinski sign is present on the right side.

Mental status is within normal limits. Motor examination and reflexes are equal bilaterally. There is a sensory level at L2 on the right and at L4 on the left. Vibration sense is impaired more on the right than on the left, as is position sense. The Romberg test is positive.

BIBLIOGRAPHY

Adams RD, Victor M: Principles of Neurology. New York, McGraw-Hill, 1985.

Brazis PW, Masdeu JC, Biller J: Localization in Clinical Neurology. Boston, Little, Brown and Company, 1985.

Chusid JG: Correlative Neuroanatomy and Functional Neurology. Los Altos, CA, Lange Medical Publishers, 1985.

Fowler TJ, May RW: Neurology. Littleton, MA, PSG Publishing Company, Inc, 1985.

Gilman S, Winans SS: Manter and Gatz's Essentials of Clinical Neuroanatomy and Neurophysiology. Philadelphia, FA Davis, 1982.

Weiner WJ, Goetz CG (eds): Neurology for the Non-Neurologist. Philadelphia, Harper and Row, 1981.

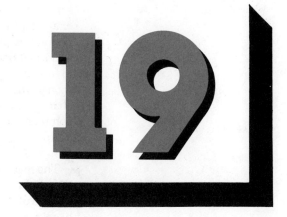

PUTTING THE EXAMINATION TOGETHER

A physician is not only a scientist or a good technician. He must be more than that — he must have good human qualities. He has to have a personal understanding and sympathy for the suffering of human beings.

**Albert Einstein
1879 – 1955**

THE TECHNIQUES

The previous chapters have dealt with the individual organ systems and the history and physical examinations related to each of them. The purpose of this chapter is to help the student assimilate each of the individual examinations into one that is complete and smoothly performed.

A complete examination is ideally performed in an orderly, thorough manner with as few movements as possible required of the patient. Most errors in performing a physical examination are due to a lack of organization and thoroughness, not to a lack of knowledge. Evaluate each part of the examination carefully before moving on to the next part. The most commonly observed errors in the physical examination are related to the following:

- Technique
- Omission
- Detection
- Interpretation
- Recording

Errors in *technique* are related to lack of order and organization of the examination, faulty equipment, and poor bedside etiquette. Errors of *omission* are common in the examination of the eye and nose, auscultation of the neck vessels, chest, and heart; palpation of the spleen; rectal and genitalia examinations; and the neurologic examination. Errors of *detection* are those in which the examiner fails to detect abnormalities that are present. Most commonly occurring errors of this type are those involving thyroid nodules, tracheal deviation, abnormal breath sounds, diastolic murmurs, hernias, and abnormalities of the extraocular muscles. Errors in the *interpretation* of findings occur most commonly with tracheal deviation, venous pulses, systolic murmurs, fremitus changes, abdominal tenderness, liver size, eye findings, and reflexes. The most common types of *recording* errors are related to the description of heart size and murmurs, improper terminology, and obscure abbreviations.

The following examination sequence is the one followed by the author. There is no right or wrong sequence. Develop your own approach. Remember that at the end of whichever technique you use, the complete examination should have been performed.

In most situations, the patient will be lying in bed when you arrive. After introducing yourself and taking a complete history, you should then inform the patient that you are ready to begin the physical examination. Start by washing your hands.

Patient Lying Supine in Bed

General Appearance

1. Inspect patient's facial expression (Chaps. 10, 11, and 14)

Vital Signs (Chap. 11)

1. Palpate blood pressure on right arm
2. Auscultate blood pressure on right arm
3. Auscultate blood pressure on left arm*

Have Patient Sit Up in Bed

Vital Signs

1. Check for orthostatic changes on left arm (Chap. 11)

Have Patient Turn and Sit with Legs Dangling Off Side of Bed

Vital Signs

1. Palpate radial pulse for rate and regularity (Chap. 12)
2. Determine respiratory rate and pattern (Chap. 10)

Head (Chap. 6)

1. Inspect cranium
2. Inspect scalp
3. Palpate cranium

---

* If the blood pressure is elevated in the upper extremity, blood pressure in the lower extremity must be assessed to exclude coarctation of the aorta. The patient is asked to lie prone, and blood pressure by auscultation is determined (see Chap. 11).

Face (Chaps. 5 and 6)

1. Inspect face
2. Inspect skin on face

Eyes (Chap. 7)

1. Assess visual acuity, both eyes
2. Check visual fields, both eyes
3. Determine eye alignment, both eyes
4. Test extraocular muscle function, both eyes
5. Check pupillary responses to light, both eyes
6. Test for accommodation, both eyes
7. Inspect external eye structures, both eyes
8. Ophthalmoscopic examination, both eyes
9. Inspect retina, both eyes

Nose (Chap. 8)

1. Inspect nose
2. Palpate nasal skeleton
3. Palpate sinuses (frontal, maxillary), both sides
4. Inspect nasal septum from both sides
5. Inspect turbinates, both sides

Ears (Chap. 8)

1. Inspect external ear structures, both sides
2. Palpate external ear structures, both sides
3. Evaluate auditory acuity, both sides
4. Perform Rinne test, both sides
5. Perform Weber test
6. Perform otoscopic examination, both sides
7. Inspect external canal, both sides
8. Inspect tympanic membrane, both sides

Mouth (Chap. 9)

1. Inspect outer and inner surfaces of lips
2. Inspect buccal mucosa
3. Inspect gingivae
4. Inspect teeth
5. Observe Stenson's and Wharton's ducts, both sides
6. Inspect hard palate
7. Inspect soft palate
8. Inspect tongue
9. Test hypoglossal nerve function (Chap. 18)
10. Palpate tongue
11. Inspect the floor of the mouth
12. Palpate floor of the mouth
13. Inspect tonsils, both sides
14. Inspect posterior pharyngeal wall
15. Observe uvula as patient says, "Ah" (Chap. 18)
16. Test gag reflex (Chap. 18)

Neck (Chap. 6)	1. Inspect neck, both sides 2. Palpate neck, both sides 3. Palpate lymph nodes of head and neck, both sides 4. Palpate thyroid gland by anterior approach 5. Evaluate position of trachea (Chap. 11) 6. Evaluate mobility of trachea (Chap. 11)
Neck Vessels (Chap. 11)	1. Inspect height of the jugular venous pulsation, right side
Neck* (Chap. 6)	1. Palpate thyroid gland by posterior approach 2. Palpate for supraclavicular lymph nodes, both sides
Posterior Chest (Chap. 10)	1. Inspect back, both sides 2. Palpate back for tenderness, both sides 3. Evaluate chest excursion, both sides 4. Palpate for tactile fremitus, both sides 5. Percuss the back, both sides 6. Evaluate diaphragmatic excursion, right side 7. Auscultate the back, both sides 8. Palpate for costovertebral angle tenderness, both sides (Chap. 14)
Sacrum (Chap. 11)	1. Test for edema
Anterior Chest† (Chap. 10)	1. Inspect patient's posture 2. Inspect configuration of chest 3. Inspect chest, both sides 4. Palpate chest for tactile fremitus, both sides
Female Breast (Chap. 13)	1. Inspect breast, both sides 2. Inspect breast during maneuvers to tense pectoral muscles, both sides
Heart (Chap. 11)	1. Inspect for abnormal chest movements 2. Palpate for point of maximum impulse 3. Auscultate for heart sounds, all four positions
Axilla (Chap. 13)	1. Inspect axilla, both sides 2. Palpate axilla, both sides 3. Palpate for epitrochlear nodes, both sides (Chap. 12)

---

* The examiner should now go to the back of the patient while the patient remains seated with his legs dangling off the side of the bed.

† The examiner should now go to the front of the patient while the patient remains seated with his legs dangling off the side of the bed.

Have Patient Lean Forward

Heart (Chap. 11)
1. Auscultate with diaphragm, base of stethoscope

Have Patient Lie Supine with Head of Bed Elevated About 30°

Neck Vessels (Chap. 11)
1. Inspect the jugular venous wave form, right side
2. Palpate the carotid artery, each side separately
3. Auscultate the carotid artery, both sides

Breasts, Male and Female (Chap. 13)
1. Inspect breast, both sides
2. Palpate breast, both sides
3. Palpate subareolar area, both sides
4. Palpate nipple, both sides

Chest (Chap. 10)
1. Inspect chest, both sides
2. Evaluate chest excursion, both sides
3. Palpate for tactile fremitus, both sides
4. Percuss chest, both sides
5. Auscultate breath sounds, both sides

Heart (Chap. 11)
1. Inspect for movements
2. Palpate for localized motion, all four positions
3. Palpate for generalized motion, all four positions
4. Palpate for thrills, all four positions
5. Auscultate heart sounds, all four positions
6. Time the heart sounds to the carotid pulse

Have Patient Turn on Left Side

Heart (Chap. 11)
1. Auscultate with bell at cardiac apex

Have Patient Lie Supine with Bed Flat

Abdomen (Chap. 14)
1. Inspect the contour of the abdomen
2. Inspect the skin of the abdomen
3. Inspect for hernias
4. Auscultate the abdomen for bowel sounds, one quadrant
5. Auscultate the abdomen for bruits, both sides
6. Percuss the abdomen, all quadrants
7. Percuss the liver
8. Percuss the spleen

9. Test superficial abdominal reflex (Chap. 18)
10. Palpate abdomen lightly, all quadrants
11. Palpate abdomen deeply, all quadrants
12. Exclude rebound tenderness
13. Check for hepatic tenderness
14. Evaluate the hepatojugular reflux (Chap. 11)
15. Palpate liver
16. Palpate spleen
17. Palpate kidney
18. Palpate aorta
19. Check for shifting dullness if ascites is suspected

Pulses (Chap. 12)

1. Palpate radial pulse, both sides
2. Palpate brachial pulse, both sides
3. Palpate femoral pulse, both sides
4. Palpate popliteal pulse, both sides
5. Palpate dorsalis pedis pulse, both sides
6. Palpate posterior tibial pulse, both sides
7. Time radial and femoral pulses, right side
8. Perform heel-to-knee test (part of neurologic examination: see Chap. 18)

Male Genitalia (Chap. 15)

1. Inspect the skin and hair distribution
2. Observe the inguinal area while instructing the patient to bear down
3. Inspect the penis
4. Inspect the scrotum
5. Palpate for inguinal nodes, both sides
6. Elevate the scrotum and inspect the perineum

Have the Man Stand in Front of Seated Examiner

Male Genitalia (Chap. 15)

1. Inspect the penis
2. Inspect the external urethral meatus
3. Palpate the shaft of the penis
4. Palpate the urethra
5. Inspect the scrotum
6. Palpate the testicle, both sides
7. Palpate the epididymis and vas deferens, both sides
8. Observe the inguinal area while instructing the patient to bear down
9. Test superficial cremasteric reflex (Chap. 18)
10. Transilluminate any masses
11. Palpate for hernias, both sides

Have the Man Turn Around and Bend over Bed

Rectum (Chap. 14)

1. Inspect the anus
2. Inspect the anus while patient strains
3. Palpate the anal sphincter

4. Palpate the rectal walls
5. Palpate the prostate gland
6. Test stool for occult blood

Woman Is Helped to Lithotomy Position

Female Genitalia
(Chap. 16)

1. Inspect the skin and hair distribution
2. Inspect the labia majora
3. Palpate the labia majora
4. Inspect the labia minora, clitoris, urethral meatus, and introitus
5. Inspect the area of Bartholin's glands, both sides
6. Inspect the perineum
7. Test for pelvic relaxation
8. Perform speculum examination
9. Inspect cervix
10. Pap smear
11. Inspect vaginal walls
12. Perform bimanual examination
13. Palpate cervix and uterine body
14. Palpate adnexa, both sides
15. Palpate rectovaginal septum
16. Test stool for occult blood

Have Patient Sit on Bed with Legs Off Side

Mental Status

1. Ask routine questions (Chap. 18)

Face (Chap. 18)

1. Test motor function of trigeminal nerve, both sides
2. Test sensory function of trigeminal nerve, both sides
3. Test corneal reflex, both eyes
4. Test facial nerve, both sides
5. Test spinal accessory nerve, both sides
6. Test double simultaneous stimulation, both sides
7. Perform finger-to-nose test

Neck

1. Test range of motion (Chap. 17)

Hands and Wrists
(Chaps. 17 and 18)

1. Inspect hand and wrist, both sides
2. Inspect nails, both sides (Chap. 5)
3. Palpate shoulder joint, both sides
4. Palpate interphalangeal joints, both sides
5. Palpate metacarpophalangeal joints, both sides
6. Test light touch, both sides
7. Test vibration sense, both sides
8. Test position sense, both sides
9. Test object identification, both sides

10. Test graphesthesia, both sides
11. Test two-point discrimination, both sides
12. Assess rapid alternating movements, both sides

Elbows (Chap. 17)

1. Inspect elbow, both sides
2. Test range of motion, both sides
3. Palpate elbow, both sides
4. Test upper extremity strength, both sides
5. Test biceps reflex, both sides (Chap. 18)
6. Test triceps reflex, both sides (Chap. 18)

Shoulders (Chap. 17)

1. Inspect shoulder, both sides
2. Test range of motion, both sides
3. Palpate shoulder joint, both sides

Shins

1. Inspect skin, both sides
2. Test for edema, both sides (Chap. 11)

Feet and Ankles
(Chaps. 17 and 18)

1. Inspect feet and ankles
2. Test range of motion, both sides
3. Palpate Achilles tendon, both sides
4. Palpate metatarsophalageal joints, both sides
5. Palpate metatarsal heads, both sides
6. Palpate ankle and foot joints, both sides
7. Test light touch, both sides
8. Test vibration sense, both sides
9. Test position sense, both sides
10. Test lower extremity strength, both sides
11. Test ankle reflex, both sides
12. Test plantar response, both sides

Knees (Chaps. 17 and 18)

1. Inspect knee, both sides
2. Test range of motion, both sides
3. Palpate patella, both sides
4. Ballotte patella if effusion is suspected
5. Test patellar reflex, both sides

Have Patient Stand with Back to Examiner

Hips (Chap. 17)

1. Inspect hips
2. Test range of motion

Spine (Chaps. 17 and 18)
1. Inspect spine
2. Palpate spine
3. Test range of motion
4. Assess gait
5. Perform the Romberg test

THE WRITTEN PHYSICAL EXAMINATION

After the examination has been completed, the examiner must be able to record objectively all the findings of inspection, palpation, percussion, and auscultation. It is very important to be precise in stating locations of abnormalities. Small drawings may be very useful to describe a shape or location better. When describing the size of a finding, it is preferable to state the size in millimeters or centimeters rather than describing it as compared to a fruit or nut, which can vary greatly in size. It is best not to use abbreviations. Abbreviations may mean different things to different readers. However, the abbreviations used in the following examples are standard and may be used. Finally, do not make diagnostic statements in the write-up; save them for the summary at the end. For example, it is better to state that *a grade III/VI holosystolic murmur at the apex with radiation to the axilla* is present, rather than *a murmur of mitral insufficiency* is present.

Patient: John Henry*

■ **General Appearance.** The patient is a 65 year old white man who is lying in bed on two pillows and is in no acute distress. He is well developed and thin and appears slightly older than his stated age. The patient is well groomed, alert, and cooperative.

■ **Vital Signs.** BP 185/65/55 right arm (lying), 180/60/50 left arm (lying), 175/65/50 left arm (sitting); heart rate 90 and regular; respirations 16.

■ **Skin.** Pink, with small hyperkeratotic papules over the face; nailbeds slightly dusky; hair thin on head; absent hair on lower portion of lower extremities; normal male escutcheon.

■ **Head.** Normocephalic without evidence of trauma; no tenderness present.

■ **Eyes.** Visual acuity with glasses using near card: OD 20/60, OS 20/40; visual fields full bilaterally; EOMs intact; PERRLA; xanthelasma present bilaterally, L > R; eyebrows normal; bilateral arcus senilis present; conjunctivae pink without injection or discharge; opacities present in both lenses, R > L; left disc sharp with normal cup-to-disc ratio; normal A-V ratio OS; no A-V nicking present OS; there is a flame-shaped hemorrhage present at 6 o'clock OS;

---

* This name is fictitious. Any similarity to a person living or dead with this name is purely coincidental.

several cotton-wool spots are also present at 1 and 5 o'clock OS; right fundus not well visualized as a result of lenticular opacity.

▪ **Ears.** Auricles in normal position; no tenderness present; small amount of cerumen in left external canal; canals without injection or discharge; Rinne, BC > AC right ear, AC > BC left ear; Weber, lateralization to the right ear; both tympanic membranes are gray without injection; normal landmarks seen bilaterally.

▪ **Nose.** Nose straight without masses; patent bilaterally; mucosa pink with a clear discharge present; inferior turbinate on the right slightly edematous.

▪ **Sinuses.** No tenderness detected over frontal and maxillary sinuses.

▪ **Throat.** Lips slightly cyanotic without lesions; patient wears an upper denture; buccal mucosa pink without injection; all lower teeth are present and are in fair condition; no obvious caries; gingivae normal; tongue midline without fasciculations; no lesions seen or palpated on tongue; mild injection of posterior pharynx with yellowish-white discharge present on posterior pharynx and tonsils; tonsils minimally enlarged; uvula elevates in midline; gag reflex intact.

▪ **Neck.** Supple with full range of motion; trachea midline and freely movable; small (1 – 2 cm) lymph nodes are present in both superficial cervical and tonsillar node chains; thyroid borders palpable; no thyroid nodules or enlargement noted; no abnormal neck vein distention present; neck veins flat while sitting upright.

▪ **Chest.** AP diameter increased; symmetrical excursion bilaterally; tactile fremitus normal bilaterally; chest resonant bilaterally; vesicular breath sounds bilaterally; coarse breath sounds with occasional crackles present at the bases.

▪ **Breasts.** Mild gynecomastia, L > R; no masses or discharge present.

▪ **Heart.** PMI 6ICS 2 cm lateral to MCL; normal physiologic splitting present; no heaves or thrills are present; S_1 and S_2 distant; a grade II/VI high-pitched holodiastolic murmur is heard at the 2ICS at the right upper sternal border; a grade I/VI medium-pitched systolic crescendo-decrescendo murmur is heard in the aortic area; the systolic murmur is mid-peaking (Fig. 19 – 1).

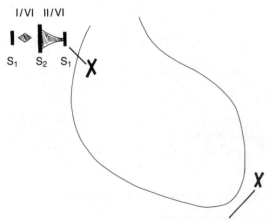

PMI 6ICS-2cm lateral MCL   **FIGURE 19 – 1.** Location of cardiac physical signs.

■ **Vascular.** A carotid bruit is present on the right; no bruits are heard over the left carotid, renal, femoral, or abdominal arteries; lower extremities are slightly cool compared with the upper extremities; 1 + pretibial edema is present on the right lower extremity; 2 + pretibial edema is present on the left; mild venous varicosities are present from midthigh to calf bilaterally; no ulceration or stasis changes are present; no calf tenderness is present.

■ **Abdomen.** The abdomen is scaphoid; a RLQ appendectomy scar as well as a LLQ herniorrhaphy scar is present; both scars are well healed; a 3 × 3 cm mass is seen in the RLQ after coughing or straining; no guarding, rigidity, or tenderness is present; no visible pulsations are present; bowel sounds are present; percussion note is tympanitic throughout the abdomen except over the suprapubic region, where the percussion note is dull; liver span is 10 cm from top to bottom in the MCL; spleen percussed in LUQ but not palpated; kidneys not felt; no CVAT present; there is an easily reducible right indirect inguinal hernia felt at the external ring.

■ **Rectal.** Anal sphincter normal; no hemorrhoids present; nontender prostate enlarged symmetrically; prostate firm without nodules felt; no luminal masses felt in rectum; stool negative for blood.

■ **Genitalia.** Circumcised male with normal genitalia; penis without induration; left hemiscrotum 4 – 5 cm below the right; palpation of left hemiscrotum reveals dilatation of the pampiniform plexus; soft testes 2 × 3 × 1 bilaterally.

■ **Lymphatic.** Nodes in anterior triangle chains already noted; two firm, 1 – 2 cm, rubbery, freely mobile nodes in left femoral area; no epitrochlear, axillary, or supraclavicular nodes felt.

■ **Musculoskeletal.** Distal IP joint enlargement on both hands causing pain on making a fist, L > R; no tenderness or erythema present; proximal joints normal; neck, arms, hips, knees, and ankles with full range of active and passive motion; muscles appear symmetrical; mild kyphosis present.

■ **Neurologic.** Oriented to person, place, and time; cranial nerves II – XII intact; gross sensory and motor strength intact; cerebellar function normal; plantar reflexes down; gait normal; deep tendon reflexes as shown in table (Table 19 – 1).

■ **Summary.** Mr. Henry is a 65 year old man in no acute distress. Physical examination reveals systolic hypertension, retinal changes suggestive of sustained hypertension, a mild cataract in his right eye, a conductive hearing loss in his right ear, tonsillopharyngitis, and gynecomastia. Cardiac examination reveals aortic insufficiency. Peripheral vascular examination reveals probable atherosclerotic disease of the right carotid artery and mild venous disease of the lower extremities. The patient has a right, easily reducible, inguinal hernia. A left-sided varicocele is present. Mild osteoarthritis of the hands is also present.

TABLE 19 – 1. Deep Tendon Reflexes of Patient John Henry

	Biceps	Triceps	Knee	Achilles
Right	1+	0	2+	1+
Left	2+	1+	3+	2+

Patient: Mary Jones*

■ **General Appearance.** The patient is a 51 year old black woman who is sitting up in bed in mild respiratory distress. She is obese and appears her stated age. She is well groomed and alert, but she constantly complains about her shortness of breath.

■ **Vital Signs.** BP 130/80/75 right arm (lying), 125/75/70 left arm (lying), 120/75/70 (sitting); heart rate 100 and regular; respirations 20.

■ **Skin.** Upper extremities slightly dusky as compared with the lower extremities; good tissue turgor; patient is wearing a wig to cover her marked total baldness; normal female escutcheon.

■ **Head.** Normocephalic without evidence of trauma; face appears edematous; no tenderness noted.

■ **Eyes.** Visual acuity using near card: OD 20/40, OS 20/30; visual fields full bilaterally; EOMs intact; PERRLA; eyebrows thin bilaterally; conjunctivae red bilaterally with injection present; lenses clear; both discs appear sharp with some nasal blurring; the cup-to-disc ratio is 1:3 bilaterally, and the cups are symmetric; the retinal veins appear dilated bilaterally.

■ **Ears.** Pinna in normal position; no mastoid or external canal tenderness; canals without injection or discharge; Rinne, AC > BC bilaterally; Weber, no lateralization; both tympanic membranes clearly visualized; normal landmarks seen bilaterally.

■ **Nose.** Straight without deviation; mucosa reddish pink; inferior turbinates within normal limits.

■ **Sinuses.** No tenderness detected.

■ **Throat.** Lips cyanotic; all teeth present except for all third molars, which have been extracted; occlusion normal; no caries seen; gingivae normal; tongue midline with markedly dilated tortuous veins on undersurface; no fasciculations of tongue noted; posterior pharynx appears within normal limits; uvula midline and elevates normally; gag reflex intact.

■ **Neck.** Full with normal range of motion; trachea midline but fixed; neck veins distended to angle of jaw while sitting upright; no adenopathy of neck noted.

■ **Chest.** AP diameter normal; symmetric excursion bilaterally; increased tactile fremitus at right base posteriorly corresponds to area of bronchial breath sounds; percussion note in this area is dull, all other chest areas are resonant; bronchophony and egophony present in area of bronchial breath sounds; crackles and wheezes present in area at right posterior base.

■ **Breasts.** Left mastectomy scar; right breast without masses, dimpling, or discharge.

---

* This name is fictitious. Any similarity to a person living or dead with this name is purely coincidental.

TABLE 19–2. Deep Tendon Reflexes of Patient Mary Jones

	Biceps	Triceps	Knee	Achilles
Right	2+	2+	2+	1+
Left	2+	1+	2+	2+

■ **Heart.** PMI 5ICS-MCL; normal physiologic splitting present; no heaves or thrills present; S₁ and S₂ within normal limits; no murmurs, gallops, or rubs present.

■ **Vascular.** There are no bruits present over the carotid, renal, femoral, or abdominal arteries; the extremities are without clubbing or edema.

■ **Abdomen.** The abdomen is obese without guarding, rigidity, or tenderness; no visible pulsations are present; bowel sounds are normal; percussion note is tympanitic throughout the abdomen; liver span is 15 cm in the MCL; spleen not percussed or palpated; kidneys not palpated; no CVAT present.

■ **Rectal.** Refused.

■ **Pelvic.** Deferred until patient more stable.

■ **Lymphatic.** No adenopathy felt in the neck chains or in the epitrochlear, axillary, supraclavicular, or femoral regions.

■ **Musculoskeletal.** Marked edema of both upper extremities, L > R; neck, arms, knees, and ankles with full range of active and passive motion; muscles appear symmetrical except for upper extremities.

■ **Neurologic.** Oriented to person, place, and time; cranial nerves II–XII intact; gross sensory and motor strength intact; cerebellar function normal; plantar reflex down bilaterally; deep tendon reflexes as shown in table (Table 19–2).

■ **Summary.** Ms. Jones is a 51 year old black woman, status post left mastectomy, in respiratory distress. She is cyanotic and has evidence of vascular engorgement of the upper half of her body. Her trachea is fixed to the mediastinum. Chest examination reveals evidence of consolidation of the right lower lobe of her lung.

BIBLIOGRAPHY

Wiener S, Nathanson M: Physical examination: Frequently observed errors. JAMA *236*:852, 1976.

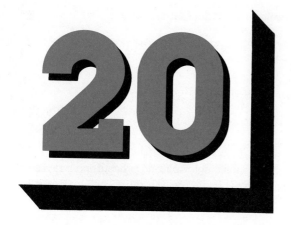

THE PEDIATRIC PATIENT

Children are not like men nor women; they are almost as different creatures, in many respects, as if they never were to be the one or the other; they are as unlike as buds are unlike flowers, and almost as blossoms are unlike fruits.

Walter Savage Landor
1775 – 1864

GENERAL CONSIDERATIONS

Over the past 50 years, there has been an increasing awareness of the importance of child health care. In addition to better infectious disease control and the great strides in technology, the importance of the behavorial and social aspects of a child's health is now recognized. Despite the many advances and the marked reduction in infant mortality, of all the infant deaths under 1 year of age, over 70% occur within the first month of life.* Of these deaths, 85% of the children die within the first week, and 40% of these die within the first day of life.

The previous chapters discuss in great detail the history and physical examination as they relate to the adult patient. This chapter discusses the differences of physical diagnosis in the pediatric age group. The field of pediatrics is very broad and encompasses children from birth through adolescence. During this period, there are enormous changes in the child's emotional, social, and physical development, all of which require thorough discussions.

This chapter is organized somewhat differently than the previous chapters. The first section is devoted to the pediatric history, which is similiar in most pediatric age groups. The sections that follow are devoted to the physical examinations of the following age groups:

---

* Data from National Center for Health Statistics, 3700 East-West Highway, Hyattsville, MD 20782.

- Newborn period (Birth – 1 week)
- Infancy (1 week – 1 year)
- Early childhood (1 – 5 years)
- Late childhood (6 – 12 years)
- Adolescence (12 – 18 years)

Most of this chapter will be devoted to the first three groups, because the examination of children from ages 6 through adolescence is similar in order and techniques to that of the adult examination.

THE PEDIATRIC HISTORY

The pediatric history, like the adult history, is obtained before the examination is performed. During this period, the child can get accustomed to the interviewer. Unlike the adult history, however, much of the pediatric history is taken from the parent or the guardian. If the child is old enough, it is very important to interview the child as well.

Good communication with the child is the key to a successful work-up just as with an adult. An infant communicates by crying. In this way, he tells us that something is wrong. Although older children can communicate through language, they often use crying as a response to pain or to express emotional unrest. This mode of communication deserves attention. Newborns often communicate by cooing and babbling. This form of communication is generally associated with contentment.

In the early stages, the child uses sounds to mimic words as well as gestures to communicate language. At about 10 – 12 months of age, the child usually speaks his first word, usually "dada" or "mama." By two years of age, the youngster may have over 200 words in his vocabulary. By three years, he is able to put together sentences of 5 or 6 words from his 1500 word vocabulary. By the time the child is 6 years old, he is able to communicate in longer sentences from his vocabulary of several thousand words.

The examiner must pay attention to everything the child says. The interactions of the child with the interviewer can be mutually beneficial. Children are very sensitive to the tone of the examiner's voice, which must be modulated with care.

A good relationship with a child begins by making friends with him. Not wearing a white coat may alleviate some of the child's fears. One of the best ways to make a child feel comfortable is through praise. When one is talking to a child, it is very useful to say, "Thank you for holding still. That makes the examination easier." The use of "You're a good boy" or "You are such a sweet girl" should be kept to a minimum, because this may only produce embarrassment. Therefore, praise should be given for a child's action and not for his personality.

While the history is being taken from the parent or child, it is often very helpful to establish physical contact with the child. Touching his arm or rubbing his back will go a long way in establishing good patient rapport.

Although most of the history is obtained from the parent or the guardian, some questions will be asked of the child. There are two simple rules in asking questions of children. These are the following:

1. Don't ask too many questions too quickly.
2. Use simple language.

The interviewer will often be amazed by how well a child can respond to questions phrased according to these rules. It is very useful for one to spend time observing the child at play while interviewing a parent. It is also rewarding to allow a toddler to play with a stethoscope, tongue blade, or penlight to "make friends" with the equipment that will be used later in the physical examination.

The pediatric history consists of the following:

- Chief complaint
- History of the present illness
- Past medical history
- Immunizations
- Birth history
- Growth and development
- Nutrition
- Social history
- Family history
- Review of systems

Basically, the *chief complaint* and the *history of the present illness* are obtained in the same manner as with the adult patient.

The *past medical history* section of the pediatric work-up contains more detailed information about *immunizations* and the severity and complications of any of the *childhood illnesses* than the adult counterpart. Ask the following questions:

> "Has the child had DPT* shots? How many? What were the dates?"
> "Has the child been given the polio vaccination by mouth? How many times? What were the dates?"
> "Has the child had shots against measles? . . . mumps? . . . German measles (rubella)? . . . HIB?" If so, record the dates for each.†
> "Has the child had any reactions to previous shots?"
> "Has he had a test for tuberculosis? When? What was the result?"
> "Has the child had any other shots? . . . BCG?‡ . . . pneumococcal? . . . hepatitis B?"
> "Has he had any other vaccinations or tests?"
> "Has your child had any of the following illnesses: . . . measles? . . . chickenpox? . . . whooping cough? . . . mumps? . . . diphtheria? . . . German measles? . . . strep diseases? . . . rheumatic

---

* Immunization against diphtheria, pertussis, and tetanus.

† *Haemophilus influenzae* type B (HIB) vaccine is now recommended for children between the ages of 2 and 6 years. HIB is the most frequent cause of meningitis and is a leading cause of epiglottitis, septic arthritis, cellulitis, pericarditis, and pneumonia in children under the age of 6 years. Children under 18 months of age demonstrate poor immunologic response to this polysaccharide vaccine; therefore, it is generally not given until 2 years of age.

‡ Vaccination with bacille Calmette-Guérin (BCG) is used for protection from the complications of primary tuberculosis. This vaccine is not given in the United States but is commonly used in Europe and in Central and South America.

fever? . . . pneumonia? . . . tuberculosis?" If so, ask about severity and complications.
"Has the child had any serious accidents? . . . surgery? . . . any other medical problem?"
"Has the child had any convulsions?"
"Has the child exhibited any unusual appetite for things such as clay, chalk, or peeling paint?"
"Does the child have asthma?"

Another important question to ask is, "Does your child have difficulty in keeping up with other children?" The answer to this question may provide valuable information about the child's development from the parent's perspective.

Allergies are pertinent to the past medical history. It is important to determine the existence of allergies to penicillin, foods, or other substances. The most common problem associated with allergies to medications is the development of a rash. Rashes, however, are very common in children and may have occurred coincidentally at the time the medication was prescribed. Therefore, it is incumbent upon the interviewer to determine if the medication was the *cause* of the rash. It is also well known that certain viral states "sensitize" a patient to a medication. The medication may be given at other times without any problems developing. Whenever a parent describes a "medication allergy," ask the following questions:

"How do you know the child is allergic to _____?"
"What was the rash like?"
"Did the child have any other problems other than the rash?"
"How long after starting the medications did the rash appear?" *
"After the medication was stopped, how long did the rash last?"
"Has the child ever had the medication again with recurrence of the rash?"

An important part of the pediatric history is the *birth history*. An opening such as "How was your pregnancy?" may be all that is needed to start this part of the past medical history. It is important to determine any maternal problems, medications taken, illnesses, bleeding, or x-rays taken during the pregnancy. Ask the following questions:

"Did you have any illnesses during your pregnancy?" If so, ask the patient to describe them.
"How much weight did you gain during your pregnancy?"
"During your pregnancy, did you . . . take any drugs, recreational or otherwise? . . . drink alcohol? . . . have any x-rays? . . . have any abnormal bleeding?"
"Were you told during your pregnancy that you had high blood pressure? . . . diabetes? . . . protein in your urine?"
"How long was your labor? Were there any problems with it?"
"What type of delivery did you have, vaginal or cesarean?" If cesarean, ask if this was a repeat cesarean related to a previous birth.
"What was the child's birth weight?"
"Did the baby come out head first or feet first?"
"Were forceps used during the delivery?"

---

* The typical *ampicillin rash* occurs around 7–8 days after starting the drug and is not considered a penicillin allergy.

"Were you told of any abnormalities at birth?"
"Were you told the Apgar* scores?"
"Did the child experience any problems in the newborn nursery, such as breathing difficulties? . . . color? . . . feeding?"
"Did the child receive oxygen in the nursery?"
"Did the child go home with the mother?" If no, ask why not.

The *child's characteristics during infancy* indicate his early developmental progress. The *developmental milestones* are useful to help determine normal patterns. These developmental milestones reflect the child's ability in the following four areas: gross motor, language, fine motor, and personal development. The following questions should be asked:

"Was the child breast fed? . . . bottle fed? For how long?"
"Would you describe your child as active, average, or quiet?"
"Has the child ever had a problem with vomiting? . . . diarrhea? . . . constipation? . . . colic?"
"Has the child ever failed to make progress or ever lost any ability he once had?"
"When did the child first sleep through the night?"
"At what age did he sit without support? . . . wave 'bye-bye'? . . . recognize objects by names? . . . walk without support? . . . learn to talk? . . . walk up and down stairs without support? . . . learn to dress himself? . . . learn to tie shoes? . . . make sentences of 3 to 5 words?"
"At what age was he toilet trained?"
"How old a child do you think he is acting like now?"

The *Denver Developmental Screening Test (DDST)* was developed to detect developmental delays in the first 6 years of a child's life, with special emphasis upon the first 2 years. It is a standardized test based upon a large group of children in the Denver area. It tests the four main areas of development indicated previously. Figure 20 – 1 illustrates this test. A line is drawn from top to bottom according to the age of the child. The examiner should test each of the milestones crossed by this line. Each milestone has a bar that indicates the percentage of the "standard" population that should be able to perform this task. Failure to perform an item passed by 90% of children is significant. Two failures in any of the four main areas indicate a developmental delay. It should be recognized that this test is a screening device for developmental delays; it is *not* an intelligence test.

The *current functioning of the child* provides insight into the present characteristics of the youngster. The child's social, motor, and language developments as well as his maturation will be reflected in his current behavior. A nice way to broach this topic is to ask, "How would you describe your child as a person?" Based upon the parent's response, it is useful to ask these questions:

"What do you enjoy the most about your child? . . . the least?"
"Does your child usually complete what he starts?"
"How does he get along with other children his age?"
"How many hours of sleep does he get each night?"
"Does he have any recurrent nightmares?"

---

* A rapid determination of the child's cardiopulmonary status at birth. This is discussed later in the chapter.

"Does he have temper tantrums?"
"What type of responsibility can he be given?"
"How old was he when he started school?"
"In what grade is he now?"
"How is he doing in school?"
"Has he ever been left back?"
"What is his grade level for reading? . . . math?"
"What does he enjoy during his free time?"
"What kinds of things scare him?"
"How does he get along with his brothers and sisters?"

It is useful to ask whether the child has any disturbing habits. This question allows the parent or guardian to vent any previously unexpressed concerns. This may be asked as follows:

"Is there anything about the child's behavior that worries you or that is different from that of other children?"

Age appropriate questions relating to *nutrition* are very important. Long-term consequences of malnutrition include defective neurologic development, stunting of growth, and decreased immunocompetence. Overeating with an unbalanced diet is equally important. Therefore, an awareness of nutrition during infancy and childhood is vital. For the newborn, it is important to determine the following:

"How many ounces of formula is the baby given a day?" *
"Is the child being breast fed?" If so, *"How often?"* *"Is supplemental fluoride being given?"*

It is important to determine how many ounces of milk and juice a toddler drinks. Inquire about the consumption of daily vegetables, fruit, and protein. In the older child and adolescent, it is important to ask these same questions in addition to asking about the consumption of "junk foods" and vitamin supplementation.

The *social history* should include the parents' occupations as well as the current living conditions. It is important to ask these questions:

"In how many rooms do you live?"
"What is the condition of the paint and plaster in your home?"
"Are there any pets?"
"Who lives in the house?"
"Does the child sleep in his own room?"
"Is the child cared for in any other house?"
"Who supervises the child during the day?"
"How does the family have fun together?"
"Do the child's parents both share in family life?"

A child with sensory deprivation will frequently go to his room and rock back and forth. A non-threatening approach to determine this would be to ask

"Some children have a habit of rocking back and forth when they are alone. Have you ever noticed your child doing this?"

---

* The normal newborn can take 15–20 ounces a day.

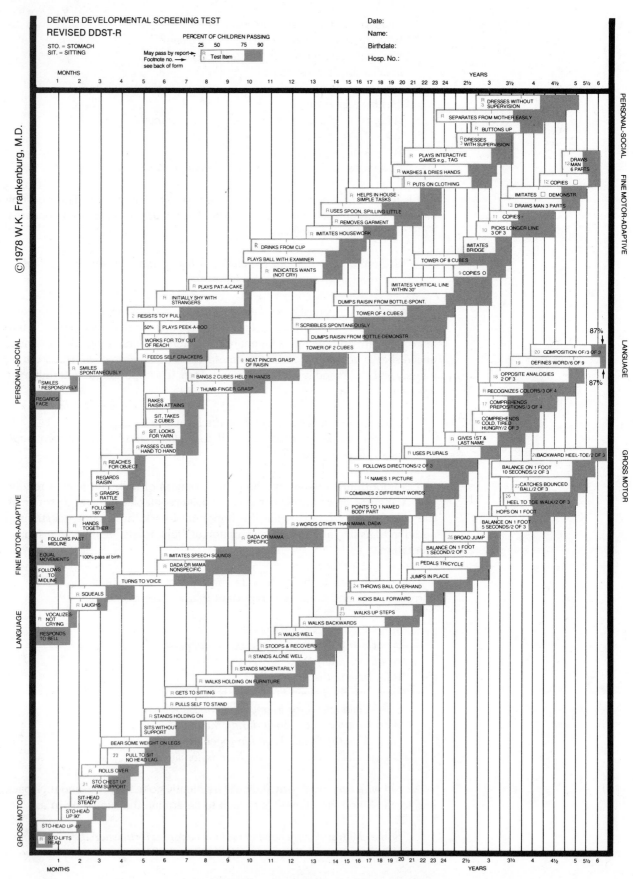

FIGURE 20–1. *See legend on opposite page*

DIRECTIONS

DATE _____

NAME _____

BIRTHDATE _____

HOSP. NO. _____

1. Try to get child to smile by smiling, talking or waving to him. Do not touch him.
2. When child is playing with toy, pull it away from him. Pass if he resists.
3. Child does not have to be able to tie shoes or button in the back.
4. Move yarn slowly in an arc from one side to the other, about 6" above child's face. Pass if eyes follow 90° to midline. (Past midline; 180°)
5. Pass if child grasps rattle when it is touched to the backs or tips of fingers.
6. Pass if child continues to look where yarn disappeared or tries to see where it went. Yarn should be dropped quickly from sight from tester's hand without arm movement.
7. Pass if child picks up raisin with any part of thumb and a finger.
8. Pass if child picks up raisin with the ends of thumb and index finger using an over hand approach.

9. Pass any enclosed form. Fail continuous round motions.

10. Which line is longer? (Not bigger.) Turn paper upside down and repeat. (3/3 or 5/6)

11. Pass any crossing lines.

12. Have child copy first. If failed, demonstrate.

When giving items 9, 11 and 12, do not name the forms. Do not demonstrate 9 and 11.

13. When scoring, each pair (2 arms, 2 legs, etc.) counts as one part.
14. Point to picture and have child name it. (No credit is given for sounds only.)

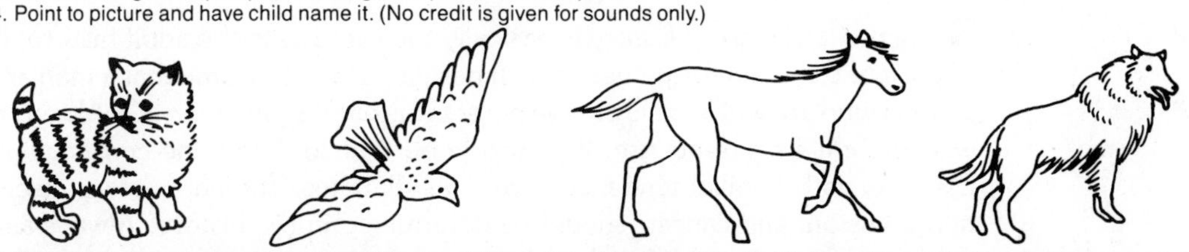

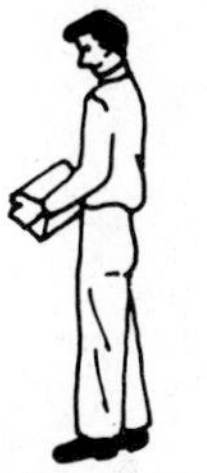

15. Tell child to: Give block to Mommie: put block on table; put block on floor. Pass 2 of 3. (Do not help child by pointing, moving head or eyes.)
16. Ask child: What do you do when you are cold? ..hungry? ..tired? Pass 2 of 3.
17. Tell child to: Put block on table; under table; in front of chair, behind chair. Pass 3 of 4. (Do not help child by pointing, moving head or eyes.)
18. Ask child: If fire is hot, ice is ?; Mother is a woman, Dad is a ?; a horse is big, a mouse is ?. Pass 2 of 3.
19. Ask child: What is a ball? ..lake? ..desk? ..house? ..banana? ..curtain? ..ceiling? ..hedge? ..pavement? Pass if defined in terms of use, shape, what it is made of or general category (such as banana is fruit, not just yellow). Pass 6 of 9.
20. Ask child: What is a spoon made of? ..a shoe made of? ..a door made of? (No other objects may be substituted.) Pass 3 of 3.
21. When placed on stomach, child lifts chest off table with support of forearms and/or hands.
22. When child is on back, grasp his hands and pull him to sitting. Pass if head does not hang back.
23. Child may use wall or rail only, not person. May not crawl.
24. Child must throw ball overhand 3 feet to within arm's reach of tester.
25. Child must perform standing broad jump over width of test sheet. (8½ inches)
26. Tell child to walk forward, ⬤⬤⬤⬤⬤ ⟶ heel within 1 inch of toe. Tester may demonstrate. Child must walk 4 consecutive steps, 2 out of 3 trials.
27. Bounce ball to child who should stand 3 feet away from tester. Child must catch ball with hands, not arms, 2 out of 3 trials.
28. Tell child to walk backward ⟵ ⬤⬤⬤⬤⬤ toe within 1 inch of heel. Tester may demonstrate. Child must walk 4 consecutive steps, 2 out of 3 trials.

DATE AND BEHAVIORAL OBSERVATIONS (how child feels at time of test, relation to tester, attention span, verbal behavior, self-confidence, etc.):

_____

_____

_____

_____

FIGURE 20–1. Denver Developmental Screening Test. (Reprinted with permission from William K. Frankenburg, M.D., Denver Developmental Materials, Inc., Denver, CO.)

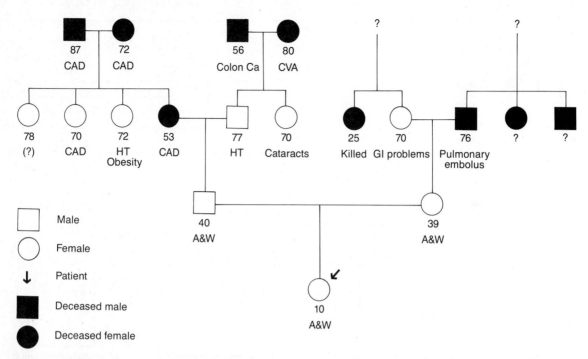

FIGURE 20–2. A family tree. *Abbreviations:* A&W = alive and well; CAD = coronary artery disease; HT = hypertension; Ca = cancer; CVA = cerebral vascular accident.

The pediatric *family history* is basically the same as in the adult history. It is important to obtain the names of both parents. Do not assume that a man and a woman who are with a child are the parents or that they are married. Always ask who the child's parents are. It is also important to determine consanguinity. Diseases with familial tendencies, such as diabetes, coronary artery disease, hypertension, and cancer, should be determined in the history. Always ask if there is a genetic or familial pattern of any disease in any relative. These diseases include hemophilia, Tay-Sachs disease, muscular dystrophy, and Huntington's chorea. If there is a positive genetic history, a complete family tree should be drawn. An example of a family tree is shown in Figure 20–2.

The health of all siblings should be ascertained. It is important to note the parents of all siblings.

The *review of systems* is essentially the same as in the adult history. In the child, however, there should be increased emphasis on the symptoms related to the *respiratory, gastrointestinal,* and *genitourinary* systems. The high incidence of symptoms and diseases related to these systems obligates the interviewer to be very methodical in these areas. It is important to ask the following questions:

> "*Does your child have frequent sore throats? . . . headaches? . . . ear infections? . . . nosebleeds? . . . draining ears? . . . cough? . . . pneumonias? . . . runny nose?"*
> "*Does your child snore? . . . wheeze?"*
> "*Have you noticed your child stop breathing for over 5 seconds?"* *
> "*Has he ever awakened from sleep gasping for breath?"*
> "*Have you noticed your child sleeping restlessly?"*

---

* Consistent with sleep apnea.

"Have you been told that your child sleeps while in school?" *
"Does he breathe through his mouth?"
"How is the child's appetite?"
"Does your child have frequent stomach aches? . . . diarrhea?
. . . constipation? . . . vomiting?"
"Has the child ever complained of burning when he urinates?"
"Has your child ever urinated red urine?"
"Does the child urinate frequently?"

The final question in the review of systems allows the parent to discuss anything that is of concern to the parent that has not already been discussed. An example of such a question might be the following:

"Is there anything else about your child that you would like to tell me?"

The adolescent patient is very special. He is too old to be considered a child, but he is too young to be considered an adult. It is during this period of adolescence that the second major growth spurt, both emotional as well as physical, occurs. The adolescent has many problems. He may be developing physically faster or slower than his friends. In either case, he is different and he is uncomfortable. He has many concerns about the changes occurring in his body. There are many psychosocial adjustments during adolescence; these include establishments of self-image and adult sexual role, achievement of independence from parents, and choosing a career. The adolescent has many questions but frequently has difficulty obtaining answers because he may be too embarrassed to ask his parents. Usually the interview and physical examination of the adolescent are performed without the parent or guardian. The interviewer should assure the patient that the interview will be strictly confidential in so far as the patient's health is not in jeopardy. With this as an introduction, most adolescents will feel comfortable to discuss their problems because confidentiality is ensured.

The interviewer should broach the major general areas of concern and allow the adolescent to respond. An approach to interviewing the adolescent might be to ask some or all of the following questions:

"Most adolescents have some concerns about the size and development of
their bodies. What thoughts do you have?"
"Do you think there is something wrong with your body development?"
"Do you think there is something seriously wrong with your health?"
"Do you think there is anything wrong with your feelings about sex?"
"How would you describe yourself? . . . your moods?"
"Stress affects everyone. What makes you feel most stressed?"

Adolescents often have many questions regarding "recreational drugs," birth control, and venereal disease but are afraid to ask their parents. The interviewer can play a key role in helping the adolescent through this trying period. Many times it is more useful to ask about birth control or sexual activity during the physical examination when the examination of the appropriate body area is being performed. The adolescent usually feels this discussion is generic to this part of the examination. It is very important to be concrete in asking questions of teenagers. The queries should be specific. The interviewer should ask these questions:

---

* Often a sign that the child may have sleep apnea and restless sleeping at night.

"Do you have any questions you would like to ask me about 'street drugs'? . . . birth control? . . . venereal disease?"
"What do your friends think about drugs? . . . sex? . . . drinking?"
"Do you have a girlfriend (boyfriend)?"
"Is it an exclusive (close) relationship?"
"Have you ever had sex?"
"What type of birth control do you use?"

Listening to the patient describe his "friend's" feelings will often reveal some of the patient's concerns. Establishing rapport and then using an open, straightforward approach will go a long way in developing a good doctor-patient relationship, one that may last several decades.

Incest and sexual abuse are not uncommon. In over 80% of all cases of sexual abuse, the molester is not a stranger. All children should be told that their bodies are very personal and that no one has the right to touch them or make them feel uncomfortable. You should listen carefully to a child who describes any type of sexual abuse. Children do not confabulate sexually explicit stories. If the child is over 3 years of age, ask him the following:

"Has anyone touched your body in any way that made you feel uncomfortable or confused?"

It is useful to ask a child to show you on his doll where the person touched him. Male and female dolls that are anatomically correct are often used by pediatricians for this purpose when asking about sexual abuse.

EXAMINATION OF THE NEWBORN INFANT

The newborn infant is assessed immediately following birth to determine the integrity of the cardiopulmonary systems. The newborn infant is placed on a warmer immediately after birth. This is where the initial examination is conducted. Start the examination by careful washing of your hands.

TABLE 20–1. The Apgar Test

Sign	Score		
	0	1	2
Color	Blue, pale	Pink body with blue extremities	Completely pink
Heart rate	Absent	Below 100	Over 100
Reflex irritability*	No response	Grimace	Sneeze or cough
Muscle tone	Flaccid	Some flexion of the extremities	Good flexion of the extremities
Respiratory effort	Absent	Weak, irregular	Good, crying

The acronym APGAR is useful for remembering the examinations of the Apgar test:

Appearance: color
Pulse: heart rate
Grimace: reflex irritability
Activity: muscle tone
Respiratory: respiratory effort

* This is determined by placing a soft catheter into the external nares.

The examination consists of five assessments:

- Color
- Heart rate
- Reflex irritability
- Muscle tone
- Respiratory effort

Dr. Virginia Apgar developed a scale for rating the newborn infant at 1 and 5 minutes after birth. The *Apgar scale* is shown in Table 20 – 1. Each of these tests has a score from 0 to 2. At one minute, a total score of 3 to 4 indicates severe cardiopulmonary depression and the infant requires immediate resuscitative measures; a score from 5 to 8 indicates mild central nervous system depression. The tests are repeated at five minutes; a score greater or equal to 8 indicates a grossly normal cardiopulmonary examination.

General Assessment

After the Apgar score has been assessed, the *gestational age* should be determined. Because menstrual dates are frequently inaccurate, it is important to make an objective determination of the gestational age, which is an indicator of the maturity of the newborn. The standardized scoring system for assessing gestational age is the *Dubowitz Clinical Assessment.* This is based on 10 neurologic signs and 11 external signs, such as skin texture, breast size, and genitalia development. The neurologic scoring system is shown in Figure 20 – 3, and the external criteria are shown in Table 20 – 2.

The total scores of the neurologic and external signs are summated. The total is then correlated with the gestational age, using the graph shown in Figure 20 – 4. A total score of 46 – 60 is associated with a gestational age of 37 – 41 weeks. A child with a gestational age between 37 and 41 weeks is denoted as a *term infant.* Gestational ages less than 37 weeks are *pre-term;* those greater than 41 weeks are *post-term.*

The newborn infant is also weighed, but weight alone does not totally relate to maturational age. The birth weight is correlated with gestational age using the standard classification of Battaglia and Lubchenco, which is shown in Figure 20 – 5. By this method, the infant is classified as being small, appropriate, or large for gestational age. If the neonate falls between the tenth and the ninetieth percentile, he is *appropriate for gestational age (AGA).* If the birth weight is less than the tenth percentile on the intrauterine growth curve, the newborn is classified *small for gestational age (SGA).* If the birth weight is greater than the ninetieth percentile, the newborn is called *large for gestational age (LGA).* Using the standard shown in Figure 20 – 5, term is defined as a gestational age between 38 and 42 weeks.

The value of weight – gestational age determination lies in its ability to predict certain risk groups. Children born in the LGA group are at risk for hypoglycemia and polycythemia. The SGA classification may be an indication of congenital anomalies, hypoglycemia, or congenital infections. *All* pre-term newborns are at risk for hyaline membrane disease, hypoglycemia, and hypocalcemia.

The remainder of the examination is usually performed in the warmed environment of the nursery. This part of the newborn examination is often performed within 24 hours after birth. *Text continued on page 550*

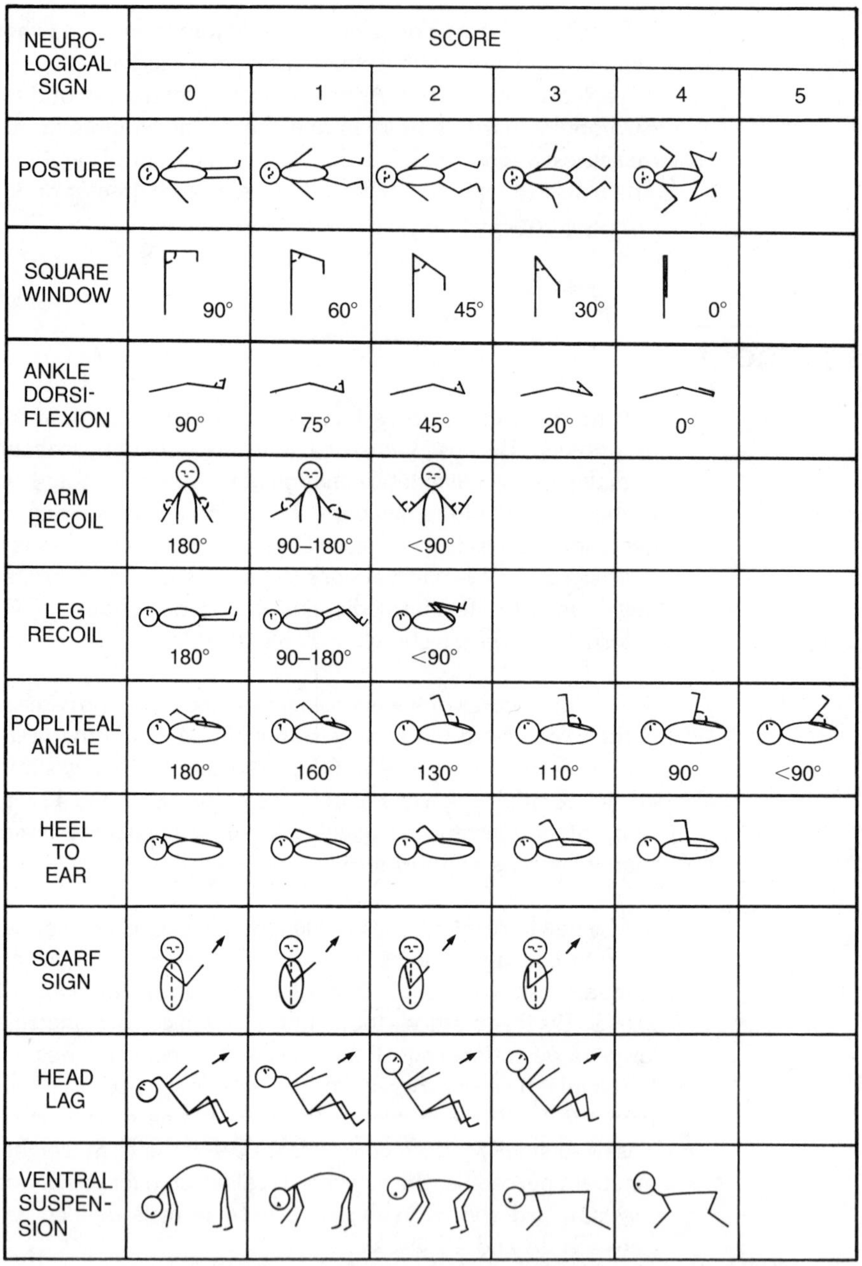

NEURO-LOGICAL SIGN	SCORE					
	0	1	2	3	4	5
POSTURE						
SQUARE WINDOW	90°	60°	45°	30°	0°	
ANKLE DORSI-FLEXION	90°	75°	45°	20°	0°	
ARM RECOIL	180°	90–180°	<90°			
LEG RECOIL	180°	90–180°	<90°			
POPLITEAL ANGLE	180°	160°	130°	110°	90°	<90°
HEEL TO EAR						
SCARF SIGN						
HEAD LAG						
VENTRAL SUSPEN-SION						

FIGURE 20–3. *See legend on opposite page*

FIGURE 20–3. The Dubowitz Clinical Assessment. Some notes on techniques of assessment of the neurologic criteria.

Posture: Observed with infant quiet and in supine position. Score 0: Arms and legs extended; 1: beginning of flexion of hips and knees, arms extended; 2: stronger flexion of legs, arms extended; 3: arms slightly flexed, legs flexed and abducted; 4: full flexion of arms and legs.

Square Window: The hand is flexed on the forearm between the thumb and index finger of the examiner. Enough pressure is applied to get as full a flexion as possible, and the angle between the hypothenar eminence and the ventral aspect of the forearm is measured and graded according to diagram. (Care is taken not to rotate the infant's wrist while doing this maneuver.)

Ankle Dorsiflexion: The foot is dorsiflexed onto the anterior aspect of the leg, with the examiner's thumb on the sole of the foot and other fingers behind the leg. Enough pressure is applied to get as full flexion as possible, and the angle between the dorsum of the foot and the anterior aspect of the leg is measured.

Arm Recoil: With the infant in the supine position, the forearms are first flexed for 5 seconds, then fully extended by pulling on the hands, and then released. The sign is fully positive if the arms return briskly to full flexion (Score 2). If the arms return to incomplete flexion or the response is sluggish, it is graded as Score 1. If they remain extended or are only followed by random movements, the score is 0.

Leg Recoil: With the infant supine, the hips and knees are fully flexed for 5 seconds, then extended by traction on the feet, and released. A maximal response is one of full flexion of the hips and knees (Score 2). A partial flexion scores 1, and minimal or no movement scores 0.

Popliteal Angle: With the infant supine and his pelvis flat on the examining couch, the thigh is held in the knee-chest position by the examiner's left index finger and thumb supporting the knee. The leg is then extended by gentle pressure from the examiner's right index finger behind the ankle, and the popliteal angle is measured.

Heel to Ear Maneuver: With the baby supine, draw the baby's foot as near to the head as it will go without forcing it. Observe the distance between the foot and the head as well as the degree of extension at the knee. Grade according to diagram. Note that the knee is left free and may draw down alongside the abdomen.

Scarf Sign: With the baby supine, take the infant's hand and try to put it around the neck and as far posteriorly as possible around the opposite shoulder. Assist this maneuver by lifting the elbow across the body. See how far the elbow will go across and grade according to illustrations. Score 0: elbow reaches opposite axillary line; 1: elbow between midline and opposite axillary line; 2: elbow reaches midline; 3: elbow will not reach midline.

Head Lag: With the baby lying supine, grasp the hands (or the arms if a very small infant) and pull him slowly towards the sitting position. Observe the position of the head in relation to the trunk and grade accordingly. In a small infant, the head may initially be supported by one hand. Score 0: complete lag; 1: partial head control; 2: able to maintain head in line with body; 3: brings head anterior to body.

Ventral Suspension: The infant is suspended in the prone position, with the examiner's hand under the infant's chest (one hand in a small infant, two in a large infant). Observe the degree of extension of the back and the amount of flexion of the arms and legs. Also note the relation of the head to the trunk. Grade according to diagrams.

If score differs on the two sides, take the mean.

(Reprinted with permission from Dubowitz LMS, Dubowitz V, Goldberg C: Clinical assessment of gestational age in the newborn period. J Pediatr *77*:1, 1970.)

TABLE 20–2. Scoring System for External Criteria of Gestational Age

External Sign	Score*				
	0	*1*	*2*	*3*	*4*
Edema	Obvious edema of hands and feet; pitting over tibia	No obvious edema of hands and feet; pitting over tibia	No edema		
Skin texture	Very thin, gelatinous	Thin and smooth	Smooth; medium thickness. Rash or superficial peeling	Slight thickening. Superficial cracking and peeling, especially of hands and feet	Thick and parchment-like; superficial or deep cracking
Skin color	Dark red	Uniformly pink	Pale pink; variable over body	Pale; only pink over ears, lips, palms, or soles	
Skin opacity (trunk)	Numerous veins and venules clearly seen, especially over abdomen	Veins and tributaries seen	A few large vessels clearly seen over abdomen	A few large vessels seen indistinctly over abdomen	No blood vessels seen
Lanugo (over back)	No lanugo	Abundant; long and thick over whole back	Hair thinning, especially over lower back	Small amount of lanugo and bald areas	At least ½ of back devoid of lanugo
Plantar creases	No skin creases	Faint red marks over anterior half of sole	Definite red marks over > anterior ½; indentations over < anterior ⅓	Indentations over > anterior ⅓	Definite deep indentations over > anterior ⅓
Nipple formation	Nipple barely visible; no areola	Nipple well defined; areola smooth and flat, diameter < 0.75 cm	Areola stippled, edge not raised, diameter < 0.75 cm	Areola stippled, edge raised, diameter > 0.75 cm	
Breast size	No breast tissue palpable	Breast tissue on one or both sides < 0.5 cm diameter	Breast tissue both sides; one or both 0.5–1.0 cm	Breast tissue both sides; one or both > 1 cm	
Ear form	Pinna flat and shapeless, little or no incurving of edge	Incurving of part of edge of pinna	Partial incurving whole of upper pinna	Well-defined incurving whole of upper pinna	
Ear firmness	Pinna soft, easily folded, no recoil	Pinna soft, easily folded, slow recoil	Cartilage to edge of pinna, but soft in places, ready recoil	Pinna firm, cartilage to edge; instant recoil	
Genitals					
Male	Neither testis in scrotum	At least one testis high in scrotum	At least one tesits right down		
Female (with hips ½ abducted)	Labia majora widely separated, labia minora protruding	Labia majora almost cover labia minora	Labia majora completely cover labia minora		

* If score differs on two sides, take the mean.

From Dubowitz LM, Dubowitz V, Goldberg C: Clinical assessment of gestational age in the newborn infant. J Pediat 77:1–10, 1970. Adapted from Farr and associates, Develop Med Child Neurol 8:507, 1966.

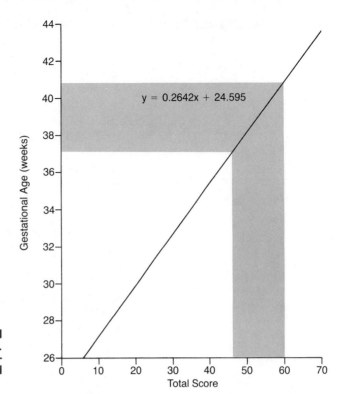

$$y = 0.2642x + 24.595$$

FIGURE 20-4. Graph for determination of gestational age based on neurologic criteria and external signs. (Reprinted with permission from Dubowitz LMS, Dubowitz V, Goldberg C: Clinical assessment of gestational age in the newborn period. J Pediatr 77:1, 1970.)

UNIVERSITY OF COLORADO MEDICAL CENTER
CLASSIFICATION OF NEWBORNS
BY BIRTHWEIGHT AND GESTATIONAL AGE

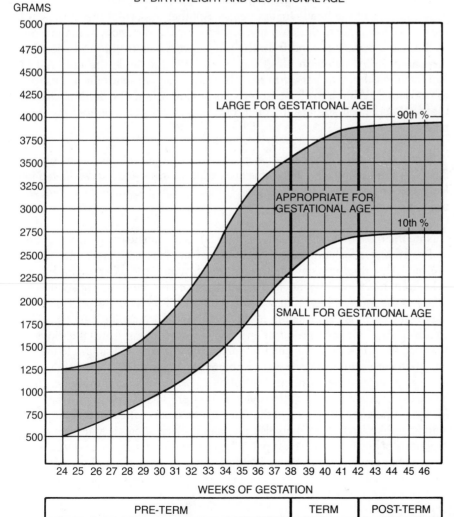

FIGURE 20-5. Classification of newborns by birth weight and gestational age. (Reprinted with permission from Battaglia FC, Lubchenco LO: A practical classification of newborn infants by weight and gestational age. J Pediatr 71:159, 1967.)

Careful assessment of the *respiratory rate* and degree of *respiratory effort* is made while the baby is undressed. The respiratory rate of a newborn varies between 30 and 50 per minute. It is important to observe the respiratory rate for 1–2 minutes, because periods of apnea and periodic breathing are common, especially in the pre-term infant. Look for grunting respirations and for retractions, each of which is evidence of respiratory distress.

Measure the *temperature* using a rectal thermometer. The infant is placed in a prone position on an examining table or in the lap. The buttocks are spread, and a well-lubricated thermometer is inserted slowly through the anal sphincter to approximately 1 inch. After 1 minute, it may be read. Newborn infants often have a relative thermal instability, and for this reason, the ambient temperature should also be determined.

Determine the *pulse* by auscultation of the heart. The average heart rate of a newborn ranges from 120 to 140 per minute. There are wide fluctuations, with the rate increasing to as fast as 190 during crying and to as low as 90 while asleep. A heart rate below 90 is of concern.

Basic *measurements of the head and chest* are taken next. The head is measured at its greatest circumference around the occipitofrontal area. Generally, three measurements are taken, the largest of which is recorded. The head circumference is usually 13.0–14.5 inches (34–37 cm). The chest circumference is normally smaller than the head circumference by 2–3 cm. The chest measurement is taken at the level of the nipples midway between inspiration and expiration. By the time the newborn is 1 year of age, the chest circumference will exceed the head circumference. Another important measurement is the *ratio of the upper to the lower* half of the body. The distances from the crown to the pubic symphysis and from the pubic symphysis to the heel should be compared. In the newborn, this ratio is 1.7 : 1; in the adult, the ratio is 1 : 1. Another measurement is the *arm span*. Normally the arm span equals the crown to heel length. Although all measurements are important, the determination of the head and chest size are the only routine measurements performed at this time.

Note the *posture*. The normal newborn lies on one side with the arms and legs flexed. A term infant who lies on his back with his arms and legs abducted in a frog position has an abnormal posture. However, this posture is consistent with prematurity.

Note the *movements*. Normally, all four limbs should be moving in a random and asymmetric fashion. Fine movements of the face and fingers are usually present. Abnormal movements include jerky, symmetric, coarse movements. All extremities should be moving, with full range of motion seen at some time. Injury to the *brachial plexus* may cause paralysis of the upper arm. This injury may result from lateral traction on the head and neck during delivery of the shoulder. An *Erb's palsy* produces an inability to abduct the arm at the shoulder, to rotate the arm externally, and to supinate the forearm. This injury to the fifth and sixth cervical nerves results in a characteristic position of arm adduction, forearm pronation, and arm internal rotation. *Klumpke's paralysis* results from injury to the seventh and eighth cervical nerves producing a paralyzed hand and forearm. The arm is held limp at the side. Involvement of the first thoracic nerve with Klumpke's paralysis may also result in ipsilateral ptosis and miosis. The prognosis of any brachial plexus palsy depends upon whether the nerve(s) were lacerated or only injured. If the palsy is related only to edema of the nerve fibers and not to actual injury, return of function usually occurs within a few months.

Skin

Skin color in newborns is partially related to the amount of fat present. Pre-term infants generally appear redder because they have less subcutaneous fat than term infants.

The newborn infant has vasomotor instability, and the color of his skin may vary greatly from time to time and from one area of the body to another. It is often noted that when the infant is lying on one side for a period of time, a sharp color demarcation appears, with the lower half of his body becoming red and the upper half being pale. This has been termed the *harlequin color change* and is benign. This color change is seen in 10–15% of infants, especially in premature infants. The attacks may persist from 30 seconds to 30 minutes.

Inspect for *cyanosis* or *acrocyanosis*. Acrocyanosis is a benign condition in which the extremities are cyanotic and cool, but the trunk is pink and warm. This condition is very common in the newborn period.

Is *plethora* present? Plethora in the newborn period usually indicates high levels of hemoglobin.

Is *pallor* present? Pallor may be associated with anemia or more commonly with cold stress and peripheral vasoconstriction. Pallor may also represent asphyxia, shock, or edema. It should be recognized that the presence of pallor may mask cyanosis in the newborn infant with circulatory failure.

Is there any evidence of *birth trauma*, manifested by petechiae, ecchymoses, or lacerations?

Physiologic jaundice is a common finding in almost 50% of all term newborns by the third or fourth day of life. This finding is even more prevalent in the pre-term infant. Icterus appearing before the third day may indicate a blood group incompatibility and hemolytic disease.

Observe the *pigmentation*. Large, slate blue, well-demarcated areas of pigmentation near the buttocks are known as *mongolian spots* and have little meaning. Within the first few years of life, these spots will usually fade and may disappear. Mongolian spots are present in over 80% of black and Asian babies. The finding of these pigmented areas in the white newborn infant is less than 10%. *Telangiectases* on the eyelids, glabella, or nape of the neck are common and frequently disappear during the first few years of life. They are often referred to as "stork bites" or "angel kisses" by the lay public.

Vascular nevi may be isolated defects or part of a syndrome. They may be flat and are commonly caused by dilated capillaries, or they may be mass lesions and consist of large, blood-filled cavities. The *port wine nevus*, also known as the *nevus flammeus*, consists of dilated capillaries and appears as a pink to purple macular lesion of variable size. It can often be as large as one half of the body. The face is a common site. If the eye is involved, *glaucoma* should be ruled out. The *strawberry hemangioma* is a bright red, protuberant lesion seen commonly on the face, scalp, or back. It may be present at birth, but it more commonly develops within the first few months of life. It may expand rapidly, reach a stationary period, and then regress. Most lesions become involuted by the time the child is 5 years of age. The *cavernous hemangioma* is a cystic lesion with a bluish hue that is more diffuse and ill-defined than the strawberry hemangioma. Like the strawberry hemangioma, the cavernous hemangioma has a growth phase followed by a period of involution. If located near the trachea, life-threatening compression may result when the hemangioma enlarges. Look at the child in Plate XV *E*. This child has a combination of a strawberry and a cavernous hemangioma. The strawberry lesion overlies the cavernous hemangioma.

Is a *rash* present? *Erythema toxicum* is a very common rash in the newborn period. It is a self-limited benign eruption of unknown etiology consisting of erythematous macules, papules, and pustules. The lesions may appear anywhere on the body except on the palms and soles. It is most commonly seen during the first 3–4 days of life but may be present at birth. The newborn shown in Plate XV *F* has erythema toxicum.

Milia on the face are commonly seen in almost 50% of all newborns. Milia appear as tiny whitish papules on the cheeks, nose, chin, and forehead and usually disappear by 3 weeks of life.

At 3–4 days of life, *staphylococcal pustulosis* may occur. This presents as pustular skin lesions found mainly around the groin and umbilicus.

Congenital infections of the fetus may present with cutaneous manifestations. *Congenital rubella* may present with purpura. Another important cutaneous sign of congenital rubella is the *blueberry muffin* lesion. These lesions are bluish-red macules ranging in size from 2 to 8 mm. They are noted at birth or within the first 24 hours and appear on the face, neck, trunk, or extremities. Look at Plate XVI *A*, showing a child with classic "blueberry muffin" rash of congenital rubella.

Congenital syphilis may present as an erythematous maculopapular rash that later becomes brown or becomes a hemorrhagic vesicular rash.

Scattered superficial bullae on the upper extremities and lips are termed *sucking blisters* and are presumed to be caused by vigorous sucking in utero. These are most commonly seen on the radial aspect of the forearms, the thumbs, and the center of the upper lip. Resolution without sequelae is the rule.

Is *hair* present? A newborn's skin may be covered with fine, soft, immature hair, known as *lanugo hair*. Lanugo hair frequently covers the scalp and brow in the premature infant but is usually absent in the term infant. Lanugo hair may be present on the ears and shoulders. Inspect the lumbosacral area for tufts of hair. Hair in this area suggests the presence of an occult spina bifida or sinus tract. Examine the *fingernails*. In the post-term infant, the fingernails are long and may be stained yellow by meconium, if meconium were present in the amniotic fluid.

Examine the *dermatoglyphics* of the fingers, palms, and soles. In addition to identification, these patterns are of importance as indicators of genetic abnormalities. Normal finger dermatoglyphic patterns are the loop, whorl, and arch. The loop is normally the most prevalent pattern. The arch is the least prevalent pattern, and the presence of more than four arches is generally abnormal. A single palmar crease, known as a *simian crease,* is frequently found in individuals with chromosomal abnormalities such as trisomy 21.

Head

Examination of the head involves a thorough assessment of its shape, symmetry, and fontanelles. The skull may be *molded,* especially if the labor was prolonged and the head was engaged for a long period. The skull of a child born by cesarean section has a characteristic roundness.

In the newborn, the *fontanelles* are frequently felt as ridges as a result of the overriding of the cranial bones by molding of the skull as it passes through the vaginal canal. Palpate the fontanelles. The *anterior fontanelle* is located at the junction of the sagittal and coronal sutures. It is usually 4–6 cm in diameter and appears diamond shaped. The *posterior fontanelle* is located at the junction of the sagittal and lambdoid sutures. The posterior fontanelle is smaller than the anterior fontanelle and measures 1–2 cm in diameter. Normally the fontanelles are flat. A bulging fontanelle may indicate increased intracranial pressure; a depressed fontanelle may be seen in dehydration. Normally during crying, the fontanelles bulge. Pulsations of the fontanelles reflect the pulse. The anterior fontanelle normally closes by 18 months, but there is a wide range of normality; the posterior fontanelle should be closed by 2 months of age. The locations of the fontanelles are shown in Figure 20–6.

A *caput succedaneum* is edema of the soft tissues over the vertex of the skull that is related to the birth process. This swelling crosses the sutures and disappears after a few days. The caput succedaneum should be differentiated from a *cephalohematoma*, which is a subperiosteal hemorrhage limited to one cranial bone, usually the parietal. There is no discoloration of the overlying scalp, and the swelling does not cross the suture line. The swelling is usually not visible until several hours after birth.

Inspect the skull for *symmetry*.

Transillumination of the skull is utilized to detect subdural effusions and congenital defects such as porencephalic cysts. These are cysts in the brain parenchyma that communicate with the arachnoid space. Transillumination is performed by using a strong light source and shining it against the skull in several areas. A soft foam collar should be placed at the lighted end. A 2–3 cm halo around the circumference of the light when placed in the frontoparietal area is normal; a 1–2 cm halo in the occipital area is also considered normal. Localized bright spots may indicate pathology. Hydrocephaly is indicated by a glow over the entire skull.

Inspect the *face* for symmetry. The eye creases should be equal. Observe the infant as he sucks or cries. The mouth should remain on a level plane. If it is

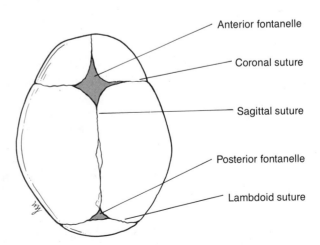

FIGURE 20–6. Location of the fontanelles.

asymmetric, suspect a facial paralysis. The face may reveal abnormal features such as *epicanthal folds, widely spaced eyes,* or *low set ears,* each of which may be associated with congenital defects.

Eyes

Several attempts to evaluate the eyes of the newborn may be necessary. Eyelid edema related to the birth process, medications, or infection makes this part of the examination difficult.

Inspect the eyes for *symmetry.* The eyes should be the same size and should be at the same depth in the orbits. Bulging eyes may be a sign of congenital glaucoma. Microcornea may result from congenital rubella.

Inspect the *eyelids* for evidence of trauma. Use a soft cloth to remove the vernix caseosa and any conjunctival exudate gently. The newborn rarely has eyebrows, but long eyelashes are frequently present. Medial epicanthal folds are seen frequently in individuals with trisomy 21.

The best method of evaluating the eyes of a newborn is to hold him at arm's length while slowly rotating him in one direction. The infant's eyes will usually open spontaneously.

Inspect the *cornea.* The cornea should be clear. Cloudiness of the cornea or a cornea that is greater than 1 cm in diameter may indicate congenital glaucoma.

Inspect the *iris.* The iris of a newborn is very pale, because full pigmentation does not occur before 10 – 12 months of life. Is an abnormal ventral cleft present in the iris? This cleft, known as a *coloboma,* is associated with defects in the lens and retina. A coloboma is commonly associated with chromosomal abnormalities such as trisomy 13 or 18. Is there a ring of whitish dots at the periphery of the iris? These dots are best seen by slit-lamp examination by the ophthalmologist, but this ring may sometimes be visible to the naked eye. These dots, called *Brushfield's spots,* may be associated with trisomy 21 or may be normal.

Inspect the *conjunctivae.* Small conjunctival hemorrhages are common. As a result of the silver nitrate drops* instilled at birth, there may be some inflammation of the conjunctivae as well as edema of the eyelids in the neonate.

The *pupils* of neonates are usually constricted until about the third week of life. Pupillary responses are not to be interpreted in this age group.

Rotate the infant slowly to one side. The eyes should turn in the direction to which he is being turned. At the end of the motion, the eyes should quickly look back in the opposite direction following a few quick, nonsustained nystagmoid movements. This is termed the *rotational response.*

Place the infant back on his back.

In order to test for *visual acuity* in the newborn, one must rely on indirect methods such as the response to a bright light known as the *optical blink reflex.*

---

* As prophylaxis against gonorrheal conjunctivitis, also known as *ophthalmia neonatorum.*

This reflex is normally observed when a bright light is shined on each eye: the newborn infant blinks and dorsiflexes his head. Although never actually tested, the visual acuity of the newborn has been estimated to be in the range of 20/600.

A careful *funduscopic examination* of all infants is important. However, very often the examination can be postponed until the infant is 3–4 months of age, when he may be more cooperative. Postponement may only be made after the presence of intraocular pathology has been excluded. In all newborns, the presence of the *red reflex* bilaterally suggests grossly normal eyes and the *absence* of glaucoma or intraocular pathology. Determine the presence of the red reflex by holding the ophthalmoscope 10–12 inches away from the eyes. The presence of the red reflex indicates that there is no serious obstruction to light between the cornea and the retina. If a red reflex is absent, funduscopic examination is required at this time.

In order to inspect the retina, you should instill a mydriatic into the eyes. Place one drop each of phenylephrine 2.5% and tropicamide (Mydriacyl) 1% into each eye and wait 15–20 minutes. At the end of this period, place the infant flat on his back and ask the parent or a nurse for assistance. Use a pacifier to help quiet the child. Hold the ophthalmoscope in the same manner as when examining an adult. The cornea can usually be visualized when the ophthalmoscope is set at + 20 diopters, the lens at + 15 diopters, and the retina at 0 diopters.

Inspect the *optic disc* and the *vessels.* In the newborn, the disc will appear paler than in the adult. The pinpoint light reflex at the fovea will be absent, because the fovea is not fully developed until 4–5 months of age. Are any *hemorrhages* present? Papilledema is rarely seen in children under the age of 2–3 years. Because the fontanelles are open until this age, any increased intracranial pressure will be dissipated by these open sutures and the optic discs will be spared. Is there any *abnormal pigmentation* present? Congenital rubella and toxoplasmosis are often associated with abnormal pigmentation of the retina. Ophthalmoscopic examination of a newborn infant is difficult. Multiple attempts may be required.

Ears

Inspect the *external ear.* An imaginary line drawn from the inner and outer canthus of the eye toward the vertex should be at the level of or below the level of the superior attachment of the ear. Low set ears are often associated with congenital kidney defects or other chromosomal disorders. Frequently, the ears may be misshapened as a result of intrauterine positioning. This usually rapidly resolves within 1–2 days.

Are any *skin tags* present? A skin tag or cleft that is present in front of the tragus often represents a remnant of the first branchial cleft.

Hearing during the newborn period may be tested by utilizing the primitive acoustic blink reflex. Blinking of the eyes in response to snapping of fingers or a loud noise indicates that the newborn infant can hear. This is a crude test with low sensitivity. A negative response should be further tested with a specific pure-tone screening device.

The *external canal* should be inspected. Hold the otoscope (as indicated in Chapter 8, The Ear and Nose) by bracing it against the child's forehead.

Because the external canal of the newborn is directed downward, insert the otoscope by pulling the pinna gently *downward.* Since the external canal is usually filled with vernix caseosa, the tympanic membrane may not be seen. If the tympanic membrane is seen, only the most superior portion is usually visualized. The tympanic membrane may appear to be bulging with amniotic fluid behind it. This is a normal condition. Rotation of the tympanic membrane to a normal anatomic position occurs within 6–12 weeks.

Nose

Inspect for a *congenitally deviated septum.*

Patency of the nasopharynx is determined by passing a soft, sterile, number 14 French catheter through each external naris and advancing it into the posterior nasopharynx. This test rules out the presence of unilateral or bilateral *choanal atresia,* which is a cause of severe respiratory distress in the newborn period. Newborn infants are nasal breathers, and obstruction to nasal flow can cause considerable distress.

Mouth and Pharynx

Test the *sucking reflex.* Put on a finger cot or glove and insert your index finger into the newborn infant's mouth. A strong sucking reflex should be present. The sucking reflex is strong at 34 weeks' gestation and disappears at 9–12 months.

Inspect the *gingivae.* The gums should be raised, smooth, and pink.

Inspect the *tongue.* The frenulum may be short or may extend almost to the tip of the tongue. Because the production of saliva is limited in the first few months of life, the presence of excessive saliva in the mouth is suggestive of *esophageal atresia.*

Inspect the *palate.* Is there a *cleft palate?* A *bifid uvula* may be associated with a submucous cleft palate. Is the palate *high arched? Petechiae* are commonly found on the hard and soft palates. Pinhead, whitish-yellow, rounded lesions on either side of the raphe on the hard palate are known as *Epstein's pearls.* These are mucous retention cysts and disappear within the first few weeks of life. Similar cysts may be present on the gingivae. A patulous white membrane on the tongue or palate may represent *thrush,* or oral candidiasis. Inspect for *neonatal teeth.* These teeth have a poor root system and may have to be removed to prevent accidental aspiration.

Inspect the *oropharynx.* This can be performed while the infant is crying. Tonsillar tissue is not visible in the newborn infant. Small ulcers or clusters of small, whitish-yellow follicles on an erythematous base are commonly seen on the anterior tonsillar pillars. The etiology is unknown, and they disappear within the first week of life.

Listen to the child's *cry.* Evaluate the cry for its nature, pitch, intensity, and effort. A healthy child will have a strong cry indicative of normal functioning airways. The cry varies in intensity with breathing. A high-pitched, shrill cry is seen in diseases associated with increased intracranial pressure. A child born to a drug-addicted mother often has a very high-pitched cry. A low-pitched, hoarse cry that is infrequent and low in intensity is often associated with hypothyroidism or hypocalcemic tetany. A "cri du chat" cry sounds like a cat mewing and may be associated with chromosomal abnormalities. Absence of crying is suggestive of severe illness or mental retardation.

Neck

The neck of a newborn appears relatively short. Is the neck *symmetric* with regard to the midline? Rotate the infant's head. The normal infant's head should be easily rotated to either side so that the chin can touch either shoulder. *Torticollis* is a condition in which the head is tilted to one side while the chin is rotated to the other shoulder. In the newborn, a hematoma of the sternocleidomastoid muscle as a result of a birth injury may produce this condition. Palpate for a mass in the area of the sternocleidomastoid muscle if torticollis is present.

Palpate the *clavicles* to rule out a fracture. You should feel for the crepitus of a fractured clavicle. Clavicular fractures as a result of a birth injury usually occur at the junction of the middle and outer third of the bone. Decreased motion in the upper extremity may be associated with a clavicular fracture.

Palpate for *masses*. A midline mass may be a thyroglossal cyst.

Is *webbing* of the neck present? Webbing is a feature of Turner's syndrome and congenital abnormalities.

Chest

Observe the *respiratory rate* while the infant is undisturbed. At several hours of age, the rate may vary from 20 to 80 per minute with an average of 30 to 40. Because of the wide variations, respirations should be counted for 1–2 minutes.

Inspect the *respiratory pattern*. The breathing pattern of the newborn is almost entirely diaphragmatic. Irregular, shallow respirations are common in the newborn. *Periodic breathing* is characterized by brief periods of apnea lasting 5–15 seconds and is not associated with bradycardia. *True apnea* has a duration of greater than 20 seconds and is associated with bradycardia. The latter is more commonly found in premature infants with pulmonary disease. Infants with true apnea are at high risk for the sudden infant death syndrome (SIDS). The presence of a *respiratory grunt, retractions* of the chest, or *flaring* of the nostrils indicates respiratory distress.

Inspect for *deformities*. The most important chest deformity in the newborn period is asymmetry that is due to unequal chest expansion on the other side. Other deformities seen in the adult, such as pectus excavatum and pectus carinatum, cannot be appreciated during the newborn period.

Percussion of the chest is performed using either one finger to tap the chest or the method discussed for the adult (see Chapter 10, The Chest). Normally, the thorax of a newborn is hyperresonant throughout. Dullness may indicate an effusion or consolidation.

Auscultate the chest with either the bell or the small diaphragm of the stethoscope. Bronchovesicular breath sounds should be easily heard throughout the lung fields and are higher in pitch than in the adult. In general, auscultation of the chest in the newborn is of low sensitivity.

Breast

Inspect the breasts. The breasts of both male and female newborns are enlarged. Not uncommonly, a milky discharge from the nipple, known as *witch's milk,* may be present. This is the effect of maternal estrogen and is present for 1–2 weeks after birth.

Supernumerary nipples may be present along the milk line. They may or may not have areolae. They may often be mistaken for congenital nevi and have no clinical significance.

Heart

Inspect for *cyanosis.* If cyanosis is present within the first hours or days of birth, suspect an atresia of one of the heart valves, transposition of the great vessels, or persistent fetal circulation.

Inspect for evidence of *congestive heart failure.* In the newborn infant, the most important signs of heart failure are persistent tachycardia of 200 beats per minute, tachypnea, and an enlarged liver. Crackles are not sensitive indicators of heart failure in the newborn. Heart failure during the first few days of life is frequently caused by a hypoplastic left heart.

Palpate for the *point of maximum impulse.* If the newborn infant is less than 48 hours old, the point of maximum impulse will often be in the xiphoid region. After this period and for several years, the point of maximum impulse should be located in the fourth left intercostal space just lateral to the midclavicular line. A right-sided point of maximum impulse suggests *dextrocardia.*

Auscultate the heart in the same locations as in the adult by using the small diaphragm and bell of the stethoscope. Because the respiratory rate is so rapid in the newborn, it is often difficult to distinguish respiratory from cardiac events. Sometimes occluding the nares for a few seconds may help to elucidate the sounds. Auscultation in the newborn period has a low degree of sensitivity in detecting congenital heart disease. There are frequently many "normal" murmurs heard in the early newborn period related to the marked changes in circulation after birth. It has been suggested that there is a less than 1 in 10 chance that the presence of a murmur heard in the newborn period is the consequence of actual congenital heart disease. The continuous machinery murmur of a *patent ductus arteriosus* is commonly heard at birth but disappears by the second or third day of life as the ductus spontaneously closes. This is frequently associated with a hyperdynamic precordium. If any murmurs are present, however, they should be noted and described as indicated in Chapter 11, The Heart.

Pulses

Palpate the femoral pulses. A delay in the femoral pulse as compared with the radial should raise the suspicion of coarctation of the aorta. Bounding pulses may indicate a patent ductus arteriosus.

Abdomen

Inspect the abdomen. The abdomen of a newborn is protuberant as a result of the poor development of the abdominal musculature. If the abdomen is scaphoid, there should be a high index of suspicion that a diaphragmatic hernia is present and the abdominal organs may be located in the chest.

Is an *umbilical hernia* present? The abdominal wall is relatively weak in the newborn, especially in the premature infant. Umbilical hernias are common in the black child. An umbilical hernia in a non-black child may be an indication of hypothyroidism.

Inspect the *umbilical cord stump.* Is there evidence of yellow staining by meconium as a result of fetal distress? The normal umbilical cord contains two ventrally placed thick-walled arteries and one dorsally placed thin-walled vein. Newborns with a single artery often have congenital renal abnormalities. Drainage of a clear discharge from the umbilicus is suggestive of the presence of a patent urachus* or a possible omphalomesenteric duct.

Auscultate the abdomen. The abdomen of newborn infants is very tympanitic, with metallic tinking sounds being heard every 15–20 seconds.

Palpate the abdomen. To relax the abdomen, use your left hand to hold the hips and knees in a flexed position while the child is sucking and palpate with your right hand. Generally, the liver edge may be felt as much as 2 cm below the right costal margin in the newborn. A liver edge more than 3 cm below the right costal margin suggests hepatomegaly. The liver span can be measured by percussion and is more accurate than abdominal measurements, because respiratory conditions could inflate the lungs and push a normal liver down into the abdominal cavity. Palpation of the spleen tip is less common.

Palpate the *kidneys.* Place your left hand under the right side of the child's back and lift upward. At the same time, place your right hand in the right upper quadrant and palpate for the right kidney. Reverse hands for the left kidney.

Unless clinically indicated, the examination of the *rectum* is not performed. Patency of the gastrointestinal tract is confirmed by the passage of meconium, which usually occurs within the first 12 hours after birth. If there is an absence of a meconium stool in the first 24 hours, consider either cystic fibrosis or Hirschsprung's disease. In either case, examine the rectum. Use your well-lubricated, gloved, right fifth finger and insert it into the rectum while the left hand holds the infant's feet together and flexes the hips. The left hand may now be used for bimanual palpation of the abdomen in conjunction with the right hand. Palpate for any masses. When the rectal finger is removed, some bleeding may occur.

---

* A canal in the fetus that connects the urinary bladder to the allantois.

Genitalia

Inspect the external genitalia for *ambiguity.*

In the full term male, the scrotum is relatively large and rugated. The foreskin of the penis is tight and adherent to the glans penis. Inspect the glans for the location of the external urethral meatus. *Hypospadias* is a condition in which the meatus is located in an abnormal ventral position. The meatus may be found anywhere from the tip of the penis to the scrotum. Hypospadias is important in the newborn period, because it represents a contraindication to circumcision. Erection is common and has no clinical significance. The testicles should be descended into the scrotum or in the inguinal canals. Palpate the testicles by a downward movement, which counteracts the active cremasteric reflex. Are any masses present? *Hydroceles* or *hernias* are not uncommon in the newborn period. A hydrocele should be evaluated until the child is 6 months of age. If by this time it is still present, the hydrocele will usually have to be repaired. A hernia should be repaired as soon as possible.

In the full term female, the labia majora should cover the labia minora and clitoris. There should be a fingertip space between the vagina and the anus. If not, the possibility of sexual ambiguity exists. A whitish serosanguineous vaginal discharge is common during the first few days of life and is due to the estrogen effect. The examiner should inspect the *urethral meatus* and *vaginal orifice* by placing his gloved thumb and index fingers on the child's perineum while pressing downward and laterally on the buttocks.

In the male or female infant born by a breech presentation, the external genitalia are often erythematous and edematous as a result of the trauma related to the birth process.

Musculoskeletal Examination

The purpose of the newborn examination is to detect gross abnormalities. The appearance of the extremities at birth usually reflects the positioning of the child within the uterus, a condition known as *intrauterine packing.*

Inspect the *extremities and digits.* Are all 4 extremities and 20 digits present?

Palpate the *clavicle* if not already performed. An area of crepitance over the distal third is suggestive of a fractured clavicle. Decreased motion in the upper extremity may also be associated with a clavicular fracture.

Check for a *brachial palsy,* which has been discussed earlier.

The most important part of the musculoskeletal examination of the newborn infant is the evaluation of the lower extremities. The *hips* are examined for the possibility of dislocation. Inspect the contours of the legs while the child is lying supine. The presence of asymmetric skin folds on the medial aspect of the thigh is suggestive of a proximally dislocated femur. The perineum should not be visible with the child in this position, because the normal position of the thighs should cover most of it. If it is visible, suspect *bilateral* hip dislocations.

Place the infant's feet side by side with the soles on the examination table, allowing the hips and knees to flex. Observe the relative height of the knees. If

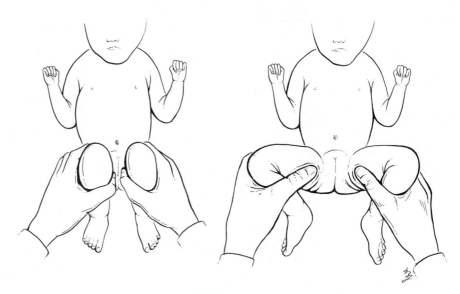

FIGURE 20-7. The Ortolani test.

one knee is at a lower level, one should suspect that the shorter knee is secondary to a dislocation of the hip on that side, a congenitally short femur, or both. If both knees are at the same height, either both hips are normal or both hips are dislocated.

After inspection of the knee heights, each hip is examined to determine joint stability. The examiner should flex the newborn's legs at the hips. The examiner holds the legs by placing his thumbs over the lesser trochanters and his index fingers over the greater trochanters and presses downward* toward the examination table. The hips are then simultaneously abducted to almost 90°. The presence of a palpable or audible "click" suggests a dislocated hip as the femoral head suddenly snaps back into the acetabulum. This test is called the *Ortolani test*. The test should be performed *gently* on a quiet infant. After the newborn period, the Ortolani test may be falsely negative. The Ortolani test is illustrated in Figure 20-7.

Inspect the *feet*. Observe the foot at the sole. An imaginary line drawn from the center of the heel through the center of the metatarsal-tarsal line should bisect either the second toe or the space between the second and third toes. If the line crosses more laterally, the forefoot is adducted (turned inward) in relation to the hindfoot. This is the common condition known as *metatarsus adductus* and is often the result of intrauterine packing. This condition may spontaneously resolve within the first few years of life but may require early casting or exercises for passive correction.

The most serious foot deformity at birth is the *clubfoot*, also known as *talipes equinovarus*. In this condition, the entire foot is deviated toward the midline. There is forefoot adduction, fixed inversion of the hindfoot, and internal tibial torsion. These deformities cannot be passively corrected. The Achilles tendon is foreshortened, and the foot assumes the position of a horse's hoof; thus, the name "equino-." The calf muscles on the affected side are also smaller than on the unaffected side. Immediate therapy is required. If not corrected by casting or splinting, surgery may be necessary at a later date. Look at the child shown in

* This downward maneuver is known as the Barlow variation. The normal hip will not dislocate by this pressure.

Plate XVI *B*. This 3 week old infant was born with bilateral club feet and bilateral hip dislocations.

Neurologic Examination

Careful inspection is the most important aspect of the newborn neurologic examination. The inspection should include the following:

- Posture
- Symmetry of extremities
- Spontaneous movements
- Facial expressions and symmetry
- Eye movements and symmetry

Notice the *position* of the newborn. Is hyperextension of the neck present? This sign is frequently present in severe meningeal or brainstem irritations. What is the position of the thumb? The *cerebral thumb* sign is the finding of the thumb curled under the flexed fingers. It is associated with many cerebral abnormalities.

The *motor* examination consists of testing the *range of motion* of all joints. Assess muscle tone and compare one side with the other. Compare the muscle sizes and strengths. Compare the resistance to passive stretch.

The *sensory* examination is generally omitted, because it has low sensitivity in the newborn age group.

Testing the *cranial nerves* is also difficult in the newborn period. A simple test for the twelfth cranial nerve consists of pinching the nostrils of the newborn. A reflex opening of the mouth with extension and elevation of the tongue in the midline is the normal response. Deviation to one side indicates a lesion on that side.

Because the corticospinal tracts are not fully developed in the newborn period, the response to testing of the deep tendon reflexes is variable and neither sensitive nor specific. *Babinski's reflex* is usually present in newborn infants and is tested as in the adult. Babinski's reflex may normally be present until about 4 years of age.

An important aspect of the newborn neurologic examination is the testing for infantile automatisms. These are primitive reflex phenomena that may be present at birth, depending upon gestational age, but that disappear soon thereafter. There are many, and not all have to be tested. The most important automatisms include the following:

- Rooting response
- Plantar grasp
- Palmar grasp
- Moro's response
- Galant's reflex
- Perez's reflex
- Placing response
- Stepping response

The rotational response, optical blinking reflex, acoustic blink response, and sucking response are also automatisms and have been discussed earlier in this chapter.

The following reflexes are elicited while the newborn infant is *lying supine* on the examination table.

The *rooting response* is elicited by having the infant lie with his hands held against his chest. The examiner should touch the corner of the newborn infant's mouth or his cheek. The normal response is turning of the head to the same side and opening of the mouth to grasp the finger. This reflex is absent in severe central nervous system disease. If only the upper lip is touched, the head will retroflex; if only the lower lip is touched, the jaw will drop. The rooting response is good at 32 weeks' gestation and usually disappears after 3–4 months. This primitive response is to ensure nursing.

The *plantar grasp* is elicited by flexing the leg at the hip and knee. The examiner should dorsiflex the foot with his hand. The normal response is plantar flexion of the toes over the hand. This response disappears after 9–12 months.

The *palmar grasp* is elicited by stabilizing the infant's head in the midline. Place your index finger into the palm of the newborn from the ulnar side. The normal response is flexion of all the fingers to grasp the index finger. If the reflex is sluggish, allow the child to suck, which normally facilitates the grasp response. The palmar grasp is usually solid by 32 weeks of gestation and usually disappears after 3–5 months. The absence of this response in the newborn period or its persistence after 5 months is suggestive of cerebral disease. The newborn commonly holds his hand in a fist. After 2 months, however, the presence of this sign suggests neurologic disease.

The infant is now picked up and *held supine* in the examiner's hands.

Moro's reflex, or *startle reflex,* is elicited by supporting the infant's body in the right hand and supporting the head by the left hand. The head is suddenly allowed to drop a few centimeters. Moro's response consists of symmetric abduction of the upper extremities at the shoulders and extension of the fingers. Adduction of the arm at the shoulder completes the reflex. The infant usually then emits a loud cry. Moro's reflex is one of the most important motor automatisms. The normal response indicates an intact central nervous system and is usually complete by 28 weeks of gestation. It normally disappears by 3–5 months of age. Persistence past 6 months may indicate neurologic disease.

The infant is now turned over and held in the *prone position* in one of the examiner's hands.

Galant's reflex is elicited by stroking one side of the back along a paravertebral line 2–3 cm from the midline from the shoulder to the buttocks. The normal response is lateral curvature of the trunk toward the stimulated side with the shoulder and hip moving toward the side stroked. Galant's reflex normally disappears after 2–3 months. The absence of this reflex is seen in transverse spinal cord lesions.

Perez's reflex is elicited by having the examiner place his thumb at the sacrum and rub his thumb firmly along the spine toward the head. The normal response is extension of the head and spine with flexion of the knees. Frequently the newborn will also urinate. This reflex is normally present until 2–3 months of age. Its absence suggests severe neurologic disease of the cerebrum or cervical spinal cord or a myopathy.

The child is now laid down on the examination table and then picked up by the examiner, holding the *infant upright*. The examiner's hands should be around the chest with the head supported.

The *placing response* and the *stepping response* are elicited by allowing the dorsum of one foot to touch the undersurface of a table top lightly. The normal placing response is for the infant to flex his knee and hip and place the stimulated foot on top of the table simultaneously. This response is then tested using the other foot. Placement of the soles of the feet on top of a table will elicit the stepping response, which is the alternating movements of both legs. Both of these responses are best observed after 4–5 days of life and disappear after a period of 2–5 months. If paresis of the lower extremities is present, these responses will be absent.

EXAMINATION OF THE INFANT

The infant of 1 week to 6 months can be examined on the examination table with the parent standing nearby. It may be easier to perform part of the examination while the infant is in his parent's arms or lap. Infants between the ages of 6 months and 1 year are best examined on the parent's lap.

Observe the infant's activity and alertness.

The more difficult portions of the examination, such as the evaluation of the pharynx and the otoscopic examination, should be performed last. Take advantage of any time when the infant is quiet to listen to his lungs and heart.

Before starting the examination, wash your hands in warm water.

General Assessment

Is any distinctive *body odor* present? Inborn errors of metabolism are associated with characteristic odors such as the odor of *maple syrup* in maple syrup urine disease, sweaty feet in isovaleric acidemia, *fish* in methionine metabolism aberrations, and *acetone* in diabetic ketoacidosis. These odors are characteristic but are rarely seen.

The average pulse of a child during the first six months of life is 130 with a range of 80–160 at rest. The average resting heart rate during the second six months of life is 110 with a range of 70–150. The normal respiratory rate varies between 20 and 40. Blood pressure is difficult to assess in this age group but may be determined by the *flush* method. In this technique, the arm is elevated while the uninflated *infant cuff* is applied to the arm. The arm is then "milked" from the fingers to the elbow so that blanching is noted. The cuff is inflated to just beyond an estimated blood pressure. The pale arm is then placed at the infant's side. The cuff pressure is then allowed to fall slowly. A sudden "flush" of color occurs at a level slightly lower than the true systolic pressure. The blood pressure determined by the flush method of a one day old infant is

50 mm Hg systolic. By the second week of life, the blood pressure has risen to 80 mm Hg systolic. By the end of the first year, the blood pressure is 95 mm Hg systolic. A more accurate Doppler blood pressure assessment is available for critical determinations.

Determine the infant's *length* and *weight*. Plot these measurements on the standard growth charts. Growth charts are used to determine whether or not a child is growing and developing according to a group of standards. More important than a single value is the use of these charts to follow the rate of change at subsequent examinations. The National Center for Health Statistics (NCHS) publishes a variety of growth charts for boys and girls of two age groups: birth to 36 months and 2–18 years. Examples of these charts are shown in Figures 20–8 and 20–9.

Somatic growth is one of the most important parts of the pediatric examination. These parameters must be determined at every visit. Deviations from the standard curves are often early sensitive indicators of a pathologic process. Children with a discrepancy between length and weight by more than two percentage lines also require further evaluation.

Skin

Inspect for dermatologic conditions. *Infantile eczema* is a type of seborrheic dermatitis that begins within the first month of life and is most troublesome during the first year of life. An initial manifestation is often a crusting of the scalp known as cradle cap. The greasy, salmon-colored, sharply delimited oval scales may also involve the face, neck, axillae, and groin. Often the entire body is involved with the dry, scaly, nonpruritic dermatitis. Seborrheic dermatitis may be differentiated from atopic dermatitis by its early onset, a lack of pruritus, and the absence of vesicles.

Atopic dermatitis is the most common cause of eczema in children. It is characterized by pruritus, erythematous papules and vesicles, serous discharge, and crusting. The atopic skin is dry and itchy. The site of predilection in the child of 6 months is the face, whereas the extensor surfaces of the arms and legs are the most common sites in the 8–10 month old infant. Patients with atopic dermatitis have a tendency toward an extra groove of the lower eyelid called the *atopic pleat*. This suggestive feature of atopic dermatitis is shown in the 6 month old child with atopic dermatitis in Plate XVI C.

Are there any *vascular lesions* present?

Palpate the skin and assess *skin turgor*. Pull up 1–2 inches of skin over the abdomen and release it. It should quickly return to its normal position. A decreased response is termed *tenting* and suggests dehydration.

Is there any evidence of physical *child abuse?* Are there any bruises, welts, lacerations, or unusual scars present? Inspect the buttocks and lower back for evidence of bruises. Paired, crescent-shaped bruises facing each other on any part of the body may represent human bite marks. Is there evidence of traumatic alopecia from pulling out of the hair? The damaged hair is broken at various lengths. Are there circular, punched-out lesions of uniform size present? These may represent cigarette burns. A circular type burn on the buttocks and thighs may result from the infant being immersed in scalding hot water. The diagnosis

Text continued on page 572

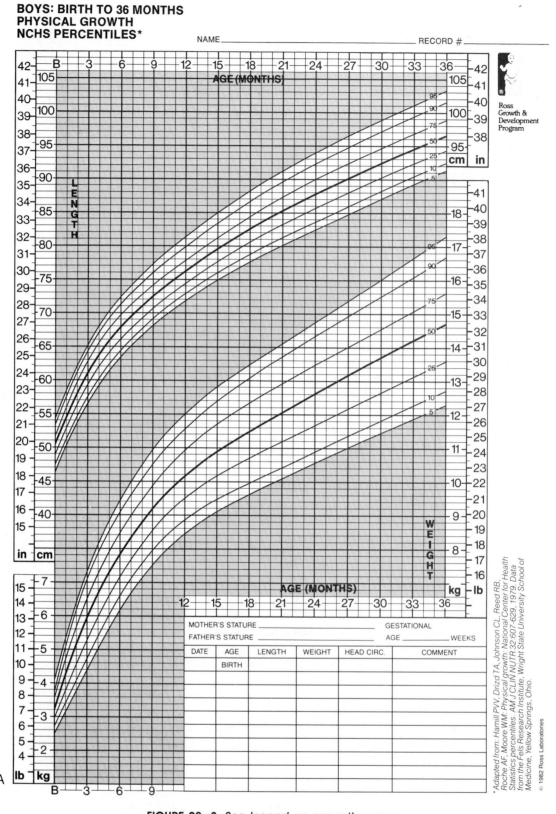

FIGURE 20-8. *See legend on opposite page*

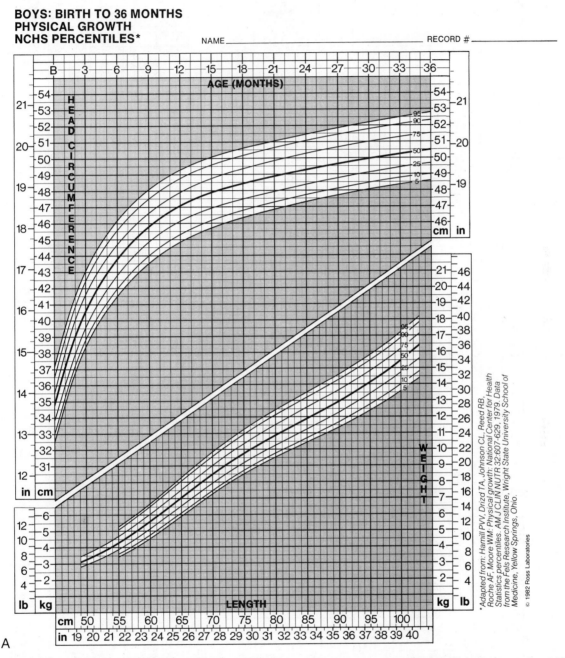

BOYS: BIRTH TO 36 MONTHS PHYSICAL GROWTH NCHS PERCENTILES*

FIGURE 20-8. National Center for Health Statistics (NCHS) growth charts, birth to 36 months. *A* shows the NCHS percentiles for boys. *B* gives the statistics for girls. (Figures provided through the courtesy of Ross Laboratories, Columbus, OH.)

Illustration continued on following page

GIRLS: BIRTH TO 36 MONTHS
PHYSICAL GROWTH
NCHS PERCENTILES*

NAME _____ RECORD # _____

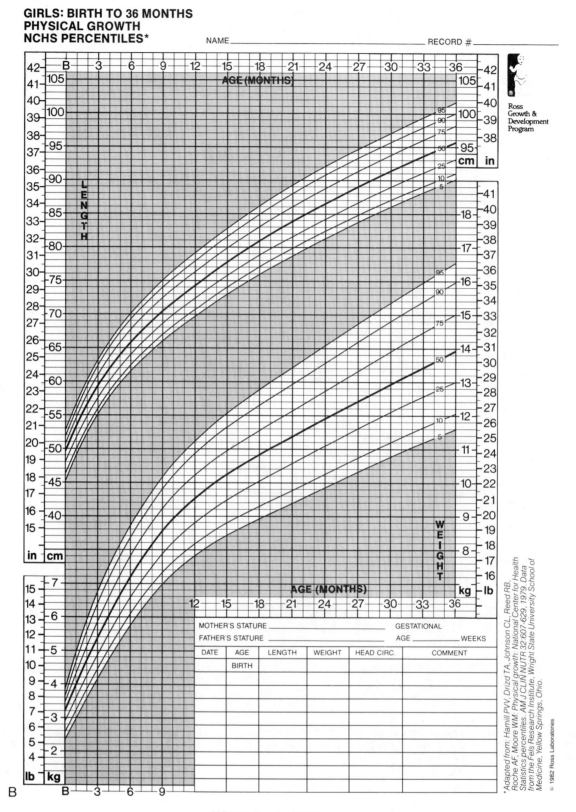

Ross
Growth &
Development
Program

*Adapted from: Hamill PVV, Drizd TA, Johnson CL, Reed RB,
Roche AF, Moore WM: Physical growth: National Center for Health
Statistics percentiles. AM J CLIN NUTR 32:607-629, 1979. Data
from the Fels Research Institute, Wright State University School of
Medicine, Yellow Springs, Ohio.

© 1982 Ross Laboratories

FIGURE 20–8. *Continued*

GIRLS: BIRTH TO 36 MONTHS
PHYSICAL GROWTH
NCHS PERCENTILES*

NAME_____ RECORD #_____

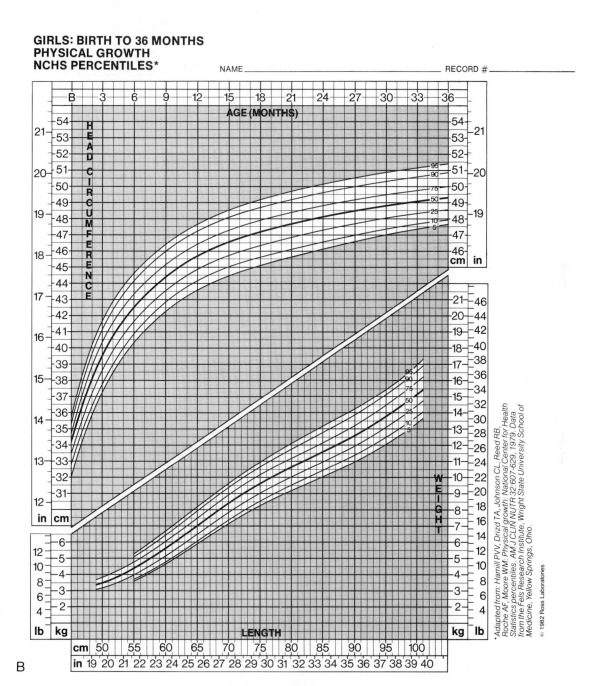

*Adapted from: Hamill PVV, Drizd TA, Johnson CL, Reed RB, Roche AF, Moore WM: Physical growth: National Center for Health Statistics percentiles. AM J CLIN NUTR 32:607-629, 1979. Data from the Fels Research Institute, Wright State University School of Medicine, Yellow Springs, Ohio.

© 1982 Ross Laboratories

B

FIGURE 20–8. *Continued*

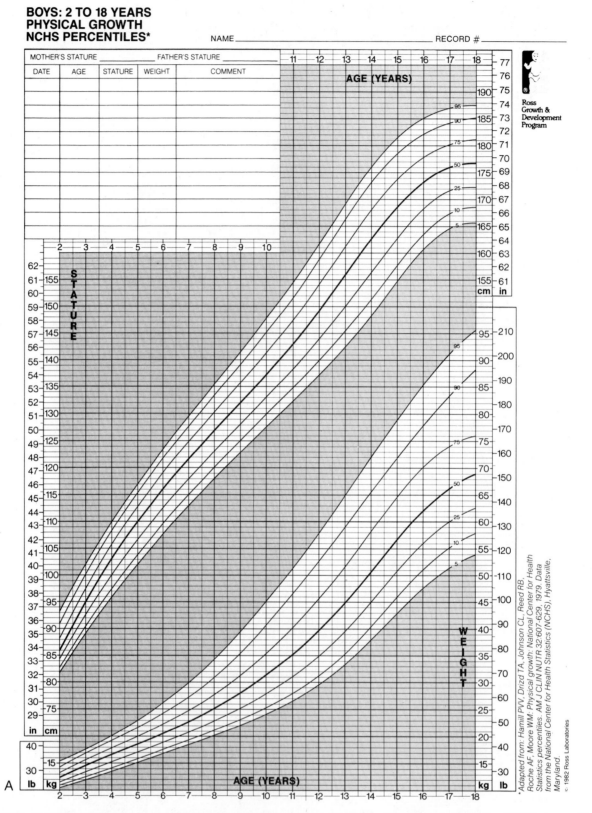

FIGURE 20-9. National Center for Health Statistics (NCHS) growth charts, 2-18 years. *A* shows the NCHS percentiles for boys. *B* gives the statistics for girls. (Figures provided through the courtesy of Ross Laboratories, Columbus, OH.)

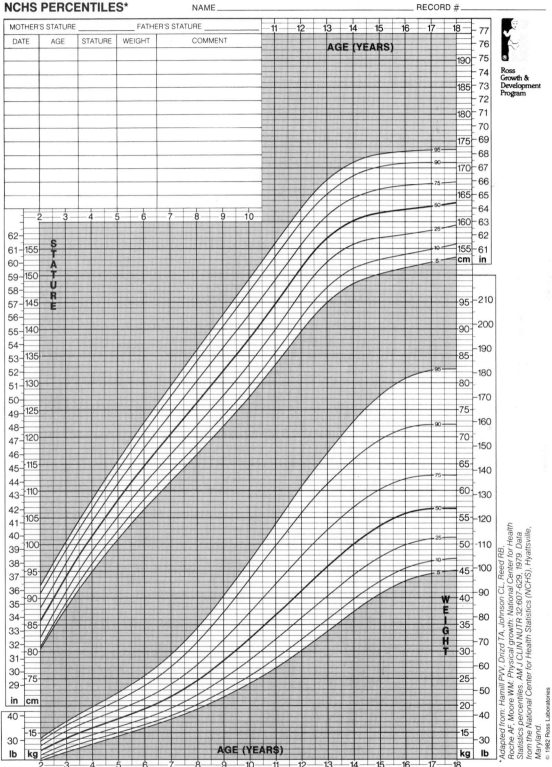

GIRLS: 2 TO 18 YEARS
PHYSICAL GROWTH
NCHS PERCENTILES*

FIGURE 20-9. See legend on opposite page

*Adapted from: Hamill PVV, Drizd TA, Johnson CL, Reed RB, Roche AF, Moore WM: Physical growth: National Center for Health Statistics percentiles. AM J CLIN NUTR 32:607-629, 1979. Data from the National Center for Health Statistics (NCHS), Hyattsville, Maryland.
© 1982 Ross Laboratories

of physical child abuse is especially important in the first 6 months of life, because the risk of a fatal outcome is very high if the diagnosis is missed. In any case of suspected child abuse, it is important to draw several laboratory tests, such as a platelet determination, to rule out any organic cause of increased bruising. If child abuse is verified, health authorities should be notified.

Head

Measure the *occipitofrontal* head circumference, as indicated previously, and chart it on the standard growth charts (see Fig. 20–8). A head that is growing too rapidly should be evaluated for *hydrocephaly*. *Microcephaly* is a defect in which the head size is 3 standard deviations below the normal mean and is related to a defect in brain growth. Check for asymmetry.

Is the *face* symmetric? An easy way to determine facial paralysis as a result of a birth injury is to observe the child when he cries. The weakened or paralyzed side will be flat compared with the normal side.

Eyes

In an infant over 3 weeks of age, check the *pupillary responses.* A sluggishly reacting pupil is suggestive of congenital glaucoma.

The production of tears begins at about 2–3 months of age, but the nasolacrimal duct is not fully patent until 5–7 months. If chronic tearing is present, the nasolacrimal duct may not be patent. In this case, massaging over the nasolacrimal sac may yield a purulent or mucoid discharge, suggesting the diagnosis of nasolacrimal obstruction.

Visual acuity is assessed by qualitative observations. By the age of 4 weeks, the infant should be capable of fixation on a target. By 6 weeks, coordinated eye movements in following an object should be present. At the age of 3 months, the normal infant can follow an object moving across the midline. Convergence is also present by this time. The presence of *optokinetic nystagmus* indicates a complete pathway from the retina to the occipital visual cortex. This response can best be elicited in the child of 3 months of age or more by using a long, striped cloth and passing it rapidly from one side to the other in the child's view. The development of nystagmus as the child attempts to maintain fixation on a stripe is the normal response, indicating normal visual pathways. At 5–6 months, the child should be able to focus on objects but is farsighted. The child should be able to reach out for an object and grasp it. Recognition of objects and faces by 4–6 months of age suggests normal visual acuity.

Observe *ocular motility* in a child 3 months of age or older. Have the child follow an object into the various positions of gaze. Alignment of the eyes is best determined by the symmetry of the *corneal light reflex* and the *alternate cover test,* which have been previously described (Chapter 7, The Eye). The child is most susceptible to *amblyopia* within the first 2 years of life, although the risk is present until age 6–7 years.

Nose

Elevate the tip of the nose to view the nasal septum, floor of the nose, and the turbinates. Are any masses or *foreign bodies* present? A foreign body should be considered in any child with a chronic nasal discharge.

Neck

Palpate for lymphadenopathy in the same areas as in the adult.

Any child with an acute illness should be examined for *nuchal rigidity* resulting from meningeal irritation. The Brudzinski and Kernig tests are described in Chapter 18, The Nervous System.

Chest

The examination of the chest is best performed while the infant is either sleeping or held by his parent.

Often the tracheal breath sounds are transmitted down to the chest. Be careful about misdiagnosing these sounds as crackles.

Is the child in *respiratory distress?* The most important signs of distress are the use of accessory muscles, head bobbing, and flaring of the nasal alae. Intercostal retractions are also commonly present.

Percuss and auscultate the lung fields.

Heart

Inspect for *cyanosis.* If cyanosis develops within the first few weeks of life, there is probably a serious anatomic anomaly such as transposition of the great vessels or *severe tetralogy of Fallot.*

Inspect for evidence of *congestive heart failure.* The most important signs are persistent tachycardia, tachypnea, and an enlarged liver. A persistent tachycardia of over 200 in newborn infants or over 150 in children up to one year of age should alert the examiner. Persistent diaphoresis or a failure to thrive is also an important sign associated with congestive heart failure. If heart failure develops within the first week or two, consider a complex defect such as a ventricular septal defect, a patent ductus arteriosus, or a coarctation of the aorta. A truncus arteriosus will also produce heart failure during this period.

---

* Tetralogy of Fallot consists of pulmonic stenosis, an overriding aorta, a ventricular septal defect, and right ventricular hypertrophy; these conditions arise from an abnormal septation of the truncus arteriosus.

Palpate for the *point of maximum impulse.*

Auscultate as in the newborn infant. An S_3 and an S_4 are very common in this age group. As previously noted, care must be taken about the clinical significance of a murmur heard, especially in the first few weeks of life. (A summary of pathologic murmurs heard in the pediatric age group is summarized in Table 20–3 in the Clinicopathologic Correlations section of this chapter.)

Abdomen

Inspect the *umbilicus.* Observe the abdomen for any masses. An umbilical hernia is not uncommon in this age group, especially in the darker-skinned child. Large peristaltic waves moving from the left to the right in the upper abdomen are occasionally seen in the infant with *pyloric stenosis.*

In the newborn after the umbilical cord has fallen off, the examiner must check for an *umbilical granuloma,* which should be cauterized with silver nitrate.

Auscultate the abdomen; percuss the abdomen; and palpate the abdomen, using light and deep palpation. Are any masses present?

Palpate for the *liver, spleen, and kidneys.* The estimated liver span of a six month old infant varies from 2.5 to 3.0 cm. At one year, the span is approximately 3 cm. The spleen is commonly palpable 1 to 2 cm below the left costal margin during the first month of life.

Genitalia

Inspect the external genitalia. Check for *ambiguous genitalia.* Is diaper rash present?

The foreskin is not fully retractable until 1 year of age. Diaper rash can cause *balanitis,* which is an acute inflammation of the glans penis. Males who are uncircumcised may develop phimosis after balanitis.

Observe the position of the *urethral meatus.*

Inspect the *scrotum.* Is unilateral swelling present? Enlargement may represent a hernia or a hydrocele. Transilluminate any mass. Remember that hydroceles will transilluminate, but hernias will not. Auscultate the mass. Listening to a hernia containing bowel may reveal bowel sounds.

Palpate the testes. Are they both in the scrotum? Can an undescended testicle be palpated in the inguinal canal? If not, while the infant is lying on the examination table, you should press on the abdomen while trying to palpate the undescended testicle in the inguinal canal with the other hand.

In the female infant, is a vaginal *discharge* present? Commonly, there is a whitish, often blood-tinged discharge lasting for 1 month after birth. This is related to the placental transfer of maternal hormones.

Inspect the *perineum* for any rashes or lesions.

Musculoskeletal Examination

Palpate the *clavicle*. At 1 month of age, the presence of a callus formation suggests a healed clavicular fracture.

The *hips* must be re-examined for dislocation at every routine visit for the first year of life. The technique has already been described under the heading Examination of the Newborn Infant.

Neurologic Examination

By the fourth month, when the supine infant is pulled into a sitting position, no head lag should be present. By the eighth month, the infant should be able to sit without support.

Coordination of the hands begins at about 5 months, when the infant can reach and grasp objects. By 7 months, he can transfer these objects from hand to hand. At 8 – 9 months, the infant should be able to use a pincer grip to pick up small objects.

Ears

The child can be either placed on the examination table or held by a parent. To examine the right ear, use your left hand to pull the pinna out, back, and down as the right hand holds the otoscope firmly against the child's forehead. Always use the largest speculum possible. The speculum is introduced slowly into the external canal. Cerumen, if present, should be removed only by someone with experience. The *tympanic membrane* should be easily visualized.

Is the tympanic membrane erythematous? Bulging? One should check for a light reflex. Its presence, however, does not exclude an otitis media. Are air-fluid levels visible behind the drum? These signs suggest otitis media.

Mouth and Pharynx

The examination of the mouth and pharynx is the last part of the examination in this age group.

The child should be seated on the parent's lap, with the parent holding the child's head. The crying infant can usually be examined without the tongue depressor. The frightened child with his mouth firmly closed can be examined by holding the child's nose; this will make him open his mouth. The tongue depressor can then be slipped between the teeth and over the tongue. Be quick if you must be forceful.

Inspect the *gingivae*. Gingival ulceration is frequently the result of *primary* herpetic infection. Small discrete whitish vesicles are also present prior to ulceration. They are found on the buccal mucosa, palate, and tongue. Severe cases can produce lesions around the mouth.

Are any *teeth* present? The first teeth to erupt are the lower centrals at about 6 months. These are followed by the lower laterals at 7 months and the upper central teeth at 7–8 months. The upper lateral teeth begin to erupt at about 9 months. Increased salivation occurs temporarily with the eruption of new teeth. (A summary of the chronology of dentition is in Table 20–4 at the end of the chapter.)

EXAMINATION OF THE YOUNG CHILD

The child of 1–5 years needs to be relaxed in order for an adequate examination to be performed. It is very important in this age group for you to speak softly to the child and to demonstrate the parts of the examination on his dolls or toy animals, on yourself, or on the parent. Allowing the child to hold the stethoscope or penlight will often distract him enough so that other parts of the examination can be performed. The child will soon learn that the light and stethoscope need not be feared. Play with the child. Have the child "blow out" the light. Let the child use the stethoscope as a telephone. Above all, *talk* to the child. It is amazing how easily an examination can often be performed by telling the young child a simple fantasy about imaginary animals. Ask the child questions about these characters. A reassuring voice will go a long way in making the child comfortable. As you proceed with the examination, describe to the child what is being done, such as, "I'm now going to listen to your heart beating." Children also seem to feel that a conversation with their parent during the examination is reassuring. Youngsters respond best to the examiner who is not wearing a white coat. Children under the age of 3 years are best examined on the parent's lap.

The child should be completely undressed for the examination. If the child is modest, remove only the clothing that is necessary for the examination. Modesty varies greatly with children in this age group. Respect the child's modesty!

Start the examination by washing your hands in warm water. In addition to cleaning, the warm hands are more comfortable for the child. If the child is on an examination table, have the parent stand at the child's feet. Any child in respiratory distress is easiest to examine in the position of most comfort, usually sitting or lying prone.

The child should always be told what to do instead of being asked to do something. For example, it is better to say, "Please turn on your back," instead of, "Would you please turn on your back?"

In a child who appears to be *uncooperative,* auscultation of the heart and lungs should be performed *first,* because this requires the child's cooperation and should be performed early when the child may be more cooperative. Because the sight of medical instruments is likely to frighten a child, use them last. Proceed with the examination in the following order for the *cooperative* child:

- Measurements
- Inspect the skin
- Examine the head
- Inspect the feet and hands
- Examine the neck
- Examine the chest
- Examine the heart

- Examine the abdomen
- Examine the genitalia
- Examine the eyes
- Examine the nose
- Examine the ears
- Examine the mouth and pharynx
- Blood pressure, if indicated
- Deep tendon reflexes, if indicated
- Temperature, if indicated

General Assessment

The heart rate of a child one to five years of age ranges from 80 to 140 with an average rate of 100. The respiratory rate varies between 30 and 40. Blood pressure assessment by auscultation is usually possible with children over the age of 3 to 4 years and should be performed on all children. It is important to inform the child that the cuff will get tight for a few moments. The size of the cuff is important. The cuff must cover two thirds of the distance between the antecubital fossa and the shoulder. A cuff that is too small will result in falsely high readings; conversely, a cuff that is too large will result in readings which are falsely low. The techniques of palpatory and auscultatory blood pressure determination are performed as in the adult. The National Heart, Lung, and Blood Institute has published standards of blood pressure measurements in boys and girls between the ages of 2 and 18. Figure 20–10A and B shows these percentile charts for boys and girls, respectively, taken in the right arm with the child seated.

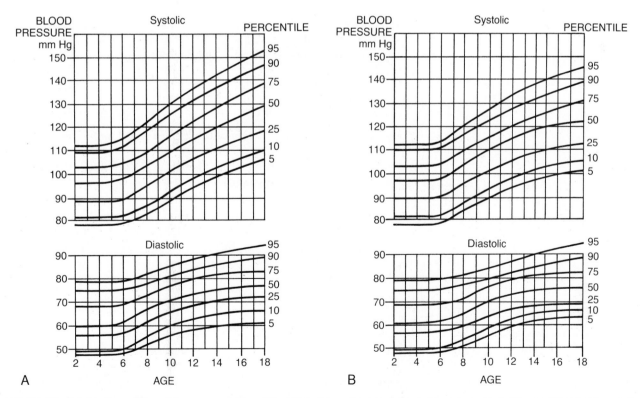

FIGURE 20–10. National Heart, Lung, and Blood Institute blood pressure measurements. *A,* Percentiles for boys. *B,* Percentiles for girls. (From the Report of the Task Force on Blood Pressure Control in Children of the National Heart, Lung, and Blood Institute. Reproduced by permission of Pediatrics (Suppl) *59:*803, 1977.)

Determine the *height, weight,* and *head circumference,* and plot these values on the standard growth charts (see Figs. 20–8 and 20–9).

Skin

The examination of the skin is the same as with the adult.

Careful descriptions of the numerous rashes seen in this age group is paramount for the diagnosis. There are many exanthematous diseases of children. These rashes may consist of macules, papules, vesicles, pustules, or petechiae. (A summary of the most important viral and bacterial diseases is given in Table 20–5 at the end of the chapter.)

Impetigo is one of the most common skin conditions of children in this age group. It presents as a superficial eruption with ulceration, oozing, and crusting, usually on the face. Look at the child shown in Plate XVI *D.* This child has the classic weeping, encrusted lesions of impetigo.

Examine the spine. Tufts of hair along the spine, especially over the sacrum, may mark the location of a *spina bifida occulta.*

Is there evidence of *trauma* or *child abuse?* The signs of physical child abuse have already been discussed in the previous section.

Head

Examine the *lymph nodes.* All of the chains (as indicated in Chapter 6, The Head and Neck) must be examined. Small (2–4 mm), movable, non-tender, discrete nodes are commonly found. Warm, tender nodes usually indicate infection.

Inspect the *shape of the head.*

Palpate the *sutures* in the 1–3 year old child. Are they depressed? Elevated?

Palpate over the *frontal* and *maxillary sinuses* in children over the age of 2 years. Tenderness may indicate sinusitis.

Inspect the area of the *parotid glands.* Localized swelling can best be detected by telling the child to look up to the ceiling while he is seated. Note any swelling below the angle of the jaw. Palpate the area. An enlarged parotid gland often pushes the pinna of the ear away from the side of the head when the child is observed from behind.

Musculoskeletal Examination

Observe the *gait* by telling the child to walk back and forth with his shoes or socks on. Having the child walk on a cold floor without socks or shoes may actually distort the gait. "In-toeing" and "out-toeing" are very common in children. Most are physiologic variants that arise from in utero positioning and correct spontaneously during the active growing period.

Tell the child to stand in front of you, and inspect the legs. Is bowing present? Commonly a child may appear "bowlegged" (genu varum) for 1 – 2 years after starting to walk. "Knock-knees" (genu valgum) are also frequently seen in children 2 – 4 years of age. The normal gait of a child 2 – 4 years of age is wide based with a prominent lumbar lordosis.

The child with a *limp* should be examined for evidence of trauma or localized bone tenderness. The presence of a limp and knee pain in a child, especially a boy, 3 – 8 years of age is suspicious for *Legg-Calvé-Perthes disease,* which is aseptic necrosis of the femoral head. The *irritable hip* syndrome, or toxic synovitis, is another cause of a limp in this age group. This condition affects both sexes equally.

The Trendelenburg test (as described in Chapter 17, The Musculoskeletal System) should be performed if weakness of the gluteus medius is suspected.

Inspect the child's shoes. Is there evidence of abnormal wear?

Neurologic Examination

The development of speech; reading abilities; and the ability to manipulate small objects, throw a ball, and understand simple directions are the best indicators of a normally developing neurologic system.

Deep tendon reflexes are generally not tested unless there is reason to suspect that there may be a developmental abnormality. If they are tested, use the same techniques as described in Chapter 18, The Nervous System.

Neck

Inspect the size and shape of the neck. Check for a *thyroglossal duct cyst.* Look at Plate XVI *E.* This young child has a midline thyroglossal duct cyst.

Palpate the anterior and posterior triangles for lymphadenopathy as in the adult. Cervical adenopathy is associated with inflammation of the sinuses, ears, teeth, or pharynx. Group A beta-hemolytic streptococci are the most frequent cause of pharyngitis in children. Streptococcal pharyngitis is also the cause of rheumatic fever. In the prediction of a positive bacterial culture, the most important diagnostic sign is reported to be tender anterior cervical lymphadenopathy (Rowe and Stone, 1977).

Palpate the *sternocleidomastoid muscle.*

Inspect the location of the *trachea.* Is it midline?

Palpate the *thyroid gland.* This is usually best felt with the child in a supine position with the examiner using his thumb and index fingers to feel for the gland.

Chest

Inspect the shape of the chest.

Determine the *respiratory rate.* The respiratory rate of a 6 year old child is 16–20 per minute.

Palpate the chest for dullness, as described earlier. Tactile fremitus is a technique of low sensitivity in childhood.

Percuss the chest, using the same technique as in the adult. Because the chest wall is thinner in the child than in the adult, the percussion notes are more resonant than in the adult. Percuss gently, because overly vigorous percussion may produce vibrations over a large area and obscure an area of dullness.

Auscultation is best performed by listening to the child when is he unaware of this portion of the examination. Telling a child to "take a deep breath" frequently results in the child holding his breath. With a cooperative child, you can hold the youngster's nose while telling him to breathe in and out. Are the breath sounds normal? Are there any adventitious sounds? Breath sounds in the child sound louder than in the adult as a result of the chest's configuration.

Heart

In the cardiac examination of the young child, follow these procedures:

1. Inspect the precordium.
2. Palpate for any lifts, heaves, or thrills.
3. Auscultate in the same areas as described in Chapter 11, The Heart. Describe any murmurs or abnormal sounds.

Abdomen

The examination of the abdomen is often one of the earlier parts of the examination of the young child, because this requires no instruments other than the stethoscope and is usually painless.

Inspect the abdomen. As the child grows older, the protuberant abdomen becomes more scaphoid, with the exception of those children who are obese.

Inspect the *umbilicus.* Tell the child to cough. Are there any bulging masses at the umbilicus?

Auscultate for peristaltic sounds. Are any *bruits* present? The presence of an abdominal bruit may suggest coarctation, especially in the presence of upper extremity hypertension and reduced or delayed femoral pulses. Use the stethoscope to listen over the kidneys posteriorly. The presence of a bruit in this location is suggestive of renal artery stenosis.

Percuss the abdomen for abnormal dullness.

Light palpation is performed as described in the adult examination. Is tenderness noted? Observe the patient's face while palpating. Facial expressions are more useful than asking the child, "Does this hurt?"

Deep palpation is also performed as in the adult examination.

Palpate the *liver and spleen* as described in Chapter 14, The Abdomen. The liver span of a 3 year old is approximately 4 cm. By 5 years of age, the span has increased to 5 cm.

The *kidneys* are frequently palpable by ballottement in the child up to 5–6 years. The examiner should place his left hand under the right costal margin at the costovertebral angle. The right hand is placed over the midposition of the right abdomen. The examiner should tap firmly on the abdomen to try to feel the size of the kidney. The hands should be reversed to feel the left kidney.

Palpate the *femoral pulses*. Place the tips of your fingers along the inguinal ligament, midway between the symphysis pubis and the iliac crest. Time the pulse with the radial pulse; they should peak at the same time.

Palpate the femoral *lymph nodes*. It is common to find several 0.5–1.0 cm nodes.

Inspect the *anus*. Is diaper rash present? Is there evidence of excoriations? Pinworm infestation commonly causes pruritus and excoriations.

Rectal examination is usually not part of the standard examination in this age group. Only children with abdominal pain or symptoms referable to the lower gastrointestinal tract require a rectal examination. Instruct the child to lie on his back and flex his knees. Tell the child that the examination will be like "taking your temperature." You should use your well-lubricated fifth finger for the examination. Tenderness and sphincter tone are determined, as well as the presence of any mass.

Genitalia

If the child is a male, inspect the *penis*. Check for *phimosis*. By the end of the first year, the foreskin can be retracted in most uncircumcised males. By the age of 4 years, the foreskin should be easily retractable in 80% of all uncircumcised males.

Inspect the *urethral meatus*.

Inspect the *scrotum*. Is there any unilateral enlargement present? Suspect a hydrocele or hernia if the scrotum appears large. Transilluminate and auscultate any scrotal mass.

Palpate the *testes*. Are both present in the scrotum? In this age group, the testicles are often retracted into the inguinal canal. If one or both testicles are not felt in the scrotum, tell the child to sit on a chair with his feet on the seat. Instruct him to grab his knees. Repeat the palpation. This additional abdominal pressure may force a retracted or undescended testicle into the scrotum. Warm hands and a warm room often make the difference.

Another useful maneuver to counteract an active cremasteric reflex is to have the child lie down and flex his leg at the knee, placing his foot on the opposite leg. This "tailor position" will bring the tendon of the sartorius muscle over the inguinal canal and prevent an active reflex from retracting the testicle.

Palpation for an *inguinal hernia* can usually be performed in a child age 4 or older. The procedure is the same as in the adult and should be performed with the child standing.

In the female, inspect the *vaginal area.* Is a *rash* present? Rashes in this area may be related to bubble baths. Is a *discharge* present? A discharge in the age group 2–6 is commonly related to a vaginal foreign body. A nasal speculum is often used to inspect the vagina for the cause of the discharge. Look for an intact hymen and a smooth vaginal opening. Be suspicious of sexual abuse. The most important signs of abuse include difficulty in walking, vaginal or anal infections, genital irritation or swelling, torn or stained underclothes, vaginal or anal bleeding, and bruises.

Eyes

Visual acuity in the child 1–3 years of age is assessed by his ability to identify brightly colored objects and by his ability to circumnavigate the examining room. Further visual acuity testing may be performed by using the Snellen E chart and asking him which way the letter faces: up, down, to the right, to the left. Visual acuity for a 3 year old is 20/40; at age 4–5, 20/30.

Confrontation visual field testing is performed only in children over the age of 4 years in whom there is a suspicion of decreased acuity. The test is conducted as in the adult except that a small toy is used instead of finger counting. The toy is brought in from the periphery, and the child is instructed to tell the examiner when he sees it.

Check *ocular motility.* Are the eyes straight? Be aware that the child with large epicanthal folds that partially cover the globe may be thought to have strabismus. The eyes should be parallel in all fields of gaze. Shine a light from 2 feet away and have the child look at it. The light should fall in the center of both pupils. Hold the patient's head and turn it to the right and then to the left while the position of the light is maintained. Is the corneal reflection symmetric in both eyes as the head is turned? If there is asymmetry, perform the *cover test* as described in Chapter 7, The Eye.

Is the *eye* red? One of the most common problems of the eyes in this age group is the *red eye.* The causes are numerous and include conjunctivitis, obstruction of the nasolacrimal duct, chalazion, local trauma, allergy, or toxin exposure.

Nose

Inspect the nostrils. Is flaring of the nostrils present? Flaring occurs in any type of respiratory distress.

Inspect the tip of the nose. Is there a permanent transverse crease near the lower part of the nose directing the tip upward? This is commonly seen in allergy sufferers. This unmistakable sign of an allergy sufferer is caused by the *allergic salute:* the child uses his palm or extended forefinger to rub his nose in an upward and outward fashion.

Elevate the tip of the nose and inspect the nasal mucosa. Are secretions present? Purulent secretions from above and below the middle turbinate suggest sinusitis. Watery discharge may indicate allergy or viral upper respiratory infections. Epistaxis is generally due to local trauma. In children with head trauma, the presence of a clear discharge from the nose suggests a cerebrospinal fluid leak.

Check for *nasal polyps.* These may be associated with allergies or cystic fibrosis.

Ears

Is any *discharge* present? Purulent discharges may be related to any bacterial infection. Eczema may cause a flaking of the ears and cracking behind the ears. A bloody discharge may be caused by irritation, injury, a foreign body, or a basilar skull fracture.

Use the otoscope to inspect the *external canal* and *tympanic membrane.* The cooperative 2–3 year old child may be either sitting or lying prone on the examination table with his head turned to one side. The uncooperative child can be held in his mother's arms or prone. The otoscope should be held as indicated previously. Use the largest-sized speculum. Insert the speculum tip to only ½ inch.

Inspect the tympanic membrane. Redness is the most common abnormality of the membrane. Infection, trauma, or even crying may be responsible. In suppurative otitis media, the drum bulges outward and becomes diffusely erythematous, hearing is decreased, and the light reflex may be lost. Is the tympanic membrane perforated? Does the tympanic membrane move with insufflation? An immobile drum is seen in suppurative or serous otitis media.

Palpate the *mastoid tip.* Is it tender? Tenderness suggests mastoiditis.

Are *posterior auricular lymph nodes* present? These nodes are classically found in children with rubella. They are also found in children with measles, roseola, chickenpox, or inflammations of the scalp.

Check *hearing.* Hearing is necessary for normal development of language beyond the one-word stage. As a screening test, occlude one ear and whisper a number into the child's ear. Ask him what number he heard. Repeat the test using the other ear. If there is a hearing loss, perform the Weber and Rinne tests as described in Chapter 8, The Ear and Nose. If a hearing loss is suspected, the child should be scheduled for audiometric testing as soon as possible.

Mouth and Pharynx

The evaluation of the mouth and pharynx is usually the last part of the examination of the small child.

Inspect the *lips* for any lesions and color.

Tell the child, "Open your mouth: I am going to count your teeth."

Inspect the *teeth* for number and caries. The first lower molars erupt at about 1 year. These are followed by the first upper molars at 14 months, lower cuspids at 16 months, upper cuspids at 18 months, second lower molars at 20 months, and finally the second upper molars at 2 years. This completes the primary dentition of 20 teeth. *Flattened edges* are seen in children who grind their teeth. (Table 20–4 at the end of this chapter summarizes the ages of tooth eruption.)

Multiple caries is often an indication of *milk caries*. This is caused by the child going to sleep with a bottle of milk or juice in the mouth. Look at the child shown in Plate XVI *F*, who has severe milk caries requiring total removal of all her primary dentition.

Inspect the *bite*. Maxillary protrusion is termed *overbite* and is the normal position; mandibular protrusion is termed *underbite*.

Have the child bite down while you inspect the occlusion. Normally, the upper teeth override the lower teeth.

Inspect the *gingivae* for any lesions.

Inspect the *buccal mucosa*. In *measles*, on the second or third day of the disease, pinpoint white spots are often seen on the buccal mucosa at the level of the lower teeth. These spots have been called *Koplik's spots* and are pathognomonic for measles. Vesicles on an erythematous base suggest *herpes simplex* infection. Similar vesicles on the soft palate suggest *herpangina* caused by Coxsackie virus infections. Red spots about 1–3 mm on the buccal mucosa and palate are an early sign of rubella.

Inspect the *tongue*. Dryness is seen in dehydration and in chronic mouth breathers. Geographic tongue is a normal variation. A strawberry tongue is associated with scarlet fever.

The child should be seated during this part of the examination for best visualization of the posterior pharynx. Tell the youngster that you are going to look in his throat and that he should open his mouth as widely as he can. If the child is uncooperative, lay him down on his back on the examination table. The parent should stand at the head of the table. The child's hands are raised over his head, and the parent squeezes the child's elbows against the head so that the head does not move. The examiner can then lean over the child holding a tongue blade in one hand and a light in the other.

Inspect the *posterior pharynx*. Inspect the size of the *tonsils*. Tonsillar size is estimated on a scale from 1+ to 4+, with 4+ indicating that the tonsils meet in the midline. "Kissing tonsils" may be associated with obstructive apnea. Is a purulent exudate present? Is a membrane present? Membranes are seen in diphtheria and Candida infections.

Are *petechiae* present? Streptococcal pharyngitis is often associated with petechiae.

Inspect the *posterior pharyngeal wall*. A "cobblestone" appearance suggests chronic postnasal drip.

EXAMINATION OF THE OLDER CHILD

The child of 6–12 years is usually a pleasure to examine. He understands the purpose of the examination and rarely presents any problems. It is often very helpful to engage the child in conversation regarding school, friends, and hobbies. Conversation will help to relax the child even if he does not appear apprehensive.

Allow the child to wear a gown or drape.

The order of the examination is essentially the same as in the adult. If the child is complaining of pain in a certain area, that area should be examined last.

As with the younger child, brief explanations about each part of the examination should be given to the older child.

It is important that you wash your hands with soap and warm water before beginning the examination.

General Assessment

In children 6 to 12 years of age, the *temperature* may be taken orally. The pulse of an average child in this age group varies from 75 to 125, and the respirations vary from 15 to 20.

Blood pressure should be obtained in all children in this age group by the methods described in Chapter 11, The Heart. It is very important to use the correct cuff size.

Measure the height and weight, and chart these on the child's record.

Skin

Inspect the skin for any evidence of fungal disease, especially between the toes.

Are any *rashes* present? Persistent dandruff may be tinea and not seborrhea. Seborrhea is most commonly seen in infancy and adolescence.

Eyes

The examination of the eyes is essentially the same as in the adult, with emphasis on *visual acuity*. A careful test using a standard Snellen chart is necessary.

Ears

The examination of the ears is as in the adult, with emphasis on *auditory acuity*. Audiometric testing should be performed on all school-aged children.

Nose

The examination of the nose is essentially the same as in the adult.

Mouth and Pharynx

The *teeth* should be carefully examined with respect to their condition and spacing. Have the child bite down, and observe the *bite*. (See Table 20–4, which summarizes the ages at which shedding of the primary teeth occurs as well as the ages of secondary teeth eruption.)

Inspect the *tongue* for dryness, size, and any lesions. Deep furrows are common and have no clinical significance.

Inspect the *palate* for petechiae.

Inspect the *tonsils* for enlargement, injection, and exudation.

Neck

Palpate the *thyroid* for nodules. The thyroid is rarely palpable in the normal child in this age group.

Palpate for *lymphadenopathy.* Anterior cervical nodes are seen in association with upper respiratory infections and dental infections. Posterior adenopathy is seen with infections of the middle ear and scalp. Generalized adenopathy is seen in viral diseases such as infectious mononucleosis, measles, and rubella.

Is the *trachea* midline?

Chest

The examination of the chest is the same as in the adult.

Heart

The examination of the heart is the same as in the adult.

Abdomen

The order of the abdominal examination is the same as in the adult. The span of the liver at age eight is 5.0–5.5 cm; at age twelve, the span is approximately 5.5–6.5 cm.

Genitalia

The age of development of the secondary sexual characteristics varies greatly. As indicated in Chapter 13, The Breast, development of the breast in the female child may begin as early as age 8 and continues for the next 5 years. The development of pubic hair in the girl occurs at the same time. Testicular development in the male child begins somewhat later, at about age 9 – 10. Pubic hair starts to develop in the boy at about age 12 and continues to develop until age 15. The growth of the penis begins about a year after the beginning of testicular enlargement, at age 10 – 11. Whereas the growth spurt of girls occurs at about age 12, this spurt is not seen until around age 14 in boys.

GENITAL DEVELOPMENT STAGES: BOYS

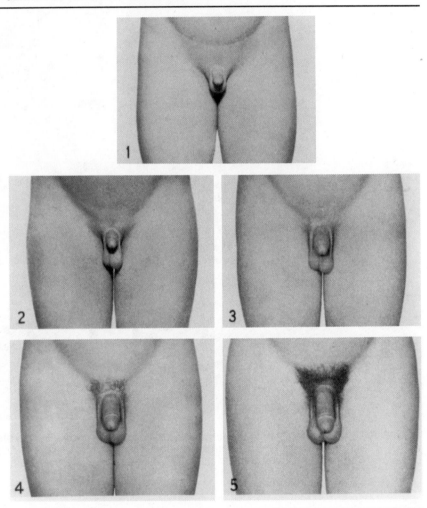

FIGURE 20 – 11. Genital development in boys. Numbers indicate sex maturity ratings. (Reprinted with permission from Tanner JM: Growth at Adolescence, 2nd ed. Oxford, England, Blackwell Scientific Publications, Ltd., 1962.)

Stage	Characteristics
1	Prepubertal. Testes, scrotum, and penis are about the same size and proportion as in early childhood.
2	Enlargement of the testes and scrotum. Scrotal skin reddens and coarsens. Little change in size of penis.
3	Enlargement of penis, which occurs mainly in length. Further growth of testes and scrotum.
4	Further enlargement of penis with growth in width and length. Enlargement of glans penis. Scrotal skin darkens.
5	Adult genitalia

PUBIC HAIR STAGES: BOYS AND GIRLS

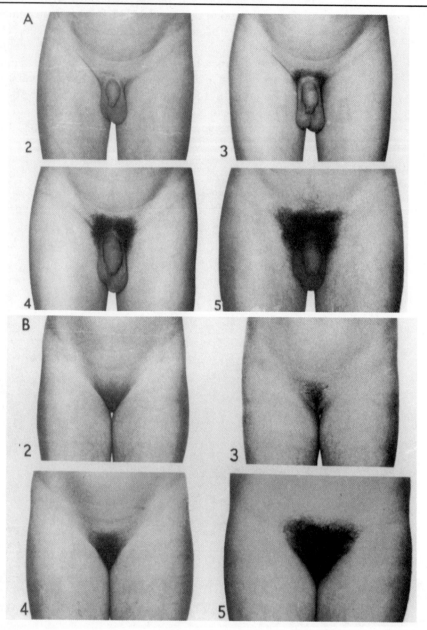

FIGURE 20–12. Pubic hair development. *A,* Development in boys. *B,* Development in girls. Numbers indicate sex maturity ratings. (Reprinted with permission from Tanner JM: Growth at Adolescence, 2nd ed. Oxford, England, Blackwell Scientific Publications, Ltd., 1962.)

Stage	Characteristics
1	Prepubertal. No true pubic hair.
2	Sparse growth of slightly pigmented, downy hair. Only slightly curled. Hair mainly at base of penis or along labia.
3	Increase in hair, which is becoming coarser, curled, and darker.
4	Adult-type hair, but limited in area. No spread to medial surface of thighs.
5	Adult-type hair with spread to thighs.

BREAST DEVELOPMENT STAGES: GIRLS

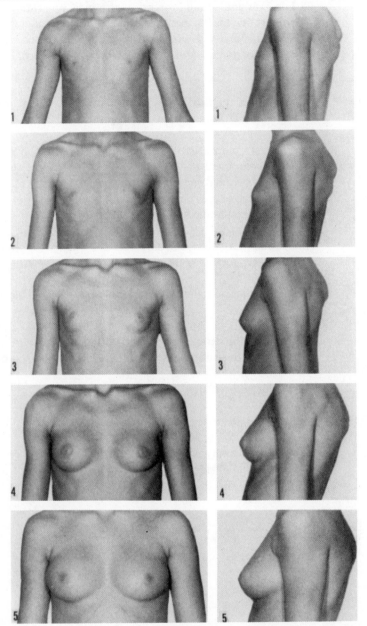

FIGURE 20–13. Breast development in girls. Numbers indicate sex maturity ratings. (Reprinted with permission from Tanner JM: Growth at Adolescence, 2nd ed. Oxford, England, Blackwell Scientific Publications, Ltd., 1962.)

Stage	Characteristics
1	Prepubertal. Elevation of only papilla.
2	Breast bud stage. Elevation of breast and papilla as a small mound. Enlargement of diameter of areola.
3	Further enlargement of breast and areola with no separation of contours.
4*	Areola projected above level of breast as a secondary mound.
5	Mature stage. Recession of areola mound to the general contour of the breast. Projection of papilla only.

* This stage does not occur in all girls. In approximately 25% of girls, it is absent. In addition, many adult women have a persistence of this stage throughout life.

Sex maturity ratings (SMR) for males and females have been established by Tanner. In the male, the growth of pubic hair and the development of the penis, testes, and scrotum are used to assign sex maturity rating in values from 1 to 5. The examiner should record two ratings, one rating for the pubic hair and the other rating for the genitalia. If the development of the penis differs from that of the testes and scrotum, the two ratings should be averaged. The sex maturity ratings for genital development in boys are illustrated and summarized in Figure 20–11.

The sex maturity ratings for the pubic hair stages for boys and girls are illustrated and summarized in Figure 20–12.

The sex maturity ratings for girls are based upon the growth of pubic hair and the development of the breasts. Five stages are also observed for each. The examiner should record two ratings, one for the breasts and the other for the pubic hair. The sex maturity ratings for breast development in girls are illustrated and summarized in Figure 20–13.

A summary of the developmental sequence for boys is diagrammed in Figure 20–14; a summary for girls is given in Figure 20–15.

The youngster should be given a gown to avoid his embarrassment in front of a parent.

Inspect the *external genitalia.* Is *pubic hair* present? What are the *sex maturity ratings?* Are any lesions present? Is there evidence of sexual abuse?

Palpate the testes.

Is an *inguinal hernia* present?

Pelvic examinations are not routine in this age group, unless clinically indicated. Vaginal bleeding in children under the age of 9 years is due to infection

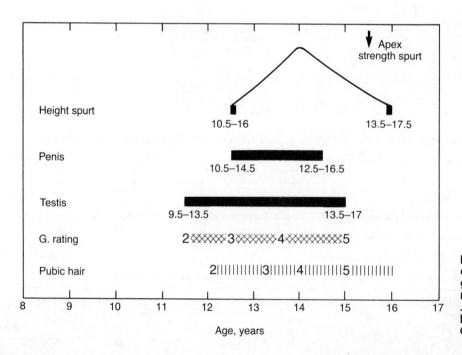

FIGURE 20–14. Developmental sequence in boys. G. rating refers to genital rating. (Reprinted with permission from Marshall WA, Tanner JM: Variations in the pattern of pubertal changes in boys. Arch Dis Child *45:22,* 1970.)

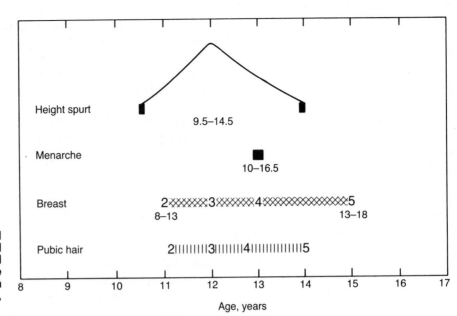

FIGURE 20–15. Developmental sequence in girls. (Reprinted with permission from Marshall WA, Tanner JM: Variations in the pattern of pubertal changes in boys. Arch Dis Child 45:22, 1970.)

from foreign objects in over two thirds of cases. Trauma accounts for an additional 16%.

Musculoskeletal Examination

The most important part of the musculoskeletal examination of the child age 6–12 is to detect *scoliosis*. Scoliosis is the most common spinal deformity, especially in pubertal girls. Have the patient stand stripped to the waist. Inspect the back. Are the shoulders or scapulae at the same height? Is the occiput aligned over the intergluteal cleft? Ask the child to bend down and try to touch his toes, allowing his arms to hang freely. A unilateral elevation of the lower ribs will be seen in the patient with scoliosis. This is demonstrated in Figure 20–16.

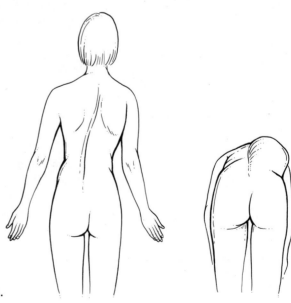

FIGURE 20–16. Technique for testing for scoliosis.

Another similar method for detecting scoliosis is for you to mark the spinous processes with a pen while the child is standing in front of you. Then ask the child to bend forward from the waist. A deviation of the marks to either side suggests scoliosis. Unfortunately, none of the methods for detecting scoliosis has been shown to have adequate sensitivity or specificity.

A limp and knee pain in a child 9 – 16 years of age must be considered to be a result of a slipped epiphysis of the hip until proved otherwise. The pathogno-monic sign of a slipped epiphysis is the hip going into external rotation as it is flexed.

Neurologic Examination

The neurologic examination is essentially the same as outlined in Chapter 18, The Nervous System. However, in the child of this age group, the complete neurologic examination is indicated only when there is evidence of developmental abnormalities.

EXAMINATION OF THE ADOLESCENT

The examination of the adolescent is exactly the same as that of the adult. It is appropriate for the examiner to ask the parent to leave during the examination, and perhaps even for the history.

Because the examination is so similiar to that of the adult, only dissimilarities are indicated in this section.

General Assessment

The average *heart rate* of the adolescent is 60 to 100 beats per minute. The respiratory rate varies from 12 to 18 per minute by age 16.

Blood pressure is important to determine by the methods already discussed in Chapter 11, The Heart.

Skin

Examination of the skin of adolescents usually reveals evidence of *pubertal changes*. These include acne, areolar pigmentation, functioning of the apocrine sweat glands, pigmentation of the external genitalia, and the development of axillary and pubic hair.

Breast

Determine the *Tanner sex maturity rating* of the breasts in the girl.

TABLE 20–3. Murmurs of Childhood

Condition	Cycle	Location	Radiation	Pitch	Other Signs
Ventricular septal defect	Pansystolic	Left sternal border at the fourth or fifth intercostal space	Over the precordium, rarely to the axilla	High	Thrill at left lower sternal border
Mitral insufficiency	Pansystolic	Apex	Axilla	High	S_1 decreased S_3
Pulmonic stenosis	Systolic ejection	Left second or third interspace	Left shoulder	Medium	Widely split S_2 Right-sided S_4 Ejection click
Patent ductus arteriosus	Continuous	Left second interspace	Left clavicle	Medium	Machinery-like, harsh Thrill
Venous hum	Continuous	Medial third of clavicles, often on the right	First and second interspaces	Low	Can be obliterated by pressure on the jugular veins

Breast development occurs in both males and females. The male with unilateral gynecomastia should be reassured that this change is part of normal puberty and will be transient.

Asymmetric breast development in the female is common. Reassure the patient that puberty is progressing normally.

Abdomen

The abdominal examination is the same as in the adult. The liver span of a 16 year old varies from 6 to 7 cm.

TABLE 20–4. Chronology of Dentition

	Deciduous Teeth			
	Eruption Maxillary (mo)	Eruption Mandibular (mo)	Shedding Maxillary (yr)	Shedding Mandibular (yr)
Central incisors	6–8	5–7	7–8	6–7
Lateral incisors	8–11	7–10	8–9	7–8
Canines	16–20	16–20	11–12	9–11
First molars	10–16	10–16	10–11	10–12
Second molars	20–30	20–30	10–12	11–13

	Permanent Teeth Eruption	
	Maxillary (yr)	Mandibular (yr)
Central incisors	7–8	6–7
Lateral incisors	8–9	7–8
Canines	11–12	9–11
First premolars	10–11	10–12
Second premolars	10–12	11–13
First molars	6–7	6–7
Second molars	12–13	12–13
Third molars	17–22	17–22

TABLE 20–5. Exanthematous Diseases of Childhood

Disease	Cutaneous Lesion	Location	Mucous Membranes	Systemic Components
Chickenpox (varicella)	Maculopapular; "tear-drop" vesicles on an erythematous base	Trunk, face, and scalp; centrifugal* spread	Yes	Mild febrile disorder; malaise; rash preceded by a 24 hr prodrome of headache and malaise; all stages and sizes of lesions found at the same time and in the same area; pruritus
Measles (rubeola)	Erythematous, maculopapular, purplish red	Scalp, hairline, forehead, behind ears, upper neck; rash starts on head and spreads rapidly to upper extremities and then to lower extremities; rash often slightly hemorrhagic; as rash fades, brown discoloration occurs and then disappears within 7–10 days	Yes†	Prodrome of 3–4 days of high fever, chills, headache, malaise, cough, photophobia, conjunctivitis; 2 days before the rash develops, Koplik'a spots may be seen
Rubella (German measles)	Rose-pink, small, irregular macules and papules; rash is the first evidence of the disease	Hairline, face, neck, trunk, extremities; centripetal‡ spread; rapidly involves body in 24 hr and tends to fade as it spreads	Yes§	Mild fever present, if any; headache, sore throat, mild upper respiratory infection; presence of suboccipital and posterior auricular lymph nodes
Erythema infectiosum	Erythematous malar blush	Face, upper arm, thighs; sudden rash in an asymptomatic child giving a "slapped cheek" appearance; maculopapular rash on upper extremities the next day; several days later, a lacy rash on proximal extremities	No	Mild fever, mild pruritus
Roseola infantum (exanthema subitum)	Macules, rose pink, 2–3 mm; rash appears at end of febrile period; duration of rash only 24 hr	Trunk	Rarely	Sudden onset; high fever
Scarlet fever	Fine, punctate, erythematous lesion that blanches on pressure	Face, along skin folds, buttocks, sternum, between scapulae	Yes‖	Disease results from toxin produced by group A streptococci as a result of pharyngeal infection; abrupt onset of fever, headache, sore throat, vomiting; 12–48 hr later, rash appears

* Moving outward from the center.
† Koplik's spots are highly diagnostic; these appear on the buccal mucosa opposite the first molar teeth; they often appear as blue-white pinpoint papules on an erythematous base.
‡ Moving toward the center.
§ Forschheimer's sign consists of petechiae or reddish spots on the soft palate during the first day of the illness.
‖ Bright red lesions, often on tonsils and soft palate.

Genitalia

Determine the *sex maturity ratings* of the pubic hair and genitalia for the male patient. Determine the sex maturity rating of the pubic hair for the female patient.

The examiner should evaluate the patient carefully and try to reassure him that the body changes are related to normal puberty.

If an internal pelvic examination is necessary for the adolescent patient, an extremely gentle approach is required. The use of a Pedersen speculum will often allow the examination to be less uncomfortable. A female nurse is always required to be present if the examiner is a male.

Musculoskeletal Examination

Knee pain in the adolescent is usually the result of trauma. Partial avulsion of the tibial tubercle associated with a painful swelling in that area is called *Osgood-Schlatter disease*. This common condition is seen more commonly in pubertal boys and is usually self-limited.

CLINICOPATHOLOGIC CORRELATIONS

Heart murmurs are common in the pediatric age group. Some are more serious than others. Table 20–3 summarizes the more common murmurs and associated findings. Table 20–4 lists the chronology of dentition. Table 20–5 lists the more common exanthematous diseases of childhood.

BIBLIOGRAPHY

Behrman RE, Vaughan VC III: Nelson Textbook of Pediatrics, 13th ed. Philadelphia, WB Saunders Co, 1987.

Green M, Haggerty RJ: Ambulatory Pediatrics 3. Philadelphia, WB Saunders Co, 1984.

Gundy JH: Assessment of the Child in Primary Health Care. New York, McGraw-Hill, 1981.

Hurwitz S: Clinical Pediatric Dermatology: A Textbook of Skin Disorders of Childhood and Adolescence. Philadelphia, WB Saunders Co, 1981.

Marshall WA, Tanner JM: Variations in the pattern of pubertal changes in boys. Arch Dis Child 45:22, 1970.

Rowe RT, Stone RT: Streptococcal pharyngitis in children. Clin Pediatr *16*:933, 1977.

Tanner JM: Growth at Adolescence, 2nd ed. Oxford, Blackwell Scientific Publications, Ltd, 1962.

21 CLINICAL DECISION MAKING

Medicine is a science of uncertainty and an art of probability. One of the chief reasons for this uncertainty is the increasing variability in the manifestations of any one disease.

Sir William Osler
1849 – 1919

ART, SCIENCE, AND OBSERVATION

The previous chapters of this book discuss the "science" of medicine by explaining the techniques for interviewing and performing the physical examination. The ability to make a correct clinical decision in the face of uncertainty is the "art" of medicine. This chapter concentrates on the rules and standards of this "art."

The student and physician are constantly faced with decision making, often about problems that can be life-threatening. Clinical decision making is the result of integrating the patient's history and physical examination with statistics and epidemiology. Each of these are elements of the decision analytic approach to problem solving in clinical medicine.

The primary steps in clinical decision making involve the following:

- Data collection
- Data processing
- Problem list development

Data collection for the student of physical diagnosis comes from the history and the physical examination. These can later be augmented with laboratory tests such as blood chemistries, complete blood count, bacterial cultures, electrocardiogram, and chest x-ray, to name a few. The history, which is the most important element of the database, accounts for over 70% of the developing problem list. The carefully performed physical examination contributes an additional 20–25% of the database, with less than 10% related to laboratory testing.

Data processing involves the clustering of pieces of data obtained from the history, physical examination, and laboratory. It is rare that a patient will have a solitary symptom or sign of a disease. He will more commonly complain of multiple symptoms, and the examiner may find several related signs during the physical examination. It is the job of the astute observer to fit as many of these clues together into a meaningful pathophysiologic relationship. This is data processing.

The interviewer obtains a history, for example, of dyspnea, cough, earache, and hemoptysis. The symptoms of dyspnea, cough, and hemoptysis can be grouped together as symptoms suggestive of possible cardiopulmonary disease. The symptom of earache does not fit with the other three symptoms and may indicate another problem. Another patient who complains of epigastric burning relieved by eating and who is found to have stool positive for blood should have this symptom and sign grouped together. It is likely that these data represent an abnormality of the gastrointestinal tract, possibly a duodenal ulcer. Although patients usually have multiple symptoms and/or signs from a pathologic condition, they may not always manifest *all* of the symptoms or signs of the disease being considered. The presence of polyuria and polydipsia in a patient with a family history of diabetes is adequate to raise the suspicion that a lateral rectus palsy may be related to diabetes, even if the patient himself has not previously been diagnosed as having diabetes. In yet another patient, the presence of a 30 pound weight loss, anorexia, jaundice, and a left supraclavicular lymph node is suggestive of gastric carcinoma with liver metastasis to the porta hepatis. This illustrates the process of data processing multiple symptoms into a single diagnosis. This has sometimes been referred to as *Occam's razor*. This rule tries to explain all the symptoms by one diagnosis. A useful rule to keep in mind, it is not always a correct one.

Problem list development results in the summary of the physical, mental, social, or personal conditions affecting the patient's health. The problem list may contain actual diagnoses or only a symptom or sign that cannot be clustered with other bits of data. The date that each problem developed is noted. The list reflects the level of understanding of the patient's problems and should have the problems listed in their order of importance. An example of a problem list is given in Table 21–1.

TABLE 21–1. Example of a Problem List

Number	Problem	Date	Resolved
1	Chest pain	6/28/87	
2	Acute inferior myocardial infarction	1/30/86	2/15/86
3	Colonic cancer	4/30/85	6/3/85
4	Diabetes mellitus	1980	
5	Hypertension	1976	
6	"Red urine"	6/10/87	
7	Problems with son's drug abuse	1/87	

The presence of a symptom or sign related to a specific problem is a *pertinent positive;* the absence of a symptom or sign that, if present, would be suggestive of a diagnosis is a *pertinent negative.* A pertinent negative may be just as important as the presence of a symptom or sign. The fact that a key finding is not present will help to rule out a certain diagnosis. For example, the presence of a history of gout and increased uric acid are pertinent positives in a patient suffering from excruciating back pain radiating to his testicle. This patient may be suffering from renal colic secondary to a uric acid kidney stone. On the other hand, the *absence* of tachycardia in a 45 year old woman with weight loss and a tremor would make the diagnosis of hyperthyroidism less likely. The presence of tachycardia would strengthen the diagnosis of hyperthyroidism; its absence suggests that the patient's symptoms may possibly be related to another condition.

An important consideration in any database is the cognizance of the patient's demographic information: *sex, age, ethnicity,* and *area of residence.* All are important in the manipulation of database information. A *man* with a bleeding disorder from birth is likely to have hemophilia. A *65 year old* person with exertional chest pain is suffering statistically from coronary artery disease. A *black* person with episodes of severe bone pain may be suffering from crises of sickle cell anemia. A person suffering from pulmonary symptoms living in the *San Joaquin valley* may have coccidioidomycosis. The use of this information often suggests a unifying diagnosis, but the absence of a "usual" finding should *never* totally exclude a diagnosis.

It has been said, "Common diseases are common." This apparently simplistic statement has great merit, because it underlines the fact that the observer should not jump to exotic diagnoses if a common one accurately explains the clinical state. Stated another way, if you hear hoof beats in Central Park in New York City, think of horses, not gazelles. On the other hand, if a common diagnosis cannot fit all the pieces together, look for another, less common, diagnosis. Apropos to common diseases, "Uncommon signs of common diseases are more common than common signs of uncommon disease." Finally, never forget, "A rare disease is not rare for the patient with the disease." If the symptoms and signs in a patient suggest an uncommon condition, that specific patient may be the 1 in 10,000 with the disease. Statistics based on population groups may be a useful guide in approaching clinical decision making for the individual patient.

MATHEMATICAL MODELS

Unfortunately, decisions in medicine can rarely be made with 100% certainty. The "odds," or probability, weight the decision. Only if the cluster of symptoms, signs, and laboratory tests are unequivocal can the physician be certain of a diagnosis. This does not occur often. How, then, can the student or physician attempt to make a correct diagnosis? The answer lies in basic logic and reasoning.

The area of mathematics used to express rational relationships is called *set theory* and *symbolic logic.* A *set* is a clustering of elements having a common defined property. Consider, for example, a set of patients with coronary artery disease, a set of patients with melena, and a set of patients with an enlarged liver. Every member of the set must have the same characteristic. A set may contain several divisions, which are called *subsets.* Each of the subsets has its own characteristic in addition to the attribute of the parent set. For example, our set of patients with coronary artery disease may have a subset of male and female patients, or patients over the age of 50 and under the age of 50. A further subdivision may include those male patients with coronary artery disease with or without hypertension.

The *universe* is a frame of reference that contains the sets. It can be thought of as the parent set. All patients with coronary artery disease, male and female, old and young, with and without hypertension, belong to the parent set or universe of all patients with coronary artery disease.

The *complement* of a set is composed of all other elements that do not belong to that set. For example, in our universe of patients with coronary artery disease, the complement of the subset of patients with hypertension is the subset of patients without hypertension.

Symbolic logic is a means of expressing set theory. *Boolean algebra,* developed by George Boole in the mid-1850s, is a branch of mathematics performed on sets. There are three main operations: union, intersection, and complementation. It is beyond the scope of this text to address Boolean algebra, but the concept as it relates to clinical decision making is important. The graphic representation of the basic Boolean theory was advanced by John Venn in the late nineteenth century. The *Venn diagrams* portray a set as the contents of a circle within a rectangle that represents the universe. Figure 21–1 illustrates this principle.

Four possible relationships may result from two sets, as shown in Figure 21–2. The sets may be

- Disjoint
- Overlapping
- Subordinate
- Identical

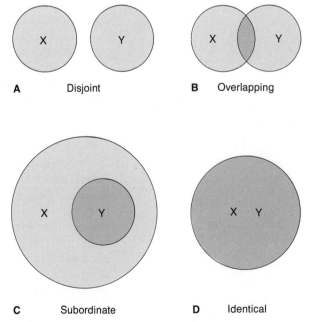

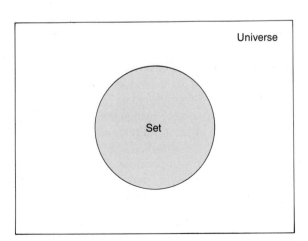

FIGURE 21–1. The Venn diagram.

FIGURE 21–2. The Venn sets. *A,* The disjoint set. *B,* The overlapping set. *C,* The subordinate set. *D,* The identical set.

The *disjoint* sets are mutually exclusive and have no members in common. An example is the set of patients with earache and the set of patients without earache (Fig. 21–2A). In this example, the two sets are also complementary.

The *overlapping* sets have some elements in common but also include elements that are distinctive to each set. Consider the universe of coronary artery disease and the subset of patients with angina and the subset of patients with hypertension. These are overlapping sets: some patients have both angina and hypertension, some have angina alone, and others have hypertension alone (Fig. 21–2B).

The *subordinate* set is a set totally contained within another set. Consider the set of patients with hypertension and the subordinate set of patients with coarctation of the aorta. All patients with coarctation of the aorta have hypertension and are contained within the set of patients with hypertension (Fig. 21–2C). There are many patients with hypertension without coarctation. These patients lie outside the coarctation subordinate set.

The *identical* sets are two sets with identical elements in that every member of one is a member of the other. Identical sets are usually not found in clinical medicine. For example, if patients require only an elevation of the creatine phosphokinase (CPK) level for the physician to make a diagnosis of myocardial infarction, the set of patients with myocardial infarction and the set of patients with elevated CPK would be identical sets (Fig. 21–2D). This, of course, is incorrect.

Venn diagrams can also illustrate a type of reasoning called *syllogisms*. A syllogism is the deductive scheme of a formal arrangement consisting of two premises, one major and one minor, and a conclusion based upon these premises. The premises are axioms or postulates that are true. Consider the famous syllogism, "All men are mortal. Socrates is a man. Therefore, Socrates is mortal." This is an example of a positive syllogism and contains only true premises and a true conclusion. This example can be expressed as in Figure 21–2C. A clinical example of a positive syllogism might be, "If a patient has cancer of the pancreas, he is very ill. This patient has cancer of the pancreas. Therefore, he is very ill."

A negative syllogism consists of a positive and negative premise and a negative conclusion. For example, "The diagnosis of acute hepatitis is made in a patient with elevation of liver function tests and the presence of jaundice. In a particular patient, the liver function tests are normal and the patient is not jaundiced. Therefore, the patient does not have hepatitis."

Deductive and inductive reasoning are part of basic logic. *Deductive reasoning* involves establishing a conclusion about an individual based upon established general facts. For example, "Gonorrhea in the male is associated with a yellowish discharge from the penis. The chance of getting gonorrhea increases with the number of sexual partners. This 32 year old man with several sexual partners has a penile discharge. He has gonorrhea." *Inductive reasoning* is based upon inference rather than upon fact. As an example, "Most patients with a myocardial infarction and ventricular irritability have suppression of the ectopic focus with lidocaine. A 48 year old man is hospitalized with an acute myocardial infarction and has frequent ventricular extrasystoles. Lidocaine is the drug of choice."

One of the major problems in assessing the probability of disease is the existence of individuals without symptoms in whom the disease is diagnosed

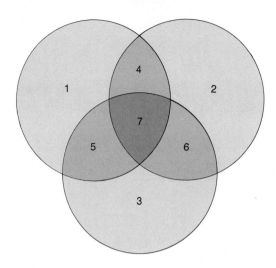

FIGURE 21-3. Three overlapping sets.

accidentally. For example, a young healthy woman without cardiac symptoms is found on routine physical examination to have a mid-systolic click and a late systolic murmur. A 65 year old patient with an acute surgical abdomen is discovered to have electrocardiographic evidence of an old anteroseptal myocardial infarction without ever having had chest pain.

Let us return to our discussion of Venn diagrams. Study the Venn diagram in Figure 21-3. In this example, we are dealing with seven subsets created by three overlapping sets. If each of the sets represents patients with a single symptom, and if all three symptoms are required for a diagnosis, only subgroup 7 would have the disease. Patients in subsets 4, 5, and 6 might have the disease but do not fulfill all the criteria. Patients in subsets 1, 2, and 3 probably do not have the disease. The *probability* of having the disease in an individual patient is highest in patients in subset 7 and lowest in subsets 1, 2, and 3.

Let us now consider the sets included in the clinical spectrum of acute rheumatic fever. The primary clinical symptoms of acute rheumatic fever are carditis, migratory polyarthritis, chorea, erythema marginatum, and subcutaneous nodules. By far, the first three symptoms are the most common. Figure 21-4 illustrates the sets and subsets of patients with the three main symptoms.

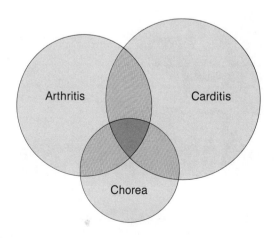

FIGURE 21-4. Clinical spectrum of acute rheumatic fever.

The presence of all three major symptoms should alert the physician of the strong possibility of acute rheumatic fever, especially if these symptoms have developed after a streptococcal pharyngitis. If any of the three symptoms occur singly, the chance, or probability, of acute rheumatic fever is markedly reduced. If none of the symptoms result in the patient seeking medical attention, the patient may still have rheumatic fever, but he is asymptomatic.

PROBABILITY

The probability of a disease varies from location to location, from inpatient to outpatient, and from medical specialty to medical specialty. No two observers or no two medical institutions will see the same type of medical population. It is well known that patients seek out physicians for a variety of reasons. The clinical spectrum of disease is distorted by where the observer is located. Epidemiologists see the asymptomatic population; the clinic physician sees the asymptomatic and mildly ill patients; the house staff member sees the very sick, hospitalized patients; and the pathologist sees the dead patients. Each must try to draw conclusions about the entire spectrum of disease from his own vantage point. This is identical to the old Indian story, depicted in Figure 21–5, of four blind men feeling different parts of an elephant. The one feeling the trunk described the elephant as a snake; the one feeling the leg described the elephant as a tree trunk; the one feeling the body described the elephant as a wall of a house; and the one feeling the tail described the elephant as a rope.

In an attempt to standardize an approach to probability, in 1763 Sir Thomas Bayes devised a set of mathematical theorems for statistical probabilities. Although primarily a mathematic method, these principles are used by physicians daily to determine the probability of disease. Throughout this text, various symptoms and signs have been described according to their *operating characteristics:* sensitivity and specificity. The higher the sensitivity and specificity of a symptom or sign, the more useful this symptom or sign will be to determine the probability that a condition actually exists. *Sensitivity,* as previously defined, is equal to the true positive rate, or the frequency of a positive test in those individuals with the disease. A symptom, sign, or test of high sensitivity is

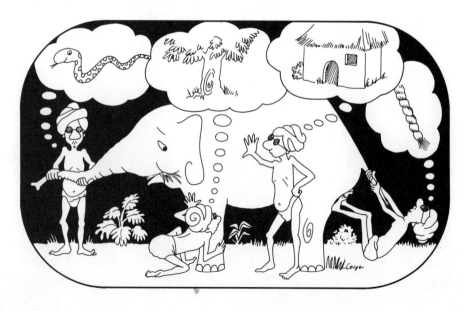

FIGURE 21–5. "Seeing" things from different vantage points.

excellent for detecting patients with the disease. Sensitivity, therefore, relates to patients with the disease. *Specificity* is equal to the true negative rate, or the frequency of a negative test in those individuals without the disease. A symptom, sign, or test of high specificity is excellent at screening out patients who do not have the disease. Specificity, therefore, relates to individuals without the disease. Because sensitivity and specificity are used to measure different attributes, a symptom, sign, or test may have both a sensitivity and a specificity value: a high sensitivity and high specificity, a low sensitivity and low specificity, a high sensitivity and a low specificity, or a low sensitivity and a high specificity.

The *2 × 2 table* is useful to express the relationship of a test, symptom, or sign to a disease. "D+" is the notation for the presence of the disease; "D—" indicates the absence of the disease; "T+" is a positive test or the presence of a symptom or sign; and "T—" is the absence of a positive test or the absence of a symptom or sign. Each of the boxes of the table represents a set of patients. Examine the following 2 × 2 table.

	WITH DISEASE D+	WITHOUT DISEASE D−
TEST POSITIVE T+	TRUE POSITIVE (TP)	FALSE POSITIVE (FP)
TEST NEGATIVE T−	FALSE NEGATIVE (FN)	TRUE NEGATIVE (TN)

Sensitivity is defined as the number of true positives divided by the total of the true positives and the false negatives. Specificity is defined as the number of true negatives divided by the total of false positives and true negatives.

$$\text{SENSITIVITY} = TP/(TP + FN)$$

$$\text{SPECIFICITY} = TN/(FP + TN)$$

Let's now put numbers into our 2 × 2 table to see how it works.

	D+	D−
T+	0.65 (TP)	0.10 (FP)
T−	0.35 (FN)	0.90 (TN)

What do these numbers mean? The left upper box indicates that 65% of individuals with a certain disease will have a certain positive test or symptom or sign. The test will have a true positive rate of 0.65 or a *sensitivity* of 65%.

The box below it indicates that the same test result, symptom, or sign will be absent in 35% of patients with the disease. The false negative rate is 0.35.

The true negative rate is 0.90, as indicated in the right lower box; this means that 90% of individuals without the disease will not have a positive test or have the symptom or sign. Therefore, the *specificity* of the test is 90%.

Finally, the false positive rate is 0.10, meaning that 10% of the population has the finding for some other reason without actually having the disease in question. This is shown in the right upper box.

The true positive rate plus the false negative rate equals 1.0; the false positive rate plus the true negative rate also equals 1.0. If the disease is aortic stenosis and the symptom is syncope in the cited table, 65% of patients with aortic stenosis have syncope and 35% do not; 90% of individuals without aortic stenosis do not have syncope and 10% do.

Although sensitivity and specificity are useful in clinical decision making, the information is often insufficient. How certain can the physician be that a patient has a disease if the test is positive or if a symptom or sign is present? This is estimated by the *positive predictive value* (PV+), which equals the number of true positives divided by the sum of the true positives and false positives.

$$PV+ = TP/(TP + FP)$$

The positive predictive value is the *frequency of disease* in those with positive test results. Stated in another way, it is the probability that a patient with a positive test actually has the disease.

How certain can a physician be that a person is healthy if a test is negative or if a symptom or sign is absent? This is determined by the *negative predictive value* (PV−) and is equal to the true negatives divided by the sum of the false negatives and the true negatives.

$$PV- = TN/(FN + TN)$$

The negative predictive value is the *frequency of nondisease* in those individuals with negative test results. Stated in another way, it is the probability of not having the disease if the test is negative or if the symptom or sign is absent.

The predictive value of a test is a function of not only the sensitivity and specificity but also the *prevalence* of the disease in a specific population. The prevalence of a disease is the frequency of disease in the population at a given point in time.

Let's look at two examples to help illustrate these points. Consider the value of the symptom of chest pain for predicting the probability of coronary artery disease. The first patient is a 65 year old man with chest pain. We know that the prevalence of coronary artery disease in a population of 65 year old men is high. Therefore, the presence of chest pain has a high positive predictive value in this patient, and it is *very probable* that coronary artery disease exists in this patient. However, the absence of chest pain has a low negative predictive value, indicat-

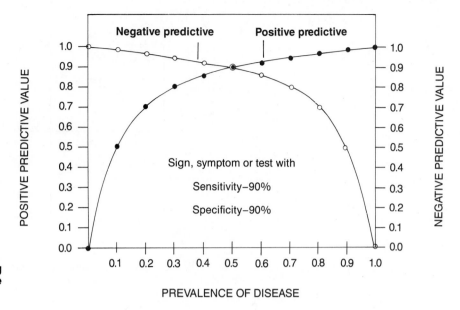

FIGURE 21-6. Effect of changing prevalence upon predictive values.

ing that because the prevalence is high, coronary artery disease may still exist even in the absence of symptoms.

On the other hand, what is the positive predictive value of chest pain in a 15 year old girl? In this age group, the prevalence of coronary artery disease is low. The probability that this patient's chest pain represents coronary artery disease is low. The presence of chest pain in a 15 year old has a low positive predictive value. However, the absence of chest pain has a high negative predictive value, indicating it is *unlikely* that coronary artery disease is present.

Study Figure 21-6. This figure illustrates the effect of changing the prevalence upon the predictive values. Notice that the most significant increase in the positive predictive value of a test, symptom, or sign occurs when the disease is less common. Small changes in prevalence, at this end of the curve, make great changes in the positive predictive value. Conversely, the most significant increase in the negative predictive value occurs when the disease is most prevalent. Slight decreases in the prevalence of common diseases produce significant increases in the negative predictive value. The higher the prevalence, the higher the positive predictive value will be and the lower will be the negative predictive value.

Unfortunately, in clinical medicine there are few 100% sensitive and 100% specific symptoms, signs, or tests. A finding that is 100% specific has no false positives. The existence of the finding carries a positive predictive value of 1.0, meaning that there is 100% probability that the condition exists. A finding that is 100% sensitive has no false negatives. Every patient with the disease has the finding. If the finding is not present, the disease does not exist. The negative predictive value is 1.0.

Let's look again at the example of syncope in patients with aortic stenosis. The following data are for use as an example only. The percentages are not necessarily accurate. Given that the prevalence of aortic stenosis is 80%, the sensitivity of syncope related to aortic stenosis is 65%, and the specificity is 90%, look at the 2 × 2 table. In a population in which the prevalence is 80%, D+ will be equal to 80 and D− will be equal to 20.

	D+ 80	D− 20
T+ With syncope	80 × 0.65 = 52 (TP)	20 × 0.10 = 2 (FP)
T− Without syncope	80 × 0.35 = 28 (FN)	20 × 0.90 = 18 (TN)

In 100 individuals, there will be $80 \times 0.65 = 52$ *true positives*, $80 \times 0.35 = 28$ *false negatives*, $20 \times 0.10 = 2$ *false positives*, and $20 \times 0.90 = 18$ *true negatives*. There are 54 positive results, 52 of which are true positives. Therefore, the positive predictive value is 52/54 = 96.3%. The presence of syncope has raised the likelihood of aortic stenosis from 80% to 96.3%. There are also 46 negative results, 18 of which are true negatives. Therefore, the negative predictive value is 18/46 = 39.1%. Because the given prevalence is 80%, there is only a 20% chance that, by prevalence alone, a given patient has the disease. When one takes into account the negative predictive value of 39.1%, the absence of syncope in this patient has reduced the likelihood of aortic stenosis from 80% to 60.9% (100% − 39.1%). Stated in another way, there is a 39.1% likelihood of aortic stenosis being absent.

When the prevalence of a disease is low, the positive predictive value of a test, sign, or symptom becomes extremely low even if the sensitivity and specificity are high. Let's calculate the predictive values when the prevalence is decreased to 20%.

	D+ 20	D− 80
T+ With syncope	20 × 0.65 = 13 (TP)	80 × 0.10 = 8 (FP)
T− Without syncope	20 × 0.35 = 7 (FN)	80 × 0.90 = 72 (TN)

There will now be 21 positive results, 13 of which are true positives. Therefore, the positive predictive value is 13/21 = 61.9%. Notice that the positive predictive value has fallen from 96.3% (when the prevalence was 80%) to 61.9% as the prevalence decreased. If the patient has syncope, the chance that this individual has aortic stenosis has increased from 20% to 61.9%. There are also 79 negative results, 72 of which are true negatives. Therefore, the negative predictive value is 72/79 = 91.1%. In this example, because the prevalence was 20%, there was an 80% chance that the patient did not have aortic stenosis. In the absence of syncope, the probability that the patient does not have the disease has been reduced from 20% to 8.9% (100% − 91.1%). Stated in another way, if the patient does not have syncope, there is a likelihood of 91.1% that this individual does not have aortic stenosis.

Differences in prevalence rates may be related either to the clinical setting in which the patient is seen or to the specific demographics of the patient. For example, a physician performing routine examinations in an outpatient clinic will find a different prevalence of disease than another physician working only with inpatients in a hospital specializing in that disease. The demographics of the patient refers to his age, sex, and race. Both the clinical setting and the characteristics of the patient help to determine the "utility" of the sign, symptom, or laboratory test, because they affect both the positive and the negative predictive values of the finding.

Let's now consider a clinical situation. Suppose a 21 year old asymptomatic woman finds a thyroid nodule on self-examination, and she is referred to an endocrinologist for evaluation. The physician describes the thyroid nodule as hard to palpation and fixed to the surrounding tissue. In *his* practice, the prevalence of thyroid cancer is 3%. What is the chance that this nodule is cancerous?

Let's construct two 2 × 2 tables, one for each finding. The prevalence of thyroid cancer is 3%. Let's first evaluate the significance of the presence of a palpable hard nodule. The presence of a hard thyroid nodule has a sensitivity of 42% and a specificity of 89% for predicting malignancy.

	D+ 3	D− 97
T+ Hard nodule	3 × 0.42 = 1.26 (TP)	97 × 0.11 = 10.67 (FP)
T− Soft nodule	3 × 0.58 = 1.74 (FN)	97 × 0.89 = 86.33 (TN)

The positive predictive value is 1.26/ (1.26 + 10.67) = 10.6%. The negative predictive value is 86.33/(1.74 + 86.33) = 98.0%.

Therefore, the probability that a hard nodule is cancer is 10.6%, and the probability that this lesion is cancerous if the nodule is not hard is 2.0% (100% − 98.0%). Notice the significant increase in probability from 3% to 10.6% if a hard nodule is found. The absence of a hard nodule has reduced the likelihood of cancer from the prevalence of 3% to 2%.

Let's now look at the other finding, namely the fixation of the nodule to the surrounding tissue. Fixation to the surrounding tissues has a sensitivity of 31% and a specificity of 94% for predicting cancer.

	D + 3	D − 97
T + Nodule fixed	3 × 0.31 = 0.93 (TP)	97 × 0.06 = 5.82 (FP)
T − Nodule not fixed	3 × 0.69 = 2.07 (FN)	97 × 0.94 = 91.18 (TN)

The positive predictive value is $0.93/(0.93 + 5.82) = 13.8\%$. The negative predictive value is $91.18/(2.07 + 91.18) = 97.8\%$.

Therefore, the probability that a fixed nodule is cancer is 13.8%. This represents a 4.6 increase in probability from 3% to 13.8% if the nodule is fixed. The probability that a nodule represents thyroid cancer if it is not fixed is 2.2% $(100\% - 97.8\%)$. However, this finding has not significantly changed the probability of thyroid carcinoma if a nodule is found to be mobile and not fixed. The likelihood of cancer in such a case has been reduced only from 3% to 2.2%.

Multiple symptoms, signs, or tests are combined to evaluate a diagnostic possibility. When one of the symptoms or signs is present or one test is positive, the combined sensitivity is higher than the most sensitive test but the specificity is lower. When all the tests are positive, the combined specificity is higher than the most specific but the sensitivity is reduced. Let's look at this principle with our example of a thyroid nodule. This can be summarized in Table 21−2.

For any given symptom, sign, or test, the sensitivity and specificity should be known prior to its performance. The use of several symptoms, signs, or tests is useful, because when all the findings are absent the disease can usually be excluded. When all the tests are positive, the presence of the disease can be confirmed.

Let us now look at the predictive values for the signs when both findings are present. The prevalence is still 3% for a malignant thyroid nodule in this office practice.

	D + 3	D − 97
T + Both signs present	3 × 0.130 = 0.39 (TP)	97 × 0.007 = 0.68 (FP)
T − Either sign present	3 × 0.870 = 2.61 (FN)	97 × 0.993 = 96.32 (TN)

TABLE 21–2. Example of Sensitivity and Specificity of Thyroid Nodule

Finding	Sensitivity (%)	Specificity (%)
Hard to palpation	42	89
Fixed	31	94
Fixed *or* hard nodule	60*	83.7†
Fixed *and* hard nodule	13.0‡	99.3§

* Combined sensitivity = 100% − (58% × 69%) = 100% − 40% = 60%
† Combined specificity = 89% × 94% = 83.7%
‡ Combined sensitivity = 42% × 31% = 13.0%
§ Combined specificity = 100% − (11% × 6%) = 100% − 0.7% = 99.3%

The positive predictive value is $0.39/(0.39 + 0.68) = 36.4\%$. The negative predictive value is $96.32/(2.61 + 96.32) = 97.4\%$.

Therefore, in answer to our original question, a thyroid nodule that is hard and fixed in an asymptomatic patient found on routine self-examination carries a probability of 36.4% that the nodule is cancer. This represents a 12.1-fold increase in probability from 3% to 36.4% over the prevalence. The chance of finding both signs in a patient without thyroid cancer is only 2.6% (100% − 97.4%).

STANDARDIZATION

A perfect test is one in which there is no overlap between patients with the disease and normal individuals. All normals do not have a symptom, sign, or positive test, whereas all patients with the condition have the finding. In clinical medicine, there are wide ranges of normality. What is *normal*? In testing, "normal" indicates that a finding falls within a predetermined range of values known as *limits* or *cutoff points*. A clinical or laboratory test is defined as normal when its range encompasses 95% of all results in individuals without the disease. The other 5% of individuals are evenly divided above and below this range.

Look at Figure 21–7A. This is a typical distribution of a perfect test. Line "X" exactly divides the diseased from the nondiseased individuals. There are no false negatives or false positives. Look at Figure 21–7B and C, which shows the distribution seen commonly in clinical medicine. In Figure 21–7B and C, line "C" represents the 50% mark of the nondiseased population, with the bell-shaped curve falling evenly around it. In Figure 21–7B, line "A" is 2 standard deviations above the mean for the normal curve. This line, however, also indicates the 60% mark for patients with the symptom, sign, or positive test. All values to the right of line "A" are considered positive. This is the limit or cutoff value. This line represents a 98% specificity and a 60% sensitivity. A test with these operating characteristics would be good for confirming a suspected diagnosis but could not be used to screen a population, owing to its low sensitivity. Compare this with Figure 21–7C. In this example, line "B" has a sensitivity of 98% and a specificity of 60%, making this a better cutoff for screening a specific population. By having moved the line to the left, sensitivity has increased at the expense of having increased the number of false positives.

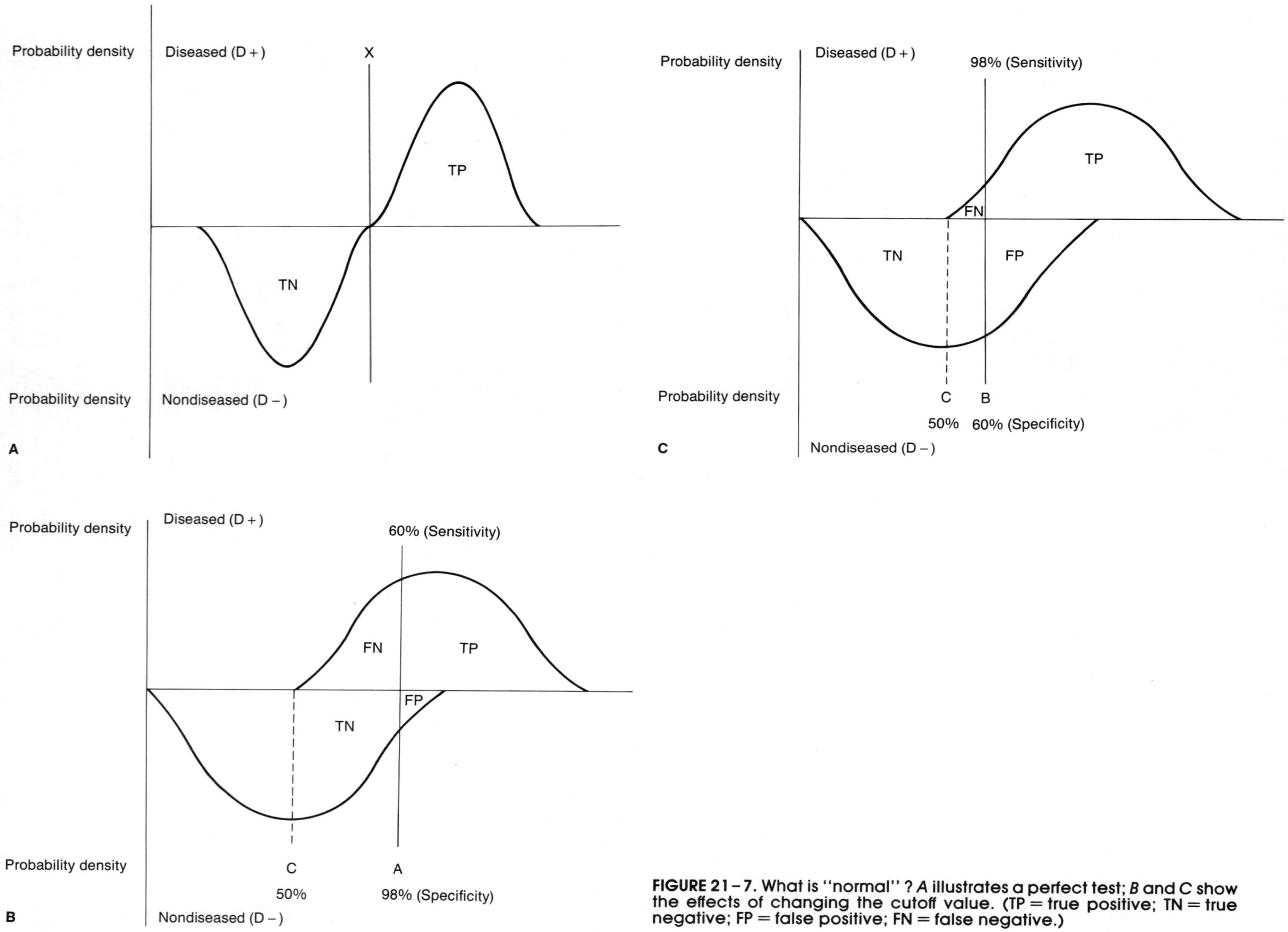

610

FIGURE 21-7. What is "normal"? A illustrates a perfect test; B and C show the effects of changing the cutoff value. (TP = true positive; TN = true negative; FP = false positive; FN = false negative.)

A laboratory value can easily be fit into a "black and white" range of normals. A symptom or sign is never as clear. Therefore, it is extremely important for the physician to gain as much experience in history taking and physical examinations as possible in order to learn what is "normal." In clinical medicine, there exists almost no satisfactory criteria for the designation of a clinical manifestation as normal or abnormal. In many cases, a finding is compared with that of the contralateral side as a frame of reference. Absolute clinical judgments are often impossible. What kind of criteria can one use to say that a patellar reflex is definitely diminished? A liver enlarged? A tympanic membrane abnormal? Dyspnea on exertion? The frame of reference is based on the individual experience of the physician; there is no universal "gold standard." There is no sharp cutoff point.

The use of several techniques or tests will often be helpful to improve predictive values. A follow-up technique or test is performed if an earlier one is "positive" or if a particular sign or symptom is present. This has the effect of raising the prevalence of disease for the group of patients for whom the second or follow-up test is performed. This enhances the predictive values of the positive test results.

Before concluding, we should address the concepts of *accuracy* and *precision*. Accuracy, also known as validity, is the proportion of all test results that are correct. This includes all the true positives and the true negatives. Accuracy reflects sensitivity and specificity. Precision, also known as reliability, refers to the ability to reproduce a measurement. Poor precision makes analyses insensitive.

Consider the example of a bathroom scale. A person can get on and off the scale several times; it always gives the same reading. The scale is precise, or reliable. The scale, however, when calibrated is found to be 10 pounds off. There is a *lack* of accuracy, or validity. An instrument must be precise to be accurate, but being precise does not imply accuracy. There is an old saying, *"We make the same mistake a thousand times over and call it clinical experience."*

BIBLIOGRAPHY

Brorsson B, Wall S: Assessment of Medical Technology: Problems and Methods. Stockholm, Swedish Medical Research Council, 1985.

Cutler P: Problem Solving in Clinical Medicine: From Data to Diagnosis. Baltimore, Williams and Wilkins, 1985.

Galen RS, Gambino SR: Beyond Normality: The Predictive Value and Efficiency of Medical Diagnosis. New York, John Wiley and Sons, 1975.

Griner PF, Panzer RJ, Greenland P: Clinical Diagnosis and the Laboratory: Logical Strategies for Common Medical Problems. Chicago, Year Book Medical Publishers, Inc, 1986.

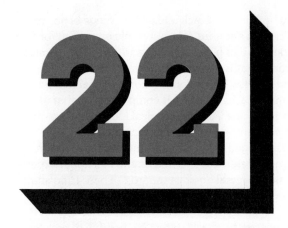

THE CLINICAL RECORD

May I never forget that the patient is a fellow human creature in pain. May I never consider the patient merely a vessel of disease.

**From the modified *Oath of Maimonides*
1135 – 1204**

PUTTING THE HISTORY AND PHYSICAL TOGETHER

Until this point, we have dealt separately with the history and the physical examination. Chapters 1 – 3 gave an in-depth analysis of the techniques of history taking. Chapters 4 – 18 discussed the many techniques of the physical examination, and Chapter 19 provided a suggested approach to performing the complete examination and its write-up. The previous chapter discussed data gathering and problem list development. In this chapter, we discuss how both the history and the physical examination can be assimilated into one succinct statement about the patient.

In writing up the history and the physical examination, the examiner should follow several rules:

- Record all pertinent data
- Avoid extraneous data
- Use common terms
- Avoid abbreviations
- Be objective
- Use diagrams where indicated

The patient's medical record is a legal document. Comments regarding the patient's behavior or attitudes should *not* be part of the record unless they are important from a medical or scientific standpoint. You should describe all parts of the examination that you have performed and indicate those that you have not. A statement such as "the examination of the *eye* is normal" is much less accurate than "the fundus is normal." In the first case, it is not clear if the examiner actually attempted to look at the fundus. If a part of the examination is not performed, state that it was "deferred" for whatever reason. Finally, it is not necessary to state all of the possible abnormalities if they are not present. It is certainly acceptable to state that "the pharynx was normal" instead of "the pharynx was not injected, and there was no evidence of discharge, erosion, masses, or other lesions." It is clear from the first statement that the examiner inspected the pharynx and felt that it was normal.

Let us now return to our patient Mr. John Doe, whom we met in Chapter 3. The following pages describe the complete history and physical examination of this 42 year old lawyer.

Patient: John Doe
Date: August 19, 1988
History

Source

Self, reliable.

Chief Complaint

"Chest pain for the past six months."

History of Present Illness

This is the first Mount Hope admission for this 42 year old lawyer with atherosclerotic coronary artery disease. The patient's history of chest pain began 4 years prior to admission. He described the pain as a "dull ache" in the retrosternal area with radiation to his left arm. The pain was provoked by exertion and emotions. On July 15, 1987, Mr. Doe suffered his first heart attack while playing tennis. He had an uneventful hospitalization in Kings Hospital in New York City. After 2 weeks in the hospital and 3 weeks at home, he returned to work. The patient suffered a second heart attack 6 months later, again while playing tennis. The patient was hospitalized in Kings Hospital, during which time he was told of an "irregularity" of his heart rate. Since then, the patient has not experienced any palpitations, nor has he been told of any further irregularities.

Over the past 6 months, Mr. Doe has had an increase in the frequency of his chest pain. The pain occurs now 4–5 times a day and is relieved within 5 minutes with 1–2 nitroglycerin tablets under his tongue. The pain is produced by exercise, emotions, and sexual intercourse. The patient also describes 1 block dyspnea on exertion. The patient relates that 6 months ago he could walk 2–3 blocks before becoming short of breath.

Although the patient shows significant denial of his illness, he is anxious and depressed.

The patient is now being admitted for elective cardiac catheterization.

Past Medical History

■ **General.** Good.

■ **Past Illnesses.** History of untreated hypertension for years (blood pressure not known); no history of measles, chickenpox, mumps, diphtheria, or whooping cough.

■ **Injuries.** None.

■ **Hospitalizations.** Appendectomy, age 15, Booth Hospital in Rochester, NY (Dr. Meyers, surgeon).

■ **Surgery.** See Hospitalizations.

■ **Allergies.** None.

■ **Immunizations.** Salk polio, tetanus, both as a child; no adverse reactions remembered.

■ **Substance Abuse.** 40 pack-year (2 packs for 20 years) history of smoking; stopped smoking after first heart attack; "pot" on rare occasions in past; drinks alcohol "socially" but also admits to having the need to have a drink as the day goes on (CAGE score, 1); denies use of other street drugs.

■ **Diet.** Mostly red meat, with little fish in diet; 3 cups of coffee a day; recent decrease in appetite, with a 10 pound weight loss in past 3 months.

■ **Sleep Patterns.** Recently, falls asleep normally but awakens around 3 AM and cannot go back to sleep.

Current Medications
Inderal 40 mg QID
Isordil 20 mg QID
Nitroglycerin 1/150 gr PRN
Chlor-Trimeton for colds
Aspirin for headaches
Multivitamins with iron daily

Family History (Fig. 22–1)

Father, 75, diabetes, broken hip
Mother died, 64, stomach cancer
Brother, 45, heart attack age 40
Sister, 37, alive and well
Son, 10, alive and well
Wife, 41, alive and well

There is no family history of congenital disease. No other history of diabetes or cardiac disease. No history of renal, hepatic, or neurologic disease. No history of mental illness.

Psychosocial History

Type "A" personality; born and raised in Middletown, NY; family moved to Rochester, NY when Mr. Doe was 13 years old; moved to New York City after high school; college and law school in New York City; works as a senior partner of a law firm for the past 17 years; married to Emily for the past 13 years; one son, age 10; patient was an active tennis player prior to second heart attack; prior to 6 months ago, enjoyed the theater and reading.

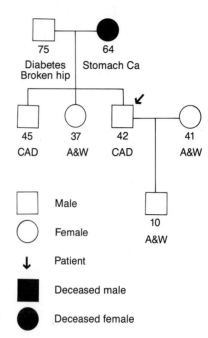

□	Male
○	Female
↓	Patient
■	Deceased male
●	Deceased female

FIGURE 22–1. Family tree of Mr. John Doe.

Review of Systems

■ **General.** Depressed for the past 6 months as a result of his ill health.

■ **Skin.** No rashes or other changes.

■ **Head.** No history of head injury.

■ **Eyes.** Wears glasses for reading; no changes in vision recently; saw ophthalmologist 1 year ago for routine examination; no history of eye pain, tearing, discharge, or halos around lights.

■ **Ears.** Patient not aware of any problem hearing; no dizziness, discharge, or pain present.

■ **Nose.** Occasional cold, 2–3 times a year, lasting 3–5 days; no hay fever, sinus symptoms.

■ **Mouth and Throat.** Occasional sore throats and canker sores associated with colds; no difficulty in chewing or eating; brushes and flosses twice a day; sees dentist twice a year; no gingival bleeding.

■ **Neck.** No masses or tenderness.

■ **Chest.** History of occasional blood-tinged sputum and cough in the morning when patient was smoking, not recently; last chest x-ray 1 year ago, told it was normal; 1 block dyspnea on exertion (as noted in *History of Present Illness*); no history of wheezing, asthma, bronchitis, or tuberculosis.

■ **Breasts.** No masses or nipple discharge noted.

■ **Cardiac.** As noted in *History of Present Illness*.

■ **Vascular.** No history of cerebrovascular accidents or claudication.

■ **Gastrointestinal.** Recent decrease in appetite with 10 pound weight loss in past few months; uses no laxatives; no history of diarrhea, constipation, nausea, or vomiting; no bleeding noted.

■ **Genitourinary.** Urinates 4−5 times a day; urine is light yellow in color, never red; nocturia × 1; no change in stream; no history of urinary infections; no sexual intercourse in past 6 months, owing to angina during sex; no history of venereal disease.

■ **Musculoskeletal.** No joint or bone symptoms; no weakness; no history of back problems or gout.

■ **Neurologic.** No history of seizures or difficulties in walking or balance; no history of motor or sensory symptoms.

■ **Endocrine.** No known thyroid nodules; no history of temperature intolerance; no hair changes; no history of polydipsia or polyuria.

■ **Psychiatric.** Depressed and very anxious about his ill health; also anxious about the results of the upcoming cardiac catheterization; asked, "What's going to happen to me?"

Physical Examination

■ **General Appearance.** The patient is a 42 year old, slightly obese white man, who is lying in bed. He appears slightly older than his stated age. He is in no acute distress but is very nervous. He is well-groomed, cooperative, and alert.

■ **Vital Signs.** BP 175/95/80 right arm (supine), 175/90/85 left arm (supine), 170/90/80 left arm (sitting), 185/95/85 right leg (prone); heart rate 100 and regular; respirations 14.

■ **Skin.** Pink; no cyanosis present; 5−7 nevi (0.5−1.5 cm each) on back, most with hair; normal male escutcheon.

■ **Head.** Normocephalic, without signs of trauma.

■ **Eyes.** Visual acuity with reading glasses using near card: OD 20/40, OS 20/30; confrontation visual fields full bilaterally; EOMs intact; PERRLA; eyebrows normal; conjunctivae pink; discs sharp; marked A-V nicking present at 1−2 disc diameters seen bilaterally; copper wiring present bilaterally; a cotton-wool spot is present at 1 o'clock (superior nasal) in the right eye and at 5 o'clock (inferior temporal) in the left eye; no hemorrhages are present.

■ **Ears.** Normal position; no tenderness present; external canals normal; Rinne AC > BC bilaterally; Weber, no lateralization; both tympanic membranes appear normal, with normal landmarks clearly seen.

■ **Nose.** Straight, without masses; patent bilaterally; mucosa pink, without discharge; inferior turbinates appear normal.

■ **Sinuses.** No tenderness present over frontal or maxillary sinuses.

■ **Throat.** Lips pink; buccal mucosa pink; all teeth in good condition, without obvious caries; gingivae normal, without bleeding; tongue midline and without masses; uvula elevates in midline; gag reflex intact; posterior pharynx normal.

■ **Neck.** Supple, with full range of motion; trachea midline and freely mobile; no adenopathy present; thyroid not felt; prominent "a" wave seen in neck veins while lying at 45°; neck veins flat while sitting upright.

■ **Chest.** Normal AP diameter; symmetric excursion bilaterally; normal tactile fremitus bilaterally; chest resonant bilaterally; clear to percussion and auscultation.

■ **Breasts.** Normal male, without masses, gynecomastia, or discharge.

■ **Heart.** PMI 5ICS-MCL; S_1 and S_2 normal; normal physiologic splitting present; a loud S_4 is present at the cardiac apex; no murmurs or rubs are heard (Fig. 22–2).

■ **Vascular.** Pulses are present and symmetric down to the dorsalis pedis bilaterally; no bruits are present over the carotids or femorals; no abdominal bruits are present; no edema is present.

■ **Abdomen.** A well-healed appendectomy scar is present in the RLQ; the abdomen is slightly obese; no masses are present; no tenderness, guarding, rigidity, or rebound is present.

■ **Rectal.** Anal sphincter normal; no hemorrhoids present; prostate slightly enlarged and soft; no prostatic masses felt; no stool in ampulla.

■ **Genitalia.** Circumcised male with normal genitalia; penis normal without induration; testes $4 \times 3 \times 2$ cm (right) and $3 \times 6 \times 4$ cm (left), with normal consistency.

■ **Lymphatic.** No adenopathy noted.

■ **Musculoskeletal.** There are several stony hard, slightly yellowish, nontender masses over the extensor tendons on the patient's hands; normal range of motion of neck, spine, and major joints of upper and lower extremities.

■ **Neurologic.** Oriented to person, place, and time; cranial nerves II–XII intact (cranial nerve I not tested); cerebellar function normal; plantar reflexes down; gait normal; deep tendon reflexes as in table (Table 22–1).

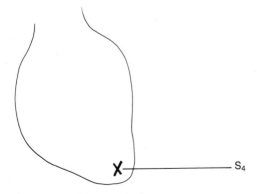

S_4

FIGURE 22–2. Diagram showing location of abnormal cardiac findings.

TABLE 22–1. Deep Tendon Reflexes of Patient John Doe

	Biceps	Triceps	Knee	Achilles
Right	2+	2+	2+	1+
Left	2+	2+	1+	1+

TABLE 22–2. Problem List for Patient John Doe

Number	Problem	Date	Resolved
1	Chest pain	1987	
2	Myocardial infarction	July 15, 1987	2 weeks later
3	Myocardial infarction	January 1988	3 weeks later
4	Hypertension	Years	
5	Smoking	1967	July 15, 1987
6	Tendinous xanthomata	?	
7	S_4 gallop		
8	Dyspnea on exertion	6 months ago	
9	Depression	3 months ago	
	Weight loss		
	Sleeping abnormality		
10	Diet modification		

Summary

Mr. Doe is a type "A" 42 year old man with a history of having had two myocardial infarctions in the past and is now admitted for elective cardiac catheterization. His risk factors for coronary artery disease are untreated hypertension and a long history of cigarette smoking. The patient also has a brother who suffered a myocardial infarction at the age of 40.

Physical examination reveals a slightly obese man with hypertension and its associated early-mid funduscopic changes. Cardiac examination reveals a loud fourth heart sound, suggestive of a non-compliant (stiff) ventricle. This may be a manifestation of ischemic heart disease or ventricular hypertrophy secondary to the hypertension. Although the patient is not aware of any lipid abnormalities, numerous tendinous xanthomata are present, which are strongly suggestive of hypercholesterolemia, an additional risk factor for premature coronary artery disease.

The problem list containing all the health problems identified with their dates of recognition and resolution for Mr. Doe might look like Table 22–2. The problems in the list are then used each time the patient is subsequently seen and examined. For each problem, the student or physician should develop a strategy for its ultimate resolution. Each problem should have the following four components:

- Subjective data
- Objective data
- Assessment
- Plan

This is the SOAP format (Weed, 1967), which contains an update of the subjective and objective data as well as the assessment of the problem and the plan for its resolution.

THE HUMAN DIMENSION

The practice of medicine is an extraordinary profession. The memory of the thrill of interviewing and examining our first patient should stay in our minds. We must always remember that even during the most trying times, we as students or physicians have been granted the enormous responsibility of caring for a patient. Common courtesy, kindness, respect, and attentiveness to the patient will go a long way in re-establishing the so-called bedside manner, which has become less evident in the past few decades. Imagine yourself in the shoes of the patient. How would you like to be treated? Each of you in medical school has the potential to develop into a devoted and compassionate physician.

Always strive for a degree of precision and accuracy. Be strict in your approach to the history and physical examination. Always follow the same basic routines. Do not take shortcuts! The development of the skills of inspection, palpation, percussion, and auscultation takes time. Only with experience can the student or physician master physical diagnosis. This textbook is only the introduction to a life of learning about patients, their problems, and their diseases. As students, you will learn much from your patients. Even the seasoned diagnostician learns daily from his patients. Just as no two individuals have the same face or body appearance, no two individuals will react the same to the same disease. This is one of the major excitements about medicine: every day offers new patients, new problems, new solutions.

BIBLIOGRAPHY

Weed LL: Medical records that guide and teach. NEJM *278*:593, 652, 1967.

Appendix
COMMONLY ABUSED DRUGS

Drug	Street Name	How Used	Symptoms and Signs
Marijuana Hashish	*Pot, Grass, Reefer, Weed, Hash, Sinsemilla, Joint*	Smoked Ingested	Loss of interest Recent memory loss Dry mouth and throat Mood changes Increased appetite
Alcohol	*Booze, Brew, Hooch*	Ingested	Impaired coordination Impaired judgment
Nicotine	*Smoke, Butt, Coffin Nail*	Smoked Chewed	Tobacco smell Stained teeth
Amphetamines	*Speed, Uppers, Pep Pills, Bennies, Dexies, Black Beauties, Meth, Crystal*	Ingested Injected Sniffed	Dilated pupils Increased energy Irritability Nervousness Needle marks
Cocaine	*Coke, Crack, Snow, White Lady, Toot*	Snorted Injected Ingested Smoked	Dilated pupils Increased energy Restlessness Intense anxiety Paranoid behavior Needle marks
Barbiturates	*Downers, Barbs, Yellow Jackets, Red Devils, Blue Devils, Double Trouble*	Injected Ingested	Constricted pupils Confusion Impaired judgment Drowsiness Slurring of speech Needle marks
Methaqualone	*Ludes, Sopors, Quaaludes*	Ingested	Slurring of speech Drowsiness Impaired judgment Euphoria Seizures
Heroin Morphine	*Junk, Scag, Dope, Horse, Smack, Dreamer*	Injected Smoked Sniffed Skin popped	Constricted pupils Needle marks Drowsiness Mental clouding

Drug	Street Name	How Used	Symptoms and Signs
Codeine	*School Boy*	Ingested Sniffed	Constricted pupils Drowsiness
Demerol Methadone Percodan Pentazocine		Ingested Injected	Constricted pupils Drowsiness Mental clouding Needle marks
PCP (phencyclidine)	*Angel Dust, Hog, Killer Weed, Supergrass*	Smoked Snorted Injected Ingested	Dilated pupils Slurring of speech Hallucinations Blurring of vision Uncoordination Agitation Confusion Aggressive behavior
LSD (lysergic acid diethylamide)	*Acid, Cubes, Purple Haze*	Ingested Injected	Dilated pupils Hallucinations Mood swings Increased alertness Acute panic reactions
Mescaline	*Mesc, Cactus*	Ingested	Dilated pupils Hallucinations Mood swings
Psilocybin	*Magic Mushrooms*	Ingested	Dilated pupils Hallucinations Mood swings
Airplane glue* Paint thinner*		Inhaled Sniffed	Poor motor coordination Impaired vision Violent behavior
Nitrous oxide	*Laughing Gas, Whippets*	Inhaled Sniffed	Hilarity Euphoria Lightheadedness
Amyl nitrate	*Poppers, Rush, Locker Room, Snappers, Amies*	Inhaled Sniffed	Hilarity Dizziness Headache Impaired thought

* The active agent in airplane glue and paint thinner is toluene. Naphtha, methyl ethyl ketone, and gasoline may produce similar symptoms.

INDEX

Note: Page numbers in *italics* indicate illustrations; page numbers followed by the letter t indicate tables.